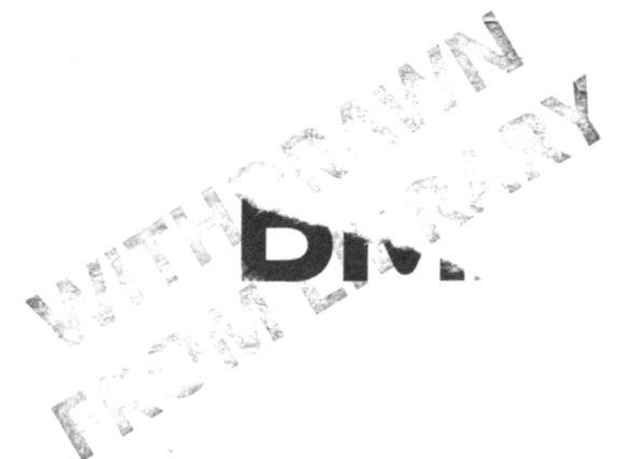

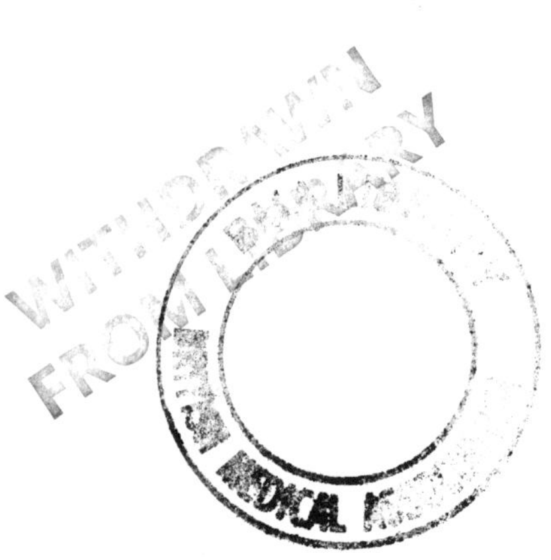

Critical Care of the Stroke Patient

Critical Care of the Stroke Patient

Edited by

Stefan Schwab

Professor and Director, Department of Neurology, University of Erlangen-Nuremberg, Erlangen, Germany

Daniel Hanley

Jeffrey and Harriet Legum Professor and Director, Division of Brain Injury Outcomes, The Johns Hopkins Medical Institutions, Baltimore, MD, USA

A. David Mendelow

Professor of Neurosurgery, Institute of Neuroscience, University of Newcastle Upon Tyne, Newcastle Upon Tyne, UK

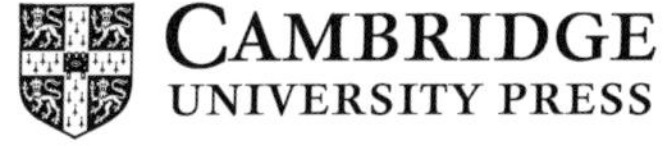

CAMBRIDGE
UNIVERSITY PRESS

University Printing House, Cambridge CB2 8BS, United Kingdom

Cambridge University Press is part of the University of Cambridge.

It furthers the University's mission by disseminating knowledge in the pursuit of education, learning and research at the highest international levels of excellence.

www.cambridge.org
Information on this title: www.cambridge.org/9780521762564

First published 2014

Printing in the United Kingdom by TJ International Ltd. Padstow Cornwall

A catalogue record for this publication is available from the British Library

Library of Congress Cataloguing in Publication data
Critical care of the stroke patient / edited by Stefan Schwab, Daniel Hanley, A. David Mendelow.
Includes bibliographical references and index.
ISBN 978-0-521-76256-4 (hardback)
I. Schwab, S. (Stefan), editor of compilation. II. Hanley, D. F. (Daniel F.), editor of compilation. III. Mendelow, A. David., editor of compilation.
[DNLM: 1. Stroke – therapy. 2. Critical Care – methods. WL 356]

ISBN 978-0-521-76256-4 Hardback

Contents

List of contributors *page* viii

Section 1. Monitoring Techniques 1

1 Intracranial pressure monitoring in cerebrovascular disease 3
Anthony Frattalone and Wendy C. Ziai

2. Cerebral blood flow 20
Rajat Dhar and Michael C. Diringer

3. Brain tissue oxygen monitoring in cerebrovascular diseases 37
Klaus Zweckberger and Karl L. Kiening

4. Cerebral microdialysis in cerebrovascular disease 44
Paul M. Vespa

5. Ultrasound and other noninvasive techniques used in monitoring cerebrovascular disease 54
Günter Seidel

6. Scales in the neurointensive care unit 66
Elise Rowan and Barbara A. Gregson

Section 2. Interventions 79

7. Antiedema therapy in cerebrovascular disease 81
Dimitre Staykov and Jürgen Bardutzky

8. Decompressive surgery in cerebrovascular disease 90
Katayoun Vahedi and François Proust

9a. Neuroradiologic intervention in cerebrovascular disease 103
Olav Jansen and Soenke Peters

9b. Neuroradiological interventions in cerebrovascular disease: intracranial revascularization 120
Martin Radvany and Philippe Gailloud

10. The use of hypothermia in cerebrovascular disease 129
Dan Holmes, Sara Pitoni, Louise Sinclair, and Peter J. D. Andrews

11. External ventricular drainage in hemorrhagic stroke 145
Mahua Dey, Jennifer Jaffe, and Issam A. Awad

12. Management of lumbar drains in cerebrovascular disease 158
Dimitre Staykov and Hagen B. Huttner

Section 3. Critical Care of Ischemic Stroke 167

13. Intravenous and intra-arterial thrombolysis for acute ischemic stroke 169
Martin Köhrmann and Stefan Schwab

14. Decompressive surgery and hypothermia 179
Rainer Kollmar, Patrick Lyden, and Thomas M. Hemmen

15. Space-occupying hemispheric infarction: clinical course, prediction, and prognosis 190
H. Bart van der Worp and Stefan Schwab

16. Critical care of basilar artery occlusion 194
Perttu J. Lindsberg, Tiina Sairanen, and Heinrich P. Mattle

17. Critical care of cerebellar stroke 206
Tim Nowe and Eric Jüttler

18. Rare specific causes of stroke 226
Alexander Beck, Philipp Gölitz, and Peter D. Schellinger

19. Blood pressure management in acute ischemic stroke 243
Sandeep Ankolekar and Philip Bath

Section 4. Critical Care of Intracranial Hemorrhage 255

20. Management of intracranial hemorrhage: early expansion and second bleeds 257
Corina Epple and Thorsten Steiner

21a. Management of acute hypertensive response in the ICH patient 274
Wondwossen G. Tekle and Adnan I. Qureshi

21b. Respiratory care of the ICH patient 286
Omar Ayoub and Jeanne Teitelbaum

21c. Nutrition in the ICH patient 297
Dimitre Staykov and Jürgen Bardutzky

21d. Management of infections in the ICH patient 306
Edgar Santos and Oliver W. Sakowitz

21e. Management of cerebral edema in the ICH patient 315
Neeraj S. Naval and J. Ricardo Carhuapoma

22a. Surgery for spontaneous intracerebral hemorrhage 320
A. David Mendelow, Barbara A. Gregson, and Patrick Mitchell

22b. Minimally invasive treatment options for spontaneous intracerebral hemorrhage 329
Andrew Losiniecki and Mario Zuccarello

22c. Image-guided endoscopic evacuation of spontaneous intracerebral hemorrhage 335
Justin A. Dye, Daniel T. Nagasawa, Joshua R. Dusick, Winward Choy, Isaac Yang, Paul M. Vespa, and Neil A. Martin

23. Intraventricular hemorrhage 348
Wendy C. Ziai and Daniel Hanley

24. Interventions for cerebellar hemorrhage 363
Jens Witsch and Eric Jüttler

25. Interventions for brainstem hemorrhage 378
Berk Orakcioglu and Andreas W. Unterberg

Section 5. Critical Care of Arteriovenous Malformations 385

26. Surgery for arteriovenous malformations 387
A. David Mendelow, Anil Gholkar, Raghu Vindlacheruvu, and Patrick Mitchell

27. Radiation therapy for arteriovenous malformations 394
Oliver Ganslandt, Sabine Semrau, and Reiner Fietkau

28. Management of cavernous angiomas of the brain 400
Mahua Dey and Issam A. Awad

Section 6. Critical Care of Subarachnoid Hemorrhage 421

29. Medical interventions for subarachnoid hemorrhage 423
Joji B. Kuramatsu and Hagen B. Huttner

30. Craniotomy for treatment of aneurysms 437
Patrick Mitchell

31. Endovascular interventions for subarachnoid hemorrhage 447
Arnd Dörfler

32. Management of vasospasm in subarachnoid hemorrhage 464
Rajat Dhar and Michael C. Diringer

33. Management of metabolic derangements in subarachnoid hemorrhage 480
Kara L. Krajewski and Oliver W. Sakowitz

34. Management of cardiopulmonary dysfunction in subarachnoid hemorrhage 490
Jan-Oliver Neumann and Oliver W. Sakowitz

Section 7. Critical Care of Cerebral Venous Thrombosis 499

35. Identification, differential diagnosis, and therapy for cerebral venous thrombosis 501
José M. Ferro and Patrícia Canhão

Section 8. Vascular Disease Syndromes Associated With Traumatic Brain Injury 515

36. Ischemic brain damage in traumatic brain injury (TBI): extradural, subdural, and intracerebral hematomas and cerebral contusions 517
A. David Mendelow

Index 538

The color plate section can be found between pages 252 and 253

Contributors

Peter J. D. Andrews
Department of Anaesthesia, Critical Care & Pain Medicine, University of Edinburgh, and Consultant, Critical Care, Western General Hospital, Lothian University Hospitals Division, Edinburgh, Scotland, UK

Sandeep Ankolekar
Division of Stroke, University of Nottingham, Nottingham, UK

Issam A. Awad
Section of Neurosurgery and Neurovascular Surgery Program, Division of Biological Sciences and the Pritzker School of Medicine, The University of Chicago, Chicago, IL, USA

Omar Ayoub
Assistant Professor of Neurology, Stroke, and Neurocritical Care, Jeddah, Saudi Arabia

Philip Bath
Division of Stroke Medicine, University of Nottingham, Nottingham, UK

Jürgen Bardutzky
Department of Neurology, University of Freiburg, Freiburg, Germany

Alexander Beck
Department of Neurology, Friedrich-Alexander-University of Erlangen-Nuremberg, Erlangen, Germany

Patrícia Canhão
Department of Neurosciences (Neurology), Hospital de Santa Maria, University of Lisbon, Lisboa, Portugal

J. Ricardo Carhuapoma
Department of Neurology, Neurosurgery and Anesthesiology & Critical Care Medicine, The Johns Hopkins Hospital, Baltimore, MD, USA

Winward Choy
Department of Neurosurgery, David Geffen School of Medicine at UCLA, Los Angeles, CA, USA

Mahua Dey
Section of Neurosurgery and Neurovascular Surgery Program, Division of Biological Sciences and the Pritzker School of Medicine, The University of Chicago, Chicago, IL, USA

Rajat Dhar
Department of Neurology, Division of Neurocritical Care, Washington University School of Medicine, Saint Louis, MO, USA

Michael C. Diringer
Department of Neurology, Division of Neurocritical Care, Washington University School of Medicine, Saint Louis, MO, USA

Arnd Dörfler
Department of Neuroradiology, University of Erlangen-Nuremberg, Erlangen, Germany

Joshua R. Dusick
Department of Neurosurgery, David Geffen School of Medicine at UCLA, Los Angeles, CA, USA

Justin A. Dye
Department of Neurosurgery, David Geffen School of Medicine at UCLA, Los Angeles, CA, USA

Corina Epple
Department of Neurology, Klinikum Frankfurt Höchst, Frankfurt, Germany

José M. Ferro
Department of Neurosciences (Neurology), Hospital de Santa Maria, University of Lisbon, Lisboa, Portugal

Reiner Fietkau
Department of Neurosurgery and Radiation Therapy, University of Erlangen-Nuremberg, Erlangen, Germany

Anthony Frattalone
Department of Neurology, Division of Neurocritical Care, The Johns Hopkins University School of Medicine, Baltimore, MD, USA

Philippe Gailloud
Department of Interventional Neuroradiology, The Johns Hopkins University School of Medicine, Baltimore, MD, USA

Oliver Ganslandt
Department of Neurosurgery and Radiation Therapy, University of Erlangen-Nuremberg, Erlangen, Germany

Anil Gholkar
The Newcastle Upon Tyne Hospitals NHS Foundation Trust, Newcastle Upon Tyne, UK

Philipp Gölitz
Department of Neuroradiology, University of Erlangen-Nuremberg, Erlangen, Germany

Barbara A. Gregson
Institute of Neuroscience, University of Newcastle Upon Tyne, UK

Daniel Hanley
Division of Brain Injury Outcomes, The Johns Hopkins Medical Institutions, Baltimore, MD, USA

Thomas M. Hemmen
Department of Neurosciences, University of California San Diego School of Medicine, San Diego, CA, USA

Dan Holmes
Department of Anaesthesia, Critical Care & Pain Medicine, University of Edinburgh, and Consultant,

Critical Care, Western General Hospital Lothian University Hospitals Division, Edinburgh, Scotland, UK

Hagen B. Huttner
Department of Neurology, University of Erlangen-Nuremberg, Erlangen, Germany

Jennifer Jaffe
Section of Neurosurgery and Neurovascular Surgery Program, Division of Biological Sciences and the Pritzker School of Medicine, The University of Chicago, Chicago, IL, USA

Olav Jansen
Institute of Neuroradiology, University of Kiel, Kiel, Germany

Eric Jüttler
Center for Stroke Research Berlin (CSB), Charité University Medicine Berlin, Berlin, Germany

Karl L. Kiening
Department of Neurosurgery, Universitätsklinikum Heidelberg, Heidelberg, Germany

Martin Köhrmann
Department of Neurology, University Hospital Erlangen, Erlangen, Germany

Rainer Kollmar
Clinic for Neurology and Neurogeriatrics, Darmstadt, Germany

Kara L. Krajewski
Department of Neurosurgery, University Hospital Heidelberg, Germany

Joji B. Kuramatsu
Department of Neurology, University of Erlangen-Nuremberg, Erlangen, Germany

Perttu J. Lindsberg
Department of Neurology, Helsinki University Central Hospital, and Molecular Neurology Research Programs Unit, Biomedicum Helsinki, and Department of Clinical Neurosciences, University of Helsinki, Helsinki, Finland

Andrew Losiniecki
Department of Neurosurgery, University of Cincinnati Neuroscience Institute and University of Cincinnati College of Medicine, Cincinnati, OH, USA

Patrick Lyden
Department of Neurosciences, University of California San Diego School of Medicine, San Diego, CA, USA

Neil A. Martin
Department of Neurosurgery, David Geffen School of Medicine at UCLA, Los Angeles, CA, USA

Heinrich P. Mattle
Department of Neurology, University of Bern, Inselspitel, Bern, Switzerland

A. David Mendelow
Department of Neurosurgery, Institute of Neuroscience, University of Newcastle Upon Tyne, Newcastle Upon Tyne, UK

Patrick Mitchell
Department of Neurosurgery, Royal Victoria Infirmary, Newcastle Upon Tyne, UK

Daniel T. Nagasawa
Department of Neurosurgery, David Geffen School of Medicine at UCLA, Los Angeles, CA, USA

Neeraj S. Naval
Department of Neurology, Neurosurgery, Anesthesiology and Critical Care Medicine, The Johns Hopkins Hospital, Baltimore, MD, USA

Jan-Oliver Neumann
Department of Neurosurgery, University Hospital Heidelberg, Germany

Tim Nowe
Center for Stroke Research Berlin (CSB), Charité University Medicine Berlin, Berlin, Germany

Berk Orakcioglu
Department of Neurosurgery, University of Heidelberg, Heidelberg, Germany

Soenke Peters
Institute of Neuroradiology, University of Kiel, Kiel, Germany

Sara Pitoni
Department of Anesthesiology and Intensive Care Unit, Policlinico Universitario 'Agostino Gemelli', Università Cattolica del Sacro Cuore of Rome, Rome, Italy

François Proust
Neurosurgery Department, Centre Hospitalier Universitaire de Rouen, Rouen, France

Adnan I. Qureshi
Zeenat Qureshi Stroke Research Center, University of Minnesota, MN, USA

Martin Radvany
Department of Interventional Neuroradiology, The Johns Hopkins University School of Medicine, Baltimore, MD, USA

Elise Rowan
Institute of Neurosciences, University of Newcastle Upon Tyne, UK

Tiina Sairanen
Department of Neurology, Helsinki University Central Hospital, Helsinki, Finland

Oliver W. Sakowitz
Department of Neurosurgery, University Hospital Heidelberg, Germany

Edgar Santos
Department of Neurosurgery, University Hospital Heidelberg, Germany

Peter D. Schellinger
Department of Neurology, Ruprechy-Karls-University, Heidelberg, Germany

Stefan Schwab
Department of Neurology, University of Erlangen-Nuremberg, Erlangen, Germany

Günter Seidel
Department of Neurology, Medical University at Lübeck, Lübeck, Germany

Sabine Semrau
Department of Neurosurgery and Radiation Therapy, University of Erlangen-Nuremberg, Erlangen, Germany

Louise Sinclair
Department of Anaesthesia, Critical Care & Pain Medicine, University of Edinburgh, and Consultant, Critical Care, Western General Hospital Lothian University Hospitals Division, Edinburgh, Scotland, UK

Dimitre Staykov
Department of Neurology, University of Erlangen-Nuremberg, Erlangen, Germany

Thorsten Steiner
Department of Neurology, Klinikum Frankfurt Höchst, Frankfurt, and Department of Neurology, Heidelberg University Hospital, Heidelberg, Germany

Jeanne Teitelbaum
Department of Neurology and Neurosurgery, Montreal Neurological Institute and MUHC, Montreal, Quebec, Canada

Wondwossen G. Tekle
Zeenat Qureshi Stroke Research Center, University of Minnesota, MN, USA

Andreas W. Unterberg
Department of Neurology, University of Heidelberg, Heidelberg, Germany

Katayoun Vahedi
Neurology Department, Lariboisière Hospital, Assistance Publique-Hôpitaux de Paris, Paris, Consultant Neurologist, Hôpital Privé d'Antony, Antony, France

H. Bart van der Worp
Department of Neurology and Neurosurgery, Brian Center Rudolf Magnus, University Medical Center Utrecht, Utrecht, The Netherlands

Paul M. Vespa
Department of Neurology and Neurosurgery, David Geffen School of Medicine at UCLA, Los Angeles, CA, USA

Raghu Vindlacheruvu
Queen's Hospital, Romford, Essex, UK

Jens Witsch
Department of Neurology, Charité University Medicine Berlin, Berlin, Germany

Isaac Yang
Department of Neurosurgery, David Geffen School of Medicine at UCLA, Los Angeles, CA, USA

Wendy C. Ziai
Department of Neurology, Division of Neurocritical Care, The Johns Hopkins University School of Medicine, Baltimore, MD, USA

Mario Zuccarello
Department of Neurosurgery, University of Cincinnati Neuroscience Institute and University of Cincinnati College of Medicine, and Mayfield Clinic, Cincinnati, OH, USA

Klaus Zweckberger
Department of Neurosurgery, Universitätsklinikum Heidelberg, Heidelberg, Germany

SECTION 1

Monitoring Techniques

1

Intracranial pressure monitoring in cerebrovascular disease

Anthony Frattalone and Wendy C. Ziai

Introduction to intracranial pressure monitoring

Intracranial pressure monitoring remains a central tenet of neurocritical care monitoring and has the potential to improve outcome (1–3). While the importance of monitoring and controlling intracranial pressure (ICP) and cerebral perfusion pressure (CPP) in traumatic brain injury is fairly well understood, its significance in acute cerebrovascular disease and the modulatory effect of therapies remain largely unexplored. This review helps to clarify basic principles and evidence for ICP monitoring and ICP-based treatment and applies these principles to the management of acute cerebrovascular disease.

Principles of intracranial dynamics

The intracranial contents (and average volumes in the adult male) contributing to the ICP are the brain (1300 mL), blood (110 mL) and cerebrospinal fluid (CSF) (65 mL) (4). In normal subjects, average ICP has been reported to be approximately 10 mmHg (5). According to the Monro-Kellie doctrine, because the intracranial contents are encased in a rigid skull and the components are relatively inelastic, change in the volume of one component must be compensated for by reduction in the volume of another component of the system or ICP will increase. Without this compensation, increased ICP may result in brain herniation by direct compression or ischemia/infarction by compromising cerebral blood flow (CBF). While arguably a simplification of the complex pathophysiology involved, the Monro-Kellie doctrine remains a helpful principle in understanding derangements in intracranial pressure.

The brain is considered a viscoelastic solid, comprising approximately 80% water, of which the extracellular compartment represents approximately 15% and the intracellular compartment the other 85% (6). Neither of these components has significant compressibility and, as a result, the brain can be displaced minimally, although it can expand under certain circumstances.

The CSF makes up about 10% of the intracranial volume and is produced predominantly by the choroid plexus, with a small amount produced as interstitial fluid from brain capillaries (7). Production is approximately 500 cc/day and is not significantly reduced by rising ICP (8). Resorption of CSF into cerebral venous sinuses occurs over a pressure gradient at the arachnoid villi by a poorly understood mechanism (9). In normal subjects, resorption increases linearly with ICP above about 7 mmHg (10). However, it is hypothesized that in cases of increased venous pressure, such as cerebral venous thrombosis, that resorption is impaired and can lead to elevated ICP (11).

As long as obstructive hydrocephalus is not present, displacement of CSF into the lumbar subarachnoid space through the foramen magnum is the initial compensatory mechanism after addition of excessive

Critical Care of the Stroke Patient, ed. Stefan Schwab, Daniel Hanley, and A. David Mendelow. Published by Cambridge University Press.

volume to the system (12). In reality, this compensation may often be insufficient in cases of low distensibility of the spinal compartment and is dependent on a normal spinal subarachnoid space and open foramen magnum. Head-up positioning to maximize this compensation and allow CSF displacement, are essential. Compensation is compromised by supine/Trendellenberg position, tonsillar herniation or pathology causing spinal epidural block (13). Another potential adaptive mechanism may be a decrease in CSF volume caused by increased absorption due to lowering of outflow resistance at the arachnoid villi (5).

Another potential compensatory mechanism for increased ICP is shunting of cerebral and dural venous sinus blood out of the cranial compartment into the central venous pool. While resistance to venous drainage by compression of the neck veins is a well-established cause of increased ICP, shift of venous blood volume in response to ICP elevation has less direct evidence (11). Nevertheless, increasing intrathoracic pressure with positive pressure ventilation and high intra-abdominal pressure have been implicated in causing ICP elevation via reduced cerebral venous drainage (14).

Once the limits of compensatory mechanisms for displacement of CSF and blood are exceeded, the slope of the intracranial pressure–volume curve increases substantially, representing decreased compliance (Fig. 1.1). Intracranial compliance ($\Delta V/\Delta P$), decreases quickly (exponential part of the curve) followed by the vertical portion where increased ICP may be irreversible and herniation occurs. Thus, in states of poor compliance, a seemingly insignificant increase in intracranial volume can result in a dramatic increase in ICP. Finally, when ICP increases beyond mean arterial blood pressure (MAP), blood is unable to enter the skull, leading to global ischemia and eventual infarction.

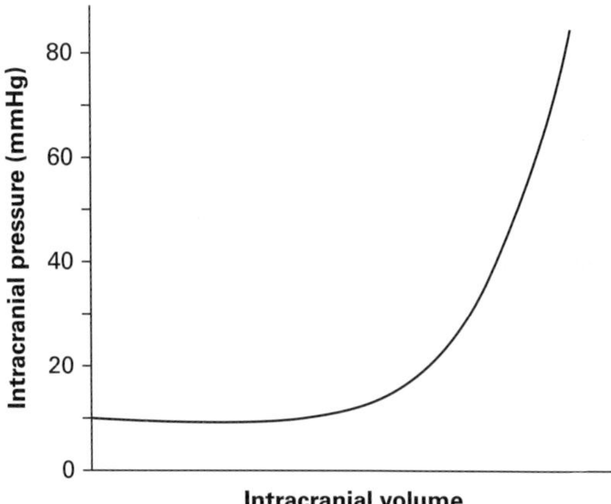

Fig. 1.1 The effect of increasing intracranial volume on intracranial pressure.

The intracranial blood volume, about 10% of the volume within the skull, is approximately 2/3 venous, 1/3 arterial. Arterial blood flow is regulated primarily by change in caliber of arterioles, which adjusts in response to systemic arterial pressure, partial pressure of oxygen (pO2), and partial pressure of carbon dioxide (pCO2). Carbon dioxide tension in arteriolar blood appears to be the most significant determinant of vessel diameter. Over the range of PCO2 usually encountered clinically, CBV decreases as PCO2 level decreases. Even though CBF (and therefore CBV) remain fairly static at physiologic levels of PO2, CBF increases rapidly if PO2 dips below 50 mmHg. Thus, hypoxia and hypercarbia may significantly increase ICP through increases in CBV. Hypocarbia, on the other hand, significantly decreases CBV and hence ICP. Overall, changes in vessel caliber at the arteriolar level allow significant alteration in total intravascular blood volume (from 15 to 70 mL) and can thus compensate for relatively large increases in intracranial volume (5). These are the principles that inform the practice of hyperventilation to lower ICP.

Cerebral autoregulation refers to the ability of the system to maintain constant CBV throughout a range of mean arterial blood pressure (MAP) from approximately 50–150 mmHg (Fig. 1.2). In normal subjects who experience a decrease in CPP, CBV remains normal due to compensatory arteriolar vasodilation. However, when the normal compensatory system is breeched such as with global ischemia (MAP below range) or malignant hypertension (MAP above range), the CBF becomes dependent on MAP. In both cases, CBF varies linearly with MAP. The main mechanism of cerebral autoregulation is vasodilatation and constriction guided by CPP induced changes in cerebral blood flow (CBF = CPP/cerebrovascular resistance). The cerebral blood vessels respond little to changes in arterial PO2 above

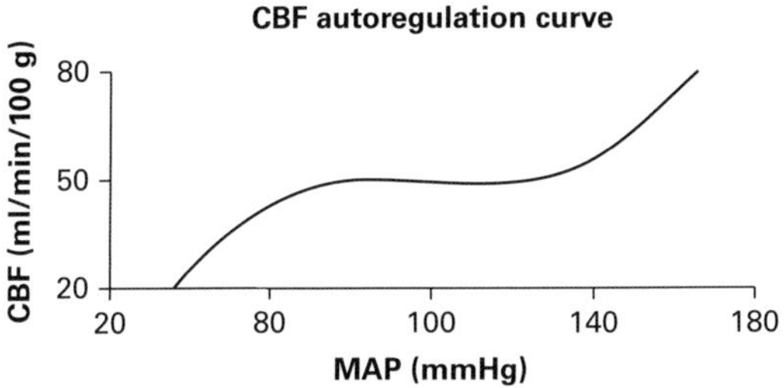

Fig. 1.2 Cerebral blood flow autoregulation curve. From: Gardner CJ, Lee K. *CNS Spectr.* **12**(1): 2007.

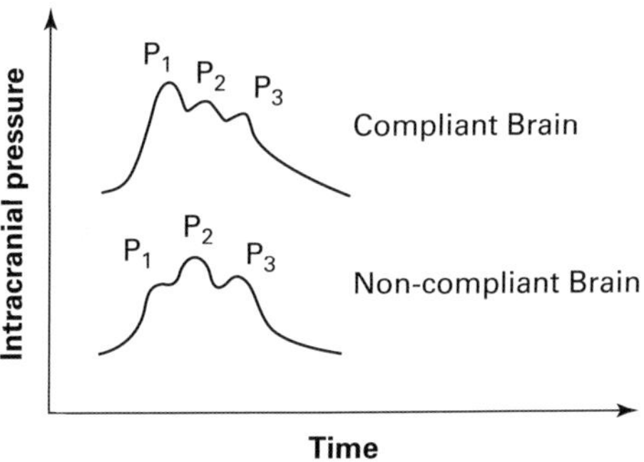

Fig. 1.3 Relationship between ICP and brain compliance

50 mmHg. Below this level, in conditions such as neurogenic pulmonary edema, status epilepticus, or pulmonary embolism, CBF increases significantly, almost doubling at PO2 30 mmHg (5). This point highlights the importance of avoiding hypoxemia and subsequent cerebral arteriolar dilation in patients with elevated ICP. Additionally, vasodilatation in response to elevated PCO2 is maximized at levels above 80 mmHg (doubling of baseline). As expected, vasoconstriction occurs with mild lowering of the PCO2 below normal; however, extremely low PCO2 (<20 mmHg) levels may cause a paradoxical increase in ICP since extreme vasoconstriction can cause tissue ischemia, triggering vasodilation (5). Elevation in ICP does not change autoregulatory responses; rather an autonomic response increases MAP with reflex bradycardia as part of the Cushing response. Acute intracranial hypertension shifts the lower limit of autoregulation towards lower CPP levels, which may be due to dilatation of small resistance vessels (15). Longstanding systemic hypertension shifts the entire curve right by 20–30 mmHg, a change that is protective against hypertensive encephalopathy when large increases in blood pressure occur.

Autoregulation may be impaired regionally in conditions such as stroke or more globally in diffuse anoxic injury or traumatic brain injury (TBI), which can result in an abnormal linear relationship between MAP and CBF. The many possible types of cerebral insults result in highly variable levels and types of impairment of autoregulation from case to case.

Cerebral perfusion pressure (CPP) is a key therapeutic target to prevent potentially fatal cerebral hypoperfusion. Defined as MAP – ICP, the CPP is dependent on both ICP and systemic blood pressure.

The ICP at equilibrium is below 10 mmHg with no pressure gradient between brain regions. The normal ICP waveform has three peaks: the percussion wave (P1), due to choroid plexus pulsation, the tidal wave (P2), a manifestation of compliance, and the dicrotic wave (P3), due to pulsations of the major cerebral arteries. When ICP increases and the slope of the pressure–volume curve rapidly increases, this is a reflection of decreased compliance. In this setting, P2 increases in magnitude and P1 is blunted, merging into P2 as compliance declines (Fig. 1.3) (16). Therefore, by examining the ICP waveform the physician can estimate the amount of compliance remaining in the system and adjust therapy to improve these parameters.

Failure of brain compliance may be accompanied by plateau, Lundberg A waves, or sudden increases in ICP up to 50–80 mmHg lasting 5–20 mins (17). Plateau waves are indicative of cerebral ischemia and may be triggered by usual ICU procedures such as tracheal suctioning, lowering the head of the bed, and routine hygiene (Fig. 1.4).

Neuromonitoring

Several studies have shown that estimation of ICP and herniation risk by clinical grounds alone is inaccurate, arguing for the need for objective ICP monitoring devices (18). Much of the data in support of intensive

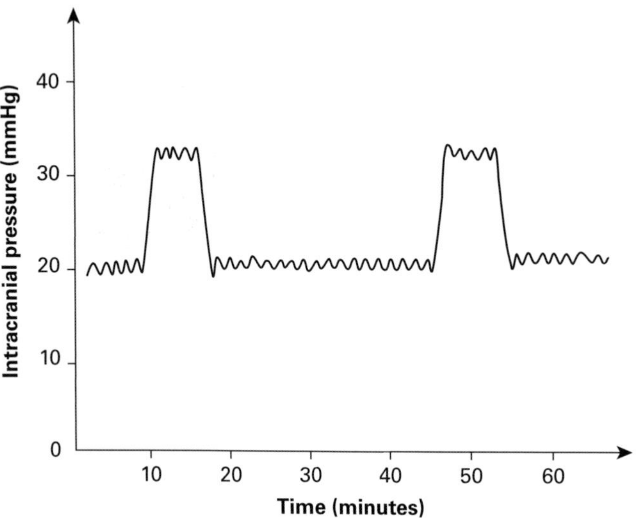

Fig 1.4 Lundberg A waves

ICP monitoring has its origin in the TBI literature. Although a randomized controlled trial of ICP monitoring with and without treatment is unlikely to ever be done, ICP monitoring is now considered standard management for patients with severe TBI and is associated with improved outcomes (18). It is clear that after brain injury of any type that ICP is not static, but instead reflective of a dynamic system with many inputs including CPP, intracranial volume changes, and the effectiveness of adaptive mechanisms. As in TBI, acute cerebrovascular events also follow stages of evolution including mass expansion, vascular changes and edema formation, which occur over several days. Without direct ICP measurement over this time period, there is no way to calculate CPP and thus no way to understand any given patient's cerebral blood flow and adaptive limitations. Finally, since there is considerable risk involved with prophylactic treatment of elevated ICP (hyperosmotic therapy, hyperventilation, hypothermia, surgery), it is imperative that ICP estimations be accurate to avoid unnecessary harm to patients.

There is evidence to support the notion that lowering ICP early is superior to an approach that relies on imaging or clinical deterioration before initiation of treatment (19). Often elevations in ICP can be an early indicator of worsening pathology, which could warrant urgent imaging and lead to timely medical or surgical treatment (18). Moreover, even though imaging assessment is essential, a significant percentage of TBI patients in coma with normal initial CT scans will later develop elevated ICP (20).

While elevated ICP can often be detected on clinical exam in conjunction with imaging and fundoscopic exam, none of these techniques provides an objective measure that can be followed frequently. Studies suggest that optic disc edema often takes at least one day to develop on fundoscopic exam, which is an unacceptable delay (21). Studies to evaluate CT scanning as a screening tool suggest that compression of the third ventricle and basal cisterns are correlated with abnormally high ICPs (22), but this method provides only a 'snap shot' in time and thus does not allow continuous monitoring. Results of studies on transcranial Doppler ultrasonography (TCD), which evaluates the basal cerebral arterial blood flow, has also been shown to correlate with high ICP in the context of changes in CPP but is not considered a sensitive screening or monitoring tool with regards to ICP (23). Some investigators have shown that the TCD pulsatility index correlates with ICP (24) while other more recent studies question the

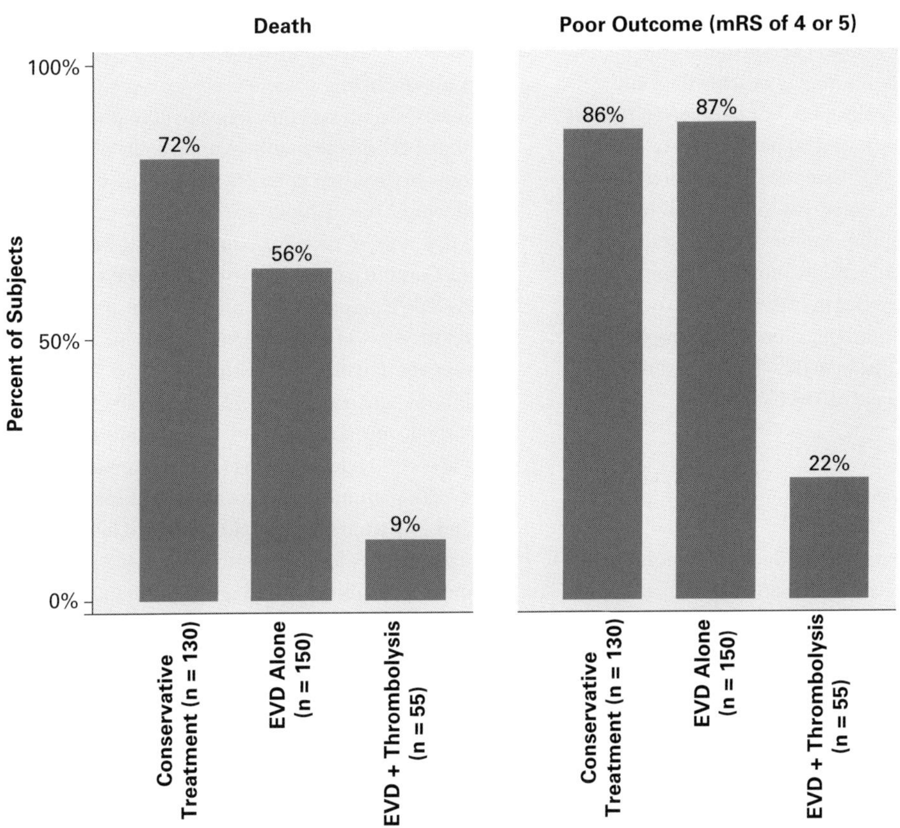

Fig 1.5 The effect of EVD on mortality as compared to traditional treatments.

accuracy of this measure (25). Interestingly, there is some promising preliminary evidence supporting the use of ultrasound of the optic nerve sheath as a screening and monitoring tool for elevated ICP, but this is not routinely available in most centers at this time (26). With this technique, ultrasound measurement of the optic nerve sheath is done rapidly at the bedside and is currently being validated as a diagnostic tool. Several studies have found the threshold optic nerve sheath diameter (ONSD) which provides the best accuracy for the prediction of intracranial hypertension (ICP >20 mmHg) is 5.7–6.0 mm, and that ONSD values above this threshold should alert the clinician to the presence of raised ICP (Fig. 1.5) (26). Unfortunately, even in the hands of a skilled physician, these noninvasive screening techniques currently determine only whether high ICP is present but most likely are not sensitive enough to gauge subtle changes in response to therapy.

In deciding whom to monitor ICP with invasive techniques, many centers use GCS <9 as a cutoff, with the assumption being that patients who are able to follow commands are likely to not have devastatingly high ICP, and the neurologic exam itself substitutes for the monitor. Still, there may be circumstances where an invasive ICP monitor is indicated in a patient with a preserved level of consciousness when the imaging suggests high likelihood of pending deterioration, when a change in the patient's care is expected to increase ICP further (such as high positive end-expiratory pressure (PEEP) or when sedation is needed and therefore the ability to follow the patient's neurologic exam will be impaired.

Duration of ICP monitoring is variable depending on the patient and the institution, but decision to remove the monitor is usually based on neurologic stabilization or normalization of ICP. Extended monitoring is unadvisable except in rare cases due to increased infectious risk over time. On the contrary, when deciding to remove the monitor, caution must be taken to avoid missing delayed increases in ICP, which can occur after a period of pseudo-normalization. For example, a secondary rise in ICP after 3–10 days has been observed in a significant percentage of TBI patients (3).

Types of monitors

All currently commercially available ICP monitors are invasive and necessitate the creation of a dural breach. While sometimes used to estimate ICP, measurements from lumbar cistern catheters (either opening pressure or drain catheter) are more dependent on patient positioning and do not reflect pressure gradients in obstructive hydrocephalus. A recent study suggests that lumbar drain pressure measurements correlate well with EVD measurements in acute post-hemorrhagic communicating hydrocephalus (27). There are several other options available for measuring ICP through the skull, allowing a more direct evaluation. The gold standard remains the intraventricular catheter, commonly referred to as an external ventricular drain (EVD) (28). An EVD is a catheter placed in the ventricle to allow transduced pressure readings as well as serving as a conduit for therapeutic drainage of CSF. Since it can be recalibrated it is felt to be more accurate and less prone to drift over time (21). However, intraventricular monitoring may not reflect compartmental increases in pressure that do not immediately result in transmission of pressure to the lateral or third ventricles, such as with the case of infratentorial masses or focal herniations. Intraventricular catheters may also be difficult to place in the context of traumatic brain injury or diffuse edema, which often causes the ventricles to shrink down to slit-like proportions. Other problems encountered with the use of EVDs include system damping from positioning of the catheter against the ventricular wall and catheter occlusion with blood or tissue clot.

Intraparenchymal monitors are extremely useful in certain cases, although they may be more prone to drift over time (21). These monitors are usually placed via a burr hole in the brain parenchyma and use a fiberoptic transducer at the catheter tip. CSF cannot be drained using this type of monitor. Some studies have shown that the Camino catheters correlate very well with IVCs, making this type of monitor preferred in some centers due to its ease of insertion, especially in the head-injured patient with small ventricles.

Subdural and subarachnoid screws are fluid-filled bolts which are screwed into a burr hole until flush with the incised dura, allowing CSF pressure to be transduced. Although they have advantages of ease of insertion and low complication rates, they are felt by many experts to be less accurate and can provide falsely low (dampened) readings with high ICP if tissue obstructs the lumen (29).

Complications of invasive ICP monitoring

Complications of ICP monitoring include hemorrhage, infection, and parenchymal brain injury. Catheter-related hemorrhages (intraparenchymal, intraventricular, subdural or along the catheter tract) occur in 1–33% of patients, many of which are small and asymptomatic (30). Risk for hemorrhage seems to be the highest with EVDs (31). Hemorrhage most often occurs at the time of catheter placement but may also be a delayed phenomenon. Malpositioning of EVDs is also not infrequent, but is clearly dependent on definition (32).

While infection is a bona fide concern due to associated morbidity, clinically insignificant catheter colonization is far more common. Neither fever, CSF pleocytosis, nor peripheral leukocytosis carry a high predictive value for infections (33). The high occurrence of these laboratory abnormalities in patients with acute brain injuries and effects of catheter placement probably explain these observations. Several series evaluating infection risk with IVCs have shown that risk is highest after five days and this complication is rare if used for three days or less (21). Level III evidence exists against routine antibiotic prophylaxis or IVC exchange, especially with newer antibiotic-coated catheters (34).

Other risk factors for IVC-related infection include ICH, SAH or IVH, ICP>20, system irrigation, leakage, open skull fractures, and systemic infection. Sterile insertion of the IVC in the ICU (rather than the operating room) has not been associated with an increased risk of infection and neither has previous IVC, drainage of CSF, or steroids)(35–37).

Intracranial pressure vs. cerebral perfusion pressure

The TBI literature is engaged with a controversy over the importance of CPP or ICP as targets for ICU management. The occurrence of brain ischemia, reduced CPP and jugular venous desaturation in the context of elevated ICP have been well described and brain ischemia after TBI is treated almost as a 'dogma' (38) . However, since severe TBI is so often accompanied by diffuse axonal injury, it may be difficult to extrapolate data from the TBI population to patients with primary cerebrovascular pathology. The Rosner protocol emphasizes preservation of cerebral blood flow to prevent cerebral ischemia (39). Although unproven by a randomized controlled study, it is argued that treatment directed at maintaining CPP > 70 mmHg is superior to traditional techniques focused on ICP management.

In Rosner's study, methods used included vascular volume expansion, cerebrospinal fluid drainage via ventriculostomy, systemic vasopressors (phenylephrine or norepinephrine), and mannitol. Barbiturates, hyperventilation, and hypothermia were specifically not used. Comparisons of outcome classification across GCS categories (survival vs. death, favorable vs. nonfavorable) with other reported series were significantly better in Rosner's series. Mechanistically, decreased CPP due to either increased ICP or low blood pressure results in vasodilatation. This vasodilation increases cerebral blood volume (CBV) and exacerbates ICP and thus further reduces CPP, which can only be improved by increasing blood pressure. The Achilles heel of this approach is that permitting a high CPP can worsen cerebral edema especially where the blood brain barrier is not intact.

The relative influence of ICP and CPP on outcome was assessed in patients who had neurological deterioration from the international, multicenter, randomized, double-blind trial of the N-methyl-D-aspartate antagonist Selfotel in patients with TBI (40). The most powerful predictor of neurological worsening was intracranial hypertension (ICP > or = 20 mmHg) either initially or during neurological deterioration. There was no correlation with CPP as long as CPP was greater than 60 mmHg. It has therefore become more common that treatment protocols for the management of severe head injury emphasize immediate reduction of elevated ICP to less than 20 mmHg. A CPP greater than 60 mmHg appears to have little influence on the outcome of patients with severe head injury. These basic tenets highlight the relative importance of ICP and CPP in the TBI population.

Intracranial pressure and ischemic stroke

Stroke has been associated with increased ICP usually in the context of major hemispheric infarction leading to cerebral edema with risk for herniation and death. Most often this phenomenon is observed after a malignant middle cerebral artery infarction, which carries 70–80% mortality if treated conservatively. Furthermore, uncal herniation complicates malignant MCA infarction in 78% of cases (41).

The value of ICP monitoring in large middle cerebral artery infarction is debated in the literature, but infrequently put into practice. Space-occupying cerebral edema can result in elevated ICP and cerebral herniation. In fact, this was the primary cause of mortality within the first week in ECASS, the European Cooperative Acute Stroke Study (42). In a study of 48 patients with clinical signs of increased ICP due to large hemispheric infarction, epidural ICP sensors were inserted ipsilateral to the primary brain injury and also contralaterally in seven patients (43). ICP was normal at the time of insertion in 74%, 20–25 mmHg in 37 patients, 25–35 mmHg in eight patients, and > 35 mmHg in three patients who all died. ICP increased in all patients during the first two days after monitor insertion and was significantly higher in patients who died compared with survivors (mean 42 vs. 28 mmHg). ICP was higher ipsilateral to the stroke in patients with bilateral monitors with a difference up to 15 mmHg. All patients with any ICP > 35 mmHg during monitoring died. However, although high ICP correlated with clinical outcome, the initial ICP did not predict outcome and clinical herniation signs preceded critical ICP elevation, casting some doubt on the ability to utilize ICP values to affect clinical outcomes in this context. Moreover, CT findings such as severe midline shift did not correlate with ICP values. Medical management of elevated ICP was initially effective, but failed beyond the first few doses of osmotic therapy. The authors concluded that ICP monitoring did not positively influence outcomes, but may serve as a predictor during therapy. These results are supported by an earlier study by Frank of 19 patients with large hemispheric infarction who underwent ICP monitoring prior to neurologic deterioration (44). In this study, ICP > 18 mmHg within the first 12 hours of clinical progression to stupor predicted 83% mortality despite maximal medical therapy. However, elevated ICP was not commonly associated with initial neurologic deterioration secondary to mass effect. Contrary to the prior study, patients with initial ICP elevation were significantly younger than those without.

Since intra-arterial recombinant tissue plasminogen activator is not an appropriate treatment for malignant MCA infarction due to high rates of brain hemorrhage, many experts have recommended decompressive craniectomy (DC). The rationale for decompressive surgery is to reduce ICP and optimize CBF in addition to minimizing further infarction from cerebral edema. In a study of 42 patients undergoing DC for malignant MCA infarction, ICP was monitored with an intraparenchymal fiberoptic sensor during and post-operatively. An anterior temporal lobectomy was performed if ICP increased > 30 mmHg, which occurred in 13/42 (31%) of patients, including three patients who underwent anterior lobectomy two to three days after initial decompression and regained consciousness promptly after operation (45). Two-thirds of such patients survived compared with no survival in patients who developed ICP > 30 mmHg, but did not undergo further anterior temporal lobectomy.

Numerous reports suggest that DC is an effective means of ICP control at least in the TBI population (46–51). This operation includes a wide range of surgical procedures, all of which involve removal of large parts of the skull with or without dural augmentation, resection of brain tissue and occasional sectioning of the tentorium or falx. A pooled analysis of decompressive craniectomy performed less than 48 hours after ictus for malignant MCA infarction has also been shown to enhance survival in three European trials, although high rates of disability and depression were still observed (52). Physiologic findings after DC include cerebral blood flow (CBF) augmentation that is likely a result of decrease in CPP, but no significant improvement in CMRO2 levels (53). In a comparison of 36 TBI patients who received DC and 86 patients who did not, CMRO2 levels were significantly lower in the operated group, even after adjustment for injury severity, and were strongly associated with poor functional outcome. CBF levels remained above the ischemic threshold suggesting that cellular energy crisis was not of ischemic origin. These data indicate that ICP reduction with CBF elevation may not improve cerebral metabolism in patients with severe mitochondrial damage and that DC should be limited to patients with refractory intracranial hypertension and GCS > 6 on admission (53). Perhaps a logical correlate of these data is the idea that the timing of DC is important, with some experts recommending 'ultra-early' surgery less than six hours after ictus, before neurologic deterioration becomes evident (45).

Overall, ICP monitoring in severe stroke syndromes may be indicated on a case-by-case basis, with the knowledge that herniation events can occur despite normal ICP values (poca), highlighting the need for careful clinical and radiologic observation.

One medical complication that not infrequently arises in the ischemic stroke patient is renal insufficiency requiring dialysis. In patients with acute brain injury (ABI) of any etiology, continuous renal replacement therapy (CRRT) is the preferred mode of renal replacement therapy (RRT) in patients with acute renal insufficiency (ARI) requiring dialysis. Intermittent hemodialysis (IHD) exacerbates intracranial hypertension in patients with ABI, usually shortly after initiation. Mechanisms implicated include osmotic or fluid shifts and rapid exchange of bicarbonate (causing 'paradoxical' intracellular acidosis) although increased ICP usually precedes significant changes in serum osmolality or pH (54–57). The more likely cause, however, is cardiovascular instability and fluctuation in cerebral perfusion pressure (CPP) in patients with impaired cerebral autoregulation (56). CRRT may provide beneficial effects on ICP control beyond just avoidance of worsening ICP. Fletcher *et al.* found a non-significant trend to reduction of ICP at 1 and 12 hours after initiation of CRRT in 4 patients with acute brain injury and refractory intracranial hypertension (3 with TBI; 1 with SAH) (58).

There was also a non-significant reduction in fluid balance over the 12 hours although this was not likely the mechanism of ICP reduction. The authors suggest that removal of cytokines and myocardial depressants, which is maximal in the first hour of therapy, as a better possible explanation (59, 60). Other studies have demonstrated ICP stability (but not ICP reduction), with CRRT, mostly in patients with fulminant hepatic failure (causing cerebral edema) and oliguric renal failure (54, 55). Remaining issues are whether venovenous ultrafiltration (UF) is superior to arteriovenous UF and whether high-intensity CRRT may have benefit for refractory intracranial hypertension in acute brain injury.

Intracranial pressure (ICP) and intracranial hemorrhage (ICH)

The assumption that there is a high risk of increased ICP after large volume ICH, especially in the presence of IVH, appears reasonable, but has limited evidence. Since some studies suggest an association with intracranial hypertension and poor outcome in ICH patients, this may suggest a role for ICP monitoring (61). In a study of 62 patients with spontaneous supratentorial ICH who had continuous ICP monitors, a relationship between high ICP and death within three days and poor Glasgow Outcome Score (GOS) at discharge was noted. However, there was no correlation between ICP within three days of ictus and GOS at six months (62). Neurologic deterioration in ICH is felt to result from mass effect from early hematoma expansion in addition to formation of edema and obstructive hydrocephalus (63). Current expert recommendations for treatment of elevated ICP include controlled hyperventilation, hyperosmolar therapy, pharmacologic coma, or decompressive craniectomy. Prophylactic mannitol and steroids have not been found to be helpful (64).

When deciding on which patients to monitor ICP, guidelines from the traumatic brain injury population may be used as a framework. Although there has not been a definitive clinical trial with ICH patients, the American Stroke Association recommends consideration for ICP monitoring in patients with a GCS score ≤ 8, those with clinical transtentorial herniation, or those with significant IVH or hydrocephalus (57). They also recommend obtaining a goal CPP of 50–70 mmHg and use of ventricular drainage as treatment for hydrocephalus in appropriate patients with a decreased level of consciousness (65). Additionally, the European Stroke Initiative guidelines advise monitoring ICP in patients requiring mechanical ventilation (66). In patients with both ICH and IVH intracranial hypertension may contribute to altered level of consciousness by acute reduction in CPP, ischemic encephalopathy (67), diffuse cerebral edema, and compression of the rostral brainstem and thalamus by an expanded third ventricle (68). Volume of intraventricular blood and degree of obstructive hydrocephalus are reported as prognostic factors in IVH (69, 70) and retrospective analyses of ICP have been performed. Adams (71) reported that emergency CSF drainage with EVD controlled initial ICP well in 20/22 patients with supratentorial ICH and hydrocephalus, but ventricular size did not decrease nor did the level of consciousness improve. Continuous ICP recordings were not analyzed. Diringe (72) found that in 81 patients with supratentorial ICH, hydrocephalus was independently associated with higher intubation rates and increased mortality, although outcomes in patients treated with EVD were not different from those not treated with EVDs. Coplin (73) reported on a cohort of 40 patients with spontaneous IVH who received EVDs. The mean initial ICP was 15.6 mmHg, and only six patients (15%) had ICP elevation (ICP > 20 mmHg) at the time of EVD placement. ICP elevation at presentation was not associated with a poor GOS. In a prospective investigation of ICP in 11 patients with IVH and small ICH (< 30 cc) who had ICP recorded every 4–6 hours while an EVD was in place, we found that both initial and subsequent ICP readings were not commonly elevated > 20 mmHg (14% of readings) despite acute obstructive hydrocephalus (74). We subsequently found in a larger prospective study of 100 patients with IVH requiring EVD that CSF drainage effectively controlled ICP over 90% of the time. However, ICP elevation > 30 mmHg, when it occurred, was an independent predictor of short-term mortality, suggesting that EVDs may play both a therapeutic and diagnostic role in this disease at least in patients with smaller ICH (unpublished data). In this study ICP elevation was a frequent occurrence during EVD closure for thrombolytic treatment, but was readily managed in most cases with conventional ICP-lowering strategies until the EVD could be reopened. While EVD placement should not be delayed in patients with severe IVH and neurologic deterioration secondary to acute hydrocephalus, retrospective studies of patients with IVH in the setting of ICH and SAH have thus far failed to show that EVD alone significantly alters mortality rates compared with conservative management (Fig. 1.6) (75). Clearly in many cases, especially in severe SAH, ICP control is likely an issue, but in others, the harmful effects may reflect the severe cognitive effects of the presence of blood in the ventricles (76) in the absence of a clear pressure problem.

Indications for ICP monitoring in severe TBI (GCS ≤ 8)

*Patient with normal head CT scan and two or more of the following:
- Motor posturing
- Age >40 years
- Arterial hypotension (systolic <90)

*Patient with abnormal head CT scan:
- Edema/swelling
- Hematoma or contusion
- Compression of basal cisterns

Fig. 1.6 Indications for ICP monitoring in severe TBI based on Brain Trauma Foundation recommendations.

Intracranial pressure (ICP) and cerebral venous thrombosis

The majority of patients diagnosed with cerebral vein thrombosis (CVT) will not require admission to an intensive care unit or ICP monitoring. Cases of increased ICP with CVT are usually complicated by extensive thrombus formation and hemorrhagic infarction. The most common cause of fatal neurologic deterioration in CVT is uncal herniation (77). Other significant complications from increased ICP in this population include optic atrophy and blindness. Since patients with CVT are almost uniformly anticoagulated, many institutions are reluctant to insert invasive ICP monitors for concern of excessive bleeding.

Treatment of presumed or measured ICP in patients with high ICP in CVT is controversial. Therapeutic anticoagulation is the mainstay of treatment for this disorder. In regards to treatment of high ICP, elevation of the bed to at least 30 degrees and avoidance of fever are well-accepted measures. Some critics question the use of hyperosmolar therapies due to concern for extensive breakdown of the blood–brain barrier as well as venous outflow obstruction, limiting the clearance of agents such as mannitol (78). Others report successfully using barbituate coma in select cases (79). Serial lumbar punctures can be carefully considered on a case-by-case basis only after imaging has verified that there is no significant mass effect and a patent ventricular system exists (21). Occasionally, CSF shunting is indicated if serial lumbar punctures have been deemed helpful. A few studies have shown a survival benefit from decompressive craniectomy in patients with CVT and life-threatening hemorrhagic infarcts (77).

Intracranial pressure (ICP) and aneurysmal subarachnoid hemorrhage (aSAH)

Multiple mechanisms of ICP elevation may coexist after aneurysmal subarachnoid hemorrhage (aSAH) including hydrocephalus, ICH, infarction, hyponatremia and seizures. Signs of high ICP in this population include bilateral sixth nerve palsies and ocular hemorrhages in addition to declining level of consciousness. Elevated ICP associated with acute hydrocephalus has been noted in approximately 20% of cases of aSAH (80).

Hydrocephalus in SAH can be characterized as communicating when there is impaired CSF resorption or non-communicating as in the case of ventricular outflow obstruction by blood clot. Hydrocephalus is usually detected clinically as decreased level of consciousness, although it may be noted on imaging alone as serial enlargement of the ventricles. Most experts agree that an external ventricular drain is warranted in patients with obstructive hydrocephalus and clear decline in level of consciousness (5). Depending on the mechanism of the hydrocephalus and other factors, a lumbar drain may also be appropriate. A lumbar drain is contraindicated in cases of significant mass effect, effacement of the basilar cisterns, obstructive clot, or significant coagulopathy (5). There is some evidence that lumbar drainage has the added benefit of reducing vasospasm risk in aSAH, although this is controversial (5).

The most appropriate method for weaning aSAH patients from ventricular drains is of considerable debate and several commonly used approaches seem reasonable. The goal of ventriculostomy weaning is to avoid complications such as infection while providing relief of hydrocephalus via CSF and clot removal while ensuring adequate CBF. Most patients will require active drainage for 7–10 days (5). Successful weaning can usually be accomplished by gradually increasing the drain's resistance against gravity over days while closely observing the clinical exam and ventricular appearance on CT for signs of deterioration. Even after lengthy periods of CSF drainage, a considerable percentage of patients will go on to develop late/chronic hydrocephalus and require a shunt. There does not appear to be an association between the type of weaning method (fast or gradual) and risk for developing shunt dependence (5). Some risk factors for the development of shunt dependency have been elucidated and are: increasing age, female sex, poor admission Hunt and Hess grade, thick subarachnoid hemorrhage on admission computed tomographic, intraventricular hemorrhage, radiological hydrocephalus at the time of admission, distal posterior circulation location of the ruptured aneurysm, clinical vasospasm and endovascular treatment (81).

Intracranial pressure (ICP) and traumatic brain injury (TBI)

Since much of the foundation for ICP monitoring and treatment in acute cerebrovascular disease was formed during investigations on TBI patients, we will briefly review the guidelines. As discussed, one may loosely apply the Brain Trauma Foundation guidelines for insertion of ICP monitors to the cerebrovascular patient (Fig. 1.7). These guidelines may oversimplify the decision-making process but provide a basic framework and emphasize both clinical and imaging characteristics. Embedded in these guidelines is the idea that low cerebral perfusion pressure is likely dangerous. CPP is generally targeted to > 70 mmHg with an ICP goal of < 20 mmHg. Clinical features such as motor posturing are also emphasized, keeping in mind that imaging cannot be relied upon as a sole predictor of high ICP (10–15 false negative rate) (82). Extremes of

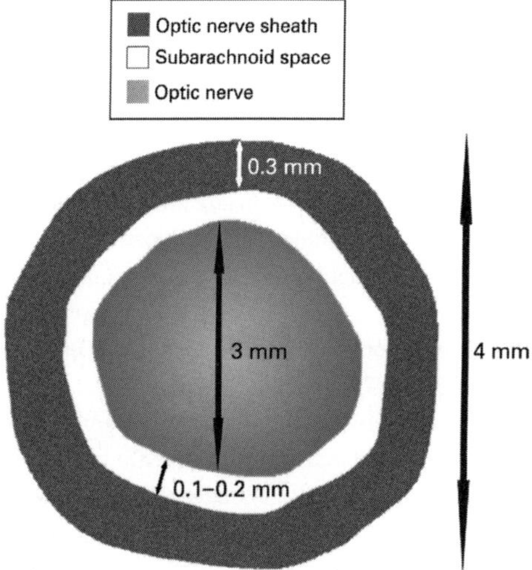

Fig. 1.7 Schematic drawing of a cross-section of the optic nerve complex. From Soldatos T *et al. Emerg Med J* (2009);**26**:630–4.

blood pressure should be avoided since the injured brain often has impaired autoregulation. Usually MAPs greater than 130 should be avoided (83). Arterial hypotension (defined as either systolic less than 90 or 100 by various sources) has also been associated with poor outcome (39).

Post-traumatic intracranial hypertension remains the leading cause of death in the ICU in brain-injured patients (84). According to the Brain Trauma Foundation Guidelines, treatment of high ICP in patients with TBI is divided into first- and second-tier options following a standardized pathway which includes sedatives and muscle relaxants (85). First-tier measures include osmotic solutions, ventricular drainage of CSF, and moderate hyperventilation; if these measures fail to control high ICP, second-tier measures are commonly used (decompressive craniectomy, barbiturate coma or therapeutic hypothermia) (85). Mannitol remains the first-line osmotic agent for treatment of intracranial hypertension attributable to TBI and other CNS insults. Mannitol is effective in decreasing ICP and was found to reduce mortality compared with barbiturates in at least one randomized trial of TBI patients, but has occasional adverse effects, including hypovolemia and renal failure (86, 87). There is also evidence that excessive administration may worsen cerebral edema due to reverse osmotic shift. Sodium-based hypertonic solutions have come into vogue in the last few decades due to their ability to reduce ICP without causing volume contraction or nephrotoxicity (88). Several small randomized clinical trials have demonstrated superiority compared to mannitol but these have been small in size and used different concentrations and formulations of hypertonic saline (89–93). Recently Kamel *et al.* performed a metaanalysis of randomized clinical trials involving humans undergoing ICP measurement with evidence of elevated ICP (94). The effect on ICP within 60 min of treatment of equimolar doses of hypertonic saline and mannitol solutions was compared and it was found that hypertonic sodium solutions were more effective than mannitol in controlling episodes of elevated ICP. A variety of CNS pathologies was represented including TBI, stroke, intracerebral hemorrhage, and subarachnoid hemorrhage. The results are compelling, although the guidelines for ICP management are unlikely to change in the near future due to the extensive experience with mannitol and because the many different regimens of HTS, in terms of concentration, dose, bolus vs. continuous infusions, and with or without supplementation of colloids make optimal use of hypertonic solutions more difficult to implement and to study.

Mechanical treatment options for elevated ICP in TBI patients include CSF removal via intraventricular or lumbar catheters, decompressive craniectomy, and evacuation of space-occupying lesions. Placement of IVCs in TBI patients is often problematic due to mass effect causing obliteration of the lateral ventricles. CSF removal through external lumbar drainage (ELD) is controversial in the adult population due to safety concerns and a lack of understanding of mechanisms underlying its efficacy in lowering long-lasting raised ICP (95–99). One recent retrospective study, however, found that the use of ELD resulted in a significant decrease in ICP in all patients with favorable long-term outcomes in 62% of patients and few complications with no associated papillary changes (100). ELD was placed after a mean of 8.6±3.9 days and CSF drainage was maintained for a mean of 6.6±3.5 days, indicating that this therapy is likely best reserved for the subacute phase.

Surgical decompressive craniectomy is increasingly performed to control intracranial pressure (101). In the multicenter, randomized, controlled Decompressive Craniectomy (DECRA) trial (102–103) to test the efficacy of bifrontotemporoparietal decompressive craniectomy in adults under age 60 years with TBI, in whom first-tier therapies failed to control ICP, early bifrontotemporoparietal decompressive craniectomy decreased ICP, number of interventions for elevated ICP and duration of both ventilator support and the ICU stay, but was associated with more unfavorable outcomes compared with standard care at six months. Several explanations for the negative result of this trial include a statistically greater number of patients with bilateral fixed dilated pupils on admission in the craniectomy group and the finding that initial ICP was not elevated > 25 mmHg in either group prior to randomization. It is also possible that the bilateral procedure has more complications that a unilateral craniectomy and expansion of the swollen brain outside the skull may cause axonal stretch (104, 105), which in vitro causes neural injury (106–108).

The role of induced hypothermia as a means to lower ICP in TBI patients is controversial, with two randomized studies showing conflicting results. The data indicate that induced hypothermia effectively reduces ICP but whether or not this affects long-term outcome compared to standard measures of ICP control remains inconclusive (109, 110). Level of hypothermia and time to reach goal temperature appear to be important factors which may partially explain these differing results. Taken as a whole, these studies suggest that active rewarming of TBI patients admitted with hypothermia should be avoided while therapeutic hypothermia is generally safe and may have a role for ICP management in select cases (111).

Recently there has been an interest in understanding the associations of markers of cerebral inflammation with commonly used clinical and radiologic indicators, including ICP. In TBI, following the initial traumatic insult, the brain experiences a secondary wave of injury in which inflammation may play an important role and potentially contribute to a poor outcome (112, 113). The endogenous neuroinflammatory response after TBI contributes to the development of cerebral edema, breakdown of the blood–brain barrier, increased ICP and ultimately to delayed neuronal death (114). Parez-Barcena *et al.* studied the relationship between the temporal pattern of cytokines known to be elevated after TBI and the behavior of ICP and brain tissue oxygenation (PBrO2) in patients with diffuse traumatic brain injury (115). Interestingly they found no clear relationship between cytokines and ICP, PBrO2, and the presence of swelling on CT scan. There appear to be a multitude of complex mechanisms and neuroinflammatory mediators involved in secondary brain injury in TBI, including probable genetic variability in the cytokine response which has yet to be investigated.

ICP management remains the gold standard largely because protocols using hypothermia, hyperbaric oxygen, CBF optimization, and pharmaceutical agents have not shown clear outcome benefits over standard ICP guided therapy (31, 35, 52, 116). However, while adherence to the BTF guidelines for TBI with aggressive ICP management has been shown to reduce mortality, benefits in terms of functional outcome are less convincing (117). Recently cerebral oxygenation or PbtO2-directed protocols aimed at limiting secondary ischemia have evolved (118). Brain tissue oximetry is another form of invasive monitoring used in many centers for TBI patients. This technology is a microsensor which is placed in peri-lesional tissue through a bolt or craniotomy defect. Use of this type of monitor is still controversial. A retrospective study comparing tissue oximetry and ICP monitoring with ICP monitoring alone found worsened rates of mortality and morbidity in the combined group (119). However, the patients receiving both monitors had more severe injuries and received more aggressive therapy than their counterparts. In a different prospective study utilizing a brain oxygen-directed protocol (rather than ICP/CPP), morbidity and mortality were reduced compared to internal historical controls. They also found correlations between low brain tissue oxygenation, high ICP, and death or poor outcome (116). A prospective, randomized study is underway. Cerebral oxygenation-directed protocols have yet to gain widespread use or acceptance because they require significant escalation in therapy intensity, and have not yet demonstrated a clear outcome advantage over ICP protocols (120). Currently only non-randomized studies have reported improved clinical outcome with the use of a PbtO2-directed protocol (116). However, in this study patients with uncontrollable ICP and persistent cerebral hypooxygenation at 48 hours both had increased risk of death and poor outcome despite maximal therapy with the PbtO2-protocol.

REFERENCES

1. Marmarou A. Traumatic brain edema: an overview. *Acta Neurochir Suppl (Wien)*. 1994;**60**:421–4.
2. Prabhakaran P, Reddy AT, Oakes WJ, *et al.* A pilot trial comparing cerebral perfusion pressure-targeted therapy to intracranial pressure-targeted therapy in children with severe traumatic brain injury. *J Neurosurg*. 2004;**100**(5 Suppl Pediatrics):454–9.
3. Unterberg. Long term observations of ICP after severe head injury. *Neurosurgery*. 1993;**32**:17–24.
4. Manz HJ. Pathophysiology and pathology of elevated intracranial pressure. *Pathobiol Annu*. 1979;**9**:359–81.

5. Wijdicks E. *The Practice of Emergency and Critical Care Neurology*. New York: Oxford University Press; 2010.
6. Doczi T. Volume regulation of the brain tissue - a survey. *Acta Neurochir (Wien)*. 1993;**121**(1-2):1–8.
7. McComb JG. Recent research into the nature of cerebrospinal fluid formation and absorption. *J Neurosurg*. 1983;**59**(3):369–83.
8. Gjerris F. Pathophysiology of cerebrospinal fluid circulation. Oxford: Blackwell Science; 2000.
9. Lyons MK, Meyer FB. Cerebrospinal fluid physiology and the management of increased intracranial pressure. *Mayo Clin Proc*. 1990;**65**(5):684–707.
10. Cutler RW, Page L, Galicich J, Watters GV. Formation and absorption of cerebrospinal fluid in man. *Brain*. 1968;**91**(4):707–20.
11. Potts DG, Deonarine V. Effect of positional changes and jugular vein compression on the pressure gradient across the arachnoid villi and granulations of the dog. *J Neurosurg*. 1973;**38**(6):722–8.
12. Wolfla CE, Luerssen TG. Brain tissue pressure gradients are dependent upon a normal spinal subarachnoid space. *Acta Neurochir Suppl*. 1998;**71**:310–12.
13. Magnaes B. Clinical studies of cranial and spinal compliance and the craniospinal flow of cerebrospinal fluid. *Br J Neurosurg*. 1989;**3**(6):659–68.
14. Apuzzo JL, Wiess MH, Petersons V, *et al.* Effect of positive end expiratory pressure ventilation on intracranial pressure in man. *J Neurosurg*. 1977;**46**(2):227–32.
15. Hauerberg J, Juhler M. Cerebral blood flow autoregulation in acute intracranial hypertension. *J Cereb Blood Flow Metab*. 1994;**14**(3):519–25.
16. Lee K. Intracranial pressure. *Neurol. Surg*. 1996;**1**:491–518.
17. Hayashi M, Handa Y, Kobayashi H, Ishii H. Intracranial hypertension and pressure waves. *No Shinkei Geka*. 1985;**13**(3):245–53.
18. Bratton S. Indications for intracranial pressure monitoring. *J Neurotrauma*. 2007;**24**(1):7.
19. Saul TG. Effect of ICP monitoring and aggressive treatment on mortality in severe head injury. *J Neurosurg*. 1982;**56**:498–503.
20. Narayan RK. ICP: To monitor or not to monitor? *J Neurosurg*. 1982;**56**:650–9.
21. Suarez J. *Critical Care Neurology and Neurosurgery*. New Jersey: Humana Press; 2004.
22. Teasdale E. CT scan in severe diffuse head injury: physiological and clinical correlations. *J Neurol Neurosurg Psych*. 1984;**47**:600–3.
23. Chan K. The effect of changes in cerebral perfusion pressure upon middle cerebral artery blood flow velocity and jugular bulb venous oxygen saturation after severe brain injury. *J Neurosurg*. 1992;**77**:55–61.
24. Bellner J. Transcranial Doppler sonography pulsatility index (PI) reflects intracranial pressure (ICP). *Surg Neurol*. 2004;**62**(1):45–51.
25. Behrens A. Transcranial Doppler pulsatility index: not an accurate method to assess intracranial pressure. *Neurosurgery*. 2010;**66**(6):1050–7.
26. Soldatos T. Optic nerve sonography a new window for the non-invasive evaluation of intracranial pressure in brain injury. *Emerg Med J*. 2009;**26**:630–4.
27. Speck V. Lumbar catheter for monitoring of intracranial pressure in patients with post-hemorrhagic communicating hydrocephalus. *Neurocrit Care*. 2010:208–15.
28. Brain Trauma Foundation. ICP monitoring technology. *J Neurotrauma*. 2007;**24**:45–54.
29. Mendelow A. A clinical comparison of subdural screw pressure measurements with ventricular pressure. *J Neurosurg*. 1983;**58**(1):45–50.
30. Maniker. Hemorrhagic complications of external ventricular drainage. *Operative Neurosurg*. 2006;**59**:419–25.
31. Lang E. Intracranial pressure: Monitoring and management. *Neurosurg Clin N Am*. 1994;**5**(4):573–605.
32. Saladino A. Malplacement of ventricular catheters by neurosurgeons: a single institution experience. *Neurocrit Care*. 2009;**10**(2):248–52.
33. Lozien AP. Ventriculostomy-related infection: A critical review of the literature. *Neurosurgery*. 2002;**51**:170–82.
34. Brain Trauma Foundation: Infection prophylaxis. *J Neurotrauma*. 2007;**24**:526–31.
35. Mayhall CG. Ventriculostomy-related infections: A prospective epidemiologic study. *N Eng J Med*. 1984;**310**:553–9.
36. Lyke KE. Ventriculitis complicating use of intraventricular catheters in adult neurosurgical patients. *Clin Infect Dis*. 2001;**33**:2028–33.
37. Paramore CG. Relative risks of ventriculostomy infection and morbidity. *Acta Neurochir*. 1994;**127**:79–84.
38. Vespa P. What is the optimal threshold for cerebral perfusion pressure following traumatic brain injury? *Neurosurg Focus*. 2003;**15**(6):1–5.
39. Rosner MJ, Rosner SD, Johnson AH. Cerebral perfusion pressure: management protocol and clinical results. *J Neurosurg*. 1995;**83**(6):949–62.
40. Juul N, Morris GF, Marshall SB, Marshall LF. Intracranial hypertension and cerebral perfusion pressure: influence on neurological deterioration and outcome in severe head

injury. The Executive Committee of the International Selfotel Trial. *J Neurosurg.* 2000;**92**(1):1–6.

41. Hacke W, Schwab S, Horn M, *et al.* 'Malignant' middle cerebral artery territory infarction: clinical course and prognostic signs. *Arch Neurol.* 1996;**53**(4):309–15.
42. Hacke W, Kaste M, Fieschi C, *et al.* Intravenous thrombolysis with recombinant tissue plasminogen activator for acute hemispheric stroke. The European Cooperative Acute Stroke Study (ECASS). *JAMA.* 1995;**274**(13):1017–25.
43. Schwab S, Aschoff A, Spranger M, Albert F, Hacke W. The value of intracranial pressure monitoring in acute hemispheric stroke. *Neurology.* 1996;**47**(2):393–8.
44. Frank, JI. Large hemispheric infarction, deterioration, and intracranial pressure. *Neurology.* 1995;**45**(7):1286–90.
45. Cho D. Ultra-early decompressive craniectomy for malignant middle cerebral artery infarction. *Surg Neurol.* 2003;**60**(3):227–32.
46. Jaeger M, Soehle M, Meixensberger J. Improvement of brain tissue oxygen and intracranial pressure during and after surgical decompression for diffuse brain oedema and space occupying infarction. *Acta Neurochir Suppl.* 2005;**95**:117–18.
47. Ho CL, Wang CM, Lee KK, Ng I, Ang BT. Cerebral oxygenation, vascular reactivity, and neurochemistry following decompressive craniectomy for severe traumatic brain injury. *J Neurosurg.* 2008;**108**(5):943–9.
48. Olivecrona M, Rodling-Wahlstrom M, Naredi S, Koskinen LO. Effective ICP reduction by decompressive craniectomy in patients with severe traumatic brain injury treated by an ICP-targeted therapy. *J Neurotrauma.* 2007;**24**(6):927–35.
49. Pompucci A, De Bonis P, Pettorini B, *et al.* Decompressive craniectomy for traumatic brain injury: patient age and outcome. *J Neurotrauma.* 2007;**24**(7):1182–8.
50. Stiefel MF, Heuer GG, Smith MJ, *et al.* Cerebral oxygenation following decompressive hemicraniectomy for the treatment of refractory intracranial hypertension. *J Neurosurg.* 2004;**101**(2):241–7.
51. Taylor A, Butt W, Rosenfeld J, *et al.* A randomized trial of very early decompressive craniectomy in children with traumatic brain injury and sustained intracranial hypertension. *Childs Nerv Syst.* 2001;**17**(3):154–62.
52. Vahedi K. Early decompressive surgery in malignant infarction of the middle cerebral artery: a pooled analyis of three randomized controlled trials. *Lancet Neurol.* 2007;**6**:215–22.
53. Soustiel J. Cerebral blood flow and metabolism following decompressive craniectomy for control of increased intracranial pressure. *Neurosurgery.* 2010;**67**:65–72.
54. Davenport A. Early changes in intracranial pressure during haemofiltration treatment in patients with grade 4 hepatic encephalopathy and acute oliguric renal failure. *Nephrol Dial Transplant.* 1990;**5**:192–8.
55. Davenport A. Continuous vs. intermittent forms of haemofiltration and/or dialysis in the management of acute renal failure in patients with defective cerebral autoregulation at risk of cerebral oedema. *Contrib Nephrol.* 1991;**93**:225–33.
56. Bertrand Y. Intracranial pressure changes in patients with head trauma during hemodialysis. *Intensive Care Med.* 1983;**9**:321–3.
57. Davenport A, Will EJ, Losowsky MS, Swindells S. Continuous arteriovenous haemofiltration in patients with hepatic encephalopathy and renal failure. *Br Med J* (Clin Res Ed). 1987;**295**(6605):1028.
58. Fletcher J. Continuous renal replacement therapy for refractory intracranial hypertension? *J Trauma.* 2010;**68**(6):1506–9.
59. De Vriese AS, Colardyn FA, Philippe JJ, *et al.* Cytokine removal during continuous hemofiltration in septic patients. *J Am Soc Nephrol.* 1999;**10**(4):846–53.
60. Bellomo R, Tipping P, Boyce N. Continuous veno-venous hemofiltration with dialysis removes cytokines from the circulation of septic patients. *Crit Care Med.* 1993;**21**(4):522–6.
61. Diringer M. Intracerebral hemorrhage: pathophysiology and management. *Crit Care Med.* 1993;**21**(10):1591–603.
62. Fernandes H. Continuous monitoring of ICP and CPP following ICH and its relationship to clinical, radiological and surgical parameters. *Acta Neurochir Suppl.* 2000;**76**:463–6.
63. Mayer S. Neurologic deterioration in noncomatose patients with supratentorial intracerebral hemorrhage. *Neurology.* 1994;**44**:1379–84.
64. Carhuapoma R. *Intracerebral Hemorrhage.* New York: Cambridge University Press; 2010.
65. Lewis B. Guidelines for the management of spontaneous intracerebral hemorrhage (American Stroke Association). *Stroke.* 2010;**41**:2108.
66. Broderick J. Guidelines for the management of spontaneous intracerebral hemorrhage. *Stroke.* 1999;**30**:905–15.
67. Naff N. Treatment of intraventricular hemorrhage with urokinase; effects on 30-day survival. *Stroke.* 2000;**31**:81–847.
68. Steinke W. Thalamic stroke: Presentation and prognosis of infarcts and hemorrhages. *Arch Neurol.* 1992;**49**:703–10.
69. Mayfrank L. Effect of recombinant tissue plasminogen activator on clot lysis and ventricular dilatation in the treatment of severe intraventricular hemorrhage. *Acta Neurochir.* 1993;**122**:32–8.

70. Tuhrim S. Volume of ventricular blood is an important determinant of outcome in supratentorial intracerebral hemorrhage. *Crit Care Med.* 1999;**27**:617–21.
71. Adams R. Response to external ventricular drainage in spontaneous intracerebral hemorrhage with hydrocephalus. *Neurology.* 1998;**50**:519–23.
72. Diringer M. Hydrocephalus: a previously unrecognized predictor of poor outcome from supratentorial intracerebral hemorrhage. *Stroke.* 1998;**29**:1352–7.
73. Coplin W. A cohort study of the safety and feasibiity of intraventricular urokinase for nonaneurysmal spontaneous intraventricular hemorrhage. *Stroke.* 1998;**29**:1573–9.
74. Ziai W. Frequency of sustained intracranial pressure elevation during treatment of severe intraventricular hemorrhage. *Cerebrovasc Dis.* 2009;**27**:403–10.
75. Nieuwkamp D. Treatment and outcome of severe intraventricular extension in patients with subarachnoid or intracerebral hemorrhage: a systematic review of the literature. *J Neurol.* 2000;**247**(2):117–21.
76. Hutter B. Cognitive deficits in the acute stage after subarachnoid hemorrhage. *Neurosurgery.* 1998;**43**:1054–65.
77. Lath R. Decompressive surgery for severe cerebral venous thrombosis. *Neurol India.* 2010;**58**(3):392–7.
78. Einhdupi K. EFNS guidelines on the treatment of cerebral venous and sinus thrombosis. *Eur J Neurol.* 2006;**13**:553–9.
79. Torbey M. *Neurocritical Care.* New York: Cambridge University Press; 2010.
80. Milhorat T. Acute hydrocephalus after aneurysmal subarachnoid hemorrhage. *Neurosurgery.* 1987;**20**:15–20.
81. Dorai Z. Factors related to hydrocephalus after aneurysmal subarachnoid hemorrhage. *Neurosurgery.* 2004;**54**(4):1031.
82. Eisenberg H. Initial CT findings in 753 patients with severe head injury. A report from the NIH traumatic coma data bank. *J Neurosurg.* 1990;**73**:688–98.
83. Czosnyka M. Cerebral autoregulation following head injury. *J Neurosurg.* 2001;**95**:756–63.
84. O'Phelan KH, Park D, Efird JT, *et al.* Patterns of increased intracranial pressure after severe traumatic brain injury. *Neurocrit Care.* 2009;**10**(3):280–6.
85. Guidelines for the management of severe head injury. Introduction. *J Neurotrauma.* 1996;**13**(11):643–5.
86. Schwartz ML, Tator CH, Rowed DW, *et al.* The University of Toronto head injury treatment study: a prospective, randomized comparison of pentobarbital and mannitol. *Can J Neurol Sci.* 1984;**11**(4):434–40.
87. Oken DE. Renal and extrarenal considerations in high-dose mannitol therapy. *Ren Fail.* 1994;**16**(1):147–59.
88. Bentsen G, Breivik H, Lundar T, Stubhaug A. Hypertonic saline (7.2%) in 6% hydroxyethyl starch reduces intracranial pressure and improves hemodynamics in a placebo-controlled study involving stable patients with subarachnoid hemorrhage. *Crit Care Med.* 2006;**34**(12):2912–17.
89. Schwarz S, Schwab S, Bertram M, Aschoff A, Hacke W. Effects of hypertonic saline hydroxyethyl starch solution and mannitol in patients with increased intracranial pressure after stroke. *Stroke.* 1998;**29**(8):1550–5.
90. Battison C, Andrews PJ, Graham C, Petty T. Randomized, controlled trial on the effect of a 20% mannitol solution and a 7.5% saline/6% dextran solution on increased intracranial pressure after brain injury. *Crit Care Med.* 2005;**33**(1):196–202; discussion 57–8.
91. Vialet R, Albanese J, Thomachot L, *et al.* Isovolume hypertonic solutes (sodium chloride or mannitol) in the treatment of refractory posttraumatic intracranial hypertension: 2 mL/kg 7.5% saline is more effective than 2 mL/kg 20% mannitol. *Crit Care Med.* 2003;**31**(6):1683–7.
92. Harutjunyan L, Holz C, Rieger A, *et al.* Efficiency of 7.2% hypertonic saline hydroxyethyl starch 200/0.5 versus mannitol 15% in the treatment of increased intracranial pressure in neurosurgical patients – a randomized clinical trial [ISRCTN62699180]. *Crit Care.* 2005;**9**(5):R530–40.
93. Ichai C, Armando G, Orban JC, *et al.* Sodium lactate versus mannitol in the treatment of intracranial hypertensive episodes in severe traumatic brain-injured patients. *Intensive Care Med.* 2009;**35**(3):471–9.
94. Kamel H, Navi BB, Nakagawa K, Hemphill JC, Ko NU. Hypertonic saline versus mannitol for the treatment of elevated intracranial pressure: a meta-analysis of randomized clinical trials. *Crit Care Med.* 2011;**39**(3):554–9.
95. Grady MS. Lumbar drainage for increased intracranial pressure. *J Neurosurg.* 2009;**110**(6):1198–9.
96. Akil H. The treatment of refractory intracranial hypertension and its control by means of external lumbar drainage (ELD). *J Trauma.* 2007;**63**(3):720–1.
97. Tuettenberg J, Czabanka M, Horn P, *et al.* Clinical evaluation of the safety and efficacy of lumbar cerebrospinal fluid drainage for the treatment of refractory increased intracranial pressure. *J Neurosurg.* 2009;**110**(6):1200–8.
98. Munch EC, Bauhuf C, Horn P, *et al.* Therapy of malignant intracranial hypertension by controlled lumbar cerebrospinal fluid drainage. *Crit Care Med.* 2001;**29**(5):976–81.
99. Abadal-Centellas JM, Llompart-Pou JA, Homar-Ramirez J, *et al.* Neurologic outcome of post-traumatic refractory intracranial hypertension treated with external lumbar drainage. *J Trauma.* 2007;**62**(2):282–6; discussion 6.

100. Llompart-Pou JA, Abadal JM, Perez-Barcena J, *et al.* Long-term follow-up of patients with post-traumatic refractory high intracranial pressure treated with lumbar drainage. *Anaesth Intensive Care.* 2011;**39**(1):79–83.
101. Sahuquillo J, Arikan F. Decompressive craniectomy for the treatment of refractory high intracranial pressure in traumatic brain injury. *Cochrane Database Syst Rev.* 2006; **1**:CD003983.
102. Cooper DJ, Rosenfeld JV, Murray L, *et al.* Decompressive craniectomy in diffuse traumatic brain injury. *N Engl J Med.* 2011;**364**(16):1493–502.
103. Vahedi K, Vicaut E, Mateo J, *et al.* Sequential-design, multicenter, randomized, controlled trial of early decompressive craniectomy in malignant middle cerebral artery infarction (DECIMAL Trial). *Stroke.* 2007;**38**(9):2506–17.
104. Cooper PR, Hagler H, Clark WK, Barnett P. Enhancement of experimental cerebral edema after decompressive craniectomy: implications for the management of severe head injuries. *Neurosurgery.* 1979;**4**(4):296–300.
105. Stiver SI. Complications of decompressive craniectomy for traumatic brain injury. *Neurosurg Focus.* 2009;**26**(6):E7.
106. Chung RS, Staal JA, McCormack GH, *et al.* Mild axonal stretch injury in vitro induces a progressive series of neurofilament alterations ultimately leading to delayed axotomy. *J Neurotrauma.* 2005;**22**(10):1081–91.
107. Staal JA, Dickson TC, Gasperini R, *et al.* Initial calcium release from intracellular stores followed by calcium dysregulation is linked to secondary axotomy following transient axonal stretch injury. *J Neurochem.* 2010;**112**(5):1147–55.
108. Tang-Schomer MD, Patel AR, Baas PW, Smith DH. Mechanical breaking of microtubules in axons during dynamic stretch injury underlies delayed elasticity, microtubule disassembly, and axon degeneration. *FASEB J.* 2010;**24**(5):1401–10.
109. Clifton G. Lack of effect of induction of hypothermia after acute brain injury. *N Eng J Med.* 2001;**344**:556–63.
110. Marion D. Treatment of traumatic brain injury with moderate hypothermia. *N Eng J Med.* 1997;**336**:540–6.
111. Schreckinger M. Contemporary management of traumatic intracranial hypertension: Is there a role for therapeutic hypothermia? *Neurocrit Care.* 2009;**11**(3):427–36.
112. Teasdale GM, Graham DI. Craniocerebral trauma: protection and retrieval of the neuronal population after injury. *Neurosurgery.* 1998;**43**(4):723–37; discussion 37–8.
113. Siesjo BK. Mechanisms of ischemic brain damage. *Crit Care Med.* 1988;**16**(10):954–63.
114. Schmidt OI, Heyde CE, Ertel W, Stahel PF. Closed head injury – an inflammatory disease? *Brain Res Rev.* 2005;**48**(2):388–99.
115. Perez-Barcena J, Ibanez J, Brell M, *et al.* Lack of correlation among intracerebral cytokines, intracranial pressure, and brain tissue oxygenation in patients with traumatic brain injury and diffuse lesions. *Crit Care Med.* 2011;**39**(3):533–40.
116. Narotam P. Brain tissue oxygen monitoring in traumatic brain injury and major trauma: outcome analysis of a brain tissue oxygen-directed therapy. *J Neurosurg.* 2009;**111**:672–82.
117. Bulger E. Management of severe head injury: institutional variations in care and effect on outcome. *Crit Care Med.* 2002;**30**:1870–6.
118. Kiening K. Brain tissue pO2-monitoring in comatose patients: implications for therapy. *Neurol Res.* 1997;**19**:233–40.
119. Martini R. Management guided by brain tissue oxygen monitoring and outcome following severe traumatic brain injury. *J Neurosurg.* 2009;**111**:644–9.
120. Haitsma I. Advanced monitoring in the intensive care unit: brain tissue oxygen tension. *Curr Opin Crit Care.* 2002;**8**:115–20.

2

Cerebral blood flow

Rajat Dhar and Michael C. Diringer

Introduction

The brain has both a high demand for energy and an inability to store important substrates for metabolism. This means that it is highly dependent on a constant supply of oxygen and glucose, provided to the tissues by capillary perfusion. Even brief interruptions in flow will trigger loss of cerebral function within seconds (e.g. syncope during cardiac arrhythmias). Cerebral blood flow (CBF), a measure of brain perfusion, is therefore a vital parameter in assessing the adequacy of substrate delivery and viability of the brain, especially in cerebrovascular disease states where flow may be impaired. It is expressed as the volume of blood reaching a defined mass of brain tissue in a given period of time (typically ml per 100 g/min). Regional reductions in CBF, usually related to mechanical obstruction (thrombosis, stenosis, vasospasm), may lead to neurological deficits and, if prolonged, focal areas of irreversible cerebral infarction.

Normal whole-brain CBF is approx. 50 ml/100 g/min [1]. This averages the more metabolically active gray matter (CBF approx. 80 ml/100 g/min), and the white matter (20 ml/100 g/min) [2]. Flow must be adequate to deliver oxygen to meet the metabolic demands of the tissue. To ensure this, flow and metabolism usually remain tightly coupled, whereas increases in cerebral metabolic demand (expressed as $CMRO_2$, or cerebral metabolic rate of oxygen) are matched by increases in CBF and oxygen delivery (DO_2). Considerable reserve is maintained, such that CBF normally delivers 2–3 times the required oxygen (e.g. DO_2 of approx. 8 ml of oxygen per 100 g/min compared to a metabolic requirement of 3 ml of oxygen/100 g/min). Therefore, the proportion of oxygen extracted (OEF) should remain constant (normally ~ 30–35%), rising only if DO_2 falls out of proportion to $CMRO_2$. The Fick principle describes the relationship between metabolism, delivery and extraction of oxygen:

$$CMRO_2 = DO_{2x}OEF$$

Where DO_2 = CBF × CaO_2 (arterial oxygen content in ml O_2 per ml blood)

Autoregulation

Given the importance of CBF to neuronal metabolic integrity, homeostatic mechanisms actively maintain stable adequate levels of CBF despite physiologic perturbations. The ability of the brain to regulate its own perfusion, independent of changes in systemic blood pressure, is known as cerebral (pressure) autoregulation. The cerebral circulation is not pressure-passive, but responds with changes in arteriolar tone, altering flow dynamics in response to systemic changes. Without autoregulation, a fall in blood pressure and cerebral perfusion pressure (CPP = MAP, mean arterial pressure minus ICP, intracranial pressure) would precipitate a drop in CBF, threatening DO_2, and could

Critical Care of the Stroke Patient, ed. Stefan Schwab, Daniel Hanley, and A. David Mendelow. Published by Cambridge University Press.

precipitate ischemia. Instead, resistance vessels (i.e. arterioles, not large arteries) increase their diameter in response to lower CPP; this reduction in cerebrovascular resistance (CVR) maintains constant CBF:

$$CBF = \frac{CPP}{CVR}$$

This model of flow is based on the Hagen–Poiseuille law of fluid dynamics. CPP (or the distal/tissue perfusion pressure, in the face of focal proximal stenosis) is the driving pressure and CVR is largely determined by the radius of the vessel (to the fourth power, so small changes in tone can induce significant changes in flow). Vasodilatation in the face of reduced CPP not only maintains CBF but will increase cerebral blood volume (CBV). Conversely, vasoconstriction protects against hyperemia and prevents hydrostatic cerebral edema as MAP/CPP rises.

However, there is a limit to the extent of this autoregulatory compensation; once a vessel is maximally dilated or constricted, autoregulation will no longer be able to preserve stable CBF. At perfusion pressures beyond these limits (typically below 50–60 mmHg at the lower end and above 150 mmHg at the upper end), CBF will fall or rise in parallel with changes in MAP and CPP. These limits are shifted to the right in the face of chronic, especially untreated, hypertension [3], making such patients more vulnerable to lowering of blood pressure to even relatively normal levels (more so if ICP is increased). At pressures above the upper limit, CBF and hydrostatic pressure will rise and hypertensive encephalopathy due to hydrostatic cerebral edema can occur.

The partial pressure of carbon dioxide (P_aCO_2) is another powerful modulator of CBF, also mediated by changes in arteriolar tone (in this case, in response to changes in local pH). A rise in P_aCO_2 by even 1 mmHg (within the range of 20–80 mmHg) induces vasodilatation sufficient to increase CBF 2–3% [4]. Conversely, lowering P_aCO_2 with hyperventilation leads to vasoconstriction, reducing CBF and CBV; this is the mechanism by which it lowers ICP. The resulting drop in CBF with hyperventilation may be hazardous if tissue is vulnerable to ischemia. Moreover, these are only transient phenomena, with vascular adaptation occurring over several hours as pH normalizes, causing CBF to return to baseline. Changes in P_aO_2 within the normal range do not affect CBF in the same way; however, once arterial saturation falls (i.e. at $P_aO_2 < 50–60$ mmHg), this will jeopardize CaO_2 and lead to compensatory vasodilatation and higher CBF to maintain constant DO_2.

A similar homeostatic response occurs in the face of anemia (as lower hemoglobin reduces CaO_2 like arterial desaturation does), with vasodilatation raising CBF to preserve DO_2 [5]. Additionally, blood viscosity, determined by red cell concentration, may be reduced with anemia. By Poiseuille's law, this may also improve CBF (CVR is proportional to viscosity). However, the autoregulatory vasomotor response to changes in blood pressure and the response to changes in hemoglobin or P_aCO_2 are not independent. If vessels are maximally vasodilated (e.g. in response to hypotension or stenosis), the ability to compensate for reductions in hemoglobin or further drops in pressure will be attenuated or lost [6].

This **cerebrovascular reserve** (ability to vasodilate further and maintain or improve CBF as needed for constant DO_2) may be an important measure of future stroke risk, as validated in those with carotid stenosis where risk was highest with impaired reserve [7]. It can be tested by applying a stimulus meant to induce vasodilatation (commonly acetazolamide or CO_2 administration) and measuring change in CBF. Pressure autoregulation can be tested by raising or lowering systemic blood pressure and evaluating whether CBF remains constant (i.e. autoregulation intact). If autoregulation is impaired and/or reserve is exhausted, CBF will vary passively with perfusion pressure. In this setting, drops in MAP even within the normal range will reduce CBF further; blood pressure may need to be monitored and maintained scrupulously in such patients to avoid worsening ischemia.

Autoregulation can either be impaired globally (e.g. after severe head trauma) or regionally (e.g. in the territory of acute focal ischemia or vasospasm [8,9] or in the hemisphere ipsilateral to severe carotid stenosis, leading to hyperemia and the hyperperfusion syndrome after revascularization [10]). Conversely, autoregulation appears preserved even within the peri-hematomal region around ICH [11], meaning that careful reductions in MAP may be tolerated without lowering CBF in these patients.

Cerebral ischemia

Ischemia occurs when CBF and supply of oxygen (i.e. DO_2) is inadequate to support cellular oxidative metabolic requirements. At CBF/DO_2 below such critical thresholds, energy failure occurs and $CMRO_2$ falls. While various CBF thresholds for ischemia have been proposed, these are not absolute [12], being affected by metabolic requirements, arterial oxygen content (i.e. hemoglobin), and other cofactors that influence supply–demand imbalance. Progression to infarction depends on both degree and duration of CBF reduction, as well as ability to compensate (cerebrovascular reserve, OEF) and the tissue involved (gray vs. white matter).

In general, as CBF falls to half of baseline (approx. 25 ml/100 g/min), EEG slowing is seen and mentation/neurological status may become altered [13]. Protein synthesis is inhibited at even higher levels [14]. At CBF below 20 ml/100 g/min there is electrical failure (i.e. EEG becomes isoelectric), and a shift to anaerobic metabolism occurs leading to increased lactate production. Once CBF falls below 10–12 ml/100 g/min, there is loss of synaptic transmission and failure of ion pumps [15]. This rapidly leads to cytotoxic edema and cell death (i.e. ischemic infarction). An **ischemic penumbra** may exist, where flow lies below the threshold for electrical failure and neurological symptoms, but above that of energy failure and inevitable infarction. The flow reductions to such tissue are fundamentally reversible, but may be recruited into the infarct if CBF is not restored.

Three stages of hemodynamic impairment have been proposed to explain the vascular and metabolic changes that occur as perfusion falls [16]. Initial drops in CPP lead to autoregulatory vasodilatation, which maintains CBF at or just below baseline levels (Fig. 2.1). CBV is increased, as is mean transit time of dye (see *Central Volume Principle*), while OEF remains normal. Once cerebrovascular reserve has been exhausted, CBF begins to fall, lowering DO_2. In response, OEF increases to maintain a steady level of total oxygen extracted for cellular metabolism (i.e. less delivered but greater proportion extracted). This stage is termed **oligemia** (or 'misery perfusion') as flow and delivery are reduced, but the volume of oxygen available for metabolism is preserved by increased OEF. This increase in extraction results in a lower saturation of oxygen in the effluent venous blood, as measured by reduced jugular venous oxygen saturation. This high-risk stage may overlap with the 'penumbra' concept of abnormal but viable tissue where metabolism is preserved despite constrained flow [15]. However, OEF can only increase up to a point (between 70–100%). Once tissue cannot extract more oxygen but CBF/DO_2 continue to fall, not enough oxygen is available and $CMRO_2$ will decrease. As CBF and $CMRO_2$ now fall in parallel, tissue reaches the threshold for ion pump and energy failure, leading to cell death. While this model provides a framework to understand how the brain responds to reductions in perfusion and CBF, it likely obscures the fact that these compensatory mechanisms overlap and act concurrently to avoid ischemia [16].

Limitations of CBF as a marker of ischemia

As described above, CBF is an integral but not absolute marker of ischemia, with no absolute thresholds valid in all situations and for all populations of neurons. There are a number of reasons why a single CBF value alone may not provide adequate information to determine the risk or presence of ischemia:

1. Reduced CBF provides information on low cerebral perfusion but not the balance between flow and the metabolic state of the tissues (which truly defines ischemia) [17]. If OEF can increase to maintain oxygen available for metabolism, then reduced CBF will not cause ischemia (i.e. compensatory state of oligemia). The point at which metabolism is jeopardized depends not only on how low CBF has fallen, but also the extent of OEF elevation possible, the metabolic requirements of the tissue, and CaO_2.
2. If metabolic demands are reduced (as has been described in hypothermia, after intracerebral hemorrhage, traumatic brain injury, and early after subarachnoid hemorrhage), then CBF may appropriately be reduced as a result of intact flow-metabolism

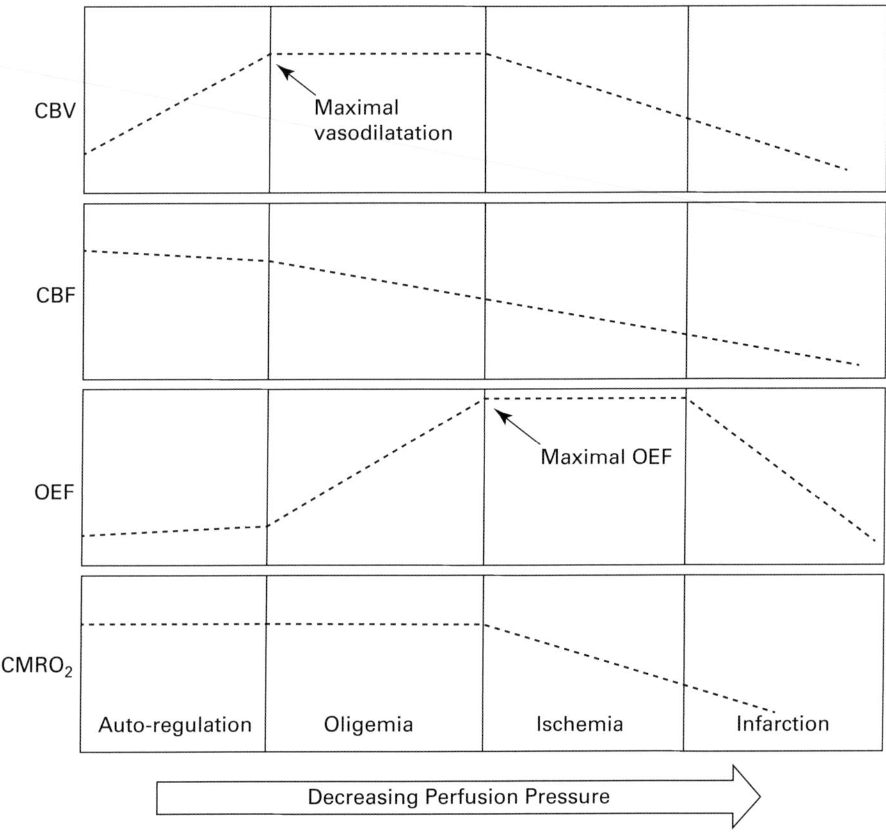

Fig. 2.1 Stages of hemodynamic impairment as cerebral tissue perfusion falls. (Modified after Powers *et al. Ann Intern Med* (1987);**106**:27–34, and Derdeyn *et al. Brain* (2002);**125**:595–607.)

coupling. In such a situation, despite an apparently low CBF measurement, OEF will be normal, and no ischemia develops. A similar effect may be seen with *diaschisis*, where sites remote from the primary injury (e.g. contralateral cerebellum) exhibit reduced metabolic demands and concordant reductions in CBF.

3. The converse can occur, when ischemia exists despite a relatively normal CBF. This can be seen with reduced CaO_2 (related to profound anemia [18] or hypoxemia), or in carbon monoxide poisoning (with inability to bind oxygen). CBF may even rise in an attempt to compensate [5]. Hypoglycemia can similarly threaten neuronal viability despite normal CBF.
4. Normal CBF can be present in the setting of significant vascular occlusion if adequate collaterals are able to maintain tissue perfusion and/or vasodilatory reserve is able to compensate for the reduction in perfusion pressure. Therefore, unless CVR testing is performed, CBF measurement will give little information on the vascular impairment present and may underestimate the imminent risk of ischemia.
5. A particular CBF value does not provide adequate information on progression to infarction; duration of ischemia is critical in determining tissue outcome. Moderately reduced CBF for prolonged durations can cause similar injury to total cessation of flow for short durations. There are also populations of neurons that are selectively vulnerable to ischemia at the same degree of hypoperfusion. Rather than an

on/off threshold, ischemia occurs along a continuum with dynamic boundaries.
6. Global measures of CBF (or jugular venous saturation, which assesses extraction) may miss small ischemic regions (e.g. in focal processes such as vasospasm).

The variability in the relationship between CBF measurement and ischemia has been demonstrated in SAH patients with delayed ischemic neurological deficits (DINDs). Patients who were clearly symptomatic had regional CBF values that ranged from less than 30 to greater than 50 ml/100 g/min [19], despite significant vasospasm.

CBF in acute ischemic stroke

The changes in flow and metabolism after ischemic stroke evolve over time from occlusion (Fig. 2.2). CBF decreases acutely after stroke onset while OEF initially rises to compensate. $CMRO_2$ may be only mildly decreased at first, but falls progressively over the next few hours in the core of the territory supplied, as tissue ischemia develops [20]. As infarction ensues and tissue is neither able to extract nor requires as much oxygen, OEF falls; it may remain elevated in the penumbra where salvageable tissue remains viable for many hours [21]. As reperfusion occurs, CBF increases above the metabolic requirements of the infarcted tissue (which remain low despite restored flow) and OEF falls below normal, a state termed *luxury perfusion*. In the subacute period, as flow-metabolism coupling returns, CBF declines to negligible values in the infarcted region and OEF normalizes. Restoring flow to the penumbra forms the rationale for attempts at reperfusion and otherwise augmenting CBF. As autoregulation may be impaired in this setting, maintaining blood pressure (e.g. permissive hypertension) is essential to avoiding extension of the infarct due to fall in CBF in this vulnerable zone. A clue to the presence of pressure-dependent penumbra is fluctuation in neurological deficits that worsen with reduction

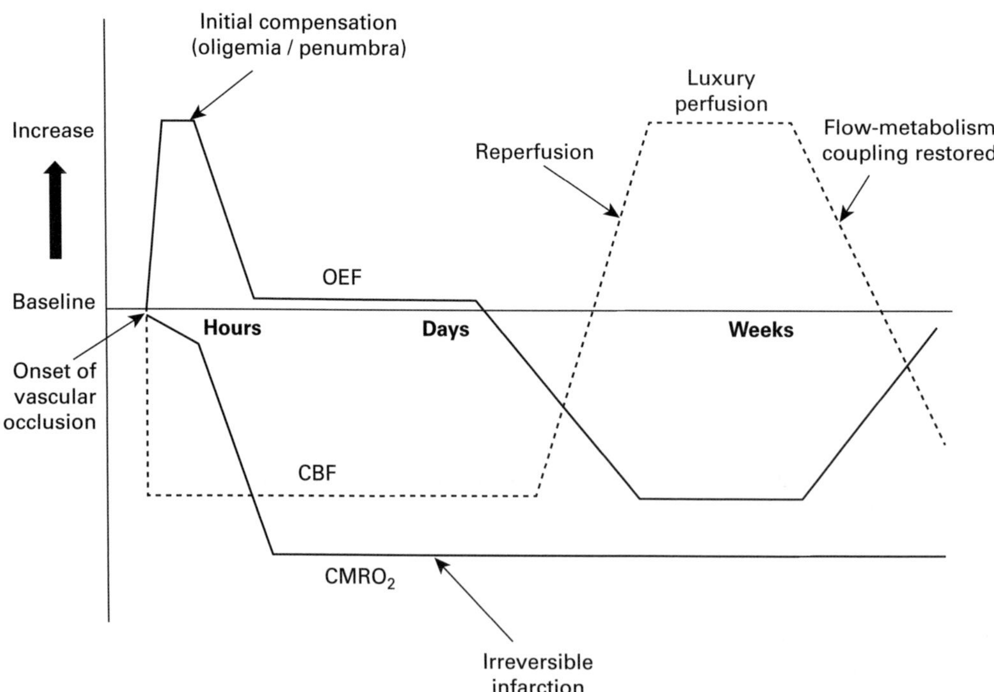

Fig. 2.2 Changes in regional CBF, OEF, and $CMRO_2$ over time after cerebrovascular occlusion (i.e. ischemic stroke).

in MAP [22]. Attempts at inducing higher blood pressure to improve CBF may be warranted when penumbra is still present, as identified clinically or by imaging [23]. Cases of early neurological deterioration after stroke have been attributed (at least partially) to hemodynamic factors, with recruitment of oligemic regions into the ischemic territory [24].

CBF in intracerebral hemorrhage

A number of studies have found reductions in CBF both globally and in the zone of tissue around the hematoma [25,26]. However, when PET imaging was performed in 19 patients within 24 hours of ICH onset, $CMRO_2$ was reduced to a greater extent than CBF (which was approx. 20 ml/100 g/min) [27]. OEF was decreased rather than increased, suggesting that rather than a zone of ischemia around ICH, there is primary metabolic down-regulation with secondary reduction in CBF. This was supported by the histopathologic description of mitochondrial dysfunction in the peri-hematomal region [28]. A preliminary study found an association between the degree of CBF (and likely $CMRO_2$) reduction, as measured by xenon-CT, and hospital discharge status [29]. However, in the absence of ischemia there should be less concern about treating severe acute hypertension after ICH. The status of autoregulation was tested by lowering MAP from a mean of 145 mmHg to 119 mmHg in 14 patients with small to moderate-sized ICH [11]. This 17% reduction in MAP was not associated with any reduction in CBF, globally or in the peri-hematomal region. This suggests that autoregulation is preserved within these bounds, and that lowering blood pressure by 15–20% does not compromise CBF in similar ICH patients. Clinical trials have suggested that acute reductions in blood pressure are safe and may result in improved critical outcomes [30].

CBF in subarachnoid hemorrhage

Many studies have documented reductions in CBF early after SAH, even prior to development of vasospasm, more severe for those with worse clinical grade [31–33]. However, this was matched by a reduction in $CMRO_2$, again suggesting primary metabolic depression (not only related to sedation) with a coupled drop in CBF; OEF was not elevated in this phase [34]. It is hypothesized that aneurysmal rupture with intense rapid rise in ICP leads to cerebral circulatory arrest, global ischemic injury, and transient 'hibernation' [35]. Alternatively, the presence of subarachnoid blood around the brainstem may directly modulate cerebral metabolic rate. The level of CBF may predict outcome and the risk of vasospasm/infarction [36,37], although this is confounded by its association with injury severity.

Narrowing of the large intracranial arteries at the base of the brain (i.e. **cerebral vasospasm**) is a common radiographic finding seen 4–14 days after SAH. This process is paralleled by a reduction in CBF that occurs both globally and in particular regions. While the magnitude of reduction in CBF roughly correlates with the severity of angiographic narrowing, it may not be restricted to or even concordant with the territory of the vessel(s) affected [38]. This suggests that the observable arterial changes may not be the sole cause of this delayed reduction in CBF. In fact, regions with significantly reduced CBF were seen even in patients and vascular territories without visible vasospasm [36], and no absolute threshold in poor-grade patients could be discerned that appeared to predict development of hypoattenuation consistent with infarction [39]. Conversely, areas that appeared 'ischemic' (with hypoattenuation on CT scans) could have CBF values that ranged from below 10 ml/100 g/min to some with values in or above the normal range [40]. Patients with apparently ischemic neurological deficits could have CBF values that were either below or above normal in the symptomatic territory [19]. This all highlights the imperfect association between degree of vasospasm, CBF values and both patient and tissue outcome.

OEF has been proposed as a more suitable marker of tissue at risk for delayed cerebral ischemia (DCI). Regional OEF was elevated, along with reduced CBF (i.e. oligemia), in MCA territories with angiographic vasospasm, and correlated with severity of vasospasm in one cohort studied with PET [33]. Measures of global extraction (i.e. jugular venous saturation) or monitors with limited spatial resolution are unlikely to detect focal areas of oligemia, and so may be less suitable to evaluate the risk of ischemia after SAH. Later in the course of DCI, OEF may fall, as does $CMRO_2$ in regions that go on to infarct (as seen in ischemic stroke), while CBF and OEF return to normal if vasospasm resolves.

Although 'Triple-H' therapy has been used for a few decades to treat DINDs, the CBF responses to hypervolemia and hemodilution are negligible. Only induced hypertension (IH) has been demonstrated to improve CBF [41], and even this is inconsistent; such ability of IH to improve CBF depends upon a loss of pressure autoregulation after SAH.

Why monitor CBF?

Hypoperfusion and ischemia are fundamental pathologic processes in the setting of acute cerebrovascular insults. The neurological examination is a relatively insensitive marker of ischemia for three reasons: 1) neurological deficits only emerge once CBF falls below fairly low critical thresholds, at which point reversibility may be limited. It is insensitive to lesser reductions in flow that may presage incipient ischemia; 2) the neurological examination is spatially insensitive, only detecting deficits when ischemia affects eloquent regions. Even significant reductions in flow to other brain regions may be asymptomatic or only accompanied by non-specific or non-focal alterations in cognition that may be easily missed. 3) Similarly, patients with severe brain injury (e.g. SAH or large ICH) are often comatose or sedated, so the neurological examination will not be accessible to detect symptomatic reductions in CBF.

The primary goal of therapy for patients with severe cerebrovascular insults is to maintain adequate flow of oxygenated blood, thus minimizing ischemia. Without a way to measure CBF or the injurious consequences of its reduction, management of these patients remains empiric. Similarly, those with vascular occlusion or stenosis (e.g. vasospasm) can have either normal or reduced perfusion (due to variable collaterals, vasodilatory reserve, blood pressure, etc.). Without measuring CBF in the affected territory, knowledge of only vascular status tells little about risk of imminent ischemia.

CBF monitoring offers a number of practical advantages in managing ICU patients:

1. Measure perfusion to determine tissue viability and prognosis (e.g. detect remaining penumbra around core of infarct that may respond to revascularization, determine the impact of vascular occlusion or stenosis on perfusion).
2. Identify emergence of new flow deficits or progression of existing disease (e.g. worsening vasospasm).
3. Allow early targeted intervention, with titration of therapies (e.g. induced hypertension) to a specific goal, aiming to prevent irreversible ischemic injury.
4. Test vasodilatory reserve/autoregulation: to predict risk of future ischemic events or ability to tolerate changes in blood pressure.
5. Avoid dangerous or unnecessary therapies that may have been used if CBF was not known (e.g. excessive hyperventilation, treating raised ICP due only to hyperemia, raising MAP in the presence of vasospasm if CBF is still normal despite significant angiographic narrowing).

Features of the ideal CBF monitor are outlined in Table 2.1.

Measuring CBF: techniques

Imaging-based measurement of CBF is based on one of two principles. Understanding the basic methodology is important in recognizing the assumptions and limitations inherent in each technique.

Fick principle

This applies the law of conservation of matter to blood flow, stating that the change in the amount of substrate in tissue is equal to the arterial flow (e.g. CBF) times the arteriovenous difference in tracer concentration. Kety and Schmidt applied this principle to measuring CBF, initially using the inert gas nitrous oxide as the tracer [1]. By measuring gas concentrations in a peripheral artery (representative of cerebral arterial blood) and the internal jugular vein after a period of gas inhalation (at steady state), and knowing the partition coefficient (the ratio of brain-to-blood levels at equilibrium) to establish uptake, they determined whole-brain CBF.

Table 2.1 Features of the ideal CBF monitor

Feature	Reason	Examples
Allows continuous monitoring	Detects changes in real-time/responds rapidly	Neuro exam (if unsedated) Transverse cardiac diameter (TCD), intracranial probes Continuous EEG
Non-invasive, portable	Used at the bedside/does not require transport	TCD, EEG, CBF probe portable CT (xenon, CTP)
Widely available, user-friendly, and inexpensive	Easily applied to wide range of patients	TCD CT perfusion
Accurate (quantitative)	Provides reliable and reproducible measure of CBF, able to detect important changes	PET Xenon CT
Repeatable	Useful to assess response to intervention	TCD, xenon CT CBF probe
Provides structural data	Recognizes infarcts, hematoma, vascular abnormalities	MRI with DWI, MRA CT with CTA
Whole brain regional coverage	Detects foci of ischemia	PET, MRI Limited in CTP, xenon
Provides information on metabolic integrity	Determines if reduced CBF is associated with ischemia	PET (OEF, $CMRO_2$) MRI - DWI?

The development of techniques using radioactive tracers that diffuse out of the blood into the brain allowed direct measurement of regional brain tissue levels (and hence perfusion) using extracranial radioactivity detectors, without invasive venous monitoring. This was first done in humans with radioactive krypton and xenon and forms the basis of modern SPECT and PET imaging. With xenon, end-tidal concentrations are used to estimate arterial levels. As SPECT does not measure arterial or end-tidal activity, it only provides qualitative relative assessments of CBF. PET, on the other hand, provides quantitative regional measures of CBF through the use of arterial blood sampling of radioactivity. Furthermore, other tracers can be used (e.g. ^{15}O-labeled carbon monoxide and oxygen) which allow measurement of CBV, OEF, and $CMRO_2$.

The Fick principle also relates the important measures, CBF and $CMRO_2$ by the ratio: $CMRO_2 = CBF \times AVDO_2$, where $AVDO_2$ is the arteriovenous difference in oxygen content ($CaO_2 \times OEF$). This means that, if metabolism remains constant (an important assumption), then any change in jugular saturation implies a parallel change in CBF.

Central volume principle

This is used to derive mean transit time (MTT), CBV and CBF in techniques that use non-diffusible intravascular tracers such as in CT and MR perfusion. A bolus of such a tracer (e.g. iodinated CT contrast) is administered and serial scans are taken as it passes through the cerebral vasculature and then washes out. The change in tissue density or susceptibility is proportional to the serum concentration of the agent, allowing a time–density curve to be constructed for each voxel [42]. MTT is the time the tracer takes to pass through the vasculature. It is related to CBF and CBV by the relationship:

$$MTT = \frac{CBV}{CBF}$$

Prolonged MTT may be seen either if CBV is increased or CBF is reduced. Further analyses (e.g. 'deconvolution' comparing density to that in a selected artery) try to tease out these individual contributions. Important limitations of techniques utilizing the central volume principle are: 1) it measures vascular perfusion (flow in vessels) not tissue perfusion, which may not be identical; 2) timing of scans with bolus arrival and selection of an arterial input function are both important. It is further discussed under the sections on CT and MR perfusion. The various types of CBF monitors are compared in Table 2.2 and discussed briefly in the subsequent sections.

Xenon CT

The use of cold (non-radioactive) xenon as a contrast agent allows noninvasive quantitative measurement of CBF. Xenon is radiodense, highly lipid soluble and freely crosses the blood–brain barrier. Subjects inhale a mixture of 28–33% xenon (an anesthetic at higher concentrations) with oxygen, over a few minutes. The change in density on subsequent serial CT images (scanning a few brain slices, relative to baseline) correlates with uptake, and along with end-tidal levels (approximating arterial concentration) and the known partition coefficient for xenon, CBF can be calculated from the modified Fick (Kety–Schmidt) principle [43]. Data processing can be done in 10 minutes, providing quantitative regional values for CBF. As half-life is short, xenon washes out rapidly, and a repeat study (e.g. post-intervention) can be performed 20 minutes after the baseline scan. While data on each voxel are calculated, regions of 1 cm^2 or larger maximize signal-to-noise, leading to measurement error of within 12%.

Despite its many advantages, limitations of xenon CT include:

1. Adverse effects of xenon: at low concentrations, sedation is minimized, but patients often experience mild sensorial alterations and paresthesias [44]. Emesis can also occur, so avoid if stomach is full. Short periods of apnea may also be seen.
2. Xenon can cause increases in CBF ('flow activation') but this phenomenon is delayed by a few minutes. With early scanning, measurement of CBF takes place before significant alterations in flow have occurred. ICP is also generally not increased by xenon.
3. Studies can be significantly limited by patient motion artifact, especially if xenon causes disturbing adverse sensations. Patients must be placed in head-immobilizing devices and stay still for over 4 minutes of inhalation. For the above reasons, best results are obtained in immobile (i.e. sedated or comatose) ventilated patients.
4. In patients with pulmonary disease, end-tidal xenon concentrations may not accurately reflect arterial levels. This may lead to an underestimation of CBF by 20% [45].
5. Radiation dose is relatively high (marginally greater than CT perfusion), limiting measurements to a few contiguous brain slices.
6. Limited availability: although the system is relatively simple and inexpensive compared to PET (it only requires a CT scanner and xenon delivery/scavenging system, both of which are now available portably), medical-grade xenon is not FDA approved and requires an IND for use.

Nonetheless, in experienced centers, xenon CT has become an established and validated tool to measure CBF in the acute setting. It provides quantitative regional CBF even at low flow rates, allowing detection of ischemic regions [46]. It has also been used to assess cerebrovascular reactivity and response to interventions, including induced hypertension and angioplasty [47,48]. If coupled with non-contrast CT and CT angiography, it can provide structural and vascular imaging data along with CBF.

CT perfusion

This technique is based on the *central volume principle*, employing bolus tracking of an intravenous contrast tracer. Major advantages include wide availability (software is available on most new high-speed spiral CT scanners), speed of acquisition and processing (in centers with experience), and ability also to image brain (non-contrast CT) and vasculature (CT angiography) in one study.

Major limitations include limited brain coverage (usually only a few brain slices can be acquired with a single bolus), inability to image the posterior fossa, risks of radiation and contrast exposure (limiting repeat studies), need for good IV access to get adequate bolus delivery, and the importance of timing image acquisition when the bolus reaches the cerebral circulation. Newer CT scanners may allow a single-pass acquisition of CTA and CTP data, limiting repeat radiation exposure and

Table 2.2 Comparison of various types of CBF monitors

Features	PET	Xenon CT	CT perfusion	MR perfusion	TCD	TD probe
Tracer	Radioisotopes (e.g. $H_2{}^{15}O$)	Stable ^{131}Xenon	Iodinated contrast dye	Gadolinium (none in ASL)	None	n/a
Based on principle	Modified Fick (Kety-Schmidt)	Kety-Schmidt	Central volume principle	Central volume principle	Flow / velocity	Thermal diffusion
Continuous	No	No	No	No	Yes	Yes
Time to acquire[1]	5–15 min	10 min	40 s	1–10 min	10–20 min	Immediate (after placement)
Processing[1]	15 min or more	10 min	5 min	5 min	Minimal	n/a
Skilled operator	Required	Required	Some experience	Some experience	Required	For insertion
Numerical CBF	Yes	Yes	Yes ±	±	No	Yes
Bedside	No	Yes[2]	Yes[2]	No	Yes	Yes
Invasive	Arterial access	No	No	No	No	Intracranial probe
Regional data	Yes	Yes	Yes	Yes	No	Around probe
Brain coverage	Whole	Limited slices	Limited (2 cm)	Whole	Vascular territories	Very focal (8 mm)
Spatial resolution	4–6 mm	4 mm	1–2 mm	2 mm	n/a	n/a
Availability	Limited (requires cyclotron and PET)	Limited (FDA IND required in US)	CT scanners widely available	Less than CT Need to be stable	Wide (but requires temporal windows)	Yes
Radiation per study (approx.)[1]	2.5 mSv	3.5–10 mSv	2–3 mSv	None	None	None
Repeat studies	Yes	Yes	Minimal	Yes	Yes	Continuous
- limited by	Radiation	Radiation	Radiation/contrast	None	None	n/a
- time between	10 min	10–20 min	10 min	5–10 min	Immediate	
CBF reproducible and accurate	Yes (Gold standard)	Yes (Caution if pulmonary pathology)	± (Depends on selection of AIF and intact BBB)	± (Semi-quantitative only)	No (Velocity not flow, affected by vessel caliber changes)	± (Minimal validation)

Table 2.2 (cont.)

Features	PET	Xenon CT	CT perfusion	MR perfusion	TCD	TD probe
Structural/ vascular data	None	Yes (CT, CTA)	Yes (CT, CTA)	Yes (MRI-DWI, MRA)	No	No
Measures of metabolism	OEF $CMRO_2$	No	No	No	No	No
Adverse effects	Arterial line	Sedation, nausea paresthesias	Contrast allergy or nephropathy	Risk of NSF if renal insufficiency	None	Probe-related
Best used for	Research	Intubated/sedated subjects if reproducible quantitative CBF values required	Hyperacute stroke, vasospasm (images flow and vasculature)	Acute stroke, vasospasm	Cerebrovascular reactivity testing Monitoring for vasospasm (not CBF)	TBI or poor-grade SAH (monitoring for low CBF/ vasospasm)

[Legend] AE = adverse effects; AIF = arterial input function; ASL = arterial spin-labeling; BBB = blood–brain barrier; CTA = CT angiography; DWI = diffusion-weighted imaging; MRA = MR angiography; NSF = nephrogenic systemic fibrosis; TBI = traumatic brain injury; TD = thermal diffusion.

[1] Some data adapted from Wintermark M, *et al. J Neuroradiol* 2005;**32**:294–314.

[2] With portable CT.

contrast requirements, while affording greater whole-brain coverage. Measurement of CBF in the most common *deconvolution method* of processing requires selection of an 'arterial input function' (e.g. a branch of the MCA or ACA) which if improperly done can significantly alter CBF results. It may also overestimate perfusion in regions with large vessels, providing a value for 'vascular perfusion', not actual capillary-level flow. CBF values obtained have been compared to xenon CT with a moderate degree of correlation (r^2=0.79).

CTP is ideally suited for studying acute ischemic stroke, helping identify core vs. penumbra (based on MTT, CBV, and CBF thresholds, or comparison to the contralateral unaffected hemisphere). However, it is also being studied in patients after SAH where it can identify vasospasm (CTA) and evaluate flow (CTP) if MTT is prolonged or CBF is reduced [49]. In fact, assessment of flow may be a more specific marker of DCI than the presence of vasospasm on angiography [50].

MR perfusion

Dynamic susceptibility-weighted MRP uses the central volume principle in a similar manner to CTP but uses changes in magnetic susceptibility as the gadolinium contrast passes through the brain to determine MTT (and from there estimate CBF). It is less widely available than CTP and more difficult to perform in unstable ICU patients or those who are claustrophobic. It allows concurrent diffusion-weighted imaging (DWI) which may detect ischemic regions with greater sensitivity than loss of gray-white differentiation on CT. While the mismatch between DWI and perfusion lesion has been suggested to represent the 'penumbra', this has not been consistently validated [51]. Its ability to provide valid quantitative CBF maps is unclear as there is a nonlinear relation between signal change and gadolinium concentration [52]. It has shown moderate agreement when compared to xenon CT (r^2=0.69) [53]. Delayed time to peak on perfusion MR (relative to the contralateral hemisphere, not absolute CBF) also correlated better with severity of vasospasm and presence of DINDs than TCD [54].

Arterial spin-labeling is a relatively new technique that applies a magnetic pulse to a slab of brain below the area of interest, labeling the inflowing water molecules. This allows flow to be determined without need for exogenous contrast (useful in patients with renal failure in whom even gadolinium exposure is relatively contraindicated). It has a low signal:noise ratio so requires a longer acquisition time and is sensitive to motion artifact. It may not detect very low flow (< 10 ml/100 g/min) and underestimates CBF at high flows. However, it is reproducible within 10%, has a high spatial resolution, and is easy to repeat. Its clinical utilization in the ICU care of stroke patients is relatively unexplored.

Thermal diffusion

Laser Doppler flowmetry is an optical method for measuring flow velocity of fluids in capillaries, and has been used in neurosurgical applications for a few decades. However, it does not measure true quantitative CBF, only allowing monitoring of trends as velocity changes. It also works optimally with a cranial window, so is better suited to the operating room (e.g. during and after aneurysm or AVM surgery). The technique of thermal diffusion flowmetry (TDF) has more recently emerged as an alternative way to provide real-time continuous measurement of CBF in the ICU.

The Hemedex™ probe (Fig. 2.3) is a flexible polyurethane catheter 1 mm in diameter that is best placed 20–25 mm below the cortical surface (i.e. in the white matter) via a small burr hole and bolt. The probe has a heat source on its distal end which generates a spherical temperature field with radius 4 mm at 2 degrees above tissue temperature. It has a second thermistor 8 mm proximal to the tip, just outside this field. As the degree of heat dissipation is proportional to blood flow, the change in temperature between the thermistors allows local tissue CBF to be derived. While clearly invasive (similar in risk to a traditional ICP monitor), its main advantage is that it allows continuous, real-time measurement of quantitative CBF at the bedside. Its greatest limitation lies in its small locus of measurement, meaning that it may miss disruptions in flow to other areas of the brain. It also may not be reliable in the setting of fever. As it is usually placed in white matter, normal values are lower (in the 20–40 mmHg range).

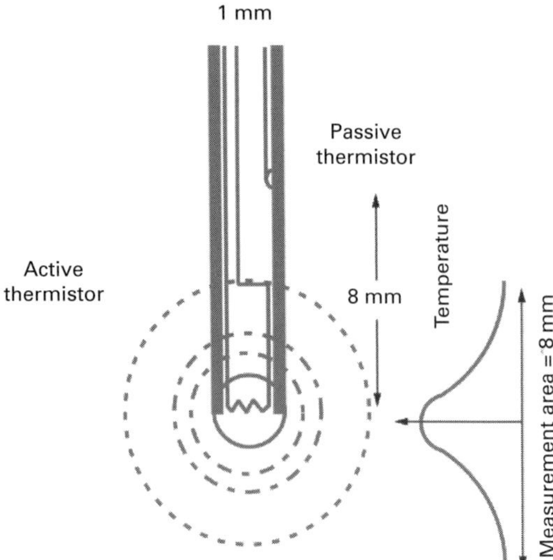

Fig. 2.3 Hemedex® thermal diffusion probe.

CBF measurement using this probe was compared to xenon CT in 16 brain-injured patients [55]. There was good agreement (r^2=0.79), with values within 5 mmHg in most cases. Changes in flow correlated well between the modalities (r^2=0.81). A subsequent study evaluated 14 patients with high-grade aneurysmal SAH, in which two probes were placed into the two vascular territories considered at highest risk for vasospasm [56]. Patients also underwent TCD, xenon CT, and angiography. The CBF probe detected a fall in CBF within territories developing vasospasm (average CBF approx. 10 mmHg vs. 20 mmHg or more in those without vasospasm). There was only weak correlation between the CBF measured at the time of developing vasospasm by xenon CT and TDF (r^2=0.32); however, the probe performed significantly better in detecting vasospasm using CBF changes than did TCD, and noted changes 2–3 days earlier. An obvious caveat lies is selecting *a priori* the high-risk territory to monitor; the authors found that even one probe (placed per protocol) would have adequately detected changes in CBF better than TCD. It may be especially useful for anterior communicating artery aneurysms where ACA vasospasm is most likely. Vasospasm in these territories is especially difficult to detect both clinically or by TCD. Other investigators have used this probe to show CBF changes with various modalities of 'Triple-H' therapy [57], and assess CO_2 reactivity with hyperventilation [58]. It was also used to demonstrate a reduction in CBF when higher PEEP (positive end-expiratory pressure) was applied to ventilated SAH patients [59], although this was related to a drop in MAP (implying that autoregulation was impaired in these patients).

Transcranial Doppler

The technique and theory of TCD are covered elsewhere (Chapter 5) but its utilization to measure CBF will be discussed briefly here. TCD has a number of major advantages as an ICU monitor. It can be performed non-invasively at the bedside and is safely repeatable. However, it is also susceptible to a number of important limitations. The angle of insonation must be kept constant otherwise flow velocity will not correlate linearly with CBF (and is thus operator-dependent). Adequate temporal bone windows must be available (which is not always the case). It also only measures large vessel flow (e.g. MCA bilaterally), thus only estimating hemispheric/territorial perfusion. It does not provide much structural data (beyond vascular patency) and depends on the assumption that the diameter of the vessel remains constant; in the setting of vascular stenosis or vasospasm, this may not be the case. Changes in flow velocity will then reflect changes in vessel caliber, and not alterations in flow itself (e.g. higher MCA flow velocities with MCA vasospasm). Conversely, when high TCD velocities are felt to reflect severe vasospasm, CBF was most often not low (as may be expected with significant narrowing), but actually hyperemic [60]. Although TCD may not reliably assess absolute CBF, it appears more accurate in gauging changes in CBF (r^2 = 0.72) [61]; it may be best suited to assess cerebrovascular reactivity and reserve.

Near-infrared spectroscopy

A number of emerging optical technologies employ specific wavelengths of light (and their reflectance after passing through the skull and cortex) to assess the ratio of oxy- to deoxyhemoglobin. A number of inferences are then applied to estimate cerebral oxygenation and CBF. These monitors are noninvasive, continuous, and can be performed easily at the bedside. A recent study in SAH and TBI patients found a positive correlation (r^2=0.53) between changes in CBF with a novel optical instrument and that measured by xenon CT [62]. However, the validity of quantitative CBF remains unclear, and further studies are required before this is widely adopted.

Indications for CBF monitoring

CBF is a fundamental measure of cerebral function and tissue viability. We now have a number of tools capable of assessing in acutely ill patients. When determining whether to utilize CBF monitoring in a particular clinical situation, three important issues must be considered. CBF measurements do not provide information about tissue metabolism and thus may not inform on the adequacy of blood flow. Secondly, virtually all technologies that assess CBF have risks: they are either invasive, require contrast and radiation exposure, and/or patient transport. Most require technical experience performing and interpreting the measurements. Finally, the available methods are either limited by being able to make relatively few discrete measurements in time (e.g. MR/CT perfusion, PET, xenon) or by sampling small regions of brain (e.g. brain TD probe).

Measurement of CBF may be considered in situations where there is risk of ongoing ischemia, especially when the neurological examination is unreliable (e.g. use of sedation, patient in coma) or insensitive to focal reductions in CBF (e.g. non-eloquent regions likely to be involved). It may also be utilized when initiating or titrating interventions directed at optimizing CBF and oxygen delivery. Two acute cerebrovascular states where CBF measurement may be helpful are delayed cerebral ischemia (DCI) after SAH, and attempts to salvage penumbral tissue from infarction after large vessel occlusion in ischemic stroke (either with reperfusion therapy or induced hypertension).

The detection of **DCI** after SAH is complex due to its heterogeneity in timing and location. It also affords the unique opportunity to detect reductions in CBF before ischemia develops, as well as monitor response to interventions, with the goal of preventing progression to infarction, a negative event most strongly correlated with poor outcome. CBF measurement is particularly helpful as symptoms correlate better with CBF than with angiographic narrowing and TCD velocities. TCD cannot distinguish between a rise in velocity due to improved flow (e.g. in response to an intervention such as induced hypertension) or that associated with a reduction in vessel diameter (i.e. worsening vasospasm) [63]. Cerebral oxygen delivery can only be assessed and optimized by measuring CBF itself.

Induced hypertension in acute ischemic stroke is an investigational therapy aimed at improving perfusion to penumbral regions and preventing recruitment into the final infarct. Anecdotal series have shown clinical response to raising blood pressure (along with improved CBF), most often in those with large vessel occlusions and significant penumbra, as assessed by mismatch between DWI lesion and perfusion defect [23]. Knowledge of CBF response as MAP is increased may allow better titration of this intervention to optimal targets.

Conclusion

CBF can now be measured by a number of modalities, each of which has advantages and disadvantages. The decision to monitor CBF must be made based on the individual patient scenario and only when that information is likely to positively impact management and prognostic decisions. Many uncertainties still exist about CBF thresholds for ischemia, which interventions best optimize CBF, and whether newer technologies can accurately and non-invasively measure it.

REFERENCES

1. Kety SS, Schmidt CF. The nitrous oxide method for the quantitative determination of cerebral blood flow in man: theory, procedure and normal values. *J Clin Invest* 1948;**27**:476–83.
2. McHenry LC, Jr., Merory J, Bass E *et al.* Xenon-133 inhalation method for regional cerebral blood flow measurements: normal values and test-retest results. *Stroke* 1978;**9**:396–9.

3. Strandgaard S, Olesen J, Skinhoj E, Lassen NA. Autoregulation of brain circulation in severe arterial hypertension. *Br Med J* 1973;**1**:507–10.
4. Kety SS, Schmidt CF. The effects of altered arterial tensions of carbon dioxide and oxygen on cerebral blood flow and cerebral oxygen consumption of normal young men. *J Clin Invest* 1948;**27**:484–92.
5. Brown MM, Wade JP, Marshall J. Fundamental importance of arterial oxygen content in the regulation of cerebral blood flow in man. *Brain* 1985;**108**(Pt 1):81–93.
6. von Kummer R, Scharf J, Back T, *et al.* Autoregulatory capacity and the effect of isovolemic hemodilution on local cerebral blood flow. *Stroke* 1988;**19**:594–7.
7. Silvestrini M, Vernieri F, Pasqualetti P, *et al.* Impaired cerebral vasoreactivity and risk of stroke in patients with asymptomatic carotid artery stenosis. *JAMA* 2000; **283**:2122–7.
8. Symon L, Branston NM, Strong AJ. Autoregulation in acute focal ischemia. An experimental study. *Stroke* 1976; **7**:547–54.
9. Yundt KD, Grubb RL, Jr., Diringer MN, Powers WJ. Autoregulatory vasodilation of parenchymal vessels is impaired during cerebral vasospasm. *J Cereb Blood Flow Metab* 1998;**18**:419–24.
10. van Mook WN, Rennenberg RJ, Schurink GW, *et al.* Cerebral hyperperfusion syndrome. *Lancet Neurol* 2005;**4**:877–88.
11. Powers WJ, Zazulia AR, Videen TO, *et al.* Autoregulation of cerebral blood flow surrounding acute intracerebral hemorrhage. *Neurology* 2001;**57**:18–24.
12. Bandera E, Botteri M, Minelli C, *et al.* Cerebral blood flow threshold of ischemic penumbra and infarct core in acute ischemic stroke: a systematic review. *Stroke* 2006;**37**:1334–9.
13. Jones TH, Morawetz RB, Crowell RM, *et al.* Thresholds of focal cerebral ischemia in awake monkeys. *J Neurosurg* 1981;**54**:773–82.
14. Siesjo BK. Pathophysiology and treatment of focal cerebral ischemia. Part I: Pathophysiology. *J Neurosurg* 1992;**77**:169–84.
15. Hossmann KA. Viability thresholds and the penumbra of focal ischemia. *Ann Neurol* 1994;**36**:557–65.
16. Derdeyn CP, Videen TO, Yundt KD, *et al.* Variability of cerebral blood volume and oxygen extraction: stages of cerebral haemodynamic impairment revisited. *Brain* 2002;**125**:595–607.
17. Powers WJ, Grubb RL, Jr., Darriet D, Raichle ME. Cerebral blood flow and cerebral metabolic rate of oxygen requirements for cerebral function and viability in humans. *J Cereb Blood Flow Metab* 1985;**5**:600–8.
18. Morimoto Y, Mathru M, Martinez-Tica JF, Zornow MH. Effects of profound anemia on brain tissue oxygen tension, carbon dioxide tension, and pH in rabbits. *J Neurosurg Anesthesiol* 2001;**13**:33–9.
19. Minhas PS, Menon DK, Smielewski P, *et al.* Positron emission tomographic cerebral perfusion disturbances and transcranial Doppler findings among patients with neurological deterioration after subarachnoid hemorrhage. *Neurosurgery* 2003;**52**:1017–22.
20. Wise RJ, Bernardi S, Frackowiak RS, *et al.* Serial observations on the pathophysiology of acute stroke. The transition from ischaemia to infarction as reflected in regional oxygen extraction. *Brain* 1983;**106** (Pt 1):197–222.
21. Baron JC, Moseley ME. For how long is brain tissue salvageable? Imaging-based evidence. *J Stroke Cerebrovasc Dis* 2000;**9**:15–20.
22. Zazulia AR, Videen TO, Powers WJ. Symptomatic autoregulatory failure in acute ischemic stroke. *Neurology* 2007;**68**:389–90.
23. Chalela JA, Dunn B, Todd JW, Warach S. Induced hypertension improves cerebral blood flow in acute ischemic stroke. *Neurology* 2005;**64**:1979.
24. Alawneh JA, Moustafa RR, Baron JC. Hemodynamic factors and perfusion abnormalities in early neurological deterioration. *Stroke* 2009;**40**:e443–e450.
25. Uemura K, Shishido F, Higano S, *et al.* Positron emission tomography in patients with a primary intracerebral hematoma. *Acta Radiol Suppl* 1986;**369**:426–8.
26. Sills C, Villar-Cordova C, Pasteur W, *et al.* Demonstration of hypoperfusion surrounding intracerebral hematoma in humans. *J Stroke Cerebrovasc Dis* 1996;**6**:17–24.
27. Zazulia AR, Diringer MN, Videen TO, *et al.* Hypoperfusion without ischemia surrounding acute intracerebral hemorrhage. *J Cereb Blood Flow Metab* 2001;**21**:804–10.
28. Kim-Han JS, Kopp SJ, Dugan LL, Diringer MN. Perihematomal mitochondrial dysfunction after intracerebral hemorrhage. *Stroke* 2006;**37**:2457–62.
29. Tayal AH, Gupta R, Yonas H, *et al.* Quantitative perihematomal blood flow in spontaneous intracerebral hemorrhage predicts in-hospital functional outcome. *Stroke* 2007;**38**:319–24.
30. Anderson CS, Heeley E, Huang Y, *et al.* Rapid blood pressure lowering in patients with acute intracerebral haemorrhage. *N Eng J Med* 2013;**368**:2355–65.
31. Grubb RL, Jr., Raichle ME, Eichling JO, Gado MH. Effects of subarachnoid hemorrhage on cerebral blood volume, blood flow, and oxygen utilization in humans. *J Neurosurg* 1977;**46**:446–53.

32. Meyer CH, Lowe D, Meyer M, *et al.* Progressive change in cerebral blood flow during the first three weeks after subarachnoid hemorrhage. *Neurosurgery* 1983;**12**:58–76.
33. Carpenter DA, Grubb RL, Jr., Tempel LW, Powers WJ. Cerebral oxygen metabolism after aneurysmal subarachnoid hemorrhage. *J Cereb Blood Flow Metab* 1991;**11**:837–44.
34. Voldby B, Enevoldsen EM, Jensen FT. Regional CBF, intraventricular pressure, and cerebral metabolism in patients with ruptured intracranial aneurysms. *J Neurosurg* 1985; **62**:48–58.
35. Grote E, Hassler W. The critical first minutes after subarachnoid hemorrhage. *Neurosurgery* 1988;**22**:654–61.
36. Geraud G, Tremoulet M, Guell A, Bes A. The prognostic value of noninvasive CBF measurement in subarachnoid hemorrhage. *Stroke* 1984;**15**:301–5.
37. Gupta R, Crago EA, Gallek M, *et al.* Reduced ipsilateral hemispheric cerebral blood flow at admission is predictive of vasospasm with infarction after aneurysmal subarachnoid hemorrhage. *Neurocrit Care* 2008;**9**:27–30.
38. Jakobsen M, Overgaard J, Marcussen E, Enevoldsen EM. Relation between angiographic cerebral vasospasm and regional CBF in patients with SAH. *Acta Neurol Scand* 1990;**82**:109–15.
39. Chieregato A, Tanfani A, Noto A, *et al.* Cerebral blood flow thresholds predicting new hypoattenuation areas due to macrovascular ischemia during the acute phase of severe and complicated aneurysmal subarachnoid hemorrhage. A preliminary study. *Acta Neurochir Suppl* 2008;**102**:311–16.
40. Fainardi E, Tagliaferri MF, Compagnone C, *et al.* Regional cerebral blood flow levels as measured by xenon-CT in vascular territorial low-density areas after subarachnoid hemorrhage are not always ischemic. *Neuroradiology* 2006;**48**:685–90.
41. Dankbaar JW, Slooter AJ, Rinkel GJ, Schaaf IC. Effect of different components of triple-H therapy on cerebral perfusion in patients with aneurysmal subarachnoid haemorrhage: a systematic review. *Crit Care* 2010;**14**:R23.
42. Harrigan MR, Leonardo J, Gibbons KJ, *et al.* CT perfusion cerebral blood flow imaging in neurological critical care. *Neurocrit Care* 2005;**2**:352–66.
43. Drayer BP, Wolfson SK, Reinmuth OM, *et al.* Xenon enhanced CT for analysis of cerebral integrity, perfusion, and blood flow. *Stroke* 1978;**9**:123–30.
44. Latchaw RE, Yonas H, Pentheny SL, Gur D. Adverse reactions to xenon-enhanced CT cerebral blood flow determination. *Radiology* 1987;**163**:251–4.
45. von Oettingen G, Bergholt B, Ostergaard L, *et al.* Xenon CT cerebral blood flow in patients with head injury: influence of pulmonary trauma on the input function. *Neuroradiology* 2000;**42**:168–73.
46. Yonas H, Sekhar L, Johnson DW, Gur D. Determination of irreversible ischemia by xenon-enhanced computed tomographic monitoring of cerebral blood flow in patients with symptomatic vasospasm. *Neurosurgery* 1989;**24**:368–72.
47. Darby JM, Yonas H, Marks EC, *et al.* Acute cerebral blood flow response to dopamine-induced hypertension after subarachnoid hemorrhage. *J Neurosurg* 1994;**80**:857–64.
48. Firlik AD, Kaufmann AM, Jungreis CA, Yonas H. Effect of transluminal angioplasty on cerebral blood flow in the management of symptomatic vasospasm following aneurysmal subarachnoid hemorrhage. *J Neurosurg* 1997;**86**:830–9.
49. Wintermark M, Ko NU, Smith WS, *et al.* Vasospasm after subarachnoid hemorrhage: utility of perfusion CT and CT angiography on diagnosis and management. *AJNR Am J Neuroradiol* 2006;**27**:26–34.
50. Dankbaar JW, de Rooij NK, Velthuis BK, *et al.* Diagnosing delayed cerebral ischemia with different CT modalities in patients with subarachnoid hemorrhage with clinical deterioration. *Stroke* 2009;**40**:3493–8.
51. Sobesky J, Zaro WO, Lehnhardt FG, *et al.* Does the mismatch match the penumbra? Magnetic resonance imaging and positron emission tomography in early ischemic stroke. *Stroke* 2005;**36**:980–5.
52. Konstas AA, Goldmakher GV, Lee TY, Lev MH. Theoretic basis and technical implementations of CT perfusion in acute ischemic stroke, part 1: Theoretic basis. *AJNR Am J Neuroradiol* 2009;**30**:662–8.
53. Hagen T, Bartylla K, Piepgras U. Correlation of regional cerebral blood flow measured by stable xenon CT and perfusion MRI. *J Comput Assist Tomogr* 1999;**23**:257–64.
54. Weidauer S, Lanfermann H, Raabe A, *et al.* Impairment of cerebral perfusion and infarct patterns attributable to vasospasm after aneurysmal subarachnoid hemorrhage: a prospective MRI and DSA study. *Stroke* 2007;**38**:1831–6.
55. Vajkoczy P, Roth H, Horn P, *et al.* Continuous monitoring of regional cerebral blood flow: experimental and clinical validation of a novel thermal diffusion microprobe. *J Neurosurg* 2000;**93**:265–74.
56. Vajkoczy P, Horn P, Thome C, *et al.* Regional cerebral blood flow monitoring in the diagnosis of delayed ischemia following aneurysmal subarachnoid hemorrhage. *J Neurosurg* 2003;**98**:1227–34.
57. Muench E, Horn P, Bauhuf C, *et al.* Effects of hypervolemia and hypertension on regional cerebral blood flow, intracranial pressure, and brain tissue oxygenation after subarachnoid hemorrhage. *Crit Care Med* 2007;**35**:1844–51.

58. Soukup J, Bramsiepe I, Brucke M, *et al.* Evaluation of a bedside monitor of regional CBF as a measure of CO_2 reactivity in neurosurgical intensive care patients. *J Neurosurg Anesthesiol* 2008;**20**:249–55.
59. Muench E, Bauhuf C, Roth H, *et al.* Effects of positive end-expiratory pressure on regional cerebral blood flow, intracranial pressure, and brain tissue oxygenation. *Crit Care Med* 2005;**33**:2367–72.
60. Clyde BL, Resnick DK, Yonas H, *et al.* The relationship of blood velocity as measured by transcranial Doppler ultrasonography to cerebral blood flow as determined by stable xenon computed tomographic studies after aneurysmal subarachnoid hemorrhage. *Neurosurgery* 1996;**38**:896–904.
61. Bishop CC, Powell S, Rutt D, Browse NL. Transcranial Doppler measurement of middle cerebral artery blood flow velocity: a validation study. *Stroke* 1986; **17**:913–15.
62. Kim MN, Durduran T, Frangos S, *et al.* Noninvasive measurement of cerebral blood flow and blood oxygenation using near-infrared and diffuse correlation spectroscopies in critically brain-injured adults. *Neurocrit Care* 2010; **12**:173–80.
63. Manno EM, Gress DR, Schwamm LH, *et al.* Effects of induced hypertension on transcranial Doppler ultrasound velocities in patients after subarachnoid hemorrhage. *Stroke* 1998;**29**:422–8.

3

Brain tissue oxygen monitoring in cerebrovascular diseases

Klaus Zweckberger and Karl L. Kiening

Introduction

Patients suffering from severe impairments to their brains are at risk of developing secondary ischemic damage. First and foremost, this is a consequence of intracranial hypertension or arterial hypotension resulting in an insufficient cerebral perfusion (CPP). This, in turn, compromises cerebral blood flow (CBF) and tissue oxygenation contributing to evolving structural and functional tissue damage and, thus, leading to negative neurological outcome. As demonstrated for healthy individuals, brain tissue oxygenation and cerebral perfusion pressure show mutual dependency [1]. Within a specific cortical unit, fractional changes in cerebral blood flow (CBF) and cerebral metabolic rate of oxygen consumption ($CMR(O_2)$) are coupled through an invariant relationship during physiological stimulation. As a consequence, any decrease in cerebral perfusion impairs oxygen supply and oxidative metabolism of the brain tissue. Thus, as shown in clinical [2,3] and experimental pathophysiological studies [4], changes in brain tissue oxygenation pO_2 ($pbrO_2$) can represent a reliable indicator to monitor evolving tissue perturbation.

Based on the facts that the mammalian brain is not equipped with sufficient oxygen, and energy depots and the activity of enzymes are regulated by $pbrO_2$, tissue oxygenation needs to be maintained within physiological limits to prevent additional and uncontrolled cell damage [5].

Experience gained within the past years has taught us that in daily clinical routine local cerebral hypoxia might develop under conditions of normal ICP, CPP, and MAP emphasizing the importance of additional tissue monitoring. Such episodes of local cerebral hypoxia can be attributed to hyperventilation-induced hypocapnia [2,6], insufficient arterial oxygenation [2] or a mismatch between oxygen delivery, i.e. cerebral blood flow (CBF), and cerebral metabolic rate of oxygen ($CMRO_2$) [7].

Since $pbrO_2$ monitoring has been extensively reported in traumatic brain injury, the following basic chapters have to refer mainly to this pathology.

Techniques to monitor cerebral partial pressure of oxygen ($pbrO_2$)

Currently, two main $pbrO_2$ systems are commercially available, the Licox® (Integra Neuroscience, Plainsboro, NJ) and the Neurovent-TO® (temperature and oxygen measurement catheter) as well as Neurovent-PTO® (parenchymal pressure, temperature and oxygen measurement catheter) from Raumedics AG (Münchberg, Germany). While the Neurovent system is a multiparameter sensor measuring temperature (and intracranial pressure) in addition to $pbrO_2$, the Licox system only allows changes in $pbrO_2$ to be assessed unless a separate temperature catheter is not inserted. The Licox system is based on the polarographic technique (modified 'Clark-typ' electrodes) [5], whereas the Neurovent oxygen

Critical Care of the Stroke Patient, ed. Stefan Schwab, Daniel Hanley, and A. David Mendelow. Published by Cambridge University Press.

microsensor works based on so-called 'oxygen quenching' (fluorescent dye molecules absorb light by entering into an excited state and return into ground state while emitting light of a certain wavelength, a process which is reduced in presence of oxygen).

In the latest Licox system design as well as in the Neurovent system, the catheters are precalibrated and therefore suitable for immediate insertion. The two systems show, however, beside the different monitoring technologies, significant different $pbrO_2$ uptake areas (Licox: 13 mm^2, Neurovent-PTO/TO: 22 mm^2). In a bench test setting, both the Neurovent-PTO and Licox probes showed accuracy in detecting different oxygen tensions, and thereby did not deviate during long-lasting recording times. The reaction time of the Neurovent-PTO probe detecting changes in pO_2 was significantly shorter in comparison to the Licox system. Furthermore, Licox probes showed an increased standard deviation with higher brain temperatures [8].

In an experimental setting, however, Orakcioglu *et al.* could demonstrate that in hypoxic and hyperoxic manoeuvres Neurovent-TO and Licox probes varied, both in their measurement of dynamic profiles and in the time of detection. Thus the Neurovent-TO probe could detect hypoxic crises of 8.5 mmHg about 1.5 minutes earlier than the Licox system [9].

Location of $pbrO_2$ catheters

As shown in experimental studies, tissue oxygenation depicts a strong heterogeneous distribution depending on the proximity of the inserted electrodes relative to vessels and the surrounding cell density. Highest $pbrO_2$ levels are found close to penetrating vessels and in neuron-rich areas (cortex and hippocampus) as opposed to white matter tracts predominantly consisting of axons [5].

To date, no consensus could be reached on the ideal placement of $pbrO_2$ catheters corresponding to the different traumatic brain lesions (e.g., focal/unilateral vs. multiple/bilateral vs. diffuse brain injury vs. generalized edema). As previously demonstrated for severely brain-injured patients, $pbrO_2$ values strongly depend on the position of the catheters applied to cerebral contusions. According to cCT controls, and in comparison to non-injured tissue, $pbrO_2$ values were significantly decreased close to cerebral lesions [10].

In clinical practice, penetrating oxygen sensors are usually placed in the contralateral ('non-injured') white matter, revealing the involvement of the uninjured hemisphere as a sign of widespread, global, energetic perturbation. Thereby, critically decreased $pbrO_2$ values might indicate depletion in arterial oxygenation, increase in ICP, impaired cerebral perfusion, or uncontrolled hyperventilation. In case of bilateral lesions, $pbrO_2$ is preferably monitored in the least injured hemisphere. On the other hand, it might be reasonable to monitor $pbrO_2$ in the pericontusional zone concentrating on the tissue which is, comparable to the penumbra in stroke, highly endangered to perish.

Hypoxic $pbrO_2$ thresholds

Likewise other established methods, e.g. jugular venous oxygen saturation ($sjvO_2$), at which oxygen saturation of 50% indicate impending cerebral ischemia, brain tissue oxygen ($pbrO_2$) monitoring has been validated for patients with severe traumatic brain injury (TBI). Thereby, a critical depletion of jugular venous oxygen saturation corresponds to an average reduction in $pbrO_2$ beneath 8.5 mmHg [11]. Owing to clinical [12] and experimental [13] studies, ischemic damage can be expected to develop below a detrimental $pbrO_2$ threshold of 8–10 mmHg. Further studies aiming to establish clinically relevant $pbrO_2$ thresholds have concentrated on the neurological outcome of patients following severe TBI corresponding to different $pbrO_2$ levels [2,7,14–19].

Clinical data revealed that any $pbrO_2$ values < 10 mmHg within the first 24 hours after TBI as well as any periods of $pbrO_2 < 10$ mmHg for longer than 15–30 minutes indicate poor prognosis [2,13,14,19,20]. Confirming these results, van Santbrink and colleagues published a series of 22 severely head-injured patients, in which five out of six patients with $pbrO_2$ values ≤ 5 mmHg died or remained in a vegetative state [21]. These results have been underlined by the same group in a large series of patients (n=101) describing a mortality rate of 50% if $pbrO_2$ levels have remained ≤ 5 mmHg for longer than 10 minutes [22].

Overall, the detrimental $pbrO_2$ threshold of 10 mmHg is adequately substantiated by the literature and confirmed by neurochemical findings (see below) [23,24].

Brain $pbrO_2$ and hyperventilation

Recent studies could clearly demonstrate that in most patients hyperventilation decreases $pbrO_2$ as a result of excessively decreased cerebral blood flow (CBF) (Δ 3% CBF/Δ 1 mmHg arterial $paCO_2$) [3,6,10,25–29] which, on the other hand, represents a potential treatment option to reduce ICP and improve CPP. Patients are especially endangered to incur cerebral hypoxia since *forced* hyperventilation ($paCO_2 \leq 30$ mmHg) [25] or if hyperventilation is used within the first 24 hours after TBI [25,29] aggravating already reduced CBF [30]. Likewise, during *moderate* hyperventilation ($paCO_2 > 30$ mmHg), critical low $pbrO_2$ levels (<10 mmHg) occur in approximately 17% of patients [6]. The extent of $pbrO_2$ changes during hyperventilation varies individually, and thus, $pbrO_2$ monitoring might guide such therapeutic interventions to preserve patients from potential critical episodes of decreased cerebral tissue oxygen saturation and might represent an option in the 'Guidelines for the Management of Severe TBI'.

Brain $pbrO_2$ and CPP

The 'Guidelines for the Management of Severe TBI' [31] recommend to maintain CPP > 50 mmHg (class III evidence). This treatment concept discloses some conflict due to the results of several $pbrO_2$ papers outlining CPP > 60 mmHg to guarantee sufficient cerebral oxygenation [3,11,14,16,27]. In detail, CPP < 60 mmHg was significantly related to critical low $pbrO_2$ levels (< 10 mmHg) [3,18,27]. Furthermore, $pbrO_2$ was not influenced by changes in CPP as long as CPP remained above the threshold of 60 mmHg [3,11,27].

In general, the above-mentioned studies highlight the importance of stable CPP for sufficient cerebral oxygenation after severe TBI; however, this may not necessarily hold true for 'traumatic vasospasm' [14]. It is unconfirmed so far if low $pbrO_2$ during traumatic vasospasm can be treated successfully by increasing CPP to the upper limit as done in the specific therapy for aneurysmal vasospasm ('triple H therapy').

Brain $pbrO_2$ and neurochemical monitoring

As recently shown [17,23,24], combining $pbrO_2$ monitoring and microdialysis measurements allow characterization of the nature of energetic perturbation (anaerobic vs. non-oxidative glycolysis) following TBI by simultaneously determining changes in tissue oxygenation and metabolic parameters. For this reason, $pbrO_2$ and microdialysis catheters are usually placed adjacent to each other.

Simultaneous monitoring of $sjvO_2$, $pbrO_2$, lactate, and glucose in patients with severe TBI revealed a close relationship between changes in tissue oxygenation and metabolic deterioration [24]. Episodes of global as well as local hypoxia reflected by decreases in $svjO_2 < 50\%$ and $pbrO_2 < 10$ mmHg coincided with a significant increase in extracellular lactate [24]. In a follow-up study, the same group reported a significant increase in lactate and decrease in glucose occurring with reversible cerebral hypoxia ($pbrO_2$ levels < 10 mmHg) [17]. These in vivo results clearly demonstrate that changes in $pbrO_2$ are essential parameters to detect anaerobic glycolysis. Metabolic changes in lactate and glucose alone could also be taken as indicators of oxidative glycolysis.

Following severe TBI, decreases in $pbrO_2$ below the ischemic threshold (< 10 mmHg) were also reported to coincide with pathologic lactate/pyruvate ratios while extracellular glutamate was found to be both normal and elevated during periods of insufficient tissue oxygenation ($pbrO_2$ <10 mmHg) [23]. Microdialysis might detect impending hypoxia early and, thus, offer the possibility for early changes in treatment [32].

Thus, microdialysis adds valuable information concerning the impact of local cerebral hypoxia on energy metabolism and thus substantiates the validity of $pbrO_2$ measurements.

Brain $pbrO_2$ in subarachnoid hemorrhage

In comparison with TBI data, in aneurysmatic subarachnoid hemorrhage (SAH) considerably less experience with $pbrO_2$ monitoring exists. Overall, however, data are robust to draw some clear conclusion for this pathology.

One experimental study on rats pointed out that aside from sudden increase of intracranial pressure (ICP) at the time of hemorrhage and delayed cerebral vasospasm, the occurrence of acute vasoconstriction and disturbed oxygen utilization may be additional factors contributing to secondary brain damage after SAH [33].

In patients, monitoring of $pbrO_2$, however, might serve as a guide during surgery (Clipping) of aneurysms [34], but it especially offers potency to detect impending vasospasm early during intensive care treatment of patients with severe SAH. The insertion of $pbrO_2$ catheters into viable tissue in the vascular territory with the highest risk for vasospasm is widely accepted. It could be clearly demonstrated that prolonged phases of brain tissue hypoxia (pbrO2 < 10 mmHg), as might occur during cerebral vasospasm, lead to cerebral infarctions. Thereby, Vath *et al.* could show that critical CPP (< 70 mmHg) as well as hypoxic $pbrO_2$ (< 10 mmHg) levels were significantly more frequent in patients who developed infarctions [35]. In ischemic areas $pbrO_2$ seemed to be dependent on CPP, suggesting both a derangement of pressure autoregulation and high regional cerebrovascular resistance (CVR). Arterial hypertension, capable of increasing CPP above normal values, thus, appeared useful in normalizing tissue oxygenation in ischemic areas [36]. For assessment of the impact on autoregulation, the index of $pbrO_2$ pressure reactivity (ORx) was calculated as a moving correlation coefficient between values of CPP and $PbrO_2$ [37]. Higher ORx values indicated disturbed autoregulation, whereas lower ORx values signified intact autoregulation. By monitoring 67 patients, Jaeger *et al.* could clearly demonstrate a close correlation between impaired autoregulation and the development of delayed infarctions [37]. While Meixenberger *et al.* could not prove critical multimodal monitoring parameters as early predictors for non-survival in 2003 [38], Ramakrishna *et al.* concluded in 2009 that patients' deaths after SAH may be associated with a lower mean $pbrO_2$ and longer periods of compromised cerebral oxygenation in comparison to survivors [39]. Furthermore, monitoring of $pbrO_2$ offers the possibility to re-evaluate effects of different treatment approaches. Administration of hypertonic saline, for example, augments CBF in patients with poor-grade SAH and significantly improves cerebral oxygenation for four hours post-infusion. A favorable outcome was associated with an improvement in brain tissue oxygenation beyond 210 minutes [40]. On the other hand, it could be demonstrated that in some patients $pbrO_2$ was reduced after the administration of nimodipine, although nimodipine use is significantly associated with improved outcome following SAH [41]. In summary, in the postoperative period, advanced monitoring techniques such as brain tissue oxygenation or microdialysis might detect harmful secondary insults, and may eventually be used as an end point for goal-directed therapy, with the aim of creating an optimal physiological environment for the comatose injured brain [42].

Brain $pbrO_2$ and ischemic stroke

Significant advancements in the field of intensive care treatment of patients with severe space-occupying stroke have led to improved care and outcome. It must be emphasized that treatment in specialized neurointensive care units improves outcome. ICP monitoring alone, however, may not be sufficient to guide therapy [43]. Multimodal monitoring thus can be used to assess anitedema drug effects and might predict pathophysiological changes considerably in advance [44]. In patients with middle cerebral artery territory stroke, administration of colloids, mannitol, or surgical decompressive therapy have been shown to increase local tissue $pbrO_2$ [44]. Furthermore, authors described a significant and critical depletion of $pbrO_2$ up to 18 hours before transtentorial herniation [44]. In stoke patients $pbrO_2$ catheters are recommended to be inserted in the penumbra region – the maximal endangered brain tissue having the chance of being rescued.

Brain $pbrO_2$ and spontaneous intracerebral hemorrhage

Monitoring of brain tissue oxygenation (pbrO2), however, has been extensively reported for traumatic brain injury and subarachnoid hemorrhage, while data concerning the use of this technique in the therapy of spontaneous intracranial hemorrhage (ICH) are only fragmentary. In an experimental set-up Hemphill *et al.* could demonstrate that a rise in ICP early after hematoma formation was accompanied by a decrease in ipsilateral and contralateral $pbrO_2$ [45]. These results could be confirmed by a series of seven patients detecting critical decreased $pbrO_2$ levels frequently after ICH [45]. In an observational pilot study both $pbrO_2$ and microdialysis catheters have been placed in the perihemorrhagic edema using neuronavigation in five nonsurgically treated patients with deep ICH. While all five patients had ORx (correlation between CPP and $pbrO_2$) indicating severely disturbed autoregulation, assessment of PRx (pressure reactivity index) only in one patient was consistent with sustained failure of cerebrovascular reactivity. At the same time this patient had the worst tissue oxygenation and metabolic derangements [46]. Although assessment of $pbrO_2$ in the perihemorrhagic penumbra seemed to be feasible, further studies have to be performed clarifying the relationship between PRx, ORx and tissue oxygenation in ICH patients.

Conclusions

The intention to monitor $pbrO_2$ continuously is to reveal acute changes suggestive of impending ischemic and energetic deterioration leading to infarctions and, furthermore, to guide therapeutic interventions aimed to prevent evolving tissue damage and neurological impairment.

One conflicting technical issue is related to the 'correct' positioning of the oxygen sensor. Since this sensor can only determine changes within a small radius of tissue surrounding the probe, the 'true' validity of this technique is limited to the monitored small tissue area. In other words, extrapolating local $pbrO_2$ data to the oxygenation status of one hemisphere or the whole brain bears the risk that regional or global ischemia may remain undetected despite normal $pbrO_2$ values in the monitored region.

A major drawback of the above cited studies conducted in the past years is the rather 'uncontrolled' nature of equally important concomitant and possibly conflicting variables in terms of sedation, analgesia, relaxation, fluid therapy, ICP and CPP management, etc. These differences in basic treatment modalities which differ from center to center need to be considered as important independent variables and have to be controlled for urgently needed prospective, randomized studies determining the importance of $pbrO_2$ guided therapy.

Taken together, monitoring of brain tissue oxygenation ($pbrO_2$) in cerebrovascular diseases offers the possibility to assess oxygen saturation of the potentially endangered brain tissue that still has the potency of being rescued. With this technique therapy can be targeted and its effects on brain tissue oxygen saturation can be controlled. Owing to the available literature concerning cerebrovascular diseases, however, monitoring of brain tissue oxygenation remains an option because of a lack of class I evidence and does not reach guideline status.

REFERENCES

1. Hoge RD, J Atkinson, B Gill, *et al.* Linear coupling between cerebral blood flow and oxygen consumption in activated human cortex. *Proc Natl Acad Sci USA* 1999;**96**:9403–8.
2. Gopinath SP, AB Valadka, M Uzura, *et al.* Comparison of jugular venous oxygen saturation and brain tissue Po2 as monitors of cerebral ischemia after head injury. *Crit Care Med* 1999;**27**:2337–45.
3. Kiening KL, R Hartl, AW Unterberg, *et al.* Brain tissue pO2-monitoring in comatose patients: implications for therapy. *Neurol Res* 1997;**19**:233–40.
4. Manley GT, LH Pitts, D Morabito, *et al.* Brain tissue oxygenation during hemorrhagic shock, resuscitation, and alterations in ventilation. *J Trauma* 1999;**46**:261–7.
5. Erecinska M, IA Silver. Tissue oxygen tension and brain sensitivity to hypoxia. *Respir Physiol* 2001;**128**:263–76.
6. Imberti R, G Bellinzona, M Langer. Cerebral tissue PO2 and SjvO2 changes during moderate hyperventilation in

patients with severe traumatic brain injury. *J Neurosurg* 2002;**96**:97–102.

7. Grohn OH, RA Kauppinen. Assessment of brain tissue viability in acute ischemic stroke by BOLD MRI. *NMR Biomed* 2001;**14**:432–40.
8. Purins K, P Enblad, B Sandhagen, *et al.* Brain tissue oxygen monitoring: a study of in vitro accuracy and stability of Neurovent-PTO and Licox sensors. *Acta Neurochir (Wien)* 2010;**152**:681–8.
9. Orakcioglu B, OW Sakowitz, JO Neumann, *et al.* Evaluation of a novel brain tissue oxygenation probe in an experimental swin model. *J Neurosurgery* 2010;**67**:1716–23.
10. Dings J, J Meixensberger, J Amschler, *et al.* Continuous monitoring of brain tissue PO2: a new tool to minimize the risk of ischemia caused by hyperventilation therapy. *Zentralbl Neurochir* 1996;**57**:177–83.
11. Kiening KL, AW Unterberg, TF Bardt, *et al.* Monitoring of cerebral oxygenation in patients with severe head injuries: brain tissue PO2 versus jugular vein oxygen saturation. *J Neurosurg* 1996;**85**:751–7.
12. Sarrafzadeh AS, KL Kiening, TF Bardt, *et al.* Cerebral oxygenation in contusioned vs. nonlesioned brain tissue: monitoring of PtiO2 with Licox and Paratrend. *Acta Neurochir suppl (Wien)* 1998;**71**:186–9.
13. Valadka AB, SP Gopinath, CF Contant, *et al.* Relationship of brain tissue PO2 to outcome after severe head injury. *Crit Care Med* 1998;**26**:1576–81.
14. Artru F, C Jourdan, A Perret-Liaudet, *et al.* Low brain tissue oxygen pressure: incidence and corrective therapies. *Neurol Res* 1998;**20** Suppl 1:S48–51.
15. Diringer MN, K Yundt, TO Videen, *et al.* No reduction in cerebral metabolism as a result of early moderate hyperventilation following severe traumatic brain injury. *J Neurosurg* 2000;**92**:7–13.
16. Filippi R, R Reisch, D Mauer, *et al.* Brain tissue pO2 related to SjvO2, ICP, and CPP in severe brain injury. *Neurosurg Rev* 2000;**23**:94–7.
17. Goodman JC, AB Valadka, SP Gopinath, *et al.* Extracellular lactate and glucose alterations in the brain after head injury measured by microdialysis. *Crit Care Med* 1999;**27**:1965–73.
18. Sarrafzadeh AS, EE Peltonen, U Kaisers, *et al.* Secondary insults in severe head injury – do multiply injured patients do worse? *Crit Care Med* 2001;**29**:1116–23.
19. van den Brink WA, H van Santbrink, CJ Avezaat, *et al.* Monitoring brain oxygen tension in severe head injury: the Rotterdam experience. *Acta Neurochir Suppl (Wien)* 1998;**71**:190–4.
20. Sheinberg M, MJ Kanter, CS Robertson, *et al.* Continuous monitoring of jugular venous oxygen saturation in head-injured patients. *J Neurosurg* 1992;**76**:212–7.
21. van Santbrink H, AI Maas, CJ Avezaat. Continuous monitoring of partial pressure of brain tissue oxygen in patients with severe head injury. *Neurosurgery* 1996;**38**:21–31.
22. van den Brink WA, H van Santbrink, EW Steyerberg, *et al.* Brain oxygen tension in severe head injury. *Neurosurgery* 2000;**46**:868–76; discussion 876–8.
23. Meixensberger J, E Kunze, E Barcsay, *et al.* Clinical cerebral microdialysis: brain metabolism and brain tissue oxygenation after acute brain injury. *Neurol Res* 2001;**23**:801–6.
24. Robertson CS, SP Gopinath, M Uzura, *et al.* Metabolic changes in the brain during transient ischemia measured with microdialysis. *Neurol Res* 1998;**20** Suppl 1:S91–4.
25. Carmona Suazo JA, AI Maas, WA van den Brink, *et al.* CO_2 reactivity and brain oxygen pressure monitoring in severe head injury. *Crit Care Med* 2000;**28**:3268–74.
26. Schneider GH, AS Sarrafzadeh, KL Kiening, *et al.* Influence of hyperventilation on brain tissue-PO2, PCO2, and pH in patients with intracranial hypertension. *Acta Neurochir Suppl (Wien)* 1998;**71**:62–5.
27. Unterberg AW, KL Kiening, R Hartl, *et al.* Multimodal monitoring in patients with head injury: evaluation of the effects of treatment on cerebral oxygenation. *J Trauma* 1997;**42**:S32–7.
28. Zhi DS, S Zhang, LG Zhou. Continuous monitoring of brain tissue oxygen pressure in patients with severe head injury during moderate hypothermia. *Surg Neurol* 1999;**52**:393–6.
29. Dings J, J Meixensberger, J Amschler, *et al.* Brain tissue pO2 in relation to cerebral perfusion pressure, TCD findings and TCD-CO2-reactivity after severe head injury. *Acta Neurochir (Wien)* 1996;**138**:425–34.
30. Bouma GJ, JP Muizelaar, WA Stringer, *et al.* Ultra-early evaluation of regional cerebral blood flow in severely head-injured patients using xenon-enhanced computerized tomography. *J Neurosurg* 1992;**77**:360–8.
31. Bratton SL, RM Chestnut, J Ghajar, *et al.* Guidelines for the management of severe traumatic brain injury. Brain oxygen monitoring and thresholds. *J Neurotrauma* 2007;**24** Suppl 1:S65–70.
32. Sarrafzadeh AS, OW Sakowitz, TA Callsen, *et al.* Detection of secondary insults by brain tissue pO2 and bedside microdialysis in severe head injury. *Acta Neurochir Suppl* 2002;**81**:319–21.
33. Westermaier T, A Jauss, J Eriskat, *et al.* Time-course of cerebral perfusion and tissue oxygenation in the first

6 hrs after experimental subarachnoid hemorrhage in rats. *J Cereb Blood Flow Metab* 2009;**29**:771–9.

34. Hoffman WE, P Wheeler, G Edelman, *et al.* Hypoxic brain tissue following subarachnoid hemorrhage. *Anesthesiology* 2000;**92**:442–6.
35. Vath A, E Kunze, K Roosen, *et al.* Therapeutic aspects of brain tissue pO2 monitoring after subarachnoid hemorrhage. *Acta Neurochir Suppl* 2002;**81**:307–9.
36. Stocchetti N, A Chieregato, M De Marchi, *et al.* High cerebral perfusion pressure improves low values of local brain tissue O2 tension (PtiO2) in focal lesions. *Acta Neurochir Suppl* 1998;**71**:162–5.
37. Jaeger M, MU Schuhmann, M Soehle, *et al.* Continuous monitoring of cerebrovascular autoregulation after subarachnoid hemorrhage by brain tissue oxygen pressure reactivity and its relation to delayed cerebral infarction. *Stroke* 2007;**38**:981–6.
38. Meixensberger J, A Vath, M Jaeger, *et al.* Monitoring of brain tissue oxygenation following severe subarachnoid hemorrhage. *Neurol Res* 2003;**25**:445–50.
39. Ramakrishna R, M Stiefel, J Udoetuk, *et al.* Brain oxygen tension and outcome in patients with aneurysmal subarachnoid hemorrhage. *J Neurosurg* 2008;**109**:1075–82.
40. Al-Rawi PG, MY Tseng, HK Richards, *et al.* Hypertonic saline in patients with poor-grade subarachnoid hemorrhage improves cerebral blood flow, brain tissue oxygen, and pH. *Stroke* 2010;**41**:122–8.
41. Stiefel MF, GG Heuer, JM Abrahams, *et al.* The effect of nimodipine on cerebral oxygenation in patients with poor-grade subarachnoid hemorrhage. *J Neurosurg* 2004;**101**:594–9.
42. Komotar RJ, JM Schmidt, RM Starke, *et al.* Resuscitation and critical care of poor-grade subarachnoid hemorrhage. *Neurosurgery* 2009;**64**:397–410;discussion 410–11.
43. Diedler J, M Sykora, E Juttler, *et al.* Intensive care management of acute stroke: general management. *Int J Stroke* 2009;**4**:365–78.
44. Steiner T, J Pilz, P Schellinger, *et al.* Multimodal online monitoring in middle cerebral artery territory stroke. *Stroke* 2001;**32**:2500–6.
45. Hemphill JC, D Morabito, M Farrant, *et al.* Brain tissue oxygen monitoring in intracerebral hemorrhage. *Neurocrit Care* 2005;**3**:260–70.
46. Diedler J, G Karpel-Massler, M Sykora, *et al.* Autoregulation and brain metabolism in the perihematomal region of spontaneous intracerebral hemorrhage: an observational pilot study. *J Neurol Sci* 2010;**295**:16–22.

4

Cerebral microdialysis in cerebrovascular disease

Paul M. Vespa

Funding acknowledgement: NINDS NS049471, P01 NS 058489-01A2, and the California Neurotrauma Initiative.

Introduction

Brain ischemia is a common reason for patients to become critically ill and end up in the neurointensive care unit. Cerebral ischemia may be easy to diagnose in the setting of acute ischemic stroke that elicits a focal neurologic deficit. Unfortunately, most patients in the intensive care unit do not have a clinical examination that can be easily or reliably followed. This is most easy to appreciate in the obtunded or comatose patient in which the examination is very difficult to interpret. There is now a substantial body of knowledge that ongoing cerebral ischemia and non-ischemic metabolic crisis occurs despite the absence of changes in the clinical exam. Hence, more sensitive and specific markers of cerebral ischemia are needed in order to understand the progression of disease and to detect ongoing ischemia. Fortunately, there are a few brain monitors that can provide this type of biomarker of ischemia. Cerebral microdialysis is one type of biomarker capable of detecting ischemia (for a comprehensive review, see 1). In this chapter, we will 1) describe the technique cerebral microdialysis monitoring, 2) describe the specific indicators of brain ischemia obtained from cerebral microdialysis, 3) provide examples of clinical scenarios in which cerebral microdialysis is used to detect brain ischemia, and 4) discuss the controversies of cerebral microdialysis monitoring.

Cerebral microdialysis technique

Cerebral microdialysis is a technique in which a chemical analysis of brain tissue is performed on a repeated basis without the actual removal of any brain tissue. The technique was developed in animal models to replace the need for whole brain tissue analysis. The cerebral microdialysis technique uses simple diffusion principles and a semipermeable membrane, very similar to the basic diffusion experiments one remembers from high school chemistry class. The basic technique involves placing a small tube, 1 mm in outer diameter, into the brain tissue that contains a dialysis system that allows for the sampling of compounds from the brain interstitial fluid using the principles of a diffusion gradient. The tube is inserted via a burr hole in a fashion similar to a parenchymal intracranial pressure monitor. The tube can be inserted via a bolt or via a removable peel-away catheter into the brain at a depth of 2–3 cm below the surface. The tube is perfused with artificial fluid that simulates normal cerebrospinal fluid in a closed loop fashion. The artificial CSF is low on concentration of glucose, lactate, pyruvate, amino acids, and other compounds but contains sodium and chloride that are isotonic to normal CSF. Based on the principles of diffusion, those chemicals that have higher concentration in the interstitium will diffuse into the tube and be collected in the effluent. This diffusion process removes only a fraction of the target chemical from the brain interstitium so as to not cause any net

Critical Care of the Stroke Patient, ed. Stefan Schwab, Daniel Hanley, and A. David Mendelow. Published by Cambridge University Press.

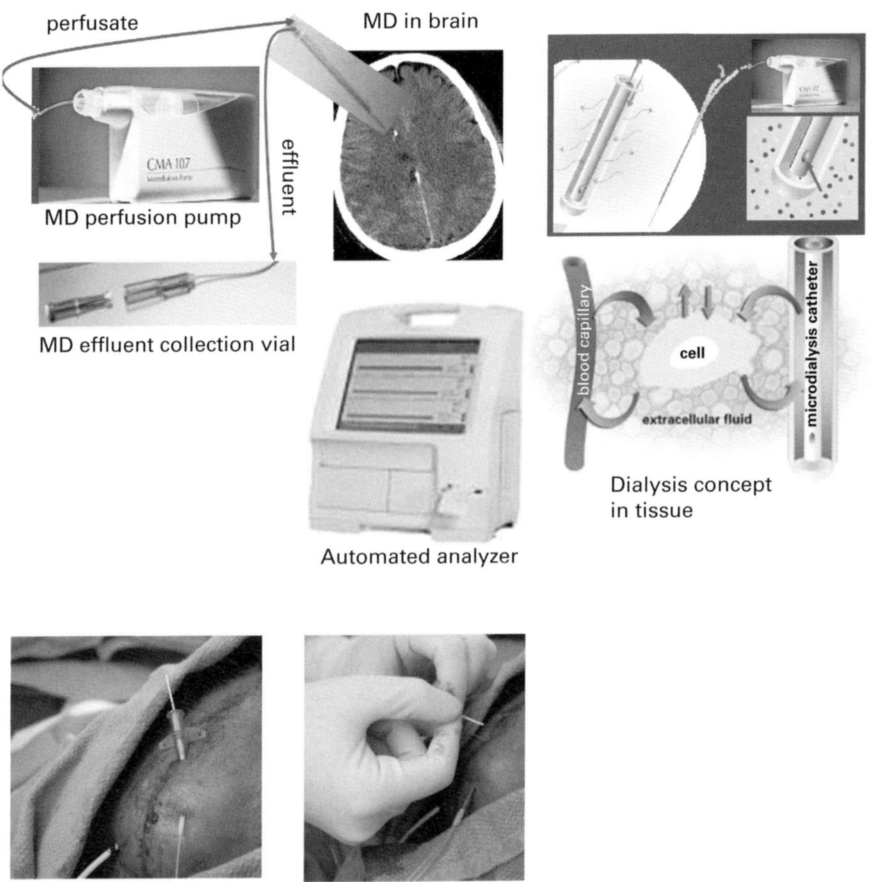

Fig. 4.1 The components of cerebral microdialysis include a perfusion pump (upper left), catheter that is inserted into the brain (highlighted enlargement, upper middle), and the analyzing system (bottom center). The fundamental method is a concentration dependent diffusion system in which molecules from the brain interstitial fluid diffuse along a concentration gradient into the microdialysis catheter (upper right). The interstitial concentration is dependent on the delivery of nutrients to the brain and the diffusion characteristics in the brain interstitium (lower right). The surgical insertion technique is shown (extreme bottom).

flux of the chemical out of the brain. The percentage of uptake of the target chemical into the effluent is called the net recovery. The net recovery of the target compound is dependent on the perfusion rate, the molecular weight of the compound, and the dialysis membrane pore size. For clinical purposes, perfusion rates range from 0.3 uL/min to 2 uL/min (Hutchinson). The slower the perfusion rate, the greater the net recovery. The effluent fluid is then collected in time-based fractions that range from 15 to 60 minutes in duration in most settings. For most clinical applications, the perfuate rate is 0.3 uL/min and the samples are collected once every hour. The effluent fluid is then analyzed using one of several methods such as high-performance liquid chromatography (HPLC) or automated enzymatic methods. Figure 4.1 shows the conceptual framework of cerebral microdialysis. Today, there is a clinical point of care testing device that performs

Table 4.1 Normal reference values for brain cerebral microdialysis from normal appearing human brain tissue

Perfusion rate	Glucose (mmol/L)	Lactate (mmol/L)	Pyruvate (μmol/L)	LPR	Glycerol (μmol/L)	Urea (mmol/L)	Glutamate (μmol/L)
0.3 μL/min	1.7 ± 0.9	2.9 ± 0.9	166 ± 47	23 ± 4	82 ± 44	4.4 ± 1.7	5 ± 10
1.0 μL/min	0.9 ± 0.6	1.4 ± 0.9	103 ± 50	21 ± 6	42 ± 29	2.5 ± 1.3	5 ± 10
2.0 μL/min	0.45 ± 0.61	0.7 ± 0.7	26 ± 19	15 ± 5	30 ± 43	2.5 ± 1.4	2.5 ± 4.7

Adapted from Hillered, 1990(3); Reinstrup *et al.*, 2000(4); and Vespa *et al.* 2007(5).

semi-automated analysis of cerebral microdialysis samples and reports values in real time.

Target biomarker chemicals

Cerebral microdialysis is capable of measuring any chemical from the brain that is small enough to pass through the microdialysis semipermeable membrane. For most clinical applications, the semipermeable membrane size is 20 kD. So, small compounds, such as metabolic substrates like glucose, can be readily sampled whereas larger compounds, such as proteins and cytokines cannot. Larger pore sizes are available, such as 100 kD, but are not yet FDA approved for clinical use. The most common target biomarker chemicals are glucose, lactate, pyruvate, glutamate, glycerol, and urea. Other biomarkers that have been less commonly measured include glycine, taurine, gama-butyric acid (GABA), arginine, citrulline, adenosine, and nitric oxide products. Infrequently measured compounds taken from clinical patients include small peptides, cytokines and amyloid, but these have mostly been obtained with larger pore size membranes. Each of these compounds is related to basic physiology of brain metabolism and the disruption of metabolism that occurs with brain injury, ischemia, or metabolic crisis. For example, during brain ischemia, brain glucose decreases, lactate increases. As such, cerebral microdialysis has focused on determining the energy state of a region of brain tissue. The sequential changes in these biomarkers during ischemia or another form of metabolic crisis have been validated by direct comparison with whole brain tissue analysis in animals (2), and further validated in human studies as we will outline below. Normal values for microdialysis biomarkers have been determined in the normal human brain (4,5). Table 4.1 shows the normal concentrations of the basic biomarkers in human brain tissue. As one can see, as the perfusion rate increases the relative recovery of the biomarker is reduced. One can use a method called the zero-flow method to detect the actual extracellular concentration of the biomarker (6), whereby the perfusion rate is lowered progressively from a high rate such as 2 μL/min to 1 μL/min and then 0.3 μL/min, and then extrapolate the regression line to 0 μL/min to estimate the actual concentration in the interstitial fluid. This concept underscores the fact that the microdialysis fluid concentration is an estimate of the brain concentration, and that slower perfusion rates provide the best estimates.

Each target biochemical is measured and reported as a concentration in the effluent. In addition, various ratios of each biochemical can be reported, such as the lactate/pyruvate ratio (LPR). Standardized reporting of these values is now commonplace. Table 4.2 shows the typical cerebral microdialysis values under the conditions of ischemia.

Location of cerebral microdialysis

Cerebral microdialysis is inserted in the brain white matter at a depth of 2–3 cm below the cortex. The non-dominant frontal lobe is the most common location for insertion of the cerebral microdialysis probes. There is debate as to what location is ideal for these probes, with some advocates for normal appearing brain and

Table 4.2 Reference values for brain microdialysis during brain ischemia

Perfusion rate	Glucose (mmol/L)	Lactate (mmol/L)	Pyruvate (μmol/L)	LPR	Glycerol (μmol/L)	Urea (mmol/L)	Glutamate (μmol/L)
0.3 μL/min	0.6 ± 0.5	4.1 ± 0.9	60 ± 47	40 ± 8	40 ± 44	4.4 ± 1.7	10 ± 10

Adapted from Persson, 1992(7); Vespa, 1998(8).

some advocates for the at-risk location, which is usually adjacent to a known brain injury or stroke (9). Few studies have compared normal and at-risk brain tissue (4,5), but those studies have reported much more abnormal values in pericontusional tissue as compared with normal tissue. The pericontusional tissue appears to be in a state of metabolic crisis more frequently and appears to have earlier changes in biomarker chemicals when changes in cerebral perfusion occur. However, these findings are not consistent across studies. Very few studies have explored the use of dual microdialysis catheters, but selected cases show regional differences between normal and pericontusional tissue. Nonetheless, most probes are placed into normal appearing brain tissue. For selected patient populations, such as aneurysmal subarachnoid hemorrhage, the normal frontal lobe represents a good sampling site, since cerebral microdialysis is meant to detect delayed cerebral ischemia from vasospasm, and this frontal lobe region represents a potential ischemic territory. For other conditions, such as focal brain hemorrhage, the most sensitive sites may be the perihematomal tissue.

Clinical indications for cerebral microdialysis

Cerebral microdialysis is a minimally invasive brain probe that is typically placed in comatose or obtunded patients who do not have a good clinical examination to follow. However, microdialysis has been used in epilepsy surgery patients, cerebrovascular surgery patients during temporary feeding vessel occlusion, and brain tumor patients during surgery. Generally speaking the clinical indications for cerebral microdialysis are: 1) comatose exam, 2) high risk of cerebral ischemia or metabolic crisis, and 3) elevated intracranial pressure or suspected intracranial hypertension. The essential concept is that the patient is at risk for silent ischemia that is not able to be detected using the basic clinical examination. The use of cerebral microdialysis in selected neurocritical care diseases is outlined below.

Brain trauma

Cerebral microdialysis has been most widely studied in severe traumatic brain injury (TBI). In TBI, elevated intracranial pressure and coma can be prolonged, during which assessment of physiology and prognosis can be difficult. Early observations using microdialysis focused on determining prognosis of comatose patients with cerebral edema (10–12). Important observations were made and can be summarized as follows: 1) There are marked disturbances of brain neurochemistry in both normal appearing and pericontusional brain tissue after TBI. 2) The neurochemical disturbances are made worse by profound elevations in intracranial pressure and reduction in cerebral perfusion pressure. 3) Herniation leading to loss of cerebral circulation results in a marked reduction in brain extracellular glucose and elevation of the lactate/pyruvate ratio and glutamate. 4) Elevation of glutamate occurs with moderate to severe reductions in cerebral perfusion. 5) Elevation in glutamate occurs with seizures. 6) Prognosis for clinical outcome is associated with reduction in extracellular glucose, and also with elevation in glutamate. 7) Neurochemistry may be more sensitive to disturbances than some other forms of brain monitoring such as brain tissue oxygen. These principles are summarized in Table 4.3.

Table 4.3 Cerebral microdialysis prognostic markers in TBI coma

Study		Main findings
Goodman	1999(13)	Low glucose and elevated lactate predict mortality
Bullock	1998(14)	Low glucose and elevated glutamate predict mortality Microdialysis is better in brain contusional injury than DAI
Vespa	1998(8)	Glutamate is elevated by reduction in CPP and seizures
Langemann	2001(11)	Very low glucose values occur with brain herniation
Vespa	2003(12)	Low glucose and elevated LPR independently associate with poor 6 month neurological outcome and mortality
Nelson	2004(15)	Patterns of variation in glucose indicate good outcome
Vespa	2007(5)	Low glucose associated with more contusional injury
Marcoux	2008(16)	Prolonged LPR independently associated with long-term atrophy
Chamoun	2010(17)	Glutamate elevation correlates with outcome after TBI
Timofeev	2011(18)	Low glucose and elevated LPR independently associated with mortality, higher pyruate associated with survival
Asgari	2011(19)	LPR elevations occur independently of elevated ICP

An example of the marked disturbances in cerebral microdialysis can be seen in this case example (Fig. 4.2). In this patient, with severe diffuse traumatic axonal injury and coma, the intracranial pressure was elevated, and she was being treated with medical therapies to enhance serum osmolarity, ensure adequate cerebral perfusion, suppression of brain activity with pentobarbital, and drainage of cerebral spinal fluid. The microdialysis neurochemistry demonstrates a progressive decrease in glucose and massive increase in the lactate/pyruvate ratio that occurred with terminal elevation of the intracranial pressure and herniation. This patient illustrates an important concept that affects the literature on microdialysis, namely that the terminal changes in microdialysis leading to marked reduction in glucose somewhat skew the data regarding outcome. The second important concept is that the pattern of changes in glucose and LPR indicate severe ischemia. This pattern provides further validation of the use of microdialysis to monitor brain ischemia. Similar patterns have been reported in other cases of terminal herniation (10,11).

The use of cerebral microdialysis in TBI has been manifold in the past 10 years. 1) The identification of prognosis continues to be done using results of microdialysis. Elevated LPR values and low glucose values are useful in this setting. 2) The use of dynamic changes in brain glucose to regulate the intensity of systemic glycemic control appears to be a new use of this technique. We will discuss this below. 3) Selection of optimal CPP using a tissue biomarker of perfusion is a frequent use of microdialysis in TBI. In this setting, the real-time response of the brain to various levels of hemodynamic support is being used. For example, increases in CPP are being tracked to determine if biomarkers such as LPR are decreasing.

Subarachnoid hemorrhage

Subarachnoid hemorrhage (SAH) is a prototypical illness in which delayed cerebral ischemia may occur due to cerebral vasospasm. Experimental primate models of reversible cerebral ischemia initially indicated that microdialysis could detect cerebral ischemia as indicated by reductions in brain glucose and elevation of LPR (20). Similar observations have been seen in humans after SAH (21). The increase in LPR is above 40, which is more than 2 standard deviations above the normal LPR range of 20–25. With reversible ischemia, the LPR decreases back to the normal range. In contrast, the LPR increases above 100 with permanent infarction. Persson and colleagues were the first to report important changes in cerebral microdialysis in delayed cerebral ischemia after SAH. In the latter study, the LPR

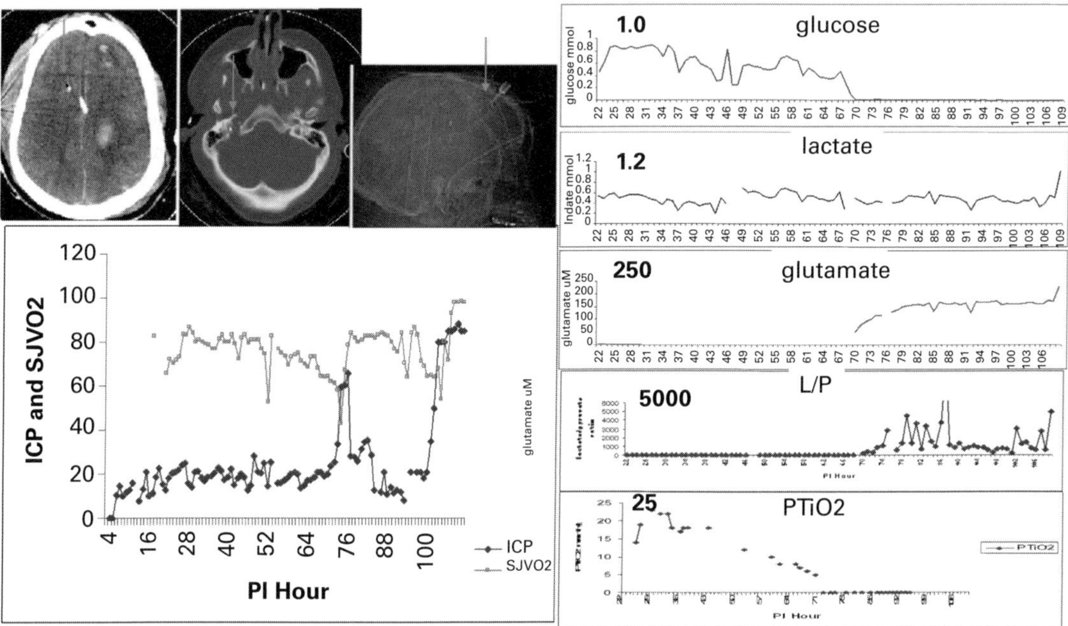

Fig. 4.2 Microdialysis changes in a comatose patient with traumatic brain injury in which the intracranial pressure increases leading to brain herniation. The microdialysis glucose values drop to undetectable levels, and the lactate/pyruvate ratio (LPR) increases into the thousands. Brain tissue oxygen drops to very low values. This is a classic pattern of severe cerebral ischemia.

increased > 40 and glucose declined to undetectable levels with cerebral ischemia. Dynamic improvements in microdialysis occurred with intra-arterial rescue therapy for vasospasm. Similar reports of the ability of microdialysis to detect cerebral ischemia and response to clinical intervention were made by Unterberg (22). Glycerol elevations have also been documented to indicate cerebral ischemia in SAH (23,24).

An example of the use of cerebral microdialysis in SAH is shown in Figure 4.3. In this example, the patient had vasospasm resulting in elevation of the LPR, and glutamate and reduction in glucose in the right frontal lobe. The angiogram confirmed severe vasospasm and the patient was treated with intra-arterial vasodilators. The microdialysis showed an early reduction in glutamate, an increase in glucose, and a slower response to LPR.

Several studies have recently been conducted in SAH using microdialysis (Table 4.4). Most studies have monitored cerebral microdialysis during critical periods in which delayed cerebral circulation occurs. Persson and Hillered (25) reported dynamic increases in glutamate, LPR and reductions in glucose with permanent infarction related to cerebral vasospasm, and reversible changes with effective treatment of vasospasm. However, this initial report also illustrates reactive increases in LPR during seizures after SAH. Thus, even with the initial report in SAH, there appears to be overlap in disruption of brain metabolism due to seizures and ischemia. This illustrates the important concept that microdialysis needs to be used in combination with other monitoring modalities in order to determine the specificity of the findings, since seizures and ischemia can give rise to similar

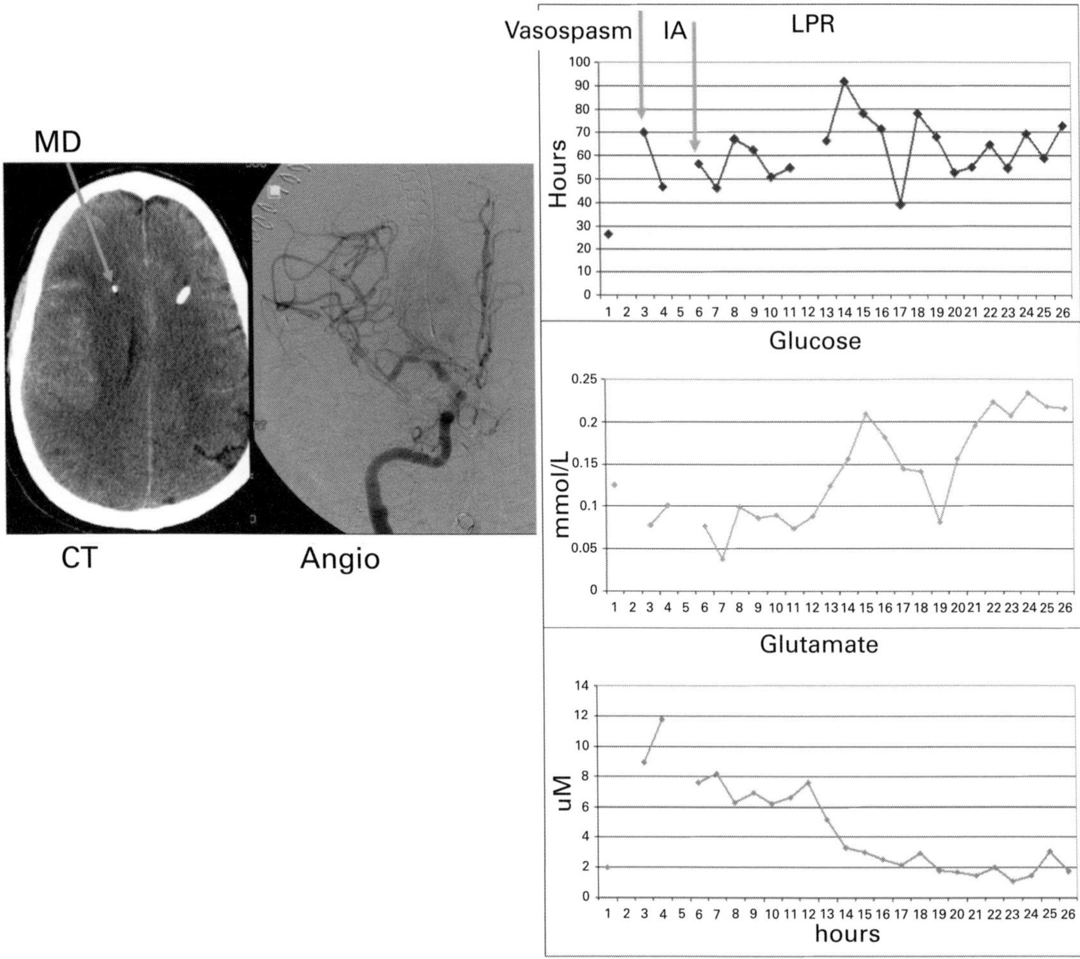

Fig. 4.3 Microdialysis changes during cerebral vasospasm after aneurysmal subarachnoid hemorrhage. The location of the probe is shown in the border zone between the anterior and middle cerebral arteries (upper left). The angiogram demonstrates severe arterial spasm (upper middle). The timing of vasospasm (left arrow) and the intervention with intra-arterial vasodilators (right arrow) are shown along with changes in glucose (increasing) and LPR (decreasing).

microdialysis findings. Several observational studies have been reported that demonstrate the feasibility of monitoring brain neurochemistry to detect delayed cerebral ischemia and to prognosticate about long-term outcome. A few observational cohort studies have demonstrated reversal of ischemic changes in microdialysis by intra-arterial vasodilators and angioplasty (22,34).

Glucose control

One of the more widely applicable uses of cerebral microdialysis is to monitor substrate delivery to the brain during coma. Generally, the brain uses glucose as the main substrate to fuel metabolic demand. Glucose is taken up by astrocytes, converted to lactate, and the lactate is consumed by neurons. A deficit of

Table 4.4 Cerebral microdialysis in subarachnoid hemorrhage

Study		Main findings
Persson Hillered	1992(25)	Elevation of glutamate, LPR, hypoxanthine with vasospasm
Persson	1992(7)	Higher glutamate, and LPR values correlate with poor outcome
Enblad	1996(21)	LPR correlates with brain ischemia on PET imaging
Unterberg	2004(22)	LPR increases with vasospasm-related brain ischemia
Samuelsson	2007(26)	Glutamine increases with reduced CPP
Samuelsson	2009(27)	Progressive hyperglycolysis occurs after SAH marked by reciprocal changes in glucose and pyruvate
Zetterling	2009(28)	Lower pyruvate with prolonged coma after SAH
Oddo	2009(29)	LPR is higher with hemoglobin < 9 mg/dl after SAH
Helbok	2010(30)	Decreased serum glucose leads to metabolic crisis after SAH
Chen	2011(31)	LPR and brain tissue oxygen are better makers of ischemia than CPP of ICP in comatose ICP patients
Helbok	2011(32)	Persistent LPR > 40 predicts the occurrence of silent DCI
Schmidt	2011(33)	CPP < 70 leads to LPR elevations in SAH

glucose therefore may trigger metabolic crisis and tissue injury. It has been widely acknowledged that hyperglycemia worsens neurologic outcome in TBI, SAH, and other diseases. Given the concern for hyperglycemia, there has been keen interest in strictly controlling glucose with the use of insulin. Tight glycemic control has become the mainstay of treating patients with acute neurologic illness. However, cerebral microdialysis has cast doubt upon the safety and wisdom of tight glycemic control. After TBI, under conditions of tight glycemic control, microdialysis glucose values drop to very low levels and LPR increases (35). The increases in LPR are associated with worsened neurologic outcome (16). A similar reduction in microdialysis glucose has been seen in SAH (28,36). Indeed, tight glycemic control leads to metabolic crisis and increased brain glycolitic rates after TBI as seen on positron emission tomography (37).

Other coma states

Cerebral microdialysis has been reported in a few case reports in other types of patients, such as meningitis patients, coma due to cardiac arrest, large ischemic stroke, and status epilepticus. The findings are similar to what have been outlined for TBI and SAH. It is intriguing to consider that multiple types of coma patients may benefit in the future from microdialysis in a way in which TBI and SAH patients are starting to now.

Future directions

Cerebral microdialysis is a minimally invasive technique that has an excellent safety record. There is a less than 1% complication rate of brain hemorrhage, infection, or stroke. Hence, the technique has the potential to be used in other coma states, and in awake patients who are at risk of brain injury. In addition to metabolic monitoring, microdialysis has been used to: 1) measure intraparenchymal drug levels (38,39); 2) measure brain-derived cytokines (40,41); 3) measure proteomics of acute brain injury (42); 4) measure amyloid and tau proteins (43); and 5) measure the effects of chemotherapy (44,45). These studies indicate the potential to use cerebral microdialysis to monitor a variety of non-metabolic based treatments, such as anti-inflammatory treatment. Hence, there is potential to improve the selectivity of our treatments for acute brain injuries and chronic diseases through direct monitoring of the tissue effects of these treatments.

REFERENCES

1. Hillered L, Vespa PM, Hovda DA. Translational neurochemical research in acute human brain injury: the current status and potential future for cerebral microdialysis. *J Neurotrauma*. 2005;**22**(1):3–41.
2. Benveniste H. Brain microdialysis. *J Neurochem*. 1989; **52**:1667–79.

3. Hillered, L, Persson L, Pontén U, Ungerstedt U. Neurometabolic monitoring of the ischaemic human brain using microdialysis. *Acta Neurochir (Wien).* 1990;**102**:91–7.
4. Reinstrup P, Stahl N, Mellergard P, Uski T, Ungerstedt U, and Nordstrom CH. Intracerebral microdialysis in clinical practice: baseline values for chemical markers during wakefulness, anesthesia and neurosurgery. *Neurosurgery.* 2000;**47**:701–9.
5. Vespa P, Ophelan K, McArthur DA, *et al.* Pericontusional brain tissue exhibits persistent elevation of lactate/pyruvate ratio independent of cerebral perfusion pressure. *Crit Care Med.* 2007;**35**(4):1153–60.
6. Hutchinson PJ, O'Connell MT, Nortje J, *et al.* Cerebral microdialysis methodology – evaluation of 20 kDa and 100 kDa catheters. *Physiol Meas.* 2005;**26**(4):423–8.
7. Persson L, Hillered L. Chemical monitoring of neurosurgical intensive care patients using intracerebral microdialysis. *J Neurosurg.* 1992;**76**:(1)72–80.
8. Vespa P, Prins M, Ronne-Engstrom E, *et al.* Increase in extracellular glutamate caused by reduced cerebral perfusion pressure and seizures after human traumatic brain injury: a microdialysis study. J *Neurosurg.* 1998;**89**:971–82.
9. Bellander BM, Cantais E, Enblad P, *et al.* Consensus meeting on microdialysis in neurointensive care. *Intensive Care Med.* 2004;**30**(12):2166–9.
10. Landolt H, Langemann H, Mendelowitsch A, Gratzl O. Neurochemical monitoring and on-line pH measurements using brain microdialysis in patients in intensive care. *Acta Neurochir* 1994;**60**:475–78.
11. Langemann H, Alessandri B, Mendelowitsch A, *et al.* Extracellular levels of glucose and lactate measured by quantitative microdialysis in the human brain. *Neurol Res.* 2001;**23**:531–6.
12. Vespa P, McArthur D, Glenn T, *et al.* Persistently reduced levels of extracellular glucose early after traumatic brain injury correlate with poor outcome at six months: A microdialysis study. *J Cereb Blood Flow Metab* 2003;**23**:865–77.
13. Goodman JC, Valadka AB, Gopinath SP, Uzura M, Robertson CS. Extracellular lactate and glucose alterations in the brain after head injury measured by microdialysis. *Crit Care Med.* 1999;**27**:1965–73.
14. Bullock R, Zauner A, Woodward JJ, *et al.* Factors affecting excitatory amino acid release following severe human head injury. *J Neurosurg.* 1998;**89**:507–18.
15. Nelson DW, Bellander BM, Maccallum RM, *et al.* Cerebral microdialysis of patients with severe traumatic brain injury exhibits highly individualistic patterns as visualized by cluster analysis with self-organizing maps. *Crit Care Med.* 2004;**32**(12):2428–36.
16. Marcoux J, McArthur DA, Miller C, *et al.* Persistent metabolic crisis as measured by elevated cerebral microdialysis lactate-pyruvate ratio predicts chronic frontal lobe brain atrophy after traumatic brain injury. *Crit Care Med.* 2008;**36**(10):2871–7.
17. Chamoun R, Suki D, Gopinath SP, Goodman JC, Robertson C. Role of extracellular glutamate measured by cerebral microdialysis in severe traumatic brain injury. *J Neurosurg.* 2010;**113**(3):564–70.
18. Timofeev I, Carpenter KL, Nortje J, *et al.* Cerebral extracellular chemistry and outcome following traumatic brain injury: a microdialysis study of 223 patients. *Brain.* 2011;**134**(Pt 2):484–94.
19. Asgari S, Vespa P, Bergsneider M, Hu X. Lack of consistent intracranial pressure pulse morphological changes during episodes of microdialysis lactate/pyruvate ratio increase. *Physiol Meas.* 2011;**32**:1639–51.
20. Enblad P, Frykholm P, Valtysson J, *et al.* Middle cerebral artery occlusion and reperfusion in primates monitored by microdialysis and sequential positron emission tomography. *Stroke* 2001;**32**:1574–80.
21. Enblad P, Valtysson J, Andersson J, *et al.* Simultaneous intracerebral microdialysis and positron emission tomography in the detection of ischemia in patients with subarachnoid hemorrhage. *J Cereb Blood Flow Metab.* 1996;**16**(4):637–44.
22. Unterberg AW, Sakotwitz OW, Sarrafzadeh AS, *et al.* Role of bedside microdialysis in the diagnosis of cerebral vasospasm following aneurysmal subarachnoid hemorrhage. *J Neurosurg,* 2001;**94**:740–9.
23. Hillered L, Valtysson J, Enblad P, Persson L. Interstitial glycerol as a marker for membrane phospholipid degradation in the acutely injured human brain. *J Neurol Neurosurg Psychiatry.* 1998;**64**(4):486–91.
24. Schulz MK, Wang LP, Tange M, Bjerre P. Cerebral microdialysis monitoring: determination of normal and ischemic cerebral metabolisms in patients with aneurysmal subarachnoid hemorrhage. *J Neurosurg.* 2000;**93**(5):808–14.
25. Persson L, Hillered L. Chemical monitoring of neurosurgical intensive care patients using intracerebral microdialysis. *Journal of Neurosurgery.* 1992;**76**:72–80.
26. Samuelsson C, Hillered L, Zetterling M, *et al.* Cerebral glutamine and glutamate levels in relation to compromised energy metabolism: a microdialysis study in subarachnoid hemorrhage patients. *J Cereb Blood Flow Metab.* 2007;**27**(7):1309–17.
27. Samuelsson C, Howells T, Kumlien E, *et al.* Relationship between intracranial hemodynamics and microdialysis markers of energy metabolism and glutamate-glutamine

turnover in patients with subarachnoid hemorrhage. Clinical article. *J Neurosurg.* 2009;**111**(5):910–15.

28. Zetterling M, Hillered L, Enblad P, Karlsson T, Ronne-Engström E. Relation between brain interstitial and systemic glucose concentrations after subarachnoid hemorrhage. *J Neurosurg.* 2011;**115**(1):66–74.
29. Oddo M, Milby A, Chen I, *et al.* Hemoglobin concentration and cerebral metabolism in patients with aneurysmal subarachnoid hemorrhage. *Stroke.* 2009;**40**(4):1275–81.
30. Helbok R, Schmidt JM, Kurtz P, *et al.* Systemic glucose and brain energy metabolism after subarachnoid hemorrhage. *Neurocrit Care.* 2010;**12**(3):317–23.
31. Chen HI, Stiefel MF, Oddo M, *et al.* Detection of cerebral compromise with multimodality monitoring in patients with subarachnoid hemorrhage. *Neurosurgery.* 2011;**69**(1):53–63.
32. Helbok R, Madineni RC, Schmidt MJ, *et al.* Intracerebral monitoring of silent infarcts after subarachnoid hemorrhage. *Neurocrit Care.* 2011;**14**(2):162–7.
33. Schmidt JM, Ko SB, Helbok R, *et al.* Cerebral perfusion pressure thresholds for brain tissue hypoxia and metabolic crisis after poor-grade subarachnoid hemorrhage. *Stroke.* 2011;**42**(5):1351–6.
34. Stuart RM, Helbok R, Kurtz P, *et al.* High-dose intra-arterial verapamil for the treatment of cerebral vasospasm after subarachnoid hemorrhage: prolonged effects on hemodynamic parameters and brain metabolism. *Neurosurgery.* 2011;**68**(2):337–45.
35. Vespa P, Boonyaputthikul P, McArthur DL, *et al.* Intensive insulin therapy reduces microdialysis glucose values without altering glucose utilization or improving the lactate/pyruvate ratio after traumatic brain injury. *Crit Care Med.* 2006;**34**(3):850–6.
36. Schlenk F, Graetz D, Nagel A, Schmidt M, Sarrafzadeh AS. Insulin-related decrease in cerebral glucose despite normoglycemia in aneurysmal subarachnoid hemorrhage. *Crit Care.* 2008;**12**(1):R9.
37. Vespa P, McArthur DL, Stein N, *et al.* Tight Glycemic Control Increases Metabolic Distress in Traumatic Brain Injury: A Randomized Controlled Within-subjects Trial. *Crit Care Med.* 2012 (in press).
38. Caricato A, Pennisi M, Mancino A, *et al.* Levels of vancomycin in the cerebral interstitial fluid after severe head injury. *Intensive Care Med.* 2006;**32**(2):325–8.
39. Dahyot-Fizelier C, Timofeev I, Marchand S, *et al.* Brain microdialysis study of meropenem in two patients with acute brain injury. *Antimicrob Agents Chemother.* 2010;**54**(8):3502–4.
40. Bouras TI, Gatzonis SS, Georgakoulias N, *et al.* Neuroinflammatory sequelae of minimal trauma in the non-traumatized human brain. A microdialysis study. *J Neurotrauma.* 2011; Nov 18.
41. Hanafy KA, Stuart RM, Khandji AG, *et al.* Relationship between brain interstitial fluid tumor necrosis factor-α and cerebral vasospasm after aneurysmal subarachnoid hemorrhage. *J Clin Neurosci.* 2010;**17**(7):853–6.
42. Lakshaman R, Loo JA, Drake T, *et al.* Metabolic crisis after traumatic brain injury is associated with a novel microdialysis proteome. *Neurocrit Care.* 2010;**12**(3):324–36.
43. Brody DL, Magnoni S, Schwetye KE, *et al.* Amyloid-beta dynamics correlate with neurological status in the injured human brain. *Science.* 2008;**321**(5893):1221–4.
44. Blakeley JO, Olson J, Grossman SA, *et al.* New Approaches to Brain Tumor Therapy (NABTT) Consortium. Effect of blood brain barrier permeability in recurrent high grade gliomas on the intratumoral pharmacokinetics of methotrexate: a microdialysis study. *J Neurooncol.* 2009;**91**(1):51–8.
45. Wibom C, Surowiec I, Mörén L, *et al.* Metabolomic patterns in glioblastoma and changes during radiotherapy: a clinical microdialysis study. *J Proteome Res.* 2010;**9**(6):2909–19.

5

Ultrasound and other noninvasive techniques used in monitoring cerebrovascular disease

Günter Seidel

Introduction

Monitoring of physiological function is an important aspect of patient care in cerebrovascular disease. Increasingly, monitoring of brain function has become of interest. Ideally, brain monitoring should be continuous, noninvasive, highly sensitive, reasonably specific, user-friendly, and not excessively expensive.

Neurosonology is an essential monitoring tool in cerebrovascular disease. Basic methods include conventional extra- and transcranial Doppler (TCD) to assess cerebral blood flow velocity and monitoring of cerebral hemodynamics, patency of vessels, and direction of flow through the circle of Willis and vasospasm (VSP) following subarachnoid hemorrhage (SAH). Advanced technologies like extra- and transcranial color-coded duplex (TCCD) sonography provide information about anatomical details, whereas TCD monitoring techniques like embolus detection and functional TCD detect changes in blood content and hemodynamics to specific stimuli over time. Advanced B-mode imaging techniques are useful in monitoring dislocation of the third ventricle, hemorrhagic transformation of an infarct, and primary hemorrhage growth. New nonlinear ultrasound technologies enable the detection of ultrasound contrast agents in the cerebral microcirculation, thus allowing the visualization of brain perfusion in real time.

Patients with cerebrovascular disease may benefit from the monitoring of brain function. *Continuous electroencephalography* (cEEG) monitoring is now an integral component of the monitoring armamentarium available to assess the cerebral function of critically ill patients. A number of studies have demonstrated the ability of cEEG to detect cerebral ischemia in a possible reversible state, thus allowing early intervention. The extensive neural pathways involved in the generation of *somatosensory evoked potentials* (SEPs) and *brainstem auditory evoked potentials* (BAEPs) provide powerful measures of neural function. Within the intensive care or stroke unit, their greatest use is that of unfavorable outcome prediction after acute stroke.

Near-infrared spectroscopy (NIRS) can be used for the noninvasive assessment of brain function through the intact skull by detecting changes in blood hemoglobin concentrations associated with neural activity. Its use is gaining acceptance in the care of patients suffering from stroke.

The use of these three noninvasive monitoring tools in gathering information on brain morphology, perfusion, metabolic state, and function is reviewed in the following sections.

Extra- and transcranial Doppler sonography

Conventional extracranial Doppler, a fast screening tool, had been used for many years to detect occlusion or stenosis of the brain-supplying arteries in acute ischemic stroke. Pulsed-wave Doppler ultrasound can identify substantial luminal narrowing based on

Critical Care of the Stroke Patient, ed. Stefan Schwab, Daniel Hanley, and A. David Mendelow. Published by Cambridge University Press.

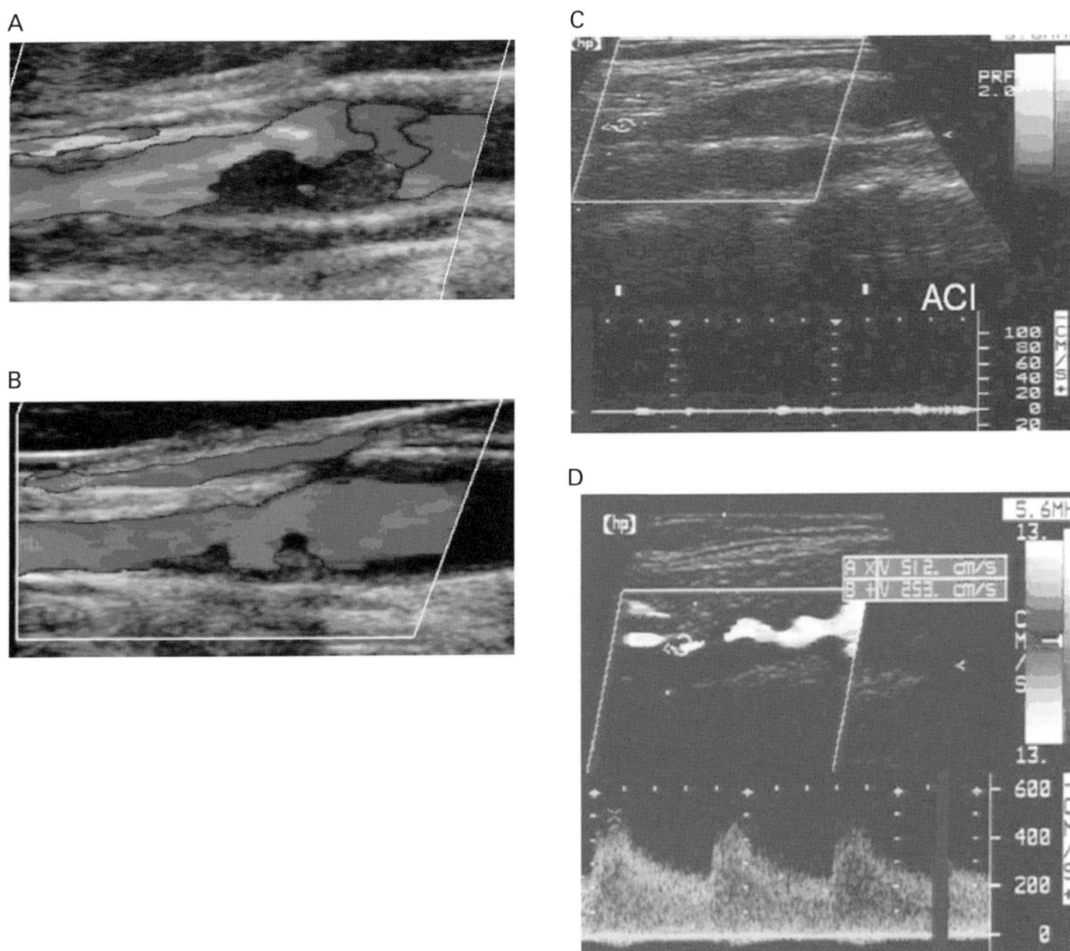

Fig. 5.1 **A–D** Thrombus at the carotid bulb of a 41-year-old female patient suffering from acute ischemic MCA stroke. **A**. initial investigation (day one), **B**. Follow-up investigation on day eight. A regression of thrombus volume is visible. **C and D**. Internal carotid artery of a 49-year-old male patient suffering from MCA ischemic stroke. **C**. Color-duplex scan two hours after symptom onset (severe MCA stroke). **D**. Follow-up investigation after 24 hours. Recanalization with a tight stenosis of the artery could be detected. (See plate section for color version).

increased velocity of blood flow across a stenotic lesion. Monitoring of blood flow velocity and waveform in acute ischemic stroke is possible. Its failure to detect certain morphological features of the arterial wall and its low reproducibility of blood flow velocity measurement (no correction of insonation angle possible) led many centers to replace this method with color-coded duplex sonography in the evaluation of patients suffering from stroke. This advanced ultrasound technology allows pathological details of the vessel wall to be visualized (Fig. 5.1) and monitored over time.

Transcranial Doppler (TCD) uses energy (2–4 MHz) to insonate cerebral vessels, typically through several bone windows in the skull. This tool can be used to identify the presence and location of an obstructive intracranial thrombus or a symptomatic stenosis in acute ischemic stroke and to obtain information on the collateral flow that is distal to the pathologic site.

Table 5.1 Recanalization rates in relation to the site of artery occlusion*†

	Prox. MCA	Distal MCA	Tandem ICA/MCA	Terminal ICA	BA
No. (%)	166 (51)	116 (35)	22 (7)	17 (5)	10 (3)
Complete recanalization ≤ 2 hours of rt-PA bolus (%)	49/163 (30)	50/113 (44)	6/22 (27)	1/17(6)	3/10 (33)
3-month mRS score ≤ 1 (%)	33/131 (25)	50/96 (52)	3/14 (21)	2/11 (18)	2/8 (25)

*Data are from Saqqur *et al.* (2)

†Prox. indicates proximal; MCA, middle cerebral artery; ICA, internal carotid artery; BA, basilar artery; rt-PA, recombinant tissue plasminogen activator; mRS, modified Rankin scale.

It is a valuable real-time bedside monitoring tool for thrombolysis, allowing patients to recover from stroke more rapidly and completely (sonothrombolysis).

Diagnosing an **intracranial artery occlusion** with TCD is difficult. For this type of diagnosis to be made, a good window of insonation must first be obtained, which in turn depends on the identification of other basal cerebral arteries with the same approach. The main finding is no detectable signals from the localization where the artery is expected to be. This is one of the major disadvantages of TCD compared with transcranial color-coded duplex sonography (TCCD). With this advanced ultrasound technology, color-coded visualization of blood flow velocity in the vessels can be superimposed on the B-mode image of the brain parenchyma. This method facilitates both the detection of the optimal acoustic bone window and the exact anatomical localization of the vessel (even if it is occluded).

The site of artery occlusion and the rate of early recanalization (Table 5.1) are important prognostic factors in acute ischemic stroke and transient ischemic attack (TIA) (1–3).

Once the arterial occlusion is located in acute ischemic stroke, the TCD probe can be fixated with a head frame, allowing blood flow monitoring in the affected artery during thrombolysis. The average rate of spontaneous complete recanalization of middle cerebral artery (MCA) occlusion is about 6% per hour during the first 6 hours after symptom onset and increases to 12.7% per hour after thrombolytic therapy (4–7).

In a recent meta-analysis of 1813 patients suffering from acute ischemic stroke, MCA occlusion by TCD was associated with a significantly increased risk for a fatal course of stroke (odds ratio [OR] 2.46, 95% confidence interval [CI] 1.33 to 4.52). Patients with patent MCA were more likely to improve clinically within 4 days than patients with MCA occlusion (OR 11.11, 95% CI 5.44 to 22.69). Full recanalization within 6 hours after symptom onset was very significantly associated with clinical improvement within 48 hours (OR 5.64, 95% CI 3.82 to 8.31) and functional independence after 3 months (OR 6.07, 95% CI 3.94 to 9.35) (8).

The presence of **microembolic signals (MESs)** in the basal cerebral arteries can be detected with the TCD. Microemboli detection has led to numerous applications of the TCD during surgical and interventional procedures. These signals are common in patients with large artery disease and are an independent marker of future stroke risk in patients with extracranial carotid disease (9,10) or intracranial stenosis (11–13). In the trial of clopidogrel and aspirin for reduction of emboli in symptomatic carotid stenosis (CARESS) (14) and the trial of clopidogrel plus aspirin versus aspirin alone for reducing embolization in patients with acute symptomatic cerebral or carotid artery stenosis (CLAIR) (15), a combination therapy with clopidogrel and aspirin was found to be more effective than aspirin alone in reducing asymptomatic embolization in patients with recently symptomatic extracranial carotid artery stenosis or MCA stenosis, as assessed by the detection of MESs with the TCD. This dual therapy led to a significant reduction in the number of clinical ischemic events, according to the meta-analysis performed for these trials. This finding indicates that TCD monitoring of MESs in early ischemic stroke in patients with macroangiopathy may identify high-risk patients who would benefit from a more intensive antithrombotic therapy.

Table 5.2 Criteria for grading proximal middle cerebral artery vasospasm with or without hyperemia*†

Mean velocity (cm/s)	Systolic BFV MCA/ICA ratio	Interpretation
< 120	≤ 3	Hyperemia
> 80	3–4	Hyperemia + possible mild spasm
≥ 120	3–4	Hyperemia + mild spasm
≥ 120	4–5	Hyperemia + moderate spasm
> 120	5–6	Moderate spasm
≥ 180	6	Moderate to severe spasm
≥ 200	≥ 6	Severe spasm
> 200	4–6	Hyperemia + moderate spasm
> 200	3–4	Hyperemia + mild spasm
> 200	< 3	Hyperemia

*Modified criteria from the data of (16), (17) and (18).
† BFV indicates blood flow velocity; MCA, middle cerebral artery; ICA, internal carotid artery.

Arterial vasospasm (VSP) is a complication of subarachnoid hemorrhage (SAH), which can lead to ischemic brain damage and delayed ischemic neurological deficit (DIND) in more than 25% of patients. Narrowing of the arterial lumen over time in the early phase of SAH produces an increase of blood flow velocity, which may affect the proximal stem and distal branches. Because many patients receive hypertension–hemodilution–hypervolemia (HHH) therapy, the differential diagnosis should always include hyperemia or a combination of VSP and hyperemia. Increased intracranial pressure and carbon dioxide tension (PCO_2) variations may also modify TCD results. Therefore, grading of VSP severity is difficult (Table 5.2 and Table 5.3), and TCD findings should be individualized. Daily TCD investigations in the first 2 weeks after SAH are necessary to detect considerable changes in velocity and pulsatility. The site of VSP influences the TCD findings. Main stem spasm leads to an increase of blood flow velocity (BFV) without an increase of velocity in the extracranial feeding artery (BFV intracranial/BFV extracranial ratio > 3), whereas distal branch VSP increases the pulsatility index (PI ≥ 1.2) of the proximal arterial segment, indicating an increased peripheral resistance. Increased intracranial pressure may also increase TCD pulsatility, which cannot be separated in every case from distal VSP.

Table 5.3 Mean flow velocity (cm/s) criteria for grading of vasospasm in basal cerebral arteries*†‡

Artery	Possible VSP	Probable VSP	Definite VSP
ICA	> 80	> 110	> 130
ACA	> 90	> 110	> 120
PCA	> 60	> 80	> 90
BA	> 70	> 90	> 100
VA	> 60	> 80	> 90

*Modified data from (19).
†Hyperemia has been mostly ruled out by the focality of the velocity increase and by an intracranial artery/extracranial ICA ratio > 3 for MCA.
‡VSP indicates vasospasm; ICA, internal carotid artery; ACA, anterior carotid artery; PCA, posterior carotid artery; BA, basilar artery; VA, vertebral artery.

In children with **sickle cell disease**, the TCD has a crucial role in predicting ischemic stroke risk. In a prospective evaluation, mean blood flow velocities greater than 170 cm/s were associated with a 44% increase in relative risk of ischemic stroke over 5 years (20). When blood transfusions were given to children with sickle cell disease who had a mean TCD blood flow velocity ≥ 200 cm/s, the relative risk of stroke was reduced by 90% (21,22).

Extra- and transcranial color-coded Duplex sonography

Color-coded Duplex sonography, an ultrasound method, is a combination of three ultrasound technologies. Color-coded, intensity-weighted mean blood flow velocity is superimposed over a gray-scale image of the tissue. Pulsed-wave Doppler ultrasound can be used in a sample volume to measure Doppler frequency spectrum. By measuring the angle of insonation, real blood flow velocity can be calculated.

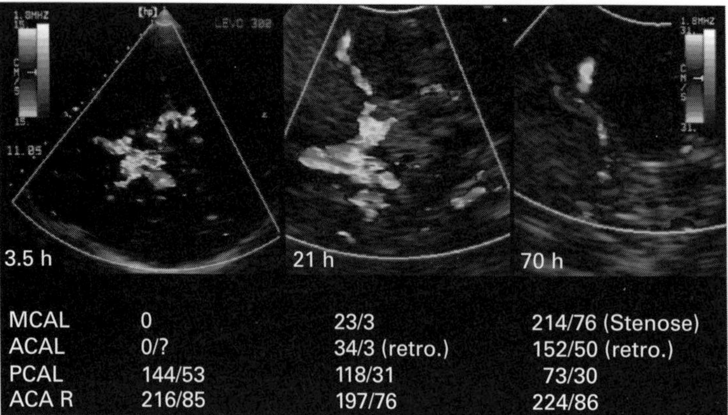

Fig. 5.2 TCCD (axial imaging plane, left side = frontal; right side = occipital) follow-up of a 76-year-old male patient suffering from acute MCA occlusion at the left side. TCCD images are given 3.5, 21, and 70 hours after symptom onset. At 3.5 hours 5 ml Levovist™ 300. Below the images blood flow velocities [cm/s] in the basal cerebral arteries are displayed. MCA reopening, and a residual stenosis could be diagnosed. ACA collateral flow improved over time and PCA collateral flow decreased.

MCA, middle cerebral artery; ACA, anterior cerebral artery; PCA, posterior cerebral artery; L, left; R, right. (See plate section for color version).

Extracranial color-coded Duplex sonography enables detailed visualization of the vessel anatomy and the measurement of angle-corrected blood flow velocity in the carotid and several segments of the vertebral artery. With this technology, we can analyze both hemodynamic and anatomic features of the vessels. For example, **thrombus formation** and regression can be visualized and monitored over time (Fig. 5.1). In some cases, these morphological changes occur without detectable changes in the hemodynamic presentation.

The site of internal carotid or vertebral artery occlusion can be localized reliably. Depending on the etiology of **internal carotid artery (ICA) occlusion**, different patterns of hemodynamic and anatomic features can be differentiated. In cases of proximal ICA occlusion resulting from atherothrombotic occlusion of a tight stenosis, inhomogeneous partial acoustic shadowing material is present at the origin of the ICA. In cases of distal carotid occlusion resulting from arterial dissection or embolic occlusion of the ICA from the heart, the artery wall at the origin of the ICA is unremarkable and pulsed-wave Doppler ultrasound of the artery shows an occlusion signal.

If an acute occlusion, particularly in an artery dissection, is diagnosed in the first 24 hours after ischemic stroke symptom onset, spontaneous recanalization may be detected in 30% to 70% of patients over time. Therefore, short- and long-term monitoring is necessary to diagnose the reopening of the artery (Fig. 5.1).

In acute ischemic stroke, **transcranial color-coded duplex sonography** (TCCD) is an imaging method that requires no indirect diagnostic criteria to identify vessel occlusion. This method has a sensitivity of up to 100% in detecting **MCA occlusions** – even in cases of poor acoustic penetration when echo contrast agents are given (23,24). With this advanced ultrasound tool, reliable follow-up of artery recanalization in the early phase of ischemic stroke can be carried out, and complex changes of the cerebral hemodynamic can be detected (Fig. 5.2).

In addition to analyzing arterial blood flow in the basal cerebral arteries, TCCD can display brain parenchyma in gray-scale imaging. An **acute cerebral hemorrhage** can be differentiated from normal and ischemic brain tissue by its hyperechogenic signal pattern. Supratentorial intracerebral hemorrhages (Fig. 5.3) can be displayed with sensitivity of up to 95% (25–27). Diagnostic problems occur in small hemorrhages (< 1 cm diameter) and in cortical localization of the hemorrhage. Data from infratentorial hemorrhages are not available. Growth of

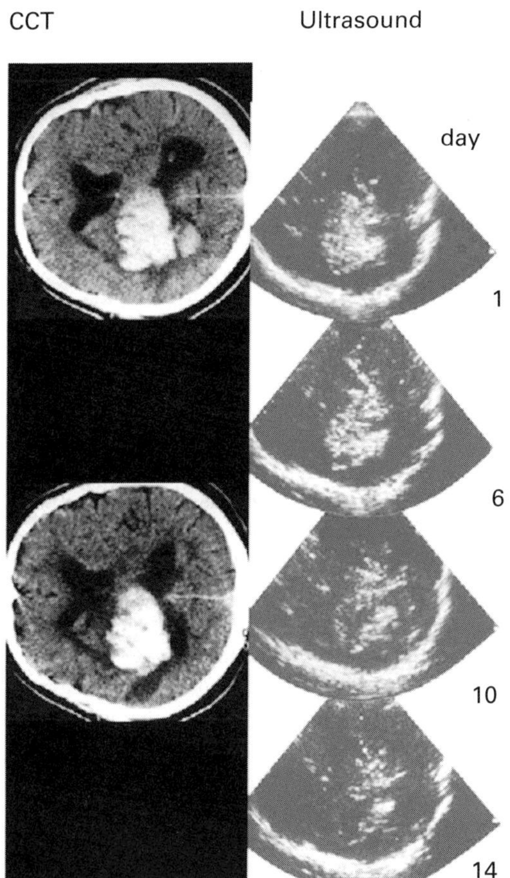

Fig. 5.3 Transcranial duplex follow-up after primary intracerebral hemorrhage from day 1 to 14 (right). Corresponding CCT scans are displayed at day 1 and 10 (left).

hyperacute supratentorial intracerebral hemorrhages can be reliably monitored by TCCD (28). In the early phase of intracerebral hemorrhage, a characteristic change in the signal pattern over time (25) has been described (Fig. 5.3). During the initial stage (day 1 to 5), the signal of the hemorrhage is strongly echogenic; during the intermediate stage (day 6 to 10), the echogenicity in the center of the clot decreases; and during the capsular stage (from day 10), the echogenicity in the center of the clot is lower than the surrounding healthy brain tissue, but the border of the clot remains hyperechogenic.

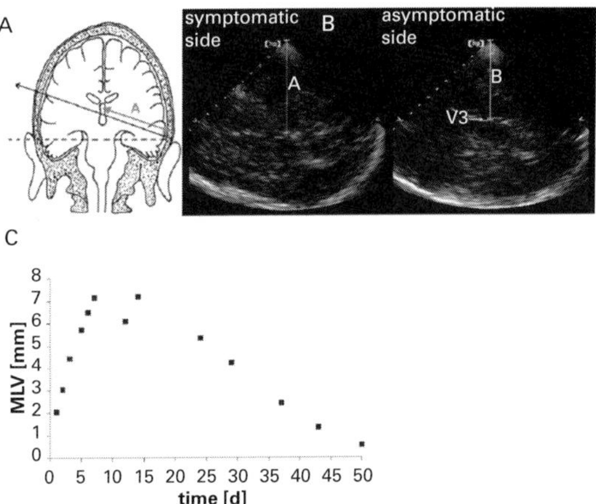

Fig. 5.4 **A**. Diagram of TCCS midline measurement (contact surface of the ultrasound probe to the third ventricle). **B**. Transcranial duplex scan of a patient suffering from space-occupying MCA infarction. Dislocation of the third ventricle (V3) is calculated by A-B / 2 (midline shift = MLS). **C**. Follow-up of MLS over time after space-occupying MCA infarction.

Hemorrhagic transformation (HT) of supratentorial ischemic stroke can be displayed by monitoring the ischemic tissue with a sensitivity of 90.0% and a specificity of 97.4% (29). In a recent study, HT was detected during the first 60 hours following the onset of supratentorial ischemic stroke in 62.5% of patients treated with tissue plasminogen activator in comparison to 33.3% of patients without thrombolysis.

Monitoring of the **dislocation of the third ventricle** in acute ischemic stroke is useful in detecting the space-occupying effects of ischemic brain edema (30–32). As early as 16 hours after stroke onset, TCCD monitoring (Fig. 5.4) can help estimate the outcome of space-occupying MCA ischemic stroke (midline shift [MLS] $\geq$ 2.5, 3.5, 4.0, and 5.0 mm after 16, 24, 32, and 40 hours from stroke onset, respectively), thus facilitating the identification of patients who are unlikely to survive without decompressive craniectomy. Because of its noninvasiveness and bedside suitability, sonographic monitoring of the MLS might be a useful tool in the management of critically ill patients who cannot undergo repeated cranial computed tomography (CCT) scans.

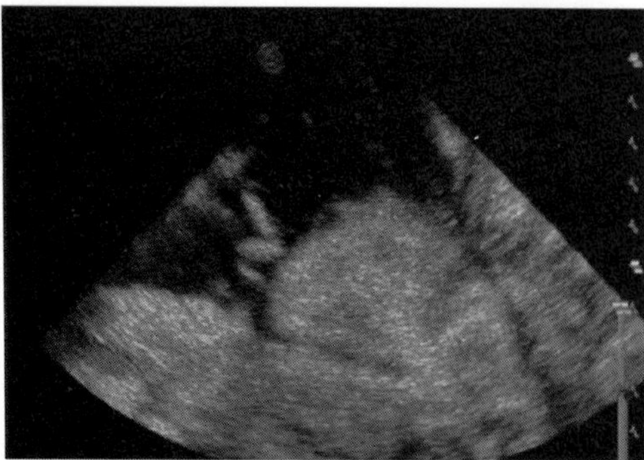

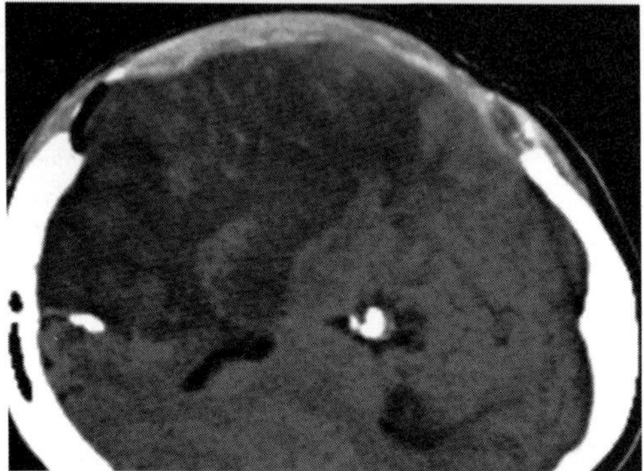

Fig. 5.5 Microvascular imaging and CCT of a patient suffering from both middle (MCA) and anterior (ACA) cerebral artery infarction. Microvascular image shows bright contrast in the perfused regions of the brain and sparing (black and light gray areas) of the ACA and MCA territory 12 hours after symptom onset. CT scan at day three, after craniectomy which was performed 36 hours after symptom onset, shows inthe investigation plane of the ultrasound image a space-occupying infarction.

During the past few years, new contrast-enhanced transcranial ultrasound technologies have been developed to assess **brain perfusion** at the bedside of patients with stroke. Sufficient insonation conditions for performing perfusion studies were reported in 76% to 84% of elderly patients who had suffered a stroke. In these studies, different parameters of the bolus kinetics curve in the ischemic region of the brain were compared with computed tomography (CT) in the acute stage and at follow-up. A combination of the signal increase and the time to peak signal proved to be most helpful in detecting the area of infarction, with a sensitivity between 75% and 86% as well as a specificity between 96% and 100% being reported (33,34). In more recent studies, parametric images were evaluated. They provided information on the time intensity curves for all pixels under evaluation, thus facilitating the visualization of the perfusion state. The areas of disturbed perfusion in the parametric images (especially the signal increase image) were found to correlate with the area of infarction in follow-up CT and the severity as well as the prognosis of stroke (35–37). More recently, real-time perfusion technologies have been developed, allowing for the contrast agent in the brain to be destroyed and the refill of the brain tissue to be analyzed (Fig. 5.5). With this advanced ultrasound perfusion technology (microvascular imaging), the evaluation of one imaging plane takes up to 7 seconds, thus permitting more than one imaging plane to be evaluated with one bolus injection of the contrast agent (38). This simple bedside investigation tool is useful in the follow-up of therapeutic procedures like thrombolysis in patients suffering from acute ischemic stroke.

Neurophysiological methods

Patients with cerebrovascular disease may benefit from the monitoring of brain function with *continuous electroencephalography* (cEEG), *somatosensory evoked potentials* (SEPs), and *brainstem auditory evoked potentials* (BAEPs). These methods are powerful measures of neural function and help to detect early deterioration and unfavorable outcome after acute stroke.

Continuous electroencephalography

Monitoring with cEEG may benefit patients suffering from stroke by detecting changes in brain function in a possible reversible state, thus allowing early intervention. The recording of EEG, according to the International 10–20 system with Ag/AgCl electrodes, with a bipolar eight-channel subset is necessary and technically feasible. Because EEG is very sensitive to ischemia, it can reveal changes at a reversible stage of reduced cerebral blood flow (CBF) and neuronal dysfunction (25–30 ml/100 g/min). The EEG progresses through predictable stages with increasing degrees of hypoperfusion, including loss of fast activity, increased slowing, and background attenuation. The parameters of cEEG are based on digital EEG data that are transformed into a quantification of the amplitude or frequency by fast Fourier transformation. The ideal quantitative EEG parameter for detecting ischemia is a matter of debate, but most options include some ratio of fast to slow activity that is displayed graphically in parallel with the raw EEG. Other options include compressed spectral array (CSA), burst suppression ratio, amplitude-integrated EEG, and the asymmetry index (39).

The brain symmetry index (BSI) is defined as the mean of the absolute value of the difference in mean hemispheric EEG power in the frequency range from 1 to 25 Hz, with values ranging from 0 (no asymmetry) to 1 (maximal asymmetry). The BSI was introduced as a measure to quantify ischemia in patients suffering from acute hemispheric stroke (Fig. 5.6). A positive correlation was found between stroke severity (as quantified by the National Institutes of Health Stroke Scale [NIHSS]) and the BSI as well as between stroke severity (as quantified by the NIHSS) and the acute delta change index (40).

Research has suggested that cEEG monitoring is useful for patients suffering from **acute hemispheric stroke** who are undergoing treatment with rt-PA (41). According to a recent study, the BSI remained constant or showed improvement during and after treatment with rt-PA. In this study, the correlation between stroke severity (as quantified by the NIHSS) and the BSI was significant and provided real-time information about the effect of thrombolysis in patients suffering from acute hemispheric stroke. Some studies have suggested that other EEG parameters (regional attenuation without delta [RAWOD]) can help select patients who would benefit from thrombolysis (42); however, clinical examination and imaging studies are likely superior to this approach.

Vasospasm after subarachnoid hemorrhage (SAH) may be clinically silent, particularly among poor grade patients. In patients with altered mental status and limited clinical examination, cEEG may reveal focal slowing that is suggestive of ischemia from vasospasm (43–45). This result may then prompt further diagnostic tests or directly lead to treatment. A number of cEEG parameters, such as relative alpha variability and post-stimulation alpha/delta ratio, have been shown to correlate with vasospasm or delayed cerebral ischemia (DCI) in good and poor grade patients. The onset of vasospasm may be detected by decreased relative alpha variability up to 2 days before clinical symptoms appear.

Evoked potentials

There is an increased awareness that predicting the further course in cerebrovascular critical care patients with acute supratentorial mass lesions is an additional domain of evoked potentials (EPs).

A recent study found that patients suffering a malignant course caused by a **space-occupying edema**, which usually occurs 48 to 72 hours after symptom onset of brain infarction, exhibited pathologic brainstem auditory evoked potentials (BAEPs) within the first 24 hours (46). Pathologic BAEP showed abnormal amplitudes, with a side-to-side difference of more than 50%, when compared to the unaffected contralateral response. No significant differences between 'malignant' and 'nonmalignant' courses were observed with regard to the results of median nerve somatosensory evoked potentials (SEPs) in the early phase. This finding is theoretically well explained: whereas the SEP reflects the functional integrity of the afferent spinal-cortical pathways, the BAEP reflects the functional integrity of mid-brainstem pathways. Lesions of the hemispheres – without compression of the brainstem – are expected to affect only the SEP, thus reflecting hemispheric damage. The life-threatening event in malignant MCA infarction, however, is not the hemispheric damage but rather the brainstem compression caused by incipient uncal herniation. This event is better reflected by the BAEP, which monitors brainstem function.

Correlations among clinical outcome, serial EPs, and intracranial pressure values have been demonstrated (47). Bilateral loss of the N20/P25 component of the SEP indicated a poor prognosis, with a probability of death in about 95% of patients. The prognostic data concerning the clinical outcome after 4 weeks were derived primarily within 24 to 96 hours from the initial examination. For patients requiring neurologic intensive care treatment, serial examination of the SEP and the BAEP during the course of disease may be valuable in detecting secondary cerebral damage (48).

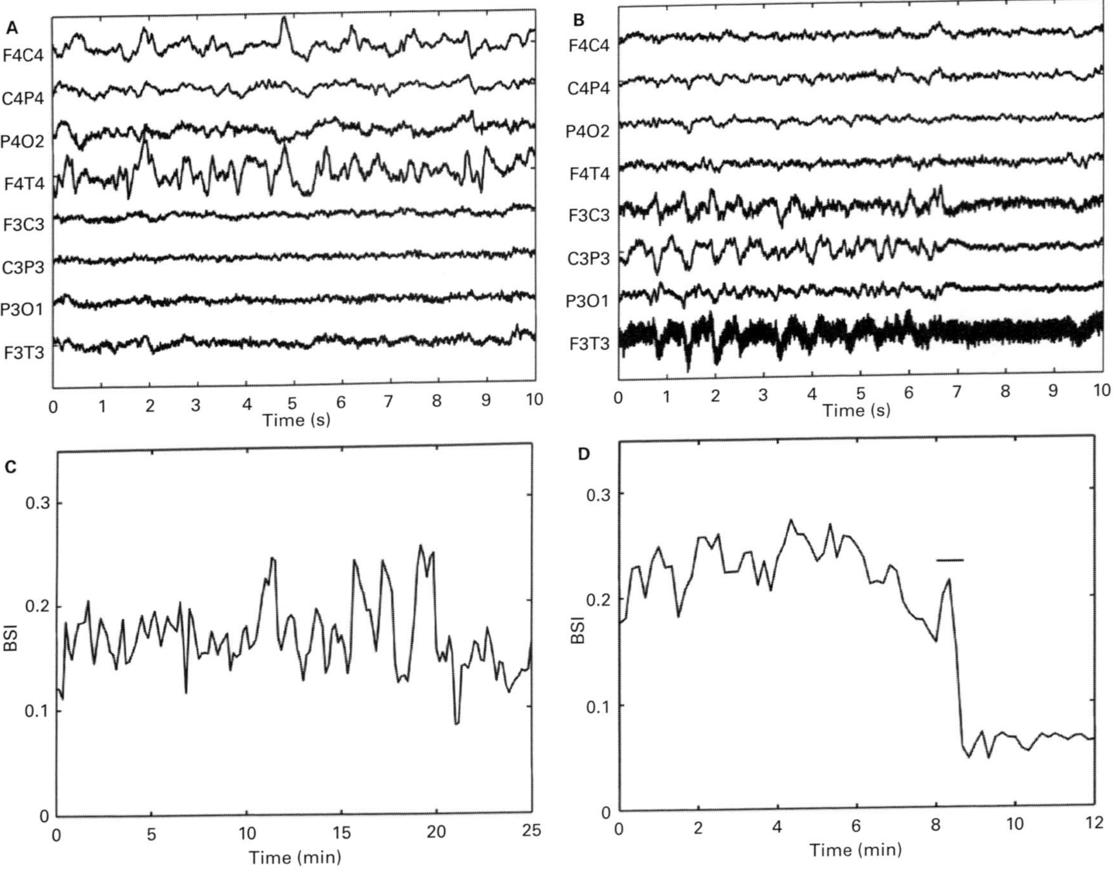

Fig. 5.6 Two examples of short segments of EEG recordings (top) and the corresponding Brain Symmetry Index (BSI) (bottom). In this example, the BSI trend was calculated for 20-second epochs, overlapping 10 seconds, to increase time resolution. The left EEG is from a patient with a right cerebral infarct (NIHSS = 13) showing polymorphic delta activity and a mean BSI ≈ 0.18. The right EEG is from a patient with a mild right-side hemiparesis (NIHSS = 3; BSI ≈ 0.06) and in whom, after several hours, subtle symptomatic focal seizures (rhythmic muscle contractions of the right facial muscles) developed. Note the abrupt decrease in BSI value from the, by now, increased BSI ≈ 0.20 to baseline when the seizure ends (indicated with the horizontal bar); this corresponds with the EEG shown at the top, showing abrupt ending of electroencephalographic seizure activity at t ≈ 7 seconds (from 40).

Near-infrared spectroscopy

Near-infrared spectroscopy (NIRS) is an emerging non-invasive modality, which provides real-time, continuous bedside sensitivity to the regional perfusion and oxygenation states of the brain. It is based on local illumination of the head by red and near-infrared light and the detection of the diffused light, which exits the tissue after propagation through the scalp, skull, and superficial layers of the cortex. By measuring changes in light reflectance at two or more wavelengths, NIRS enables the spectroscopic resolution of oxyhemoglobin (HbO_2) and deoxyhemoglobin (HbR) concentration changes. Consequently, variations in oxygen saturation and total hemoglobin, which are directly proportional to cerebral blood volume, can be measured. Typically, NIRS has been applied in measuring cerebral hemodynamic changes associated with brain activation during functional studies, as well as in assessing variations in brain oxygenation during cardiac surgery, neurovascular interventions, and stroke.

The crucial importance of monitoring both the infarcted and noninfarcted hemispheres in the management of space-occupying MCA infarction is increasingly recognized, but the debate regarding the optimal technique continues. In a recent study (49), the potential of NIRS to provide relevant information noninvasively on intracranial oxygenation was demonstrated. Bilateral NIRS may provide more useful information on cerebral oxygenation than unilateral measurements. Although NIRS is potentially useful in monitoring cerebral oxygenation, it does not, at present, effectively predict the outcomes of stroke or vascular death in patients with carotid artery occlusion (50).

REFERENCES

1. Allendoerfer J, Goertler M, von Reutern GM, for the Neurosonology in Acute Ischemic Stroke (NAIS) Study Group. Prognostic relevance of ultra-early Doppler sonography in acute ischaemic stroke: a prospective multicentre study. *Lancet Neurol* 2006;**5**:835–40.
2. Saqqur M, Uchino K, Demchuk AM, *et al.* for CLOTBUST Investigators. Site of arterial occlusion identified by transcranial Doppler predicts the response to intravenous thrombolysis for stroke. *Stroke* 2007;**38**:948–54.
3. Meseguer E, Lavallé PC, Mazighi M, *et al.* Yield of systematic transcranial Doppler in patients with transient ischemic attack. *Ann Neurol* 2010;**68**:9–17.
4. Molina CA, Montaner J, Abilleira S, *et al.* Timing of spontaneous recanalization and risk of hemorrhagic transformation in acute cardioembolic stroke. *Stroke* 2001; **32**:1079–84.
5. Furlan A, Higashida R, Wechsler L, *et al.* Intra-arterial prourokinase for acute ischemic stroke. The proact II study: A randomized controlled trial. Prolyse in acute cerebral thromboembolism. *JAMA* 1999;**282**:2003–11.
6. Uchino KMC, Saqqur M, Demchuk AM, *et al.* Likelihood of early arterial recanalization with intravenous tpa and its predictors: A multicenter transcranial Doppler study. *Stroke* 2003;**34**:347 (abstract).
7. Molina CA, Rubiera M, Montaner J, *et al.* Predictors of early arterial reocclusion after TPA-induced recanalization. *Stroke* 2004;**35**:250 (abstract).
8. Stolz E, Cioli F, Allendoerfer J, *et al.* Can early neurosonology predict outcome in acute stroke? A metaanalysis of prognostic clinical effect sizes related to the vascular status. *Stroke* 2008;**39**:3255–61.
9. King A, Markus HS. Doppler embolic signals in cerebrovascular disease and prediction of stroke risk: a systematic review and meta-analysis. *Stroke* 2009;**40**:3711–17.
10. Markus HS, MacKinnon A. Asymptomatic embolization detected by Doppler ultrasound predicts stroke risk in symptomatic carotid artery stenosis. *Stroke* 2005; **36**:971–5.
11. Gao S, Wong KS, Hansberg T, *et al.* Microembolic signal predicts recurrent cerebral ischemic events in acute stroke patients with middle cerebral artery stenosis. *Stroke* 2004;**35**:2832–6.
12. Wong KS, Li H, Chan YL, *et al.* Use of transcranial Doppler to predict outcome in patients with intracranial large-artery occlusive disease. *Stroke* 2000;**31**:2641–7.
13. Wong KS, Gao S, Chan YL, *et al.* Mechanisms of acute cerebral infarctions in patients with middle cerebral artery stenosis: a diffusion-weighted imaging and microemboli monitoring study. *Ann Neurol* 2002;**52**:74–81.
14. Markus HS, Droste DW, Kaps M, *et al.* Dual antiplatelet therapy with clopidogrel and aspirin in symptomatic carotid stenosis evaluated using Doppler embolic signal detection: the clopidogrel and aspirin for reduction of

emboli in symptomatic carotid stenosis (CARESS) trial. *Circulation* 2005;**111**:2233–40.

15. Sing K, Wong L, Chen C, *et al.*, for the CLAIR study investigators. Clopidogrel plus aspirin versus aspirin alone for reducing embolisation in patients with acute symptomatic cerebral or carotid artery stenosis (CLAIR study): a randomised, open-label, blinded-endpoint trial. *Lancet Neurol* 2010;**9**:489–97.
16. Bragoni M, Feldmann E. Transcranial Doppler indices of intracranial hemodynamics. In: Tegeler CH, Babikian VL, Gomez CR (eds.). *Neurosonology*, St Louis: Mosby, 1996.
17. De Chiara S, Mancini M, Vaccaro O, *et al.* Cerebrovascular reactivity by transcranial Doppler ultrasonography in insulin-dependent diabetic patients. *Cerebrovasc Dis* 1993;**3**:111–15.
18. Sugimori H, Ibayashi S, Irie K, *et al.* Cerebral hemodynamics in hypertensive patients compared with normotensive volunteers. A transcranial Doppler study. *Stroke* 1994;**25**:1384–9.
19. Sloan MA. Transcranial Doppler monitoring of vasospasm after subarachnoid hemorrhage. In: Tegeler CH, Babikian VL, Gomez CR (eds.) *Neurosonology*, St. Louis: Mosby, 1996.
20. Adams R, McKie V, Nichols F, *et al.* The use of transcranial ultrasonography to predict stroke in sickle cell disease. *N Engl J Med* 1992;**326**:605–10.
21. Adams RJ, McKie VC, Hsu L, *et al.* Prevention of a first stroke by transfusions in children with sickle cell anemia and abnormal results on transcranial Doppler ultrasonography. *N Engl J Med* 1998;**339**:5–11.
22. Adams RJ, Brambilla D. Optimizing Primary Stroke Prevention in Sickle Cell Anemia (STOP 2) Trial Investigators. Discontinuing prophylactic transfusions used to prevent stroke in sickle cell disease. *N Engl J Med* 2005;**353**:2769–78.
23. Alexandrov AV, Burgin S, Demchuk AM, *et al.* Speed of intracranial clot lysis with intravenous tissue plasminogen activator therapy. Sonographic classification and short-term improvement. *Circulation* 2001;**103**:2897–902.
24. Seidel G, Meairs S. Ultrasound contrast agents in ischemic stroke. *Cerebrovasc Dis.* 2009;**27** Suppl 2: 25–39.
25. Seidel G, Kaps M, Dorndorf W. Transcranial color-coded duplex sonography of intracerebral hematomas in adults. *Stroke* 1993;**24**:1519–27.
26. Seidel G, Kaps M, Gerriets T. Potential and limitations of transcranial color-coded sonography in stroke patients. *Stroke* 1995;**26**:2061–6.
27. Mäurer M, Shambal S, Berg D, *et al.* Differentiation between intracerebral hemorrhage and ischemic stroke by transcranial color-coded duplex-sonography. *Stroke* 1998;**29**:2563–7.
28. Pérez ES, Delgado-Mederos R, Rubiera M, *et al.* Transcranial duplex sonography for monitoring hyperacute intracerebral hemorrhage. *Stroke* 2009;**40**:987–90.
29. Seidel G, Cangür H, Albers T, *et al.* Sonographic evaluation of hemorrhagic transformation and arterial recanalization in acute hemispheric ischemic stroke. *Stroke* 2009; **40**:119–23.
30. Seidel G, Gerriets T, Kaps M, *et al.* Dislocation of the third ventricle due to space-occupying stroke evaluated by transcranial duplex sonography. *J Neuroimaging* 1996; **6**:227–30.
31. Stolz E, Gerriets T, Fiss I, *et al.* Comparison of transcranial color-coded duplex sonography and cranial CT measurements for determining third ventricle midline shift in space-occupying stroke. *AJNR Am J Neuroradiol* 1999; **20**:1567–71.
32. Gerriets T, Stolz E, König S, *et al.* Sonographic monitoring of midline shift in space-occupying stroke: an early outcome predictor. *Stroke* 2001;**32**:442–7.
33. Seidel G, Albers T, Meyer K, *et al.* Perfusion harmonic imaging in acute middle cerebral artery infarction. *Ultrasound Med Biol* 2003;**29**:1245–51.
34. Federlein J, Postert T, Meves SH, *et al.* Ultrasonic evaluation of pathological brain perfusion in acute stroke using second harmonic imaging. *J Neurol Neurosurg Psychiatry* 2000;**69**:616–22.
35. Seidel G, Meyer-Wiethe K, Berdien G, *et al.* Ultrasound perfusion imaging in acute middle cerebral artery infarction predicts outcome. *Stroke* 2004;**35**:1107–11.
36. Seidel G, Cangür H, Meyer-Wiethe K, *et al.* On the ability of ultrasound parametric perfusion imaging to predict the area of infarction in acute ischemic stroke. *Ultraschall Med* 2006;**27**:543–8.
37. Meyer-Wiethe K, Cangür H, Schindler A, *et al.* Ultrasound perfusion imaging: determination of thresholds for the identification of critically disturbed perfusion in acute ischemic stroke – a pilot study. *Ultrasound Med Biol* 2007;**33**:851–6.
38. Seidel G, Roessler F. Microvascular imaging in acute ischemic stroke. *Cerebrovasc Dis* 2010;**29** Suppl 2.

39. Kurtz P, Hanafy KA, Claassen J. Continuous EEG monitoring: is it ready for prime time? *Curr Opin Crit Care* 2009;**15**:99–109.
40. van Putten MJ, Tavy DL. Continuous quantitative EEG monitoring in hemispheric stroke patients using the brain symmetry index. *Stroke* 2004;**35**:2489–92.
41. de Vos CC, van Maarseveen SM, Brouwers PJ, *et al.* Continuous EEG monitoring during thrombolysis in acute hemispheric stroke patients using the brain symmetry index. *J Clin Neurophysiol* 2008;**25**:77–82.
42. Schneider AL, Jordan KG. Regional attenuation without delta (RAWOD): a distinctive EEG pattern that can aid in the diagnosis and management of severe acute ischemic stroke. *Am J Electroneurodiagnostic Technol* 2005;**45**:102–17.
43. Claassen J, Hirsch LJ, Kreiter KT, *et al.* Quantitative continuous EEG for detecting delayed cerebral ischemia in patients with poor-grade subarachnoid hemorrhage. *Clin Neurophysiol* 2004;**115**:2699–710.
44. Claassen J, Mayer SA, Hirsch LJ. Continuous EEG monitoring in patients with subarachnoid hemorrhage. *J Clin Neurophysiol* 2005;**22**:92–8.
45. Vespa PM, Nuwer MR, Juhász C, *et al.* Early detection of vasospasm after acute subarachnoid hemorrhage using continuous EEG ICU monitoring. *Electroencephalogr Clin Neurophysiol* 1997;**103**:607–15.
46. Burghaus L, Liu WC, Dohmen C, *et al.* Evoked potentials in acute ischemic stroke within the first 24 h: Possible predictor of a malignant course. *Neurocrit Care* 2008;**9**:13–16.
47. Krieger D, Jauss M, Schwarz S, *et al.* Serial somatosensory and brainstem auditory evoked potentials in monitoring of acute supratentorial mass lesions. *Crit Care Med* 1995; **23**:1123–31.
48. Haupt WF, Pawlik G, Thiel A. Initial and serial evoked potential in cerebrovascular critial care patients. *J Clin Neurophysiol* 2006;**23**:389–94.
49. Damian MS, Schlosser R. Bilateral near infrared spectroscopy in space-occupying middle cerebral artery stroke. *Neurocrit Care* 2007;**6**:165–73.
50. Palazzo P, Tibuzzi F, Pasqualetti P, *et al.* Is there a role of near-infrared spectroscopy in predicting the outcome of patients with carotid artery occlusion? *J Neurol Sci* 2010;**292**:36–9.

6

Scales in the neurointensive care unit

Elise Rowan and Barbara A. Gregson

Introduction

Requirements to diagnose and monitor ITU patients accurately have resulted in the development of scales of relevance in stroke and head injury. Diagnostic classification scales assist with identifying stroke/head injury types whilst severity scales are useful for quantifying deficits/symptoms and monitoring changes. One severity scale may incorporate other severity scales as subcomponents. When well-designed severity scales are applied to patient populations, they reveal a range of abnormal scores for each relevant item/symptom examined. Additionally, the score for each item changes whenever a patient improves or deteriorates with regard to that item.

It is beyond the scope of this chapter to discuss every scale in existence. We therefore focus on some of the more common ones. This chapter aims to give the reader an overview of each scale (see Table 6.1) and draws attention to recent updates and current opinions.

We begin with the Glasgow Coma Scale (GCS) which is usually the first scale to be applied by emergency medical services to stroke or head injured patients. Following this, other common scales are described which document generic features such as conscious state and severity of injuries. We also consider scales for describing/categorizing the specific neurological deficits of stroke or particular stroke subtypes before discussing some outcome/handicap scales.

Glasgow Coma Scale

When was it developed and why?

GCS was developed in 1974 as a quick means of recording/grading the conscious state of a head injured patient both for initial and subsequent assessment [1]. Today, GCS has been translated into many languages and is used by emergency paramedic services, first aiders and doctors and is applied to all acute medical and trauma patients as well as chronic patients in ICUs. GCS assists medical staff with making clinical decisions about specialist referral, CT scans, and even surgery after a brain injury/insult.

What does it measure?

Originally GCS was a 14 point scale; however, the version normally used today is a modified 15 point version [2]. The 15 point GCS assesses three components indicative of conscious state; best eye opening response ('E', scored 1–4), best verbal response ('V', scored 1–5) and the best motor response ('M', scored 1–6). For each GCS component, 1 represents the worst score (no response). The term 'best' is used so that the highest level attained during each assessment is recorded. This is important because during a single assessment a patient may improve as they become more awake.

The three component scores can be summed giving a total score; total scores can range from 3 (coma or death) to 15 (fully conscious). GCS total allows categorization of

Critical Care of the Stroke Patient, ed. Stefan Schwab, Daniel Hanley, and A. David Mendelow. Published by Cambridge University Press.

Table 6.1 Key features of the scales discussed

Name of scale	Year first published	What it measures	Notes
Glasgow coma scale	1974	Conscious state.	Used by emergency services. Most recent version is 15-item.
FOUR Score	2005	Unresponsiveness/consciousness.	New scale. Overcomes some limitations of the GCS.
APACHE	1981	Likelihood of in-hospital mortality.	Three versions of the scale now exist. GCS is a subcomponent.
Marshall classification	1991	Severity of brain injury.	A CT scale.
OCSP classification	1991	Anatomically based stroke categorization scale.	Can be used with and without CT to describe stroke type.
Scandinavian stroke scale	1985	Neurological stroke scale.	Captures items of functional significance to patients.
NIHSS	1989	Neurological stroke scale.	A modified version of this now exists. Useful in stroke therapy trials.
Canadian neurological scale	1986	Neurological stroke scale.	Good overall indicator of stroke severity.
WFNS grading system	1987/1988	Consciousness and motor deficit in SAH.	GCS is a subcomponent.
Fisher grade	1980	Categorizes the appearance of SAH blood.	A CT scale.
Hunt and Hess	1968	Meningeal inflammatory reaction, severity of neurological deficit, associated diseases in patients with aneurysm.	Useful for determining surgical risk and timing of surgery when treating patients with aneurysm.
European stroke scale	1994	Neurological scale for MCA stroke.	Useful in clinical trials for measuring therapeutic effects.
Rankin scale	1957	Handicap.	A modified version of this scale (mRS) is used today.
Barthel ADL index	1965	Assesses requirements for assistance with personal care.	10- and 15-item versions available.
Glasgow outcome scale	1975	Assesses outcome after head injury/neurosurgery/stroke.	Useful in clinical and surgical trials for measuring effects on quality of life.

brain injuries as severe (GCS total ≤ 8), moderate (GCS total 9–12) or minor (GCS total ≥ 13). A GCS total score < 8 is regarded as 'critical' and generally applies to patients in coma or comatose. Patients emerging from coma generally score > 8.

Has it been validated and what are the pros and cons?

GCS predicts mortality, coma, amnesia, and longer term outcome after brain injury [3]. GCS is easy to apply, however, inter-rater reliability can be affected by rater experience and the timing and setting can also influence overall score which can be skewed towards motor components [4]. Although most researchers today use the 15 point version, many still erroneously cite the 14 point version [5].

Full GCS score cannot be assigned in patients with severe facial swelling, aphasia or intubation where eye and/or verbal responses are un-testable. In these situations, codes have been devised; eye score would be expressed as 'E = 1c' if eyes were closed and verbal score would be expressed as 'V = 1t' where a patient was intubated. To avoid using these codes, a shortened version of GCS (eliminating the verbal component) can be applied to acute stroke patients [6] or predictive statistical methods can be used in intubated patients [7].

GCS data are categorical and not normally distributed therefore statistical analyses should involve the use of non-parametric tests [8].

FOUR Score (Full Outline of UnResponsiveness Score)

When was it developed and why?

FOUR Score measures unresponsiveness [9]. It was developed in 2005 to overcome shortcomings in the GCS; namely failure to assess verbal score in intubated patients and inability to test brainstem reflexes. It is too early to report whether it will become as popular as GCS; however, early indications are positive because it exists in a number of languages.

What does it measure?

This scale has four components: eye, motor, brainstem, and respiration. Each is scored between 0 and 4, with 4 indicating most responsiveness. For the eye component, the best response to three trials is recorded taking into account whether the eyelids are open or respond to voice or pain and whether the eyes track. The motor component records the best response from the arms. The brainstem component records brainstem reflex responses, taking into account pupil, corneal, and cough responses. The respiration component records breathing patterns and intubation.

Has it been validated and what are the pros and cons?

Inter-rater reliability has been assessed in ICU, and also by intensive care nurses [9–12]; inter-rater agreement is excellent and exact inter-rater agreement is better for FOUR Score than GCS [12]. There is also a high degree of internal consistency. FOUR Score is a good predictor of prognosis. In particular, the mortality rate of patients with the lowest FOUR Score is higher than the mortality rate in patients with the lowest GCS [10]. It provides more information than GCS because it differentiates locked-in syndrome and can recognize stages of herniation [9]. FOUR score does not include a verbal component and is not limited in intubated patients.

Acute physiology and chronic health evaluation (APACHE) score

When was it developed and why?

APACHE estimates the likelihood of mortality in ITU or during hospitalization taking into account physiological and chronic health status. It was first published in 1981 [13] and records 34 variables categorized into eight classes: cardiovascular, respiratory, renal, gastrointestinal, hematological, septic, metabolic, and neurologic. Each variable is rated 0–4 (0 being normal, 4 being most abnormal). Total scores are derived for each of the classes (by summing the variable scores within each class) and these are then summed to give the overall APACHE score. A pre-admission health status classification (coded A to D; A being in good health, D being in very poor health) is also determined by asking about the patient's health in the 3–6 months prior to hospitalization. APACHE can estimate %mortality rate, while a combination of APACHE and pre-admission health status classification can estimate the probability of a particular patient dying in the ICU/hospital as an overall estimate or in the case of them being an operative/non-operative patient.

Has it been validated and what are the pros and cons?

APACHE score was validated in the original publication which demonstrated good agreement between the APACHE score and the following therapeutic effort and mortality in a broad range of patients.

In 1985 a second simpler version of APACHE (APACHE II) was published and was well received by the medical community [14]. APACHE II takes 3.7 ± 1.0 minutes – three times longer than the GCS [15]. In 1995, APACHE II was applied to neurosurgical patients in HDU and did not significantly improve prediction of outcome above and beyond the routinely used GCS [16]. It was concluded that it may not be worth investing extra time/resources in collecting data for APACHE II for neurosurgical patients in HDU or for patients outside ITUs.

APACHE III was published in 1991 [17] and was the result of efforts to improve the overall precision of the scale and also included a differential weighting of neurological assessment of traumatic and non-traumatic coma cases. Research suggested that APACHE III may be more accurate than APACHE II and GCS in terms of predicting severe morbidity in head-injured patients [18]. At release, APACHE III was ahead of its time technologically speaking because it was developed with a view to embedding it in a user-friendly graphical computer interface that would allow clinicians to link it directly to monitoring devices and electronic medical records. It remains to be seen whether current technological advances will facilitate the widespread use of APACHE III.

Marshall CT classification of head injury

When was it developed and why?

Severity of head injury and resulting prognosis is frequently related to features observed on CT scans which include midline shift, compression of basal cisterns, and subarachnoid hemorrhage as a result of trauma. The Marshall classification was developed in 1991 in order to standardize the reporting of such CT features in traumatic brain injury (TBI) [19].

What does it measure?

The Marshall classification divides injuries into six categories on the basis of CT evidence. The first four categories document diffuse injuries in increasing severity. The first category, 'Diffuse Injury Type I' indicates no pathology visible on CT. The second category, 'Diffuse Injury Type II' is for patients in whom the cisterns are present with midline shift from 0–5 mm but with no lesions > 25 ml. 'Diffuse Injury Type III' is for patients who have swelling where cisterns are compressed or absent with midline shift from 0–5 mm but again with no lesions > 25 ml. 'Diffuse Injury Type IV' is for patients who demonstrate a midline shift > 5 mm who do not have lesions > 25 ml. The final two categories require retrospective knowledge of the patient's clinical course/treatment and are for patients who have significant lesions; the 'Evacuated Mass Lesion' category is for patients who receive surgical evacuation and the 'Non-evacuated Mass Lesion' category is for non-surgical patients who have lesions > 25 ml.

Has it been validated and what are the pros and cons?

The Marshall classification can predict mortality and is widely used by the clinical community and in clinical trials. Despite wide acceptance, limitations have been summarized in a recent review [20]. These include inter-observer variability and the need for retrospective knowledge regarding clinical course/treatment. The requirement to measure/estimate lesion volume has potential to increase inter-observer variability in the absence of standardized measurement procedure guidelines. Additionally, the Marshall scale does not allow us to subcategorize patients who have no visible CT pathology according to the severity of their clinical symptoms and this limits its usefulness in mild TBI patients. Recent research suggests that individual CT features including intraventricular and traumatic subarachnoid hemorrhage may actually be more useful than the Marshall classification for predicting outcome after TBI [21].

Stroke scales

Oxfordshire community stroke project classification (OCSP)

When was it developed and why?

The OCSP classification was described in 1991 [22]. It was developed for use in epidemiological studies and clinical trials of acute stroke and was designed to be quick and easy to use.

What does it measure?

OCSP allocates patients with cerebral infarction (confirmed by imaging) into one of four subtypes depending on presenting symptoms and signs. The subtypes have an anatomical basis and are as follows: lacunar infarcts (LACI), total anterior circulation infarcts (TACI), partial anterior circulation infarcts (PACI), and posterior circulation infarcts (POCI).

Conversely, where hemorrhage has been confirmed by imaging, patients can also be categorized as: lacunar hemorrhage (LACH), total anterior circulation hemorrhage (TACH), partial anterior circulation hemorrhage (PACH), and posterior circulation hemorrhage (POCH).

Under circumstances where patients have not received imaging, the scale can still be used and patients can be categorized simply by syndrome: LACS, TACS, PACS, and POCS.

Has it been validated and what are the pros and cons?

A recent publication investigated the accuracy of OCSP in predicting sites and sizes of infarcts [23]. Patients were classified by OCSP syndrome before brain imaging and then a neuroradiologist evaluated subsequent scans. Seventy-five per cent of patients with visible infarcts were classified correctly. OCSP may thus be a useful classification tool in situations where imaging is not feasible (e.g. in epidemiology studies and reviews of old case notes) or where infarcts are not seen on CT. A drawback is that it is possible to misclassify patients during the period when their symptoms are still evolving and further work needs to be done in order to evaluate accuracy of the OCSP with respect to timing.

Scandinavian stroke scale (SSS)

When was it developed and why?

The SSS was created and published in 1985 for a specific multicentre study on hemodilution [24]. At that time, the investigators wanted a simple scale that could be applied by non-neurologists in both neurological wards and general medical wards. The aim of the scale was to capture items of functional significance to patients.

What does it measure?

SSS measures nine neurological 'functions': consciousness, eye movement, affected arm motor power, affected hand motor power, affected leg motor power, orientation, speech, facial palsy, and gait (walking ability). Two scores are derived by summing the appropriate 'function' scores; a prognostic score and a long-term score. Functions contributing to the prognostic score include consciousness, eye movement, affected arm motor power, and affected leg motor power, giving a potential maximal score of 22 (22 indicating no problems, 0 indicating problems in all functions). Functions contributing to the long-term score include affected arm motor power, affected hand motor power, affected leg motor power, orientation, speech, facial palsy, and gait. This gives a maximal score of 48 for the sum of these functions (48 indicating no problems, 0 indicating problems in all functions).

Has it been validated and what are the pros and cons?

SSS can be used prospectively and estimated retrospectively from medical records [25]. It is useful in observational studies and audit. The prognostic value of SSS has been assessed in mild ischemic stroke where it predicted death and dependence [26].

The National Institutes of Health stroke scale (NIHSS)

When was it developed and why?

The NIHSS was developed and validated in 1989 [27] as a simple scale that could be used prospectively as an efficacy measure in stroke therapy trials.

What does it measure?

NIHSS is a quantitative measure of neurological deficits relating to stroke and the original version is broken down into 15 items assessed during a quick (6–7 minutes) bedside examination. The items are as follows: 1) level of consciousness (subdivided into items 1a–1c); 2) pupillary response; 3) gaze; 4) visual fields; 5) facial palsy; 6) best motor arm; 7) best motor leg; 8) plantar reflex; 9) limb ataxia; 10) sensory; 11) neglect; 12) dysarthria; 13) best language; 14) any change from a previous examination; and 15) any change from the baseline examination. Items 1 to 13 inclusive are rated from 0–2 or 0–3 (a score of 0 being normal) and a total score is derived. Changes from baseline/previous exams are graded as 'same', 'better', or 'worse'.

Has it been validated and what are the pros and cons?

In the original publication [27] the authors validated the 15-item NIHSS in terms of inter-rater reliability, test-retest reliability, and correlation to infarction volume as measured by CT scan and functional outcome. The scale performed satisfactorily in all of these aspects. A modified 11-item version (mNIHSS) has now been developed [28]. The mNIHSS is considered simpler and easier to use than the 15-item version and has eliminated some of the items that were considered less reliable. The mNIHSS has excellent reliability and validity in prospective research studies and may be more powerful than the original version when subjected to statistical analysis. The mNIHSS can be accurately abstracted from medical records [29].

NIHSS correlates with infarction volumes in ischemic stroke; however, patients who have left-sided strokes are likely to score about four more points on average than patients with right-sided strokes due to an over representation of left hemisphere items in the NIHSS [30].

Canadian neurological scale

When was it developed and why?

The Canadian neurological scale was first described in 1986 [31]. It was developed as a simple practical method of documenting neurological status in acute stroke. The scale was developed for patients who were alert or drowsy for whom the Glasgow coma scale would probably be too insensitive.

What does it measure?

The Canadian neurological scale is split into two sections, namely mentation and motor function. The mentation section records the level of consciousness, orientation, and speech. There are two versions of the motor function section: for patients who are or are not able to comprehend instructions. The motor function section assesses asymmetry in the face and any weaknesses in the limbs. The components within each section are summed (maximum score of 5 in each section) and an overall total score is derived (maximum score of 10). A score of 10 indicates no detectable deficits and a score of 0 indicates maximal deficits.

Has it been validated and what are the pros and cons?

The Canadian neurological scale is very simple and quick to use (it takes only 5–10 minutes) and compares well with the NIHSS in predicting 3-month post-stroke outcome [32].

The disadvantage is that, unlike NIHSS, it does not record details such as sensory loss, visual acuity/neglect, and dysarthria. It may therefore be more useful as an overall clinical indicator of acute stroke severity which can be easily applied by a variety of medical personnel of differing specialities and may not be quite so suitable for clinical trials/research where more detailed information is required.

Scales for specific subtypes of stroke

World Federation of Neurosurgical Societies (WFNS) grading system for subarachnoid hemorrhage scale

When was the scale developed and why?

The WFNS grading system was developed in 1987/1988 to provide a simple, reliable method for grading subarachnoid hemorrhage (SAH) patients [33].

What does it measure?

It is based on assessments of consciousness and motor deficits. The scale combines total Glasgow coma score (GCS) with an assessment of motor deficit and, depending on the combination of these assessments, a grade can be assigned. Grades range from I through to V. Grade I represents a patient with GCS 15 and no motor deficit whereas Grade V represents a patient with a GCS between 3 and 6 and a presence/absence of motor deficits. Interpretation guidelines suggest that SAH patients who score GCS ≥ 8 have a good chance of recovery whereas patients scoring GCS 3–5 are more likely to die.

Has it been validated and what are the pros and cons?

The WFNS scale is easy and quick to use. Nevertheless, one study [34] suggested that although it was effective at predicting discharge Glasgow outcome score, mortality and length of hospital stay, it may still not be as effective as a graded version of the GCS in this regard. NIHSS can actually reveal subtle abnormal neurological signs even in patients with good WFNS grade [35]. Patients with these abnormal signs would not be expected to have such good outcome at 3 months and this demonstrates that WFNS grading should not be relied upon as an outcome predictor and should not be performed in the absence of further detailed neurological assessment.

Despite this, the WFNS scale has been shown to be well correlated with SAH clot volume in SAH patients [36]. The scale is therefore still helpful in analysis of retrospective clinical data where imaging details are scant.

Fisher grade (FG)

When was it developed and why?

This scale was developed in 1980 to predict cerebral vasospasm, the major cause of delayed ischemia in patients with SAH [37].

What does it measure?

The scale classifies the appearance of SAH blood on CT into four groups. Group 1 is for scans without subarachnoid blood, Group 2 is for diffuse or thin layers of blood < 1 mm thick, Group 3 is for localized clots or layers $\geq$ 1 mm thick, while Group 4 is for patients with diffuse or no SAH who have intraventricular or intraparenchymal clots.

Has it been validated and what are the pros and cons?

The original publication of the scale examined only 47 cases but nevertheless demonstrated good correlation between FG and vasospasm. Since that time the scale has become the standard for predicting delayed ischemia in SAH. The predictive validity of FG in today's patients has, however, been questioned in the light of improvements in availability and resolution of CT scanning and in the treatment/management of vasospasm [38].

Hunt and Hess

When was it developed and why?

The Hunt and Hess scale was described in 1968 [39]. It was developed to describe surgical risk for patients with intracranial aneurysms.

What does it measure?

The scale quantifies the intensity of the meningeal inflammatory reaction, the severity of neurological deficit, and the presence/absence of noteworthy associated diseases (e.g. vascular risk factors). Meningeal inflammatory reaction is evaluated by assessing degree of headache, neck stiffness, and level of consciousness. The scale has five categories labeled grade I through to grade V. Grade I represents patients who are asymptomatic/have minimal headache and slight neck rigidity while grade V represents patients who are in deep coma, have decerebrate rigidity, and appear close to death. Presence of any significant systemic disease in addition to the criteria set out in the standard five-category scale (e.g. hypertension) would place a patient into the next most severe category.

Has it been validated and what are the pros and cons?

In the original publication, 275 cases of intracranial aneurysm were evaluated. Eleven per cent of cases who were grade I at admission died, whilst 26%, 37%, 71%, and 100% of cases with grades II, III, IV, and V respectively at admission died. Patients who were grade I and II at admission were taken to surgery as soon as they received diagnosis. In patients who were grade I and II at the time of surgery, 5.5% and 25% died respectively. Patients who were grade III or below were treated conservatively until they improved to either grade I or grade II when they were considered for delayed surgery. Interestingly, 55% of patients who were grade III at admission later improved to grades I and II. This paper elegantly demonstrates the potential for using scales to evaluate surgical risk and optimize timing of surgical intervention.

The Hunt and Hess scale has been used extensively, particularly in North America; however, it is gradually being superseded by the WFNS scale.

European stroke scale (ESS)

When was it developed and why?

The ESS was developed in 1994 [40]. It was designed to assess impairments in middle cerebral artery stroke and also to be used as an instrument to match treatment groups and measure therapeutic effect.

What does it measure?

ESS covers 14 aspects: level of consciousness, comprehension, speech, visual field, gaze, facial movement, outstretched arm position, arm raising, wrist extension, finger grip, maintained leg position, leg flexing, dorsiflexion, and gait. Completion of the scale takes between 4 and 14 minutes.

Has it been validated and what are the pros and cons?

Inter-rater and intra-rater reliability and internal consistency are good. ESS has high correlation with NIHSS and SSS as well as other lesser known stroke scales. ESS is more sensitive than some other scales as it covers a range of neurological deficits and distinguishes between proximal and distal parts of limbs. It can be more sensitive than the SSS and is a good predictor of outcome although it has not been widely used outside Europe.

Scales measuring outcome, handicap, and activities of daily living

Modified Rankin scale (mRS)

When was it developed and why?

The Rankin scale was a five-point ordinal scale developed in 1957 as a measure of handicap [41]. The scale was expanded to six points in 1988 and is now known as the modified Rankin scale or mRS [42].

What does it measure?

The mRS requires careful observation of the patient and derivation of a general opinion about their level of impairment, disability, and dependence on others. Attention must be given as to whether the patient has any symptoms which relate to their medical crisis, whether they can carry out all their previous duties/activities, the level of assistance they need with activities of daily living, and whether they can walk. Patients are graded as 0–5 (i.e. six categories), with 0 representing those with no symptoms and 5 representing those who are severely disabled requiring constant care or nursing. More often than not, an additional seventh category called '6' is also added – to account for death (in clinical and surgical trials this is necessary in order to account for all participants).

Has it been validated and what are the pros and cons?

The mRS is the most popular functional outcome measure in stroke research and has been studied extensively with regard to reliability. The main advantage is that it is very simple. It is practical to perform the mRS in neuro ICU in order to inform health professionals involved with subsequent rehabilitation and out-patient care. A systematic review of ten mRS reliability studies has, however, confirmed a general suspicion that there is potential for inter-observer variability which can be considered as 'moderate' [43].

Barthel ADL index (BI)

When was the scale developed and why?

BI was published in 1965 [44]. It was developed to assess whether patients could live independently and determine whether they need supervision/assistance with personal care in their everyday lives. The scale is therefore useful in planning practical care during a hospital stay or social support and care after discharge.

What does it measure?

BI measures what patients actually do at a given point in time – in terms of activities of daily living. It includes ten items: feeding, bathing, grooming, dressing, bowels, bladder, toilet use, transfers (bed to chair), mobility, and stairs. Each item is scored according to whether the patient is able to perform the task independently or not (the use of aids is acceptable if they mean that a patient does not require assistance from a carer). For each item values are assigned according to the amount of physical assistance the patient requires to do the task. If a patient is completely unable to meet any of the criteria set out for each item then that item is scored as zero. The maximal score is 100 and this indicates a patient who can feed him- or herself, dress, get out of a bed/chair, bath, walk, and negotiate stairs independently. This does not necessarily mean that the patient can actually live alone (they may still be unable to cook, shop or do housework) but it does indicate that an attendant is not required for personal care.

Has it been validated and what are the pros and cons?

BI is easy and convenient to complete. It can be conducted quickly with input from the patient, carers, friends, and relatives in combination with direct observation; direct testing is not required.

The Barthel score can be affected by the environment and this is useful since one purpose of the test is to measure changes in independence effected by the provision of adaptive aids during rehabilitation. For example, a patient who is in a wheelchair may not be capable of being independent in a house where there is no stair lift and the bathroom is upstairs, whereas they may be almost fully independent in a bungalow with wide doorways and grab handles in the bathroom. In order to get the full value from a Barthel assessment, one should therefore record details about when and where the assessment was performed and identify any special environmental requirements that may improve the situation.

Despite the fact that the full ten-item BI is simple, a shorter five-item version has been developed [45] containing the following original items: transfers, bathing, toilet use, stairs, and mobility. A recent validation study suggested that whilst the five-item scale is useful, it is perhaps less accurate at discriminating patients with severe disabilities at admission than the ten-item scale [46].

Glasgow outcome scale (GOS and GOSE)

When was it developed and why?

The Glasgow outcome scale was first described in 1975 and was developed to describe outcome after head injury [47]. It was considered important to have a measure which reflected the impact of brain injury on a patient's quality of life and independence which would be useful in epidemiological studies and for research into patient management.

What does it measure?

In order to make an accurate assessment, a standardized structured interview should be performed with the patient and/or their carer(s) [48]. The results of the interview allow the clinician to grade outcome. The most common form of the scale (known as the five-item GOS or GOS) is broken down into five possible outcomes: good recovery (no symptoms and capable of resuming previous activities with only minor complaints),

patients with large strokes. *Arch Neurol.* 2004;**61**(11): 1677–80.

31. Cote R, Hachinski VC, Shurvell BL, Norris JW, Wolfson C. The Canadian Neurological Scale: a preliminary study in acute stroke. *Stroke.* 1986;**17**(4): 731–7.
32. Muir KW, Weir CJ, Murray GD, Povey C, Lees KR. Comparison of neurological scales and scoring systems for acute stroke prognosis. *Stroke.* 1996;**27**(10): 1817–20.
33. Teasdale G, Drake C, Hunt W. A universal subarachnoid hemorrhage scale: report of a committee of the World Federation of Neurosurgical Societies. *J Neurol Neurosurg Psychiatry.* [Letter]. 1988;**51**:1.
34. Oshiro EM, Walter KA, Piantadosi S, Witham TF, Tamargo RJ. A new subarachnoid hemorrhage grading system based on the Glasgow Coma Scale: a comparison with the Hunt and Hess and World Federation of Neurological Surgeons Scales in a clinical series. *Neurosurgery.* 1997;**41**(1): 140–7; discussion 7–8.
35. Leira EC, Davis PH, Martin CO, *et al.* Improving prediction of outcome in 'good grade' subarachnoid hemorrhage. *Neurosurgery.* 2007;**61**(3): 470–3; discussion 3–4.
36. Rosen DS, Amidei C, Tolentino J, Reilly C, Macdonald RL. Subarachnoid clot volume correlates with age, neurological grade, and blood pressure. *Neurosurgery.* 2007;**60**(2): 259–66; discussion 66–7.
37. Fisher CM, Kistler JP, Davis JM. Relation of cerebral vasospasm to subarachnoid hemorrhage visualized by computerized tomographic scanning. *Neurosurgery.* 1980;**6**(1): 1–9.
38. Smith ML, Abrahams JM, Chandela S, *et al.* Subarachnoid hemorrhage on computed tomography scanning and the development of cerebral vasospasm: the Fisher grade revisited. *Surg Neurol.* 2005;**63**(3): 229–34; discussion 34–5.
39. Hunt WE, Hess RM. Surgical risk as related to time of intervention in the repair of intracranial aneurysms. *J Neurosurg.* 1968;**28**(1): 14–20.
40. Hantson L, Deweerdt W, Dekeyser J, et al. The European Stroke Scale. *Stroke.* 1994;**25**(11): 2215–19.
41. Rankin J. Cerebral vascular accidents in patients over the age of 60. III. Diagnosis and treatment. *Scott Med J.* 1957;**2**(6): 254–68.
42. United Kingdom transient ischaemic attack (UK-TIA) aspirin trial: interim results. UK-TIA Study Group. *Br Med J* (Clin Res Ed). 1988;**296**(6618): 316–20.
43. Quinn TJ, Dawson J, Walters MR, Lees KR. Reliability of the modified Rankin Scale: a systematic review. *Stroke.* 2009;**40**(10): 3393–5.
44. Mahoney FI, Barthel DW. Functional evaluation: The Barthel Index. *Md State Med J.* 1965;**14**: 61–5.
45. Hobart JC, Thompson AJ. The five item Barthel index. *J Neurol Neurosurg Psychiatry.* 2001;**71**(2): 225–30.
46. Hsueh IP, Lin JH, Jeng JS, Hsieh CL. Comparison of the psychometric characteristics of the functional independence measure, 5 item Barthel index, and 10 item Barthel index in patients with stroke. *J Neurol Neurosurg Psychiatry.* 2002;**73**(2): 188–90.
47. Jennett B, Bond M. Assessment of outcome after severe brain damage. *Lancet.* 1975;**1**(7905): 480–4.
48. Wilson JT, Pettigrew LE, Teasdale GM. Structured interviews for the Glasgow Outcome Scale and the extended Glasgow Outcome Scale: guidelines for their use. *J Neurotrauma.* 1998;**15**(8): 573–85.
49. Wilson JT, Edwards P, Fiddes H, Stewart E, Teasdale GM. Reliability of postal questionnaires for the Glasgow Outcome Scale. *J Neurotrauma.* 2002;**19**(9): 999–1005.
50. Govan L, Langhorne P, Weir CJ. Categorizing stroke prognosis using different stroke scales. *Stroke.* 2009;**40**(10): 3396–9.

SECTION 2

Interventions

7

Antiedema therapy in cerebrovascular disease

Dimitre Staykov and Jürgen Bardutzky

Introduction

Pathophysiology of brain edema in cerebrovascular disease

Ischemic brain edema

Severe middle cerebral artery or hemispheric infarctions are commonly associated with a high mortality rate, reaching approximately 80% in intensive care based series, despite maximal conservative treatment [1]. The development of brain edema in the clinical course of such patients is a major factor leading to a fatal outcome [1]. The patients typically present with a severe hemispheric syndrome including eye deviation, hemiplegia, and aphasia or dysarthria. Progressive brain edema, usually manifesting between the second and fourth day after stroke onset, then leads to neurological deterioration caused by tissue shifts compressing the midline structures, eventually leading to transtentorial and uncal herniation.

Two major types of edema generation are distinguished in ischemic stroke, namely cytotoxic (intracellular) and vasogenic (extracellular) edema. Cytotoxic edema develops within minutes in the ischemic core and is mainly mediated by energy failure and anoxic membrane depolarization with accumulation of intracellular sodium, leading to influx of water and cellular swelling. The classical conception of vasogenic edema suggests disruption of the blood-brain barrier (BBB), leading to increased permeability and movement of proteins and fluid from the intravascular space into the intercellular compartment [2]. However, experimental data show that abnormal sodium transport into the extracellular space may also contribute to interstitial swelling, rather than structural changes to the BBB. Those changes in electrolyte balance are probably caused by the shift of ions and water into the cells during the formation of cytotoxic brain edema [3]. Other mechanisms, including aquaporins, free radicals, matrix metalloproteinases, nitric oxide synthase, also seem to play a role in this process. An inflammatory component of BBB damage and edema formation, mediated by inflammatory cells and their mediators, possibly adds to the already mentioned mechanisms in the course of edema formation [3,4]. Different pathophysiological mechanisms, acting during reperfusion of ischemic tissue, may also contribute to aggravation of post-ischemic brain edema.

Posthemorrhagic brain edema

The role of perihemorrhagic edema (PHE) as a cause of morbidity and mortality in intracerebral hemorrhage (ICH) has not been satisfactorily elucidated yet. The recently reported INTERACT study [5] did not show any influence of absolute or relative PHE development on morbidity and mortality. Another study paradoxically showed improved outcome in ICH patients with larger relative PHE in the first hours after ICH [6]. However, the interpretation of this finding is difficult, because PHE

Critical Care of the Stroke Patient, ed. Stefan Schwab, Daniel Hanley, and A. David Mendelow. Published by Cambridge University Press.

seems to reach its maximum mass effect much later [7]. Clinical data on the longitudinal course of PHE are scarce, indicating that it develops immediately after ICH and peaks several days later [5,7–9]. Edema formation may lead to a significant additional mass effect and increase in intracranial pressure, especially in large hematomas, eventually causing herniation and possibly playing a role as a predictor of mortality [7,9,10].

After ICH, products of coagulation and clot breakdown initiate a secondary cascade of damage to perihematomal brain tissue, mainly mediated by thrombine and iron toxicity, blood-brain-barrier damage, inflammation and oxidative stress [10,11]. An inflammatory response in the brain tissue surrounding the hematoma occurs soon after ICH and peaks several days later [12]. The complement system plays a central role in inflammation following ICH, and it is possibly capable of brain injury mediated by cell lysis [13]. Matrix metalloproteinases have also been associated with inflammatory brain injury after ICH [14]. Blood-brain-barrier damage mediated by inflammatory mechanisms, or hydrostatic pressure with consecutive increased permeability and vasogenic edema formation, seems to occur already several hours after ICH [15]. Thrombin, an essential component in the clotting cascade, has also been shown to cause an inflammatory reaction, i.e. inflammatory cell infiltration, microglia activation, proliferation and edema, after injection into the brains of animals [16,17]. Finally, erythrocyte lysis and release of hemoglobin and its breakdown products, mainly iron, seems to further contribute to the pathogenesis of perihematomal damage after ICH [18,19]. Because erythrocyte lysis occurs several days after the hemorrhagic event [20], it is held responsible for the development of late edema and midline shift after ICH [7,9]. All those mechanisms possibly contribute to the formation of perihemorrhagic brain edema.

Medical antiedema therapy

Several conservative treatment strategies have been proposed to reduce brain edema and control intracranial pressure after ischemic stroke. Those strategies include mechanical ventilation and hyperventilation, osmotherapy, thromethamine, and barbiturate administration. However, to date, the efficacy of those conventional therapies to improve clinical outcome has not been tested in a randomized controlled trial [2]. The available data on conservative treatment options for brain edema are reviewed below. Novel promising treatment modalities as hypothermia and decompressive craniectomy are described in detail elsewhere (Chapters 8, 9B, and 14); therefore, they are not addressed within the present chapter.

Osmotherapy

Mannitol

The use of osmotic agents for treatment of brain edema is based on the idea of creating an osmotic pressure gradient across the semipermeable BBB and thereby drawing interstitial and intracellular water from the swollen brain into the intravascular compartment. Mannitol is one of the most widely used osmotic agents for antiedema treatment [2]. In addition to its osmotic effect, mannitol may improve microvascular cerebral blood flow by hemodilution and increased deformability of erythrocytes with a subsequent reduction of cerebral blood volume (CBV) and intracranial pressure (ICP) via vasoconstriction. Mannitol may also cause an increase of cerebral perfusion pressure (CPP) by augmentation of mean arterial pressure, thereby leading to vasoconstriction and reduction in CBV and ICP [21]. On the other hand, usage of hypertonic solutions in stroke patients may have negative effects. Theoretically, the effectiveness of osmotherapy depends on an intact BBB and osmotic agents may cause a preferential shrinkage of the hemisphere not affected by stroke, where the BBB is still intact, thereby leading to a worsening of tissue shifts [22]. Moreover, accumulation of mannitol in damaged brain tissue after repeated boluses may cause a reversal of the osmotic gradient and aggravation of brain edema, as demonstrated in an animal study [23]. However, the quantification of those different mechanisms in both the experimental and the clinical setting is difficult.

The results of animal studies, investigating the effects of mannitol on focal cerebral ischemia and edema formation, have been inconsistent. Most studies found beneficial effects of intravenous mannitol, considering infarct volume, edema formation and elevated ICP [24,25]. Effective mannitol doses varied markedly, ranging between a single bolus of 1 g/kg and repeated boluses of 2.5 g/kg, applied every 4 hours [25]. Other studies could not demonstrate any significant effect of mannitol on brain edema [26], and some studies even found negative effects [23].

Although mannitol has been used for over 40 years, and is the most widely administered osmotic agent for treatment of brain edema worldwide, surprisingly few clinical trials have been performed to investigate its effects on outcome after ischemic stroke and ICH. In a recent Cochrane report [27], a total of 16 studies on this matter have been identified, and only three were found to be unconfounded, truly randomized trials. The only available randomized trial investigating the usage of mannitol after ischemic stroke [28] found no significant effects and was criticized because of methodological issues. The two trials on patients with ICH [29, 30] also could not identify any beneficial effects of mannitol on outcome. However, it should be noted that all three trials used mannitol in a dose lower than 1 g/kg, a dosage below which mannitol did not always reduce ICP [31]. This evidence certainly does not allow a general recommendation of routine mannitol usage in all patients with acute stroke. Nevertheless, the use of mannitol in certain clinical conditions, in carefully selected patients with stroke, e.g. those with reduced level of consciousness and ICP elevation, may be appropriate. However, the use of mannitol in such cases is solely based on small nonrandomized case series, e.g. [32] and experimental data.

Hypertonic saline

Hypertonic saline solutions are considered an alternative to mannitol for antiedema treatment in various underlying conditions [2]. Several mechanisms are held responsible for the ICP-lowering properties of hypertonic saline, the main mechanism being, as in the case with mannitol, osmotic withdrawal of fluid from the brain. Hypertonic saline is considered a more favorable osmotic agent, because the intact BBB is completely impermeable for sodium ions. Moreover, hypertonic saline has the effect of expanding the intravascular volume and increasing mean arterial pressure, leading to improved CPP. In contrast, mannitol rather induces diuresis, thereby leading to secondary volume depletion. Other proposed beneficial mechanisms of action include modulation of inflammatory response and neuron excitation, and improved oxygenation [33]. Adverse effects of hypertonic saline include congestive heart failure, pulmonary edema, hyperchloremic acidosis, hypokaliemia, and hypomagnesemia. The most feared complication of severe hypernatriemia and pontine myelinolysis has been rarely observed in the clinical setting, thereby remaining rather hypothetical [33].

Experimental studies of hypertonic saline in different models of brain injury other than ischemia have brought up conflicting results with regard to antiedema and ICP-lowering properties [34]. In stroke animal studies, results have also been inconsistent. Hypertonic saline (7.5%) has been shown to worsen infarct volume in a rat stroke model, when given as a bolus immediately after reperfusion, with following continuous infusion [35]. In the same stroke model, the authors found a beneficial effect on brain edema when infusion was started 6 or 24 hours after induction of ischemia [36,37].

Most of the currently available clinical studies on usage of hypertonic saline for ICP control have been performed on patients with traumatic brain injury and subarachnoid hemorrhage [38]. The majority of studies utilized a bolus of hypertonic saline rather than continuous infusion, and sodium chloride concentrations varied markedly from 1.7% [39] to 30% [40]. Hypertonic saline has been found to reduce ICP significantly in most of the studies on patients with traumatic brain injury [38,41,42], and there has been also some support that it might be more effective than mannitol [34,43,44]. Studies on patients with subarachnoid hemorrhage have also revealed a significant reduction in ICP [38,45]. Two small case series (n = 9 and 8, respectively) report on the use of hypertonic saline in patients with large middle cerebral artery infarction [46,47]. Those studies also described a significant ICP-lowering effect. One more recent and larger study investigated the use of early continuous hypertonic saline infusions (3%, target sodium 145–155 mmol/l, target osmolality 310–320 mOsm/kg) over a median of 13 (4–23) days in patients with severe cerebrovascular disease (aneurysmal SAH, n = 19; ischemic stroke, n = 29; and ICH, n = 52) [48]. In line with previous research, this study found a reduction in the number of episodes with elevated ICP, as compared to a historical control group with equal underlying disease. There was no difference between the two groups considering adverse events. Interestingly, the authors reported a significantly lower mortality in the group of patients treated with hypertonic saline (17 versus 29.6%, p = 0.037). The same workgroup published an analysis demonstrating reduced PHE edema evolution in ICH patients treated with continuous hypertonic saline, as compared to controls [49]. Despite many limitations and methodological issues being subject of criticism in those studies, the effect of hypertonic saline on ICP decrease seems to be reproducible across different underlying conditions. Unfortunately, randomized controlled trials and thereby convincing evidence of a beneficial effect of this therapy on mortality and clinical outcome are still lacking [38].

Glycerol

The sugar glycerol may have several advantages over other osmotic agents used for antiedema therapy in cerebrovascular disease. First, glycerol has almost no major side effects [50]. Second, although the occurrence of a rebound effect has been controversial [51], glycerol has the theoretical advantage of being metabolized in the brain after passage of the BBB, thereby reducing the risk of rebound brain edema. Third, glycerol administration after stroke has been associated with increase of blood flow to ischemic territories and consecutive improvement in ischemic brain energy metabolism [52].

Glycerol has been evaluated in numerous clinical trials of acute stroke, including patients with ischemic stroke and intracerebral hemorrhage. A Cochrane systematic review identified ten randomized controlled studies comparing a total of 482 glycerol-treated patients with 463 controls [50]. Glycerol treatment was associated with a non-significant reduction in mortality within the scheduled treatment period (odds ratio [OR] 0.78, 95% confidence interval [CI] 0.58–1.06). When looking at patients with probable or definite ischemic stroke, this reduction was significant (OR 0.65, 95% CI 0.44–0.97). There was, however, no evidence of any effect of glycerol on mortality at the end of scheduled follow-up. Functional outcome could be compared in only two of ten trials, and there was a non-significant reduction in odds for death or dependency with glycerol treatment (OR 0.73, 95% CI 0.37–1.42). A major limitation of this meta-analysis becomes obvious at this point, namely, most of the included trials were performed in the pre-CT era, and very few patients received cranial imaging in order to confirm the diagnosis of stroke. Furthermore, only one study considered the extent of brain edema in its inclusion criteria.

In summary, glycerol seems to have a beneficial effect on short-term mortality after acute ischemic stroke, but no long-term efficacy. Based on that data, a general recommendation for its routine usage in patients with acute stroke cannot be made.

Barbiturates

The main effect of barbiturates is based on a decrease in cerebral metabolism. Reduced metabolic rate and consecutively decreased cerebral blood flow and blood volume is believed to contribute to reduction of edema formation and ICP [2]. However, barbiturates may also cause severe side effects such as hypotension, hepatic dysfunction, decreased cardiac performance, or severe infections [53].

Barbiturates have been used in a variety of clinical conditions to control elevated ICP, especially in traumatic brain injury, and case series suggest that this treatment may be helpful in acute ICP crisis; however, the ICP lowering effect of barbiturates appears to be relatively inconsistent [54–56]. A comparative study on 95 head-injured patients has shown that the ICP-lowering properties of barbiturates may be inferior to those of mannitol, and there have been indications that barbiturates may even exert harmful effects in head-injured patients without cerebral hematoma [57]. The use of barbiturates for antiedema treatment in patients with ischemic stroke is based on limited data. In a case series of 21 patients with elevated ICP after middle cerebral artery infarction, barbiturate treatment led to a temporary decrease in ICP; however, there was also a persistent reduction in cerebral oxygen pressure and CPP in all patients [32]. Another study prospectively investigated the use of barbiturates in 60 consecutive patients with middle cerebral artery ischemia and elevated ICP after failure of osmotherapy and hyperventilation [58]. Only five of those patients survived. Although effective ICP lowering was initially reached in 50 patients, sustained ICP control could be achieved only in the five survivors. In addition, a significant reduction in CPP was observed in all patients during barbiturate infusion.

As far as no randomized controlled studies on that matter exist up to date, the usage of barbiturates for ICP lowering seems to offer limited and short-lasting success, which often does not lead to sustained ICP control. The benefit of this treatment may be outweighed by severe adverse effects, especially hypotension with consecutive decline in CPP.

Hyperventilation

Hypocapnia (achieved with hyperventilation) induces ICP decrease by reduction in cerebral blood volume via cerebral arterial vasoconstriction. The effects of hyperventilation on CBV and CBF are potent: CBF decreases by approximately 3% per mmHg decrease in PaCO2, as demonstrated in patients with head trauma [59]. The ICP lowering potential of hyperventilation has been shown in numerous case series of traumatic brain-injured patients, with duration of hyperventilation ranging between 10 and 30 minutes [60]. Although hyperventilation is still being widely used, especially in the management of head-injured children and adults, there is no proof beyond clinical experience with incipient herniation that hyperventilation improves neurological outcome [61]. On the contrary, hyperventilation can even be harmful by causing or worsening cerebral ischemia [62]. Apart from vasoconstriction, mechanisms like impairment of cerebral oxygenation and metabolism have been suggested to play a role in this process [2,62,63]. Considering the large body of evidence indicating the possible deleterious effects of hyperventilation (hypocapnia) on cerebral blood flow, oxygenation and metabolism, and the lack of evidence of any beneficial effects on outcome, this treatment cannot be recommended in a setting other than the emergent management of life-threatening intracranial hypertension, or to facilitate intraoperative neurosurgery [61].

Tromethamine

Tromethamine, a cerebrospinal fluid penetrating agent, is believed to neutralize acidosis-induced vasodilation of cerebral vessels, thereby reducing ICP. Beyond ICP-lowering properties, animal studies on traumatic brain injury have suggested beneficial effects of tromethamine on edema formation and cerebral energy metabolism [64]. In animal models of focal cerebral ischemia, tromethamine infusion was associated with a significant reduction of infarct size, brain edema and lactate concentration [65]. To date, clinical studies have failed to demonstrate a beneficial effect of tromethamine treatment on outcome. However, a prospective, randomized, placebo controlled trial on 149 patients with traumatic brain injury has confirmed the ICP-lowering properties of tromethamine, showing a significantly lower incidence of ICP elevation episodes and requirement of barbiturate coma [66].

Although there is a lack of controlled studies on tromethamine in the setting of acute stroke, some authors consider it as an option for treatment of elevated ICP and brain edema after large middle cerebral artery infarction [51].

Elevated head position

Moderate elevation of the head is considered standard practice in the management of increased ICP, although this technique has not been investigated in randomized, controlled trials. The mechanism of ICP decrease is thought to be based on reduction of venous hydrostatic pressure and volume, and increase of venous outflow at the cranial level [2]. Therefore, stroke patients are traditionally nursed in a moderately elevated head position (15 to 45°). Such recommendations are mainly derived from pathophysiological considerations and some studies on patients with head trauma.

Head elevation, however, may result in sustained reduction in mean arterial pressure and CPP with the risk of ischemic brain damage [67], an issue of particular importance in patients with ischemic stroke. A small case series of 12 patients with large supratentorial stroke investigated the effects of upper body position on ICP and CPP and could demonstrate that mean ICP decreased only slightly from 13 mmHg in the horizontal position to 11.4 mmHg at 30° backrest elevation, whereas CPP markedly declined from 77 to 64 mmHg [68]. Another study investigated the influence of body position on the residual blood flow velocity in affected vessels in patients with acute stroke (n = 20) [69]. Return to flat position led to a significant increase in residual flow velocity in all patients and immediate neurological improvement in three patients [69].

Based on those data, the routine use of elevated head positioning cannot be recommended for patients with stroke, because the increase in ICP in the horizontal position is probably not of clinical significance, whereas reduction of CPP with head elevation may be harmful.

Steroids

A Cochrane database systematic review evaluated the available evidence on corticosteroid treatment in acute ischemic stroke [70]. A total of 22 trials on patients with presumed ischemic stroke were identified, seven of which were considered acceptable for further analysis, comprising in total 453 patients. Notably, in only one study, computed tomography was used to exclude hemorrhagic stroke. The authors concluded that the analyzed trials do not provide any evidence of a beneficial effect of steroid treatment on mortality or functional outcome in those patients. Another Cochrane review addressed corticosteroid treatment after subarachnoid or intracerebral hemorrhage, including 256 SAH and 206 ICH patients [71]. Analyzing eight trials, the authors found no sufficient evidence of a beneficial or adverse effect of steroids in SAH or ICH patients, whereas there were indications that steroids may increase the risk of serious adverse events. Based on those data of overall poor quality, steroids cannot be recommended for routine treatment of acute ischemic or hemorrhagic stroke.

Given the mode of action of steroids, namely their antiedematous effect on vasogenic edema, it has been hypothesized that patients with significant vasogenic edema secondary to large ischemic infarction could theoretically benefit from such a treatment, whereas steroids would rather be ineffective in patients with small strokes [2,70]. However, this issue has not yet been addressed specifically in a clinical trial.

Emerging specific approaches in intracerebral hemorrhage

Anti-inflammatory treatment

The inflammatory response in the perihemorrhagic zone causes damage to brain tissue and plays an important role in the pathogenesis of PHE after ICH [10,13]. Various mediators of inflammation act within the perihemorrhagic zone, and some of them represent potential treatment targets in ICH. Animal studies have demonstrated an effect of the direct thrombin inhibitor argatroban for reduction of secondary brain injury after ICH [72,73]. Antithrombin treatment for ICH seems somewhat paradoxical, because of the central role of thrombin in coagulation and thereby prevention of hematoma expansion. However, ICH growth most frequently occurs within 24 hours of the initial bleeding event and thrombin is released from the intracerebral clot for two weeks after bleeding onset [74]. Therefore, there might be a time window after the hematoma has stopped expanding, when thrombin inhibitors could be administered [10,74]. The complement cascade plays an important role in secondary brain injury after ICH by triggering leukocyte infiltration, microglial activation, disruption of the BBB, and development of PHE [13]. On the other hand, this response is central for the clearance of erythrocytes and posthemorrhagic cellular debris and thereby beneficial for recovery after ICH. Animal studies suggest that those different effects are possibly mediated by different components of the complement system [75]. Attenuation of PHE development by means of complement depletion or selective deactivation has also been demonstrated in experimental ICH [76,77]. Therefore, selective complement inhibition represents an attractive strategy for reducing inflammation after ICH and should be the subject of further research.

Deferoxamine

As iron toxicity plays an important role in perilesional brain damage and PHE formation after ICH, it represents a logical treatment target with a strong pathophysiological background. Until now, there is extensive experimental evidence showing that deferoxamine, an iron chelator, can reduce hemoglobin induced neurotoxicity after ICH [78]. This has been demonstrated in rat ICH models, where deferoxamine could reduce PHE formation and improve functional outcome [79,80]. Initial clinical data from an ongoing study (www.clinicaltrials.gov, NCT00598572) indicate that deferoxamine probably reduces oxidative stress in ICH patients [78].

REFERENCES

1. Hacke, W., *et al.*, 'Malignant' middle cerebral artery territory infarction: clinical course and prognostic signs. *Arch Neurol*, 1996;**53**(4): 309–15.
2. Bardutzky, J., S. Schwab, Antiedema therapy in ischemic stroke. *Stroke*, 2007;**38**(11): 3084–94.
3. Simard, J. M., *et al.*, Brain oedema in focal ischaemia: molecular pathophysiology and theoretical implications. *Lancet Neurol*, 2007;**6**(3): 258–68.
4. Ayata, C., A. H., Ropper, Ischaemic brain oedema. *J Clin Neurosci*, 2002;**9**(2): 113–24.
5. Arima, H., *et al.*, Significance of perihematomal edema in acute intracerebral hemorrhage: the INTERACT trial. *Neurology*, 2009;**73**(23): 1963–8.
6. Gebel, J. M. Jr., *et al.*, Relative edema volume is a predictor of outcome in patients with hyperacute spontaneous intracerebral hemorrhage. *Stroke*, 2002;**33**(11): 2636–41.
7. Staykov, D., *et al.*, Natural course of perihemorrhagic edema after intracerebral hemorrhage. *Stroke*, 2011;**42** (9): 2625–9.
8. Inaji, M., *et al.*, Chronological changes of perihematomal edema of human intracerebral hematoma. *Acta Neurochir Suppl*, 2003;**86**:445–8.
9. Zazulia, A. R., *et al.*, Progression of mass effect after intracerebral hemorrhage. *Stroke*, 1999;**30**(6): 1167–73.
10. Xi, G., R. F. Keep, J. T. Hoff, Mechanisms of brain injury after intracerebral haemorrhage. *Lancet Neurol*, 2006;**5**(1): 53–63.
11. Nakamura, T., *et al.*, Iron-induced oxidative brain injury after experimental intracerebral hemorrhage. *Acta Neurochir Suppl*, 2006;**96**: 194–8.
12. Xue, M., M. R. DelBigio, Intracerebral injection of autologous whole blood in rats: time course of inflammation and cell death. *Neurosci Lett*, 2000;**283**(3): 230–2.
13. Ducruet, A. F., *et al.*, The complement cascade as a therapeutic target in intracerebral hemorrhage. *Exp Neurol*, 2009;**219**(2): 398–403.
14. Xue, M., V. W. Yong, Matrix metalloproteinases in intracerebral hemorrhage. *Neurol Res*, 2008;**30**(8): 775–82.
15. Yang, G. Y., *et al.*, Experimental intracerebral hemorrhage: relationship between brain edema, blood flow, and blood-brain barrier permeability in rats. *J Neurosurg*, 1994;**81**(1): 93–102.
16. Lee, K. R., *et al.*, Edema from intracerebral hemorrhage: the role of thrombin. *J Neurosurg*, 1996;**84**(1): 91–6.
17. Lee, K. R., *et al.*, Mechanisms of edema formation after intracerebral hemorrhage: effects of thrombin on cerebral blood flow, blood-brain barrier permeability, and cell survival in a rat model. *J Neurosurg*, 1997;**86**(2): 272–8.
18. Huang, F. P., *et al.*, Brain edema after experimental intracerebral hemorrhage: role of hemoglobin degradation products. *J Neurosurg*, 2002;**96**(2): 287–93.
19. Wagner, I., *et al.*, Radiopacity of intracerebral hemorrhage correlates with perihemorrhagic edema. *Eur J Neurol*, 2012;**19**(3): 525–8.
20. Enzmann, D. R. *et al.*, Natural history of experimental intracerebral hemorrhage: sonography, computed tomography and neuropathology. *AJNR Am J Neuroradiol*, 1981;**2** (6): 517–26.
21. Diringer, M. N., A. R. Zazulia, Osmotic therapy: fact and fiction. *Neurocrit Care*, 2004;**1**(2): 219–33.
22. Videen, T. O., *et al.*, Mannitol bolus preferentially shrinks non-infarcted brain in patients with ischemic stroke. *Neurology*, 2001;**57**(11): 2120–2.
23. Kaufmann, A. M., E. R. Cardoso, Aggravation of vasogenic cerebral edema by multiple-dose mannitol. *J Neurosurg*, 1992;**77**(4): 584–9.
24. Karibe, H., G. J. Zarow, P. R. Weinstein, Use of mild intraischemic hypothermia versus mannitol to reduce infarct size after temporary middle cerebral artery occlusion in rats. *J Neurosurg*, 1995;**83**(1): 93–8.
25. Paczynski, R. P., *et al.*, Multiple-dose mannitol reduces brain water content in a rat model of cortical infarction. *Stroke*, 1997;**28**(7): 1437–43; discussion 1444.
26. Oktem, I. S., *et al.*, Therapeutic effect of tirilazad mesylate (U-74006F), mannitol, and their combination on experimental ischemia. *Res Exp Med (Berl)*, 2000;**199**(4): 231–42.
27. Bereczki, D., *et al.*, Mannitol for acute stroke. *Cochrane Database Syst Rev*, 2007;(3): CD001153.

28. Santambrogio, S., *et al.*, Is there a real treatment for stroke? Clinical and statistical comparison of different treatments in 300 patients. *Stroke*, 1978;**9**(2): 130–2.
29. Kalita, J., *et al.*, Effect of mannitol on regional cerebral blood flow in patients with intracerebral hemorrhage. *J Neurol Sci*, 2004;**224**(1–2): 19–22.
30. Misra, U. K., *et al.*, Mannitol in intracerebral hemorrhage: a randomized controlled study. *J Neurol Sci*, 2005;**234**(1–2): 41–5.
31. James, H. E., Methodology for the control of intracranial pressure with hypertonic mannitol. *Acta Neurochir (Wien)*, 1980;**51**(3–4): 161–72.
32. Steiner, T., *et al.*, Multimodal online monitoring in middle cerebral artery territory stroke. *Stroke*, 2001;**32**(11): 2500–6.
33. Kempski, O., Hypertonic saline and stroke. *Crit Care Med*, 2005;**33**(1): 259–60.
34. Rabinstein, A. A., Treatment of cerebral edema. *Neurologist*, 2006;**12**(2): 59–73.
35. Bhardwaj, A., *et al.*, Hypertonic saline worsens infarct volume after transient focal ischemia in rats. *Stroke*, 2000;**31**(7): 1694–701.
36. Toung, T. J., *et al.*, Osmotherapy with hypertonic saline attenuates water content in brain and extracerebral organs. *Crit Care Med*, 2007;**35**(2): 526–31.
37. Toung, T. J., *et al.*, Global brain water increases after experimental focal cerebral ischemia: effect of hypertonic saline. *Crit Care Med*, 2002;**30**(3): 644–9.
38. Strandvik, G. F., Hypertonic saline in critical care: a review of the literature and guidelines for use in hypotensive states and raised intracranial pressure. *Anaesthesia*, 2009;**64**(9): 990–1003.
39. Simma, B., *et al.*, A prospective, randomized, and controlled study of fluid management in children with severe head injury: lactated Ringer's solution versus hypertonic saline. *Crit Care Med*, 1998;**26**(7): 1265–70.
40. Murphy, N., *et al.*, The effect of hypertonic sodium chloride on intracranial pressure in patients with acute liver failure. *Hepatology*, 2004;**39**(2): 464–70.
41. Munar, F., *et al.*, Cerebral hemodynamic effects of 7.2% hypertonic saline in patients with head injury and raised intracranial pressure. *J Neurotrauma*, 2000;**17**(1): 41–51.
42. Schatzmann, C., *et al.*, Treatment of elevated intracranial pressure by infusions of 10% saline in severely head injured patients. *Acta Neurochir Suppl*, 1998;**71**: 31–3.
43. Kamel, H., *et al.*, Hypertonic saline versus mannitol for the treatment of elevated intracranial pressure: a meta-analysis of randomized clinical trials. *Crit Care Med*, 2011;**39**(3): 554–9.
44. Mortazavi, M. M., *et al.*, Hypertonic saline for treating raised intracranial pressure:literature review with meta-analysis. *J Neurosurg*, 2012;**116**(1): 210–21.
45. Tseng, M. Y., *et al.*, Enhancement of cerebral blood flow using systemic hypertonic saline therapy improves outcome in patients with poor-grade spontaneous subarachnoid hemorrhage. *J Neurosurg*, 2007;**107**(2): 274–82.
46. Schwarz, S., *et al.*, Effects of hypertonic (10%) saline in patients with raised intracranial pressure after stroke. *Stroke*, 2002;**33**(1): 136–40.
47. Schwarz, S., *et al.*, Effects of hypertonic saline hydroxyethyl starch solution and mannitol in patients with increased intracranial pressure after stroke. *Stroke*, 1998;**29**(8): 1550–5.
48. Hauer, E. M., *et al.*, Early continuous hypertonic saline infusion in patients with severe cerebrovascular disease. *Crit Care Med*, 2011;**39**(7): 1766–72.
49. Wagner, I., *et al.*, Effects of continuous hypertonic saline infusion on perihemorrhagic edema evolution. *Stroke*, 2011;**42**(6): 1540–5.
50. Righetti, E., *et al.*, Glycerol for acute stroke. *Cochrane Database Syst Rev*, 2004;(2): CD000096.
51. Steiner, T., P. Ringleb, W. Hacke, Treatment options for large hemispheric stroke. *Neurology*, 2001;**57**(5 Suppl 2): S61–8.
52. Meyer, J. S., *et al.*, Circulatory and metabolic effects of glycerol infusion in patients with recent cerebral infarction. *Circulation*, 1975;**51**(4): 701–12.
53. Juttler, E., *et al.*, Clinical review: Therapy for refractory intracranial hypertension in ischaemic stroke. *Crit Care*, 2007;**11**(5): 231.
54. Woodcock, J., A. H. Ropper, S. K. Kennedy, High dose barbiturates in non-traumatic brain swelling: ICP reduction and effect on outcome. *Stroke*, 1982;**13**(6): 785–7.
55. Rockoff, M. A., L. F. Marshall, H. M. Shapiro, High-dose barbiturate therapy in humans: a clinical review of 60 patients. *Ann Neurol*, 1979;**6**(3): 194–9.
56. Cormio, M., *et al.*, Cerebral hemodynamic effects of pentobarbital coma in head-injured patients. *J Neurotrauma*, 1999;**16**(10): 927–36.
57. Schwartz, M. L., *et al.*, The University of Toronto head injury treatment study: a prospective, randomized comparison of pentobarbital and mannitol. *Can J Neurol Sci*, 1984;**11**(4): 434–40.
58. Schwab, S., *et al.*, Barbiturate coma in severe hemispheric stroke: useful or obsolete? *Neurology*, 1997;**48**(6): 1608–13.
59. Cold, G. E., Cerebral blood flow in acute head injury. The regulation of cerebral blood flow and metabolism during the acute phase of head injury, and its significance for therapy. *Acta Neurochir Suppl (Wien)*, 1990;**49**: 1–64.

60. Stocchetti, N., *et al.*, Hyperventilation in head injury: a review. *Chest*, 2005;**127**(5): 1812–27.
61. Curley, G., B. P. Kavanagh, J. G. Laffey, Hypocapnia and the injured brain: more harm than benefit. *Crit Care Med*, 2010;**38**(5): 1348–59.
62. Marion, D. W., *et al.*, Effect of hyperventilation on extracellular concentrations of glutamate, lactate, pyruvate, and local cerebral blood flow in patients with severe traumatic brain injury. *Crit Care Med*, 2002;**30**(12): 2619–25.
63. Imberti, R., G. Bellinzona, M. Langer, Cerebral tissue PO2 and SjvO2 changes during moderate hyperventilation in patients with severe traumatic brain injury. *J Neurosurg*, 2002;**96**(1): 97–102.
64. Yoshida, K., A. Marmarou, Effects of tromethamine and hyperventilation on brain injury in the CAT. *J Neurosurg*, 1991;**74**(1): 87–96.
65. Nagao, S., *et al.*, Effect of tris-(hydroxymethyl)-aminomethane on experimental focal cerebral ischemia. *Exp Brain Res*, 1996;**111**(1): 51–6.
66. Wolf, A. L., *et al.*, Effect of THAM upon outcome in severe head injury: a randomized prospective clinical trial. *J Neurosurg*, 1993;**78**(1): 54–9.
67. Rosner, M. J., I. B. Coley, Cerebral perfusion pressure, intracranial pressure, and head elevation. *J Neurosurg*, 1986;**65**(5): 636–41.
68. Schwarz, S., *et al.*, Effects of body position on intracranial pressure and cerebral perfusion in patients with large hemispheric stroke. *Stroke*, 2002;**33**(2): 497–501.
69. Wojner-Alexander, A. W., *et al.*, Heads down: flat positioning improves blood flow velocity in acute ischemic stroke. *Neurology*, 2005;**64**(8): 1354–7.
70. Qizilbash, N., S. L. Lewington, J. M. Lopez-Arrieta, Corticosteroids for acute ischaemic stroke. *Cochrane Database Syst Rev*, 2002;(2): CD000064.
71. Feigin, V. L., *et al.*, Corticosteroids for aneurysmal subarachnoid haemorrhage and primary intracerebral haemorrhage. *Cochrane Database Syst Rev*, 2005;(3): CD004583.
72. Nagatsuna, T., *et al.*, Systemic administration of argatroban reduces secondary brain damage in a rat model of intracerebral hemorrhage histopathological assessment. *Cerebrovasc Dis*, 2005;**19**(3): 192–200.
73. Kitaoka, T., *et al.*, Delayed argatroban treatment reduces edema in a rat model of intracerebral hemorrhage. *Stroke*, 2002;**33**(12): 3012–18.
74. Matsuoka, H., R. Hamada, Role of thrombin in CNS damage associated with intracerebral haemorrhage: opportunity for pharmacological intervention? *CNS Drugs*, 2002;**16**(8): 509–16.
75. Wu, G., F. P. Huang, Effects of venom defibrase on brain edema after intracerebral hemorrhage in rats. *Acta Neurochir Suppl*, 2005;**95**: 381–7.
76. Xi, G., *et al.*, Brain edema after intracerebral hemorrhage: the effects of systemic complement depletion. *Acta Neurochir Suppl*, 2002;**81**: 253–6.
77. Rynkowski, M. A., *et al.*, C3a receptor antagonist attenuates brain injury after intracerebral hemorrhage. *J Cereb Blood Flow Metab*, 2009;**29**(1): 98–107.
78. Selim, M., Deferoxamine mesylate: a new hope for intracerebral hemorrhage: from bench to clinical trials. *Stroke*, 2009;**40**(3 Suppl): S90–1.
79. Nakamura, T., *et al.*, Deferoxamine-induced attenuation of brain edema and neurological deficits in a rat model of intracerebral hemorrhage. *J Neurosurg*, 2004;**100**(4): 672–8.
80. Okauchi, M., *et al.*, Effects of deferoxamine on intracerebral hemorrhage-induced brain injury in aged rats. *Stroke*, 2009;**40**(5): 1858–63.

8

Decompressive surgery in cerebrovascular disease

Katayoun Vahedi and François Proust

Introduction

In the acute phase of stroke, brain herniation secondary to elevated intracranial pressure (ICP) is the major cause of death. In ischemic stroke, elevated ICP is the consequence of either hemorrhagic transformation or progression of brain ischemic edema. Both situations are the consequences of cerebral capillary dysfunction and progressive alteration in the permeability of the blood-brain barrier [1]. Brain ischemic edema has a progressive course during the first hours and days after a focal ischemia with a maximum on days three to five [2]. It causes mass effect with midline shift, raised intracranial pressure, alteration of cerebral perfusion pressure, damages to normal brain tissues and finally brain herniation and brain death in some cases of large middle cerebral artery (MCA) infarction (Fig. 8.1). This type of stroke has been called malignant MCA infarction with a mortality ranging between 50% and 80% in observational studies and 70% in randomized trials that included patients less than 60 years of age [2,3]. Almost all deaths are related to brain herniation and occur during the first days after stroke onset, particularly in younger patients.

In the same way, space-occupying edematous cerebellar infarction may lead to death or severe disability by brainstem compression, obstructive hydrocephalus and brain transforaminal or transtentorial herniation secondary to ischemic edema. Some patients may deteriorate as late as 10 days after stroke onset.

In hemorrhagic stroke elevated ICP results from the growing hematoma and its surrounding edema. Ultimately other complications such as brainstem compression and hydrocephalus occur and lead to brain death. Hospital mortality is up to 30% and about 50% of patients survive at 1 year and mostly with residual disability.

Antiedematous drugs such as osmotic agents, corticosteroids and diuretics have failed in clinical studies to show benefit in preventing brain herniation or reducing mortality or improving outcome in the acute phase of stroke, although some may temporarily reduce ICP.

In recent years more interest has come from decompressive surgery to treat elevated ICP in the acute phase of different varieties of cerebrovascular diseases with poor prognosis. The aim of such an invasive neurosurgical procedure is to save lives but also to enable survival with acceptable residual disability. Enthusiasm came from the results of a pooled analysis of three randomized trials of hemicraniectomy in malignant MCA infarction showing a considerable benefit of surgery on mortality, with the majority of survivors living with moderate to moderately severe disability.

The procedure of decompressive hemicraniectomy

Historically, in the last part of the nineteenth century, the indication of decompressive hemicraniectomy

Critical Care of the Stroke Patient, ed. Stefan Schwab, Daniel Hanley, and A. David Mendelow. Published by Cambridge University Press.

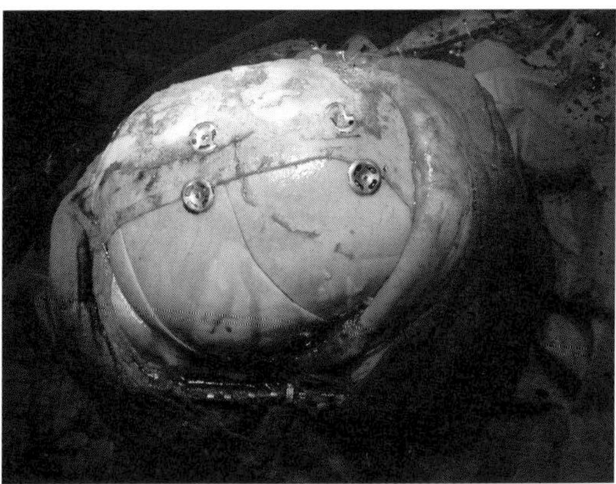

Fig. 8.1 Perioperative view showing a bilateral autologous osseous graft of the cranial vault.

(DC) was inoperable brain tumors. Progressively, this surgical procedure has been used to manage other patients with uncontrollably high ICP. The procedure consists of the removal of a large bone flap from either one or both sides of the skull, followed by a large opening of the dura mater to relieve the ICP [4,5]. The main aim is to allow the outward brain expansion and to avoid compromising the healthy brain areas by midline shift. In addition, normalization of ICP results in an improvement of the cerebral pressure perfusion and a raise in the cerebral blood flow which leads to better oxygenation of the brain tissue [6,7].

Extended bone decompression

There are many variations in the surgical procedure of decompressive craniectomy (DC). The main factors to be considered include the involved hemisphere, the location of the lesion and its size. The bone flap must be sufficiently large to prevent additional ischemic lesions and may be uni- or bilateral. A unilateral bone flap must expose the length of the cranium, including parts of the frontal, parietal, temporal and occipital squama [8]. Under general anesthesia, the patient has to be placed in supine position, a block under the shoulder with head in rotation to expose the side of the craniectomy, in straightness above the heart in order to facilitate venous drainage. A skin 'crossbow' incision allows a large exposition of the whole length of the cranium (Fig. 8.1). The scalp has to be tipped forward and separated from the pericranium. The size of craniectomy is of crucial importance, with an antero-posterior diameter of at least 12 cm recommended for adequate gain in cranial volume. A minimum diameter of 10 cm enables a gain in cranial volume of 50 ml [9]. The bone flap, of oval shape, must expand into the temporal base and reach 3 cm away from the midline along the superior longitudinal sinus, and avoid the frontal sinus. The margins of the craniectomy may be subject to refinement by placing vascular channels around the major vessels, or by its inclination in order to avoid acute angle between the brain surface and the bone limits [10].

In case of bilateral craniectomy, the patient has to be placed in supine position under general anesthesia, with head in straightness above the heart in order to facilitate venous drainage [11]. The skin incision is cut posterior to the frontal hairline from zygoma to zygoma. The scalp is tipped forward and separated from the pericranium to preserve the two supra orbital nerves. A bifrontal flap is performed from the floor of the anterior cranial fossa to the coronal suture posteriorly and to the pterion laterally. It is not necessary to leave an osseous bridge in the midline over the superior sagittal sinus.

According to the ICP monitoring, the management of the large bone flap may be either an immediate cranioplasty or a secondary cranioplasty. The preservation in place of the bone flap – immediate cranioplasty – uses the procedure of hinge cranioplasty or slack sutures allowing a cerebral hernia without midline shift [12]. For a secondary cranioplasty, the removed bone flap should be stored either frozen in a bone bank or in a subcutaneous cavity in the abdominal fat or in the controlateral subgaleal space of the head.

Large dural opening

In the past, craniectomies were performed without dural opening, but now it is recognized that the dura mater must be largely opened as scarification of the dura mater alone is not sufficient to achieve brain decompression [13,14]. The dural incision, after intraoperative osmotic therapy, follows the limits of the bone flap at 1 cm from the osseous margins. Small peripheral incisions orthogonal to the dural opening prevent the pia mater trauma of the expanding brain. But the recommendations as regards the dura mater envelope are variable: cruciform incision or sectioning of the falx [15,16].

Expansive duraplasty is recommended for maximum expansion of the brain. This operative procedure is performed under ICP monitoring. The dural patch, using an autologous large flap of pericranial tissue or temporal fascia, is inserted on the dural margin by sutures; many types of dural graft have been proposed such as periosteum, fascia lata or miscellaneous substitutes. The aim of the duraplasty is to allow an easy cleavage plane for the cranioplasty. However, the habits as regards the duraplasty are variable. The dura mater may also be left open, resting on top of the brain and lined with a surgical sheet without increasing the risk of cerebrospinal fluid (CSF) leak [11]. This technique of rapid closure appears safe by comparison with the watertight suturing of dural graft [17].

Intracranial pressure monitoring

ICP monitoring helps the management of uncontrollably high ICP in patients who undergo DC, by taking into account the new cerebral perfusion pressure and compliance [18]. We recommend the routine insertion of a pressure probe in the contralateral side either in the preoperative period for proper indication of DC or at the start of the surgical procedure to follow the ICP at each step of the DC from the skin incision to the management of cranioplasty and in the immediate postoperative period.

Decompressive craniectomy of the posterior fossa

For decompressive surgery of the small infratentorial space, the principle is to combine an external ventricular derivation to a large posterior fossa craniectomy with or without cerebellar resection. The dura mater, opened in Y-shape, must be left largely suspended into the muscles and the duraplasty should be avoided because of the major risk of infection. For this location, a secondary cranioplasty is not necessary.

Indications of surgical decompression

Acute ischemic stroke

Hemispheric infarction

The earliest studies on the relevance of decompressive surgery in malignant MCA infarction were observational studies (either retrospective or more recently prospective) that suggested that hemicraniectomy could be associated with higher survival and acceptable outcome [19]. The surgical procedure consists of removing, ipsilateral to the stroke, a bone flap as large as possible but with no resection of swollen ischemic brain tissue (see above and Fig. 8.2). It aims at decreasing intracranial pressure by means of an increase in the intracranial volume, therefore preventing brain temporal herniation and subsequent brain death.

Although it is essential to prevent brain death in this severe form of stroke, it is also of crucial importance to leave survivors with no extremely severe residual disability.

Until recently data from randomized controlled trials were missing for non-biased comparison between surgery and no surgery. Thus the decision of hemicraniectomy was extremely controversial since questions regarding the outcome of patients were considered unanswered, particularly whether patients could have 'acceptable' residual disability and good quality of life. In addition, because of the very sudden onset of a malignant MCA infarction, it is impossible to consider the preference of the patient at the time of the decision.

Recently the effect of early decompressive surgery on functional outcome in patients with malignant hemispheric infarction has been studied in three European randomized controlled trials: the French DECIMAL (DEcompressive Craniectomy In MALignant middle cerebral artery infarcts), the German DESTINY (DEcompressive Surgery for the Treatment of malignant INfarction of the middle cerebral arterY), and the Dutch HAMLET (Hemicraniectomy After Middle

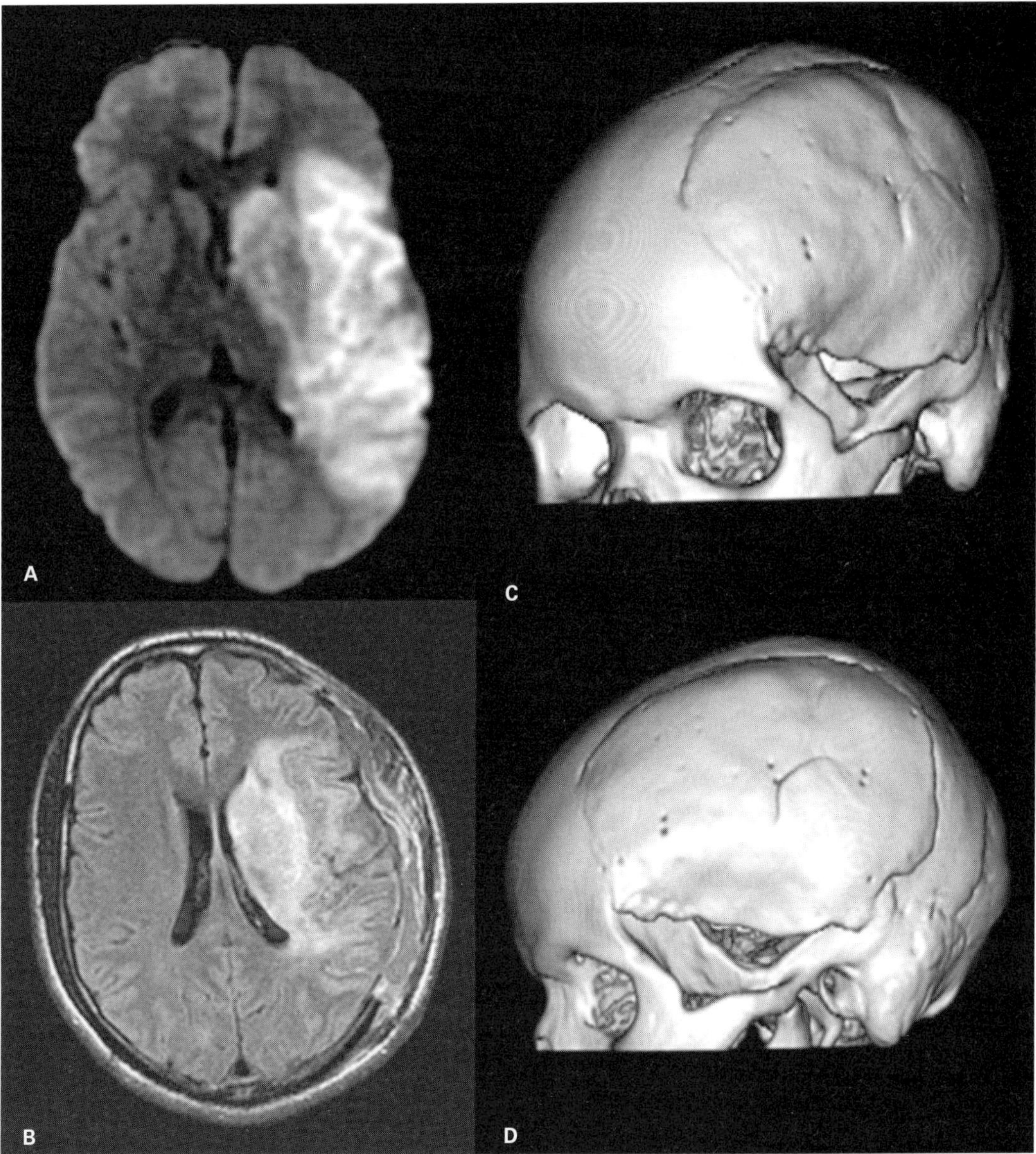

Fig. 8.2 Right malignant middle cerebral artery infarction on diffusion-weighted imaging in a 24-year-old man (A), emergency large decompressive hemicraniectomy on axial FLAIR (B), and secondary cranioplasty on CT scan 3D volume (C and D).

cerebral artery infarction with Life-threatening Edema Trial) [20–22a].

After about half of the calculated sample size had participated in each of the three trials (between 2002 and 2007), they stopped prematurely for different reasons (difficulty with recruitment, results of interim analyses, ethical concerns). However, while the three trials were still recruiting and their final results strictly unknown, the principal investigators decided on a novel protocol of prospective pooled analysis of the individual data from the three trials by an independent research group. This was possible as all three trials shared a common methodology with identical primary hypothesis and primary outcome measure (i.e. significantly fewer patients alive with severe disability at 1 year in the surgery group). Importantly, this pooled analysis would allow the necessary statistical power by sharing individual data and thus reducing the number of patients needed in each therapeutic group.

Indeed the pooled analysis included a total of 93 patients and showed very significantly more patients alive with a moderate residual disability (modified Rankin score of 2 or 3 at 1-year follow-up) in the surgery group compared to the medical group with an absolute risk reduction of 23% (2–41) [3] (Table 8.1 and Table 8.2). In total mortality was reduced by 50% (33–67) by surgery. There were also more patients alive with a moderately severe residual disability (Rankin 4) after surgery, whereas the number of patients with a severe residual disability was not increased and remained small (about 5%) [3].

In the DECIMAL trial, which included younger patients than the two other trials, younger age was correlated with better outcome on the modified Rankin scores in the surgery group [20]. But without surgery the best predictor of bad outcome (death) was the volume of infarction measured on baseline diffusion weighted imaging (DWI) within 24 hours of symptom onset. No patients with a volume more than 210 cm^3 survived, whereas all patients screened but not included because of a DWI infarct volume less than 145 cm^3 survived [20]. In the

Table 8.1 Score description of the modified Rankin scale (MRS)

0 = No symptoms at all
1 = No significant disability despite symptoms; able to carry out all usual duties and activities
2 = Slight disability; unable to carry out all previous activities, but able to look after own affairs without assistance
3 = Moderate disability; requiring some help, but able to walk without assistance
4 = Moderately severe disability; unable to walk without assistance and unable to attend to own bodily needs without assistance
5 = Severe disability; bedridden, incontinent and requiring constant nursing care and attention
6 = Dead

Table 8.2 Randomized controlled trials of decompressive hemicraniectomy versus standard medical treatment in malignant middle cerebral artery infarction

Authors	Timing of surgery from stroke onset	No. of patients	Follow-up	Absolute risk reduction, % (95% CI) for MRS 4–6	Absolute risk reduction, % (95% CI) for MRS 5–6	Absolute risk reduction, % (95% CI) for death
Vahedi *et al.* 2007 [3]	< 30 hours	38	1 year	28 (− 1 to 57)	53 (26 to 80)	53 (26 to 80)
Juttler *et al.* 2007 [7]	< 36 hours	32	1 year	20 (−12 to 53)	43 (12 to 74)	36 (5 to 67)
Hofmeijer *et al.* 2009 [22b]	< 99 hours	64	1 year	0 (−21 to 21)	19 (−5 to 43)	38 (15 to 60)
Prospective pooled analysis [3]	< 48 hours	91	1 year	23 (5 to 41)	51 (34 to 69)	50 (33 to 67)
Pooled analysis [12]	< 48 hours	109	1 year	16 (−0 to 33)	42 (25 to 59)	50 (34 to 66)

MRS = modified Rankin score; CI = confidence interval

surgery group, baseline infarct volume on DWI was also a prognostic factor with a non-significant trend toward better outcome with smaller infarct volume [20].

After the results of the pooled analysis, HAMLET was the only trial that continued patient recruitment for those randomized after 48 hours (and before 96 hours) of stroke onset, but finally it had to completely stop inclusions as interim analyses suggested that the initial calculated sample size of 112 patients would lack statistical power to show significant differences between the two groups [22b]. At the time of the premature end of the HAMLET trial, 64 patients were randomized. The final results showed no benefit of late surgery (< 99 hours) over medical management for the functional outcome (survival with no severe disability) but significant benefit on survival with an absolute risk reduction of 38%, p = 0.002.

It should be noted that in all three randomized trials any serious co-existent disorder that may interfere with the short-term and long-term outcome after hemicraniectomy, as well as any significant pre-existing disability that may interfere with functional outcome and rehabilitation, were exclusion criteria. This should be considered whenever an individual decision of hemicraniectomy has to be taken. Indeed a favorable outcome after decompressive hemicraniectomy does not mean complete recovery but recovery with disability. The debate is ongoing about what is an 'acceptable' disability and who should decide, the patient him or herself, the relatives or the physicians? Is a modified Rankin 4 (moderately severe disability) an 'acceptable' disability [23]? This will depend on many individual and subjective factors that can hardly be evaluated in randomized trials. In addition, quantitative measurements of quality of life are lacking validation in severe stroke patients. Residual neuropsychological disability including aphasia, hemineglect and frontal executive dysfunction may over-or underestimate health-related quality of life in such patients. In this specific form of severe stroke, it is crucial to maintain rehabilitation for a long period of time (at least 5–10 years after stroke).

In malignant MCA infarction, it is not easy to predict outcome in all cases and it is often impossible to consider the preferences of the patient except if they have been expressed in advance. Therefore in the decision of surgery, prognostic factors such as young age (< 50 years), absence of pre-existing disability or severe co-morbid disease, as well as pragmatic predictive factors such as strong family support, should be considered each time. More studies on patients' and relatives' perception of surviving with a substantial disability would improve patients' management and follow-up.

Cerebellar infarction

According to case series, mainly of retrospective design, decompressive surgery improves survival in patients who deteriorate because of space-occupying edematous cerebellar infarction [24]. In two recent clinical retrospective studies, bilateral suboccipital craniectomy at the time of neurological deterioration due to edematous compression or hydrocephalus, showed 40% death and 35–40% of patients alive with good functional outcome (mRS 0–2) at follow-up [25,26]. However there are several limitations to these studies as regards the heterogeneity of the surgical procedures (suboccipital craniectomy only, external ventricular drainage only or both, with or without evacuation of necrotic tissue), the timing of surgery from stroke onset and the clinical presentation at the time of the decision of surgery. Overall surgery was performed late at the time of deterioration, whereas earlier prophylactic surgery may be much more effective as it has been shown in malignant hemispheric infarction. By comparison with hemispheric infarction, clinical outcome after cerebellar decompressive surgery may even be better, with a higher proportion of patients alive with mild residual disability.

Predictive factors of good outcome after suboccipital craniectomy in space-occupying or malignant edematous cerebellar infarction may be younger age, lower delay to surgery, absence of clinical signs of brainstem compression, and normal level of consciousness, but in the absence of confirming data from controlled trials none of these factors can be accepted as definitely predictive or their absence be a source of rejection of surgery.

Hemorrhagic stroke

In acute intracerebral hemorrhage (ICH), the leading cause of death is the increased intracranial pressure resulting from the growing hematoma and its surrounding edema. Hospital mortality is up to 30% and in many patients, because of the severity of the mass effect, the absence of evidence-based treatments and the overall unfavorable prognosis of ICH (50–60% mortality at 1 year), a care limitation strategy is preferred to more aggressive therapeutics of the elevated ICP. However, considering the results of randomized trials of hemicraniectomy in malignant MCA infarction and as hematoma evacuation has failed to show a benefit in ICH, large hemicraniectomy has been recently suggested as a life-saving procedure in cases of large deep hemispheric hematoma at the level of the basal ganglia. However, the reports are mainly individual cases or small case series with no comparative groups and some patients had, in addition to hemicraniectomy, hematoma evacuation [27].

In experimental ICH, decompressive hemicraniectomy performed up to 24 hours after the initial ICH showed significant benefit over no hemicraniectomy on mortality with better neurological scores [28]. The final ICH volume was, however, only non-significantly larger in the ICH and no craniectomy group compared with the ICH and craniectomy groups ($p = 0.065$) [28]. These data are encouraging but need confirmation in clinical trials. Thus the routine indication of DC in hemorrhagic stroke is currently very limited.

Subarachnoid hemorrhage

Decompressive hemicraniectomy has been proposed in poor-grade aneurysmal subarachnoid hemorrhage (SAH) to treat elevated ICP secondary either to brain edema or intrapenchymal hemorrhage or brain infarction. In a large case series, among 787 consecutive patients with aneurysmal SAH, 43 underwent decompressive hemicraniectomy [29]. Twenty-five per cent (11 patients) achieved good outcome with no influence of the pre-operative clinical presentation (brain edema alone or with additional parenchymal lesions either hemorrhagic or ischemic). The results were less evident in other studies but they were all retrospective [30]. Very early emergency prophylactic decompressive hemicraniectomy may be more interesting to prevent secondary damage to brain tissue [31]. Because of the heterogeneity of the clinical presentation (edema, infarction, parenchymal hemorrhage, hydrocephalus) and the course of deterioration in aneurysmal SAH, larger prospective case series are needed to identify the best selection criteria and timing of decompressive hemicraniectomy in SAH. Currently the best indication is poor grade cerebral aneurysms with intracerebral hematoma.

Cerebral venous thrombosis

Although mostly of favorable outcome, cerebral venous thrombosis may lead to death by transtentorial herniation despite the use of anticoagulants. The underlying mechanism of deterioration is the hemodynamic changes that lead to elevated intracranial pressure and brain edema. At the time of deterioration most patients reported in case series had hemorrhagic parenchymal lesions with mass effect and midline shift [32]. The term 'malignant CVT' has been proposed to designate a subset of severe CVT involving cortical veins, with or without sinus thrombosis, with edematous or hemorrhagic supratentorial parenchymal lesions and signs of transtentorial herniation (4.5% of an academic hospital-based registry of CVT) [32]. Compared to malignant MCA infarction, malignant CVT has a much more heterogeneous clinical and radiological presentation. Some patients deteriorate early whereas some have an unfavorable course later during the first days after symptoms onset even under anticoagulants. In such circumstances of 'malignant' CVT with high risk of brain herniation, decompressive surgery may be life saving. It consists either of a large hemicraniectomy with opening of the dura or an intra-parenchymal hematoma evacuation, or both (Fig. 8.3). Although available data come from small cases series or individual cases, the benefit of surgery seems important in terms of reduction of mortality and good functional recovery [33]. It is important to note that most reported patients had surgery at the time of

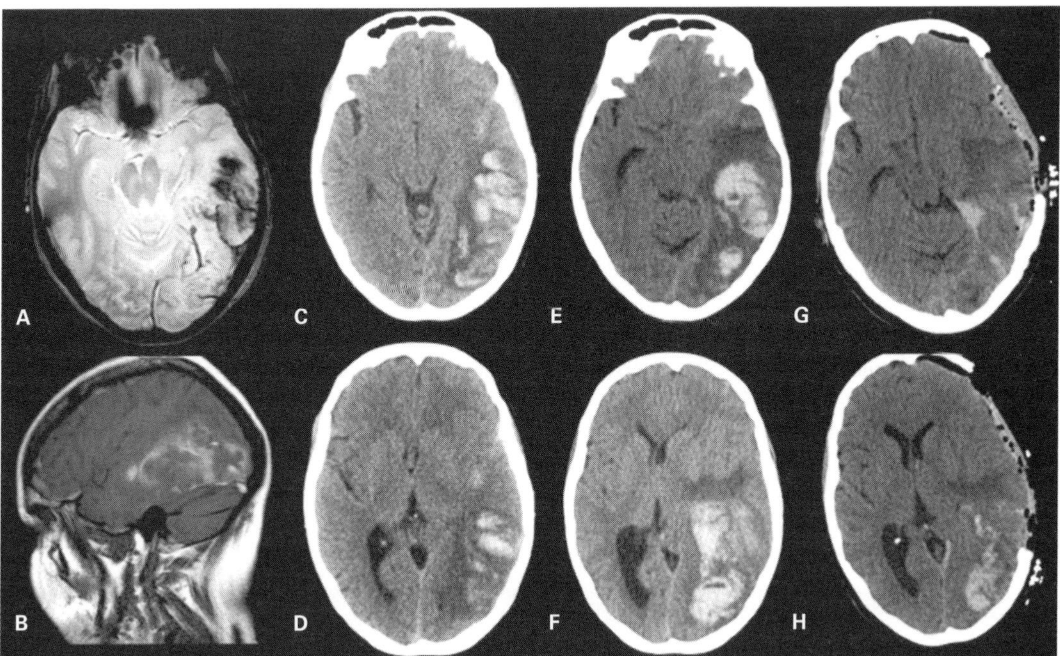

Fig. 8.3 Axial T2 echo-gradient (A), sagittal T1 (B) and axial CT scan (C–D) of a 50-year-old woman at admission showing a large left temporal hemorrhagic lesion and a thrombosed left lateral sinus (arrow). Axial CT scan (E–F) at the time of clinical worsening on day 10 while the patient was on anticoagulation, showing hydrocephalus, subfalcine and temporal herniation. Axial CT scan (G–H) the same day after emergency decompressive hemicraniectomy showing no more signs of herniation.

deterioration. The question remains whether the benefit of decompressive surgery in CVT would not be much better in the case of early prophylactic surgery done before signs of imminent herniation, which has been shown for malignant MCA infarction [3]. Indeed in CVT as in malignant MCA infarction, timing of surgery may be crucial. There is no animal model of hemicraniectomy in CVT but in pig models of superior sagittal sinus thrombosis there is a stepwise progression of intracranial pressure depending on thrombus progression to cortical and bridging veins [34]. A multidisciplinary management with early and collegial discussion between stroke neurologists, neurosurgeons and anesthesiologists is warranted in such cases of malignant CVT. The aim of any treatment strategy should be complete or near complete recovery.

The timing of use of anticoagulants after decompressive surgery is not yet well defined. Anticoagulants should be restarted as soon as possible during the 6–8 post-operative days with the consideration of the underlying cause of the CVT.

Complications of surgical decompression

Complications following DC may occur at different operative periods from immediate bleeding to late CSF hydrodynamic alterations.

Infectious process

Under intraoperative prophylactic antibiotic agents, the post-operative infectious rate is between 3% and 5% [35]. The risk factors of infection that have been identified are: the large skin incision with long scalp pedicle, the sacrifice of the pedicle artery, the opening of the frontal sinus or air cells in the middle fossa and the frequent contamination of surgical fields in emergency surgery. Post-operative infection is also increased by using dural substitute for expansive duraplasty, and after cranioplasty with frozen bone implant.

Perioperative complications

Hemorrhagic expansion of contusions is observed in approximately 40% of patients after hemicraniectomy for severe traumatic brain injury [36,37].

The external cerebral herniation is defined by expansion of the brain through the bone defect due to an increasing brain swelling [38]. This complication is related to the combination of several mechanisms: cortical hypoperfusion, transcapillary leakage fluid due to a higher hydrostatic pressure gradient which may lead to venous ischemia by compression of cortical veins within the herniated segment of the brain [38,39]. This complication may be prevented by a large skull opening and the use of vascular channels at the edge of flap.

Early post-operative complications

Subdural effusion or hygroma is defined by an accumulation of CSF usually at the level of craniectomy within eight days after DC and may lead to mass effect [38]. The underlying mechanism is an alteration of the CSF dynamic or an increasing cerebral perfusion pressure [40]. It may be prevented by duraplasty but in most cases it resolves spontaneously.

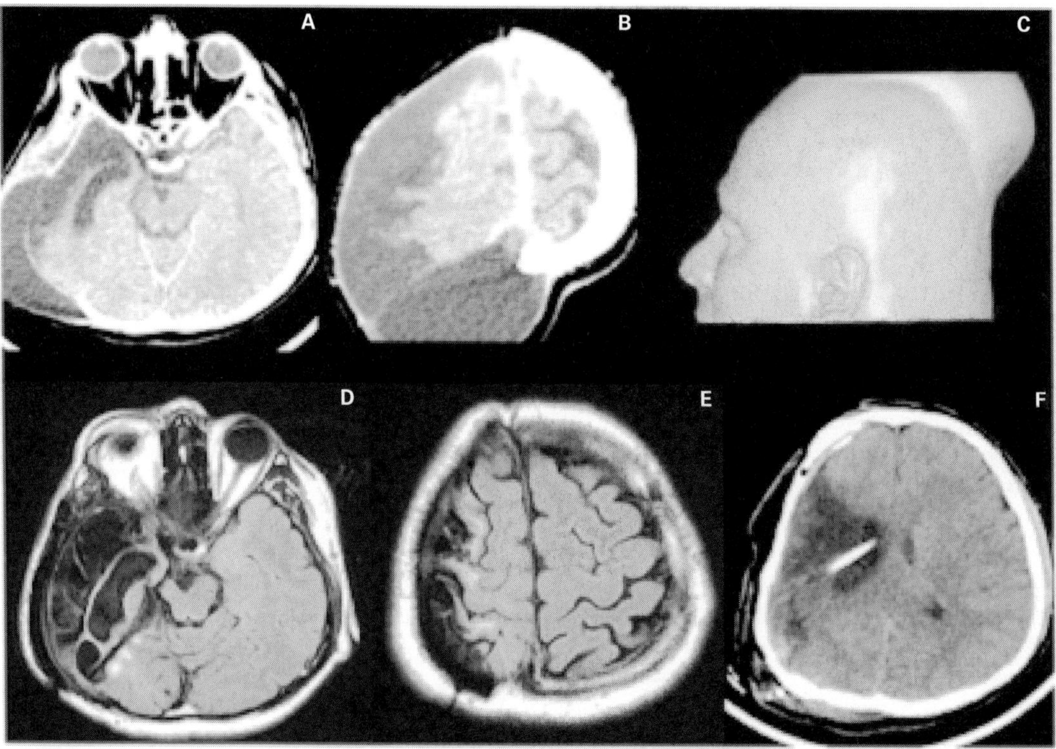

Fig. 8.4 Cerebrospinal fluid collection under the scalp in a 40-year-old man following hemicraniectomy for malignant middle cerebral artery infarction. Axial and 3D volume CT scan (A–C): right hemisphere hypodensity and large CSF collection under the scalp; Axial FLAIR and CT scan (D–F) after peritoneal ventricular drainage and cranioplasty with no more CSF collection.

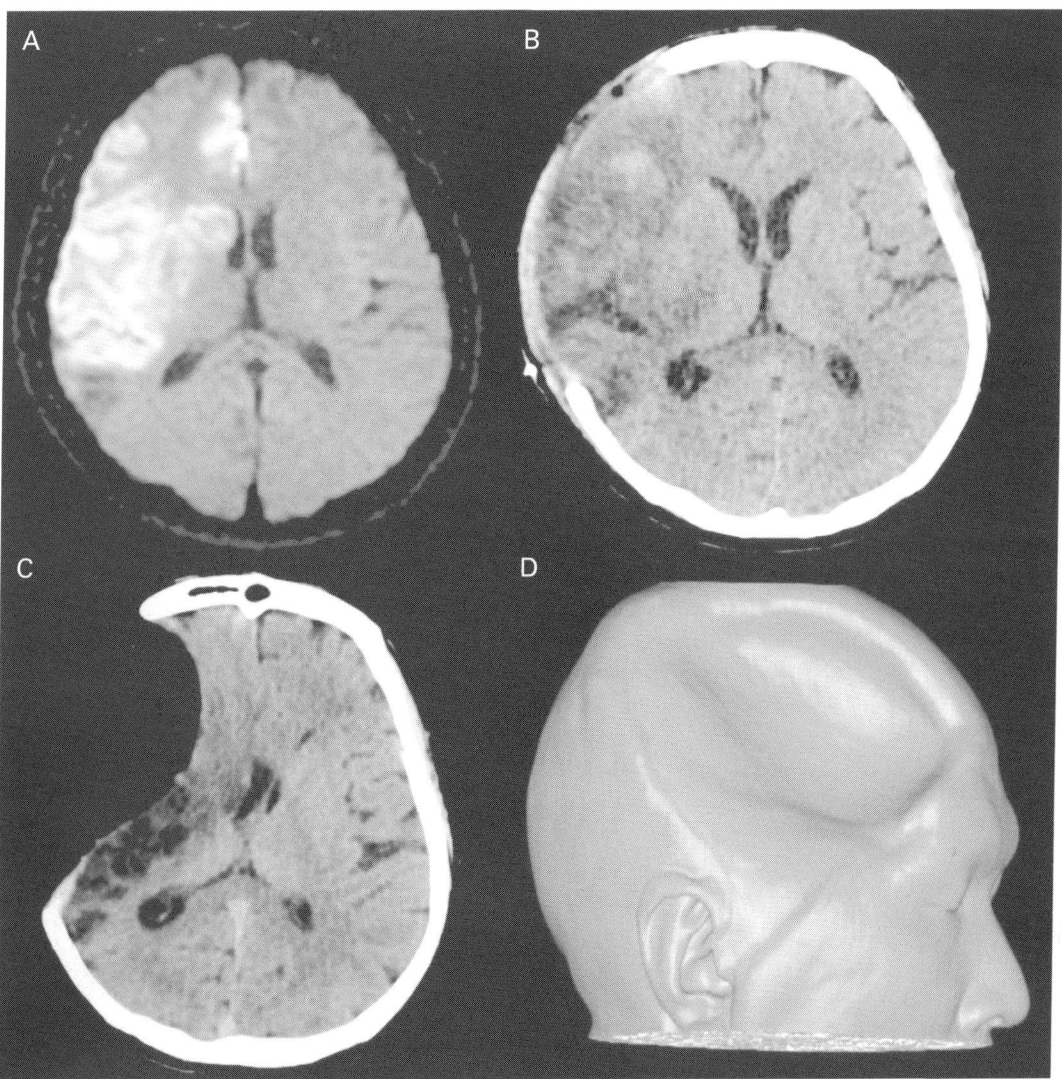

Fig. 8.5 Sinking skin flap syndrome and paradoxical herniation in a 45-year-old man: axial DWI (A): right total MCA and partial ACA infarction; axial CT scan 10 days later (B): right hemicraniectomy; axial CT scan 4 months after stroke at the time of clinical signs of brain herniation (right hemicrania, vomiting and apathy exacerbated by sitting or standing up and improved by lying down) (C): depressed and severe compression of right hemisphere with lateral ventricular and subfalcine herniation; CT scan 3D volume (D): profound skin depression at the site of craniectomy.

Paradoxical herniation with compression of the brainstem and neurological deterioration is secondary to a negative pressure gradient between the cranial and spinal compartments [41]. In case of spinal leak of the CSF, clamping of lumbar drainage is necessary. Other symptomatic treatments consist of hyperhydratation or discontinuation of hyperosmolar therapy, Trendelenburg position, blood patch or cranioplasty.

Delayed complications

Other complications related to CSF dynamic alterations are hydrocephalus and the syndrome of the trephined or sinking skin syndrome (Fig. 8.4 and Fig. 8.5). Sinking skin flap syndrome may be more prevalent than expected as shown in a prospective study of 27 malignant MCA patients followed until cranioplasty who had at three to five months post-hemicraniectomy either symptomatic or asymptomatic (one out of four patients) scalp depression which progressed to a 'paradoxical' brain herniation in two patients as the consequence of atmospheric pressure exceeding intracranial pressure [42]. Orthostatic hemicrania and seizures were the two other main symptoms of sinking skin flap syndrome which was more prevalent in older patients and those who have a smaller surface of craniectomy [42]. It can be prevented by early cranioplasty for restoration of normalization of cerebral hemodynamics and intracranial pressure.

Resorption of the bone plate occurs commonly in about 50% of cases [43,44]. To prevent this adverse event, there are several possibilities: 1) a thigh approximation of the free bone flap to a lengthy surface of the native craniectomy margin using rigid plate and screw fixation to minimize movement of the flap; 2) a hinge craniotomy as an alternative to classical hemicraniectomy under ICP monitoring, allowing the native plate to remain in place [15]; and 3) the use of osteoclast inhibitors in the future.

Cranioplasty

After hemicraniectomy, the repositioning of the bone flap – cranioplasty – is carried out at variable timing. The cranioplasty is recommended to satisfy cosmetic concerns, to lessen the risk of direct trauma to the craniectomy site, to decrease the barotraumas to the brain, to improve regional cerebral blood flow, to prevent the trephined or sinking skin flap syndrome, and to reduce the alterations of CSF dynamics [45,46]. The stored bone flap must be replaced as early as possible because of the osseous resorption process that reduces the flap size [47]. Autogenous bone graft is the treatment of choice but the difficulties of storage, the anatomical conditions, and the infectious complications frequently lead to the loss of the bone flap [48]. Otherwise several qualities appear essential for the skull vault repair: 1) resistance; 2) biocompatibility, i.e. with maximal reduction of the inflammatory reaction and rejection; and 3) integrability with the surrounding living bone in order to become a part of it [49]. Several alloplast graft cranioplasties are available such as polymethylene methacrylate (PMMA), titanium, acrylic resins or hydroxyapatite in cement or ceramics [49]. Moreover, the computer-assisted design and manufacturing of the cranioplasty improves the cosmetic result, reduces the operative time for implantation and is associated with a 34% reduction of the immediate complication rate [49,50].

Conclusion

Emergency decompressive surgery is a life-saving procedure in the acute phase of stroke with clear benefit in functional outcome in selected patients and thus should be part of the acute stroke treatment strategy as necessary. Ideally, the decision should be made with the family informed about overall prognosis of the patient without surgery and about what is expected from decompressive surgery and its modality in the presence of stroke neurologists, neurosurgeons, neuroradiologists and intensivists.

REFERENCES

1. Simard JM, Kent TA, Chen M, *et al.* Brain oedema in focal ischaemia: molecular pathophysiology and theoretical implications. *Lancet Neurol* 2007;**6**:258–68.
2. Hacke W, Schwab S, Horn M, *et al.* 'Malignant' middle cerebral artery territory infarction: clinical course and prognostic signs. *Arch Neurol* 1996;**53**:309–15.
3. Vahedi K, Hofmeijer J, Juettler E *et al.* Early decompressive surgery in malignant infarction of the middle cerebral artery: a pooled analysis of three randomised controlled trials. *Lancet Neurol* 2007;**6**:215–22.
4. Hutchinson P, Timofeev I, Kirkpatrick P. Surgery for brain edema. *Neurosurg Focus* 2007;**22**:E14.

5. Park J, Kim E, Kim GJ, Hur YK, Guthikonda M. External decompressive craniectomy including resection of temporal muscle and fascia in malignant hemispheric infarction. *J Neurosurg* 2009;**110**:101–5.
6. Jaeger M, Soehle M, Meixensberger J. Effects of decompressive craniectomy on brain tissue oxygen in patients with intracranial hypertension. *J Neurol Neurosurg Psychiatry* 2003;**74**: 513–15.
7. Juttler E, Schellinger PD, Aschoff A, *et al.* Clinical review: Therapy for refractory intracranial hypertension in ischaemic stroke. *Crit Care* 2007;**11**:231.
8. Kenning TJ, Gandhi RH, German JW. A comparison of hinge craniotomy and decompressive craniectomy for the treatment of malignant intracranial hypertension: early clinical and radiographic analysis. *Neurosurg Focus* 2009;**26**:E6.
9. Wagner S, Schnippering H, Aschoff A, *et al.* Suboptimum hemicraniectomy as a cause of additional cerebral lesions in patients with malignant infarction of the middle cerebral artery. *J Neurosurg* 2001;**94**:693–6.
10. Csokay A, Egyud L, Nagy L, Pataki G. Vascular tunnel creation to improve the efficacy of decompressive craniotomy in post-traumatic cerebral edema and ischemic stroke. *Surg Neurol* 2002;**57**:126–9.
11. Hutchinson P, Timofeev I, Kirkpatrick P. Surgery for brain edema. *Neurosurg Focus* 2007;**22**:E14.
12. Schmidt JH, Reyes BJ, Fischer R, Flaherty SK. Use of hinge craniotomy for cerebral decompression. Technical note. *J Neurosurg* 2007;**107**:678–2.
13. Jaeger M, Soehle M, Meixensberger J. Effects of decompressive craniectomy on brain tissue oxygen in patients with intracranial hypertension. *J Neurol Neurosurg Psychiatry* 2003;**74**:513–15.
14. Yoo DS, Kim DS, Cho KS, *et al.* Ventricular pressure monitoring during bilateral decompression with dural expansion. *J Neurosurg* 1999;**91**:953–9.
15. Kenning TJ, Gandhi RH, German JW. A comparison of hinge craniotomy and decompressive craniectomy for the treatment of malignant intracranial hypertension: early clinical and radiographic analysis. *Neurosurg Focus* 2009;**26**:E6.
16. Sahuquillo J, Arikan F. Decompressive craniectomy for the treatment of refractory high intracranial pressure in traumatic brain injury. *Cochrane Database Syst Rev* 2006: CD003983.
17. Guresir E, Vatter H, Schuss P, *et al.* Rapid closure technique in decompressive craniectomy. *J Neurosurg* 2010;**114**(4): 954–60.
18. Timofeev I, Czosnyka M, Nortje J, *et al.* Effect of decompressive craniectomy on intracranial pressure and cerebrospinal compensation following traumatic brain injury. *J Neurosurg* 2008;**108**:66–73.
19. Schwab S, Steiner T, Aschoff A *et al.* Early hemicraniectomy in patients with complete middle cerebral artery infarction. *Stroke* 1998;**29**:1888–93.
20. Vahedi K, Vicaut E, Mateo J, *et al.* Sequential-design, multicenter, randomized, controlled trial of early decompressive craniectomy in malignant middle cerebral artery infarction (DECIMAL Trial). *Stroke* 2007;**38**:2506–17.
21. Jüttler E, Schwab S, Schmiedek P, *et al.* Decompressive Surgery for the Treatment of Malignant Infarction of the Middle Cerebral Artery (DESTINY): a randomized, controlled trial. *Stroke* 2007;**38**:2518–25.

22a. Hofmeijer J, Amelink GJ, Algra A, *et al.* Hemicraniectomy after middle cerebral artery infarction with life-threatening edema trial (HAMLET). Protocol for a randomised controlled trial of decompressive surgery in space-occupying hemispheric infarction. *Trials* 2006;**7**:29.

22b. Hofmeijer J, Kappelle LJ, Algra A, *et al.* Surgical decompression for space-occupying cerebral infarction (the Hemicraniectomy After Middle Cerebral Artery infarction with Life-threatening Edema Trial [HAMLET]): a multicentre, open, randomised trial. *Lancet Neurol* 2009;**8**:326–33.

23. Puetz V, Campos CR, Eliasziw M, Hill MD, Demchuk AM; Calgary Stroke Program. Assessing the benefits of hemicraniectomy: what is a favourable outcome? *Lancet Neurol* 2007;**6**:580; author reply 580–1.
24. Jauss M, Krieger D, Hornig C, Schramm J, Busse O, for the GASCIS study centers. Surgical and medical management of patients with massive cerebellar infarctions: results of the German–Austrian cerebellar infarction study. *J Neurol* 1999;**249**:257–64.
25. Jüttler E, Schweickert S, Ringleb PA, *et al.* Long-term outcome after surgical treatment for space-occupying cerebellar infarction: experience in 56 patients. *Stroke* 2009;**40**:3060–6.
26. Pfefferkorn T, Eppinger U, Linn J, *et al.* Long-term outcome after suboccipital decompressive craniectomy for malignant cerebellar infarction. *Stroke* 2009;**40**:3045–50.
27. Ramnarayan R, Anto D, Anilkumar TV, Nayar R. Decompressive hemicraniectomy in large putaminal hematomas: an Indian experience. *J Stroke Cerebrovasc Dis* 2009;**18**:1–10.
28. Marinkovic I, Strbian D, Pedrono E, *et al.* Decompressive craniectomy for intracerebral hemorrhage. *Neurosurgery* 2009;**65**:780–6.
29. Güresir E, Raabe A, Setzer M, *et al.* Decompressive hemicraniectomy in subarachnoid haemorrhage: the influence

of infarction, haemorrhage and brain swelling. *J Neurol Neurosurg Psychiatry* 2009;**80**:799–801.

30. D'Ambrosio AL, Sughrue ME, Yorgason JG, *et al.* Decompressive hemicraniectomy for poor-grade aneurysmal subarachnoid hemorrhage patients with associated intracerebral hemorrhage: clinical outcome and quality of life assessment. *Neurosurgery* 2005;**56**:12–19.
31. Smith ER, Carter BS, Ogilvy CS: Proposed use of prophylactic decompressive craniectomy in poor-grade aneurysmal subarachnoid hemorrhage patients presenting with associated large sylvian hematomas. *Neurosurgery* 2002;**51**:117–24.
32. Théaudin M, Crassard I, Bresson D, *et al.* Should decompressive surgery be performed in malignant cerebral venous thrombosis? A series of 12 patients. *Stroke* 2010;**41**:727–31.
33. Coutinho JM, Majoie CB, Coert BA, Stam J: Decompressive hemicraniectomy in cerebral sinus thrombosis: consecutive case series and review of the literature. *Stroke* 2009;**40**:2233–5.
34. Fries G, Wallenfang T, Hennen J, *et al.* Occlusion of the pig superior sagittal sinus, bridging and cortical veins: multistep evolution of sinus-vein thrombosis. *J Neurosurg* 1992;**77**:127–33.
35. Aarabi B, Hesdorffer DC, Ahn ES, *et al.* Outcome following decompressive craniectomy for malignant swelling due to severe head injury. *J Neurosurg* 2006; **104**:469–79.
36. Flint AC, Manley GT, Gean AD, Hemphill JC, Rosenthal G: Post-operative expansion of hemorrhagic contusions after unilateral decompressive hemicraniectomy in severe traumatic brain injury. *J Neurotrauma* 2008; **25**:503–12.
37. Oertel M, Kelly DF, McArthur D, *et al.* Progressive hemorrhage after head trauma: predictors and consequences of the evolving injury. *J Neurosurg* 2002;**96**:109–16.
38. Stiver SI. Complications of decompressive craniectomy for traumatic brain injury. *Neurosurg Focus* 2009;**26**:E7.
39. Olivecrona M, Rodling-Wahlstrom M, Naredi S, Koskinen LO. Effective ICP reduction by decompressive craniectomy in patients with severe traumatic brain injury treated by an ICP-targeted therapy. *J Neurotrauma* 2007; **24**:927–35.
40. Yang XF, Wen L, Shen F, *et al.* Surgical complications secondary to decompressive craniectomy in patients with a head injury: a series of 108 consecutive cases. *Acta Neurochir (Wien)* 2008;**150**:1241–7; discussion 1248.
41. Vilela MD. Delayed paradoxical herniation after a decompressive craniectomy: case report. *Surg Neurol* 2008;**69**:293–6; discussion 296.
42. Sarov M, Guichard JP, Chibarro S, *et al.* Sinking skin flap syndrome and paradoxical herniation after hemicraniectomy for malignant hemispheric infarction. *Stroke* 2010;**41**:560–2.
43. Iwama T, Yamada J, Imai S, *et al.* The use of frozen autogenous bone flaps in delayed cranioplasty revisited. *Neurosurgery* 2003;**52**:591–6; discussion 595–6.
44. Posnick JC, Goldstein JA, Armstrong D, Rutka JT. Reconstruction of skull defects in children and adolescents by the use of fixed cranial bone grafts: long-term results. *Neurosurgery* 1993;**32**:785–91; discussion 791.
45. Staffa G, Nataloni A, Compagnone C, Servadei F. Custom made cranioplasty prostheses in porous hydroxy-apatite using 3D design techniques: 7 years experience in 25 patients. *Acta Neurochir (Wien)* 2007;**149**:161–70; discussion 170.
46. Stiver SI, Wintermark M, Manley GT. Reversible monoparesis following decompressive hemicraniectomy for traumatic brain injury. *J Neurosurg* 2008;**109**:245–54.
47. Shoakazemi A, Flannery T, McConnell RS. Long-term outcome of subcutaneously preserved autologous cranioplasty. *Neurosurgery* 2009;**65**:505–10.
48. Edwards MS, Ousterhout DK. Autogeneic skull bone grafts to reconstruct large or complex skull defects in children and adolescents. *Neurosurgery* 1987;**20**:273–80.
49. Gooch MR, Gin GE, Kenning TJ, German JW. Complications of cranioplasty following decompressive craniectomy: analysis of 62 cases. *Neurosurg Focus* 2009;**26**:E9.
50. Staffa G, Nataloni A, Compagnone C, Servadei F. Custom made cranioplasty prostheses in porous hydroxy-apatite using 3D design techniques: 7 years experience in 25 patients. *Acta Neurochir (Wien)* 2007;**149**:161–70; discussion 170.

9a

Neuroradiologic intervention in cerebrovascular disease

Olav Jansen and Soenke Peters

Interventional stroke treatment

An ischemic stroke is a common cause of death or disability. The symptoms depend on the localization of the occluded vessel and the individual collaterals. Two-thirds of strokes occur in the anterior circulation, mostly involving the middle cerebral artery. Occlusion of the basilar artery is less common but has a mortality rate of 80–90% if it remains untreated. The main causes for vessel occlusion are embolism of cardiac or arterial origin, e.g. from carotid bifurcation. Intracranial stenosis or paradox venous embolism at persisting oval foramen are less common causes.

In order to analyse the results of stroke treatment, the time-frame from symptom onset until therapy and of course successful recanalization are essential [1]. In the absence of contraindications, intravenous thrombolysis is still the principal therapy, being easy and fast to practice, widely accessible, non-invasive, and relatively low cost. However, intravenous thrombolysis is often contraindicated, mostly because of an elapsed (< 4.5 h) or unknown time-frame, and IV-thrombolysis is limited in cases with high clot burden. In these cases the interventional treatment is an alternative opportunity. Because of lower thrombolytic medication doses and therefore a lower bleeding risk, local intra-arterial thrombolysis is approved in a prolonged time-frame. The mechanical thrombectomie, a newer interventional treatment, surrenders thrombolytic medication, which also lowers the risk of bleeding. The successful reopening rates of large vessel occlusions with mechanical thrombectomy are up to 80% [2]. To secure a clinical benefit of this more invasive and more expensive treatment a critical patient selection is necessary. Furthermore, a well-trained interventionalist should perform this procedure to avoid complications and to ensure a fast recanalization.

Treatment indication

For every patient with symptoms of a stroke it is necessary to acquire pictures of the brain to exclude an intracerebral hemorrhage or other causes for the clinical symptoms. Depending on the hospital infrastructure CT or MRI is used, in both cases a fast and standardized approach is essential. Native parenchymal imaging, vascular imaging and a measurement of the cerebral perfusion should be part of the protocol in both cases. Besides the infarct demarcation, which is expected as irreversible damaged tissue, the tissue at risk, also called penumbra, can be measured here. This tissue at risk areas is supposed to be affected functionally but still structurally intact. The aim of therapy is to rescue this poorly perfused but not yet irreversibly damaged tissue. If too much infarct core is seen on the initial CT or MRI scan an interventional treatment is contraindicated because the reperfusion of large irreversibly damaged tissue areas might lead to intracerebral bleeding, with no clinical benefit expected. For the territory of the middle cerebral artery the 'one-third rule' is an approach for drawing the line. If more than one-third of the area is damaged, a reopening of the vessel is not

Critical Care of the Stroke Patient, ed. Stefan Schwab, Daniel Hanley, and A. David Mendelow. Published by Cambridge University Press.

indicated. A more subtle graduation for the territory of the middle cerebral artery is the Alberta stroke program early CT score (ASPECTS) [3]. The consequences are similar if too much tissue is damaged (ASPECT ≤ 4), as a reopening of the vessel does not improve the clinical outcome. In particular, the combination of relatively large demarcated infarction and a long time-frame is not promising, so an interventional treatment is not indicated. Due to the high mortality rates of the untreated, the indication for interventional treatment of the occluded basilar artery is less strict and local intra-arterial therapy should be discussed as first line therapy.

A further scenario where interventional therapy should be discussed, even if less than 4.5 h since symptom onset have passed, is a thrombus length over 8 mm. Here the thrombolytic agent largely fails to reopen the vessel so an early interventional treatment is advisable [4]. Besides these exceptions, intravenous thrombolysis is the first therapy of choice. If contraindications for intravenous thrombolysis exist, mostly elapsed or unknown time-frame, or if the symptoms remain 1 h after intravenous thrombolysis, an interventional treatment should be enforced.

The patient's age is less important in the treatment decision. If possible the circumstances of everyday life should be considered. Whereas some older people in their eighties live on their own, others in their seventies may live in residential care pre-stroke. Even though the patient's wishes and those of their family are mostly unknown in the emergency setting, they should be respected where possible.

To summarise, interventional treatment is indicated for big vessel occlusion with a contraindication for intravenous thrombolysis if symptoms persist 1 h after intravenous lysis or if the thrombotic mass is high. Interventional treatment should be discussed as first line treatment for occlusions of the basilar artery. Interventional treatment is contraindicated if too much tissue is damaged irreversibly, while the time-frame and patient age play a minor role.

Treatment

In accordance with the saying 'time is brain', therapy should be started as soon as possible. If the patient is in the time-frame for intravenous thrombolysis and the decision for an interventional treatment is made, the lysis can be given prior to the IA-approach. This is supposed to soften the thrombus and make the following extraction easier. In particular, if the patient has to be transferred to a hospital with interventional neuroradiology, an intravenous lysis should be started if not contraindicated ('drip and ship'). This is meant to lower the thrombus burden and avoid a thrombus growth. In addition, a softening of the thrombus is expected, as mentioned previously. After transfer a current neurological examination and a CT or MRI are usually needed to confirm the indication for an interventional treatment.

Because most stroke patients are agitated or have aphasia if the left middle cerebral artery is involved, a general anesthesia is often needed. The intubation takes time so the anesthesiologist should do just basic preparation, e.g. a urinary catheter will be passed to start the intervention as early as possible. Furthermore, the anesthesiologist needs to keep the blood pressure in a high normal range. Collateral perfusion is essential for the patient as a drop in blood pressure may endanger the tissue at risk and therefore compromise the clinical outcome. Excessively high blood pressure of course elevates the risk of cerebral bleeding, especially if thrombolytic medication is given. An intervention with sedation is a possible alternative to save time and to lower the risk of blood pressure drops during intubation. Of course a calm patient needs to be guaranteed for this scenario, otherwise the risk of intervention-related complications is too high.

The interventional options are a local intra-arterial thrombolysis, a mechanical thrombectomy or a combination of both. For the local thrombolysis mostly rtPA is used, which will be applied over a microcatheter placed directly in front of the thrombus. The local use of thrombolytic medication guarantees higher concentrations at the thrombus with lower systemic doses, which leads to a decreased bleeding risk compared to the intravenous thrombolysis. Urokinase is less commonly used. Intra-arterial rtPA leads to slightly higher recanalization rates but it also seems to be accompanied by a higher rate of intracerebral hemorrhages than urokinase [5].

Mechanical thrombus extraction can be done with different devices. The stent-retriever has recently become a widely used device (Fig. 9a.1). Stent-retrievers

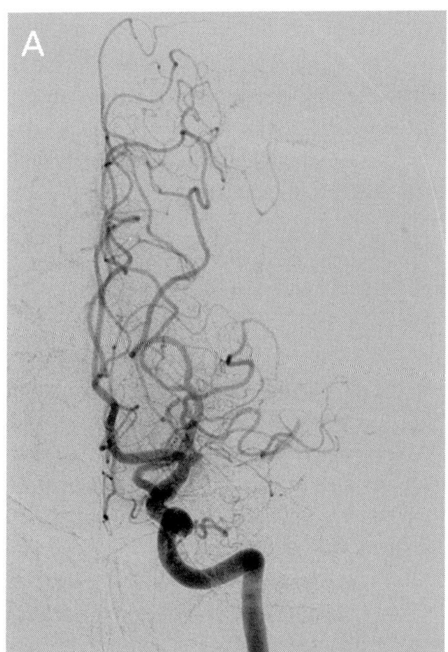

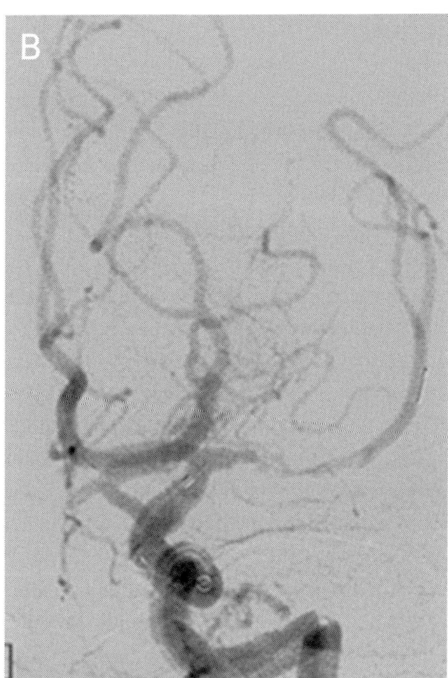

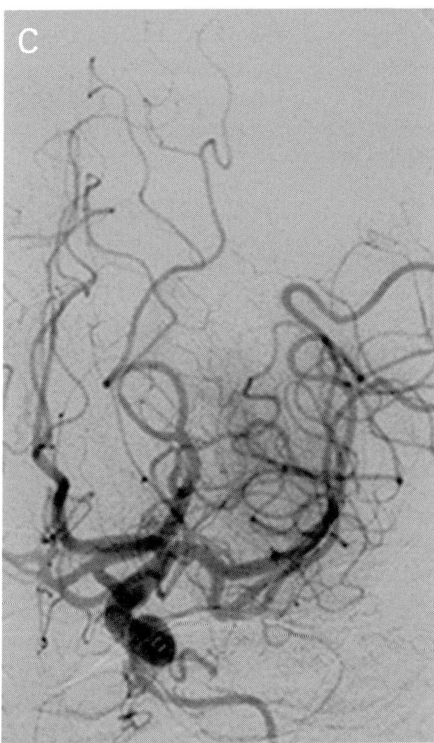

Fig. 9a.1 Thrombectomy of acute occlusion of the proximal medial cerebral artery (M1). Initial diagnostic angiogram of the left internal carotid artery (ICA) shows complete occlusion of left proximal M1 (A). Via an intermediate catheter a microcatheter is navigated through the M1 occlusion and a stent-like retriever is deployed, which partially opens the thrombosed M1 (B). After one retraction maneuver the M1 is totally reopened resulting in a TICI III result (C).

are self-expanding closed-cell stents which can be pulled back after deploying. After passing the thrombus with a microcatheter the stent-retriever gets developed at the thrombus position by pulling back the microcatheter. The first intended effect is a temporary bypass caused by the radial force of the stent. It is recommended to wait three to four minutes so that the thrombus can migrate into the meshes of the stent. Afterwards the stent gets pulled back to extract the thrombus. For this maneuver an aspiration over a catheter placed in front of the thrombus is needed, firstly to avoid a scattering of thrombus fragments and secondly to support the thrombus extraction. This procedure might need to be repeated if the parts of the vessel are still occluded. Other thrombectomy devices with a corkscrew-like shape or a brush-like shape are less commonly used. Recent studies have shown significantly lower recanalization rates and worse clinical outcomes in comparison to stent-retrievers [2,6]. A different approach is the use of fragmentation devices, i.e. microwires, snares, separators or soft balloons, in combination with an aspiration over a catheter placed in front of the thrombus. The idea is to destroy the thrombus mechanically and to remove the fragments by suction. However, at the moment stent-retrievers are the most frequently used devices. With up to 80–90 % they have the highest reopening rates and because of the fast reopening of the vessel and the high success rates they can lead to a good clinical outcome in about 50% of patients [7,8].

The combination of mechanical thrombectomy and intra-arterial thrombolysis might become necessary if the thrombectomy device fails to extract the whole thrombus or if fragments of the thrombus occlude vessels not reachable with the thrombectomy device. In cases where reachable thrombus fails to be extracted, the thrombectomy devices can be used to enlarge the surface of the thrombus. This leads to a better effect of the thrombolytic medication. If all attempts for recanalization fail or if a stenosis is accompanied with the vessel occlusion, a permanent stenting might be necessary. However, because of the relatively high morbidity and mortality rates after intracranial stenting and the need for antiplatelet medication, a permanent stenting should be considered only as the second line of treatment.

In cases of very high clot amount (i.e. thrombotic occlusion of the whole extra- and intracranial ICA), primarily thrombus fragmentation and aspiration show the best results (penumbra system).

Extra- and intracranial stenting

Stenoses of the brain-supplying arteries are related with a high risk of experiencing an ischemic stroke, and the risk of a stroke rises with the grade of the stenosis [9,10]. Stenting of vessels is an elegant method to treat stenoses and therefore to lower the risk of stroke. When considering alternative treatment methods, the treatment risks and the results are relevant to the treatment indication and the choice of treatment. Here extra- and intracranial stenting has to be discriminated strictly. Beside the different indications, the treatment itself differs in some not irrelevant aspects.

A further indication for stenting of brain-supplying vessels is a dissection with a hemodynamic relevant narrowing of the vessel or the failure of medical treatment. Dissections might occur as spontaneous, traumatic or iatrogenic during an angiography.

Treatment indication

In most cases, arteriosclerotic stenoses of the extracranial brain-supplying arteries are located in the internal carotid artery directly distal to the carotid bifurcation. This procedure must differ if the stenosis is symptomatic with a stroke or a TIA, or if the stenosis is asymptomatic. In symptomatic patients the stenosis should be treated if it is higher than 50% measured with the NASCET method or if the stenosis is symptomatic during antiplatelet medication. For patients with symptomatic stenoses less than 50% (NASCET), the best medical treatment with antiplatelet medication and lowering of risk factors is recommended [11]. An intervention or operation on a carotid stenosis should only be done if the symptoms persist or if the stenosis is progressive.

For patients with asymptomatic stenoses the treatment criteria are less well defined. Stenoses under 60% (NASCET) should be treated with the best medical treatment, as mentioned above. For the other patients an operative or interventional treatment can be discussed.

When choosing between an operation and interventional treatment, the medical history, age, and wishes of the patient must be considered. Both methods lead to comparable results, assuming experienced doctors in both cases [12,13]. Besides this aspect it seems that elderly patients benefit more from an operation, whereas younger patients benefit more from the intervention. Also patients with heart disease seem to have fewer complications if treated with a stent because no general anesthesia is needed [14]. Further scenarios such as tandem stenoses, radiogenic stenoses, stenoses after neck dissection, surgical poorly accessible stenoses and stenoses with bad collateralization by the circle of Willis benefit from carotid artery stenting. In summary, for extracranial stenoses, stenting is an alternative option to an operation, where the interventionalists have shown their quality with low complication rates. For symptomatic stenoses the complication rates should be under 6% [15], whereas the complication rates for stenting of asymptomatic stenoses should be under 3%.

Intracranial stenoses are less frequent and a stricter indication for stenting is necessary. Because of the relatively high morbidity and mortality rate after intracranial stenting, the medical treatment with antiplatelet medication and lowering of risk factors is the first line of therapy [16–18]. Only if the symptoms persist under medication, if the stenosis is hemodynamic relevant with a bad collateralization, or a progressive stenosis is documented, is treatment with a stent justified. Because of the intracranial localization, an operation is always complicated and only in rare cases represents an alternative option.

Treatment

For both intra- and extracranial stenting, the patient needs to be prepared with dual antiplatelet therapy including aspirin (100 mg/day) and clopidogrel (75 mg/day) at least three days before the stenting. For urgent or emergency cases higher loading doses can be given. Especially for the intracranial stenting a preinterventional testing for the clopidogrel response should be done. In addition to the antiplatelet medication a weight-adjusted intravenous heparin bolus to the start of the angiography should increase the activated clotting time (ACT) to 250–350 seconds.

Stenting of the extracranial brain-supplying arteries can be done under local anesthetic, mostly by inguinal access. The advantage of a conscious patient is that clinical testing during the procedure is possible. All stents used for the cervical arteries must be self expandable, so that external pressure does not deform the stent. Different stent designs are available. Closed-cell stents with small cells should be used if possible to minimize the risk of embolisms out of the plaque [19,20]. For very elongated vessels open-cell stents, which are more flexible, are favored. In these cases the risk of periprocedural embolization rises slightly and the use of a protection filter can be discussed, although the use of a protection system itself includes a slightly elevated treatment risk [19,21]. The stent size needs to be chosen depending on the local anatomy. After passing the stenosis with a microwire in high-grade stenoses a predilatation with a small balloon might be necessary to afterwards pass the stenosis with the microcatheter and the stent. After placing the stent a dilatation with a bigger balloon is necessary (Fig. 9a.2). Before doing this at the carotid bifurcation, where pressure receptors are located, atropine needs to be given to counter the parasympathetic response. For proximal stenoses of the internal carotid artery the stent begins in the common carotid artery, the 'overstenting' of the external carotid artery is not a problem. After successful stenting the double antiplatelet medication needs to be continued, clopidogrel for 6 weeks and aspirin for at least 6 months. After this time the stent struts should be covered by the intima and therefore will be less thrombogenic. In cases of a persistent stenosis or stenoses in other vessels aspirin should be taken over the lifetime.

When treating intracranial vessels, a general anesthetic is essential to prevent patient movement during catheterization of the smaller vessels. Here self-expandable stents can be used as well as balloon-mounted stents. The balloon-mounted stents are less flexible, so that passing of curved vessels might be harder. Using self-expandable stents requires a predilatation, which includes an exchange maneuver and therefore prolongs the procedure. This more flexible

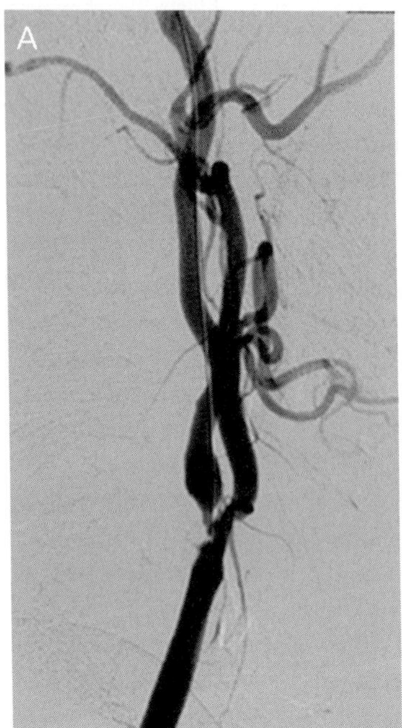

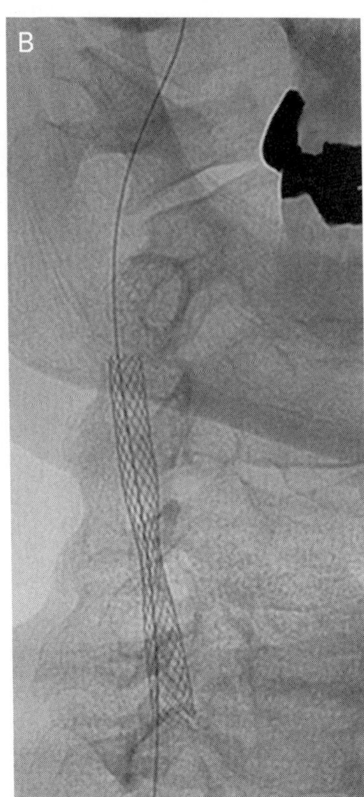

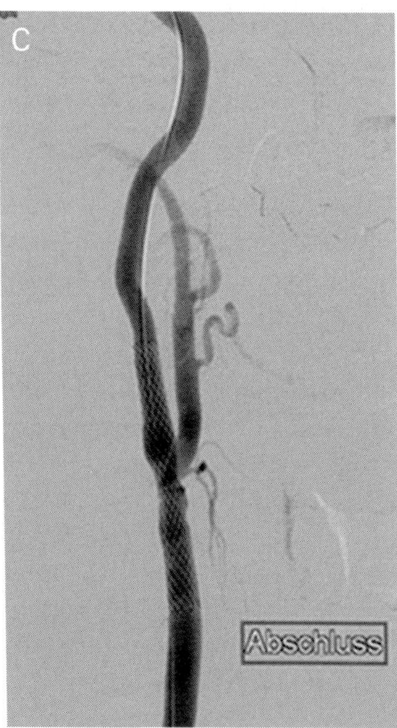

Fig. 9a.2 Stent protected angioplasty of ICA stenosis (SPAC). Initial angiogram demonstrates a severe stenosis of the origin of the right ICA (A). After pre-dilatation a self-expanding closed-cell stent is deployed (B). Postdilatation results in total reconstruction of the vessel lumen (C).

system might be useful for longer or inaccessible stenoses. A third option is a balloon agioplasty without a stent, but here the protection of the stent, especially for dissections, is missing. Again a continuing post-interventional antiplatelet medication is needed. Clopidogrel should be maintainted for 3–6 months and aspirin should be taken over the lifetime.

Regardless of where the stenting was performed the patient should be kept on an intensive care unit or at least an intermediate care unit afterwards. Especially for high-grade stenoses and elderly patients a normotensive blood pressure after the intervention is needed to prevent a hyperperfusion syndrome. Besides the antiplatelet therapy, follow-up examinations are essential to ensure good results. For the case of re-stenoses, re-interventions can be discussed.

Therapy for vasospasm

Neurological deficits incurred as a result of cerebral vasospasm after subarachnoid hemorrhage (SAH) can sometimes be more devastating than those resulting from the initial aneurysmal rupture. Although triple-H therapy which includes hypervolemia, hypertension, and hemodilution is the first-line mode of treatment, endovascular treatment of vasospasm can sometimes be successful in cases in which medical management is not effective.

Endovascular treatment in patients with vasospasms can generally be performed in two ways, angioplasty to treat vasospasm of the more proximal vessels, and the intra-arterial chemical method in the smaller, more distal arteries. For the latter much interest has emerged regarding the intra-arterial selective application of calcium channel blockers during cerebral angiographic studies [22]. Compared with papaverine, for example, calcium channel blockers appear to have a more prolonged effect on arterial dilation and have not been associated with increases in ICP [23].

Treatment indication

One of the major problems is the early diagnosis of vasospasm in patients after SAH. Transcranial Doppler examinations are routine and are mostly performed daily in these patients; however, this technique has several potential pitfalls, including under- and overestimation of blood flow in the arteries of the circle of Willis. Major factors which can cause incorrect interpretation of Doppler results are triple H-therapy with consecutive general increase of blood flow, missing or minor approach to the intracranial artery due to thick skull-bone, or the interindividual low reproducibility of Doppler findings by different investigators. The major drawback of the Doppler technique is, however, that vasospasms of peripheral vessels cannot usually be detected. Cerebral perfusion techniques with CT-perfusion or MR-perfusion may help to optimize the early diagnosis of vasospasms [24,25]; however, these techniques cannot be applied and, besides, repeated perfusion studies with CT result in increased radiation of the patients and MR-perfusion studies in ventilated patients are logistically difficult. Nevertheless, in patients who are at high risk of developing vasospasms and/or Doppler findings and/or clinical findings suggest vasospasms perfusions studies should be performed early.

In SAH patients with vasospasms or with pathologic perfusion studies conventional four-vessel-angiography should be performed to show proximal or distal vasospasms and to initiate endovascular therapy.

In general proximal vasospasms are suitable for mechanical spasmolysis while distal vasospasms are a target for chemical spasmolysis.

Treatment

Mechanical spasmolysis is performed by *angioplasty* and has demonstrated permanent reversal of vasospasm in treated vessels [25,26], but it can be applied to only proximal vessel segments, and it must be performed by experienced interventional neuroradiologists (Fig. 9a.3). Owing to the invasive nature of the procedure this treatment is nearly always performed under general anesthetic. Via a transfemoral approach a guiding catheter is placed in the cervical artery. In severe vasospasms an initial chemical spasomolysis can be done first to make the direct endovascular approach easier. The angioplasty is performed with non-compliant balloons to provide the possibility to

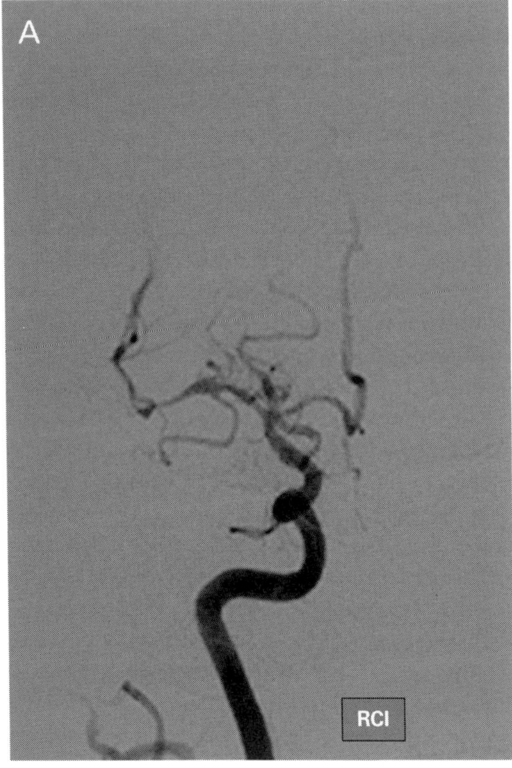

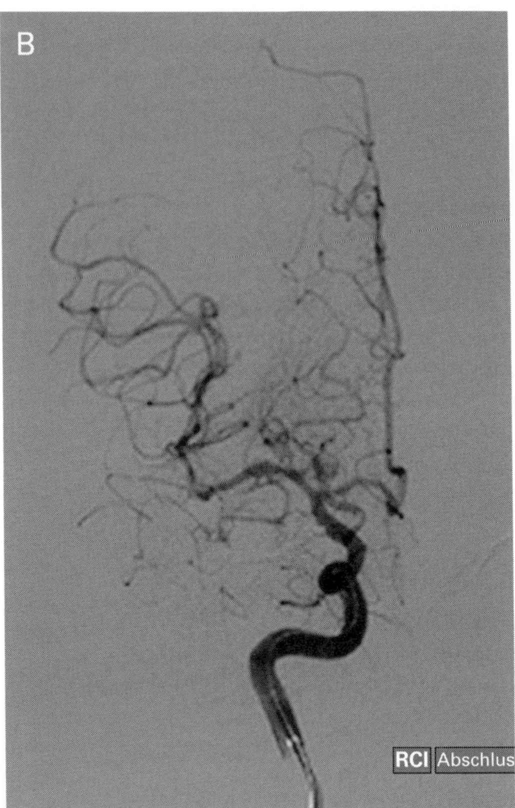

Fig. 9a.3 Mechanical spasmolysis after SAH. Initial angiogram demonstrates severe vasospasm of right M1 (lateral segment) and disturbed flow in the media territory (A). Dilatation with a micro-balloon results in a nearly complete normalization of vessel lumen and flow (B).

dilate more proximal spasms as well (internal carotid artery) and also spasms in the M1 segment without changing the balloon. Mechanical spasomolysis is limited to vessels of the proximal part of the circle of Willis (C1, M1, V4, basilar artery). The dilatation of the A1 is possible but often technically difficult.

The advantage of the mechanical spasmolysis is the immediate positive effect on the cerebral perfusion and the almost permanent reversal of vasospasm in treated vessels. However, in a few cases reversal of vasospasms within 24–48 hours after angioplasty may occur.

While the mechanical approach is limited to the proximal part of the circle of Willis, more distal and diffusely located vasospasm can be treated with chemical spasmolysis [22]. This attempt is technically less invasive and can be performed under local anesthetic. A guiding or even diagnostic catheter is placed in the cervical part of the brain-supplying artery and a calcium channel blocker is injected or infused into the cerebral territory. The total amount of the drug depends on the angiographic proven effect of the intra-arterial infusion; generally a maximum of 5–10 mg is applied in each territory while more than one territory can be treated in each session.

While the effect of the chemical spasmolysis is often only temporary and spasms may occur within 6–12 hours, some interventional groups favor a permanent intra-arterial chemical spasmolysis. For this, smaller catheters (4F) are placed into the cervical artery and the calcium channel blocker is permanently (up to 48 hours) intra-arterially infused in a lower concentration. Very particular attention is necessary to avoid thrombotic complications and a full heparinization of the patients is recommended during the procedure.

Aneurysm therapy

Besides presentation with an acute subarachnoid hemorrhage, intracranial aneurysms are often diagnosed incidentally, especially in MRIs performed for other reasons. The supposed prevalence is about 2–3%, if a direct relative has an aneurysm the prevalence rises to 6–10% or up to 19% if two or more relatives have a cerebral aneurysm [27]. The incidence of subarachnoid hemorrhages is about 6–9 per 100 000 per year [27,28]. Even though there are other reasons for a subarachnoid hemorrhage, aneurysm rupture is the main cause. Considering the aneurysm prevalence and the subarachnoid hemorrhage incidence it is understandable that not all aneurysms rupture. Therefore the treatment indication for incidental aneurysms has to be discussed closely in every individual case.

Treatment indication

Subarachnoid hemorrhage is a severe event correlated with a high rate of morbidity and mortality. In the first 12 hours the risk of a rebleeding, which is associated with a worse outcome, is at its maximum [29]. Therefore an early treatment of an acute aneurysmal subarachnoid hemorrhage is necessary. Besides the high morbidity and mortality after subarachnoid bleeding, in asymptomatic patients the treatment recommendation should consider the individual rupture risk and the risk of treating the aneurysm.

The operation risk of clipping an aneurysm is about 6–7% [30], whereas the interventional treatment risk is under 5% and decreases with constantly developing techniques [31]. A precondition for this relatively low interventional treatment risk is an experienced interventionalist. In some rare cases, if an aneurysm bleeding is accompanied by a critical intracerebral hemorrhage that needs to be operated on, clipping of the aneurysm is the immediate treatment option. Because of the localization some aneurysms are almost exclusively treated interventionally whereas others are almost exclusively operated on. In summary, aneurysms should be treated primarily interventionally if possible, if indicated and if the patient does not need an operation because of an associated critical intracerebral bleeding [32].

The estimated 5-year-bleeding-risk of an incidental aneurysm is about 5% [27], although it has to be considered that different factors influence the individual rupture risk. One of the most important factors is the aneurysm size, as aneurysms lager than 7 mm have a higher bleeding risk [33]. Additionally, increasing size over time and wall irregularities like 'baby aneurysms' are correlated with an increased rupture risk as well as an aneurysm bleeding from another aneurysm in the medical history. If the aneurysm is located vertebrobasilar, including the posterior communicating artery, the rupture risk is elevated too [28]. Other factors raising the rupture risk are female gender, smoking, Japanese or Finnish nationality and a high patient age [34]. In contrast to the elevated rupture risk in elderly patients, in younger patients the cumulative rupture risk might indicate that treatment is appropriate. Finally, the individual wish of the patient has to be considered. Some patients are affected psychologically through knowledge of the aneurysm and a fear of bleeding. In these cases a treatment has to be discussed too.

All these individual risk factors and the wish of the patient should be compared with the expected treatment risk to see if the treatment is recommendable or not. If no indication for therapy is seen, follow-up examinations with MRI might be reasonable.

Treatment

As mentioned above the interventional treatment is the first choice of treatment if possible. Besides the treatment indication, the procedure for treating a ruptured or an unruptured aneurysm is the same. The commonly practised endovascular method is the coil embolization, where the aneurysm is stuffed with detachable platinum coils.

For the embolization the aneurysm has to be entered with a microcatheter. This is a critical part of the intervention with the risk of rupturing the aneurysm. To ensure no unexpected movements of the patient all interventions usually have to be performed under general anesthetic. In the next step the aneurysm is filled stepwise with detachable coils. To reach an optimum result the coils can be replaced or removed before becoming detached if necessary. Depending on the aneurysm size, different coil sizes and lengths exist. Optimally, coils are placed inside the aneurysm until no more inflow is detectable. This mostly requires multiple coils. The coils can be differentiated between framing, filling, and finishing coils, where the filling coils and especially the finishing coils are softer. The idea is to form a 'coil-cage' with the framing coils in the aneurysm to prevent a prolapse of the softer filling coils into the vessel. The softer filling coils can be packed more densely to fill out the aneurysm completely.

Some technical tricks, called remodeling, exist to prevent a prolapse of coils in cases with a broad aneurysm neck. One possibility is to inflate a small balloon in front of the aneurysm ostium after placing the microcatheter inside the aneurysm. In the next step the aneurysm is coiled with framing and filling coils. After deflating the balloon the coils are fixed in the densely packed aneurysm. Because of the temporary vessel occlusion, the treating interventionalist must work quickly. The advantage of this technique is that in the case of a perforation the vessel can be occluded with the balloon immediately. The alternative, often practised technique to treat aneurysms with a broad neck is to use a stent to prevent the coils from prolapsing into the parent vessel (Fig. 9a.4). In such cases the microcatheter is placed in the aneurysm either before releasing the stent (jailing) or afterwards through the stent-meshes. To prevent a compression of the stent struts only soft coils are used for the stent-assisted coiling. After the coiling the catheter can be pulled back in both cases. If a stent is used, sufficient double antiplatelet medication is necessary to avoid thrombembolic complications.

The use of flow-reducing stents with narrow meshes (so-called flow-diverter stents) is controversial. The benefit of such stents is that they offer an opportunity to treat otherwise untreatable broad neck or even fusiform aneurysms. High recurrence rates in extremely large aneurysms or broad neck aneurysms have been observed after conventional coiling or coiling and stenting and it is suspected that the long-term results of these large aneurysms treated with flow diverters is better. However, secondary rupture of aneurysms only treated with flow diverters are observed in up to 2% of cases. The general recommendation nowadays is that flow diverters should only be used in those cases that cannot be treated otherwise [35].

Other forms of interventional aneurysm treatment such as small woven plugs or glue are not routinely used now.

Endovascular therapy for arterial malformations (AVMs and fistulas)

Brain arterial malformations (BAM) are generally symptomatic by hemorrhage or seizures. While there is little doubt that BAVM after hemorrhage need to be treated because of higher risk of rebleeding there is an open discussion on the necessity of treatment in unsymptomatic patients with BAVM or in BAVM patients with seizures who can be treated sufficiently by medical treatment.

Owing to the increased use of brain imaging, especially MRI, nowadays two and a half times more BAVM cases are diagnosed with an unruptured malformation as compared with those detected after intracranial hemorrhage. The overall incidence of unruptured BAVM patients is suspected to be about 1.27/100 000 persons per year with an incidence of AVM hemorrhage of 0.50/100 000 persons per year [36].

Beside these general data there are specific hemodynamic attributes thought to be of relevance for an increased risk of hemorrhage. These factors are probably a deep location of the AVM, a deep venous drainage, intranidal aneurysms and/or aneurysms of the brain feeding AVM and severe fistula components.

Current invasive treatment strategies for brain arteriovenous malformations (BAVMs) are varied and include endovascular procedures, neurosurgery, and radiotherapy alone and in combination, often dependent on the decisions of the local clinical team. All of these invasive treatments are administered on the

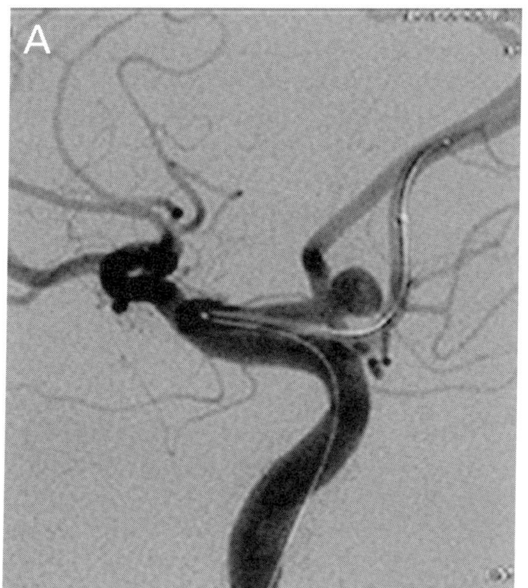

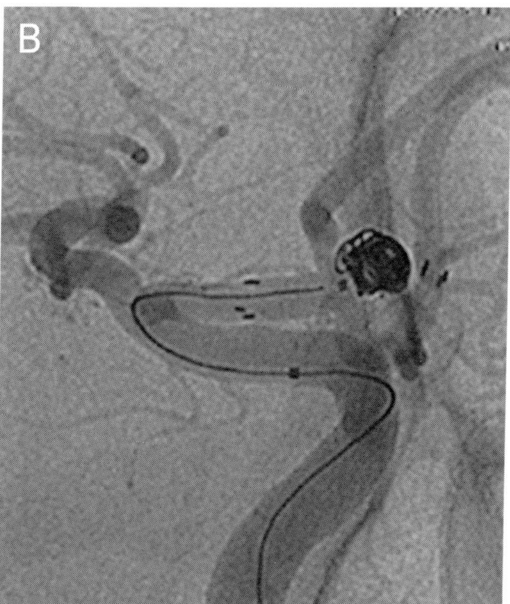

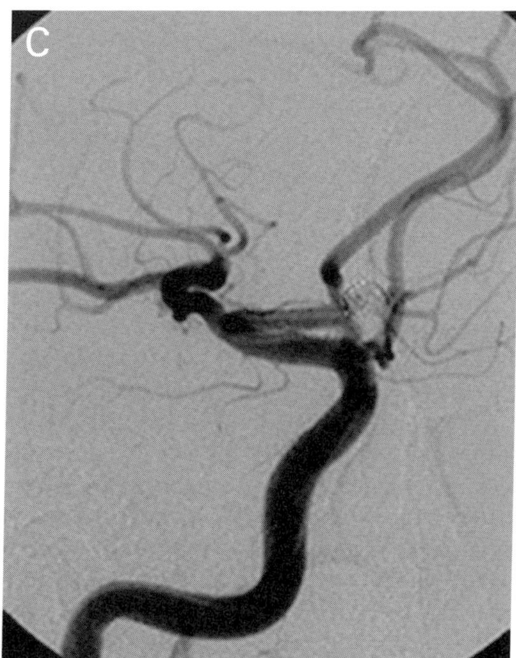

Fig. 9a.4 Stent-assisted coiling of a right A1 aneurysm. Right ICA angiogram documents a broad neck aneurysm of the right A1, a microcatheter is navigated into the left A2 to deploy a self-expanding aneurysm stent (A). A microcatheter is navigated through the stent-cells into the aneurysm and detachable coils are deployed into the aneurysm (B). Final angiogram demonstrates complete occlusion of the aneurysm (C).

assumption that they will decrease the risk of hemorrhage and lead to better long-term outcomes.

Endovascular treatment is able to finally cure BAVM patients by embolization alone only in 15–20% of cases. Even with the availability of modern liquid embolization materials most of the BAVM cannot be totally occluded and additional surgical operation or radiotherapy is requested.

Therefore the indication for interventional AVM management and the way, why, and how embolization is performed should be based on a multidisciplinary decision in a neurovascular team of neuroradiologists, neurosurgeons, neurologists and radiotherapists.

Embolization strategy can focus on the treatment of flow-related aneurysms at the AVM feeding vessels and/or the occlusion of the BAVM itself. For the latter an interdisciplinary strategy is strongly recommended to open or optimize the way for the following therapy (operation or radiotherapy).

Embolization of the AVM can be done to perform a downstaging of the malformation and make the final therapy possible or more comfortable. However, worldwide the different neurovascular centers follow different strategies in terms of timing, mono- or multistage approach, and intensity of this approach for endovascular therapy [36].

Embolization technique

An intensive imaging work-up is necessary prior to any therapeutic approach. MRI has the key role in this concept and high-resolution MRI is needed to demonstrate the anatomy in cross-sectional technique. FMRI is helpful to demonstrate the relation between eloquent territories and the nidus of the angioma to avoid neurological deficits after therapy. Several non-invasive angiographic MRI techniques (including 4D-MRA, ASL) are available to supply more hemodynamic information prior to invasive diagnostic or therapeutic approaches or for non-invasive follow-ups.

Nevertheless the gold standard for detailed therapy planning is selective catheter-based DSA, which helps to identify the main feeders of the angioma, detects flow-associated aneurysms either on the feeding vessels or in the nidus itself, shows the hemodynamic in the angioma and helps to define the venous drainage. Classification of the angiomas is done with the Spetzler–Martin classification, which was originally developed to describe the operative risk of AVMs [37]. However, this classification is also helpful to support interdisciplinary communication. The WADA test is normally no longer required while fMRI usually helps to answer the question of hemispheric dominance. In selective cases a superselective WADA test performed via a microcatheter injection in selective pial branches may be helpful to localize functional eloquent territories. Superselective ASL angiography or perfusion may be a non-invasive alternative for a superselective WADA test.

Endovascular therapy of angiomas is usually done under general anesthetic, to increase the patient's safety and comfort. Flow-related aneurysms at the AVM feeding vessels or located directly intranidal should be embolized first, usually with coil embolization, to avoid aneurysm rupture, because any therapeutic manipulation (embolization, surgery, radiation) on the AVM may change the hemodynamic characteristics of the angioma in an unpredictable way.

High-flow components (fistulas) in the AVM can be treated with coils, glue or Onyx, depending upon how far a microcatheter can be navigated into the fistula and the fistula volume. Today, the endovascular treatment of the angioma itself is performed mostly with Onyx injection (Fig. 9a.5). Onyx is a glue developed specifically for the endovascular treatment of angiomas and aneurysms. It can be injected via a microcatheter into the AVM vessels to perform a glue-casting of the angioma-nidus. For this it is important to guide the embolization catheter as far as possible into the nidus. With controlled injection of the Onyx, sufficient occlusion of the AVM or of parts of the AVM can be performed in a safe way, either to perform a final occlusion of the AVM (which is possible only in about 20% of cases) or to prepare for additional therapy with surgery or radiation. A controlled medical periembolization strategy is important to avoid break-through hemorrhage (i.e. blood pressure management).

Controlled outcome data on different therapeutic strategies are not available. In a meta-analysis from 25 sources of 2425 patients of Castel and Kantor [38], no reports of any of the treatment modalities were free from

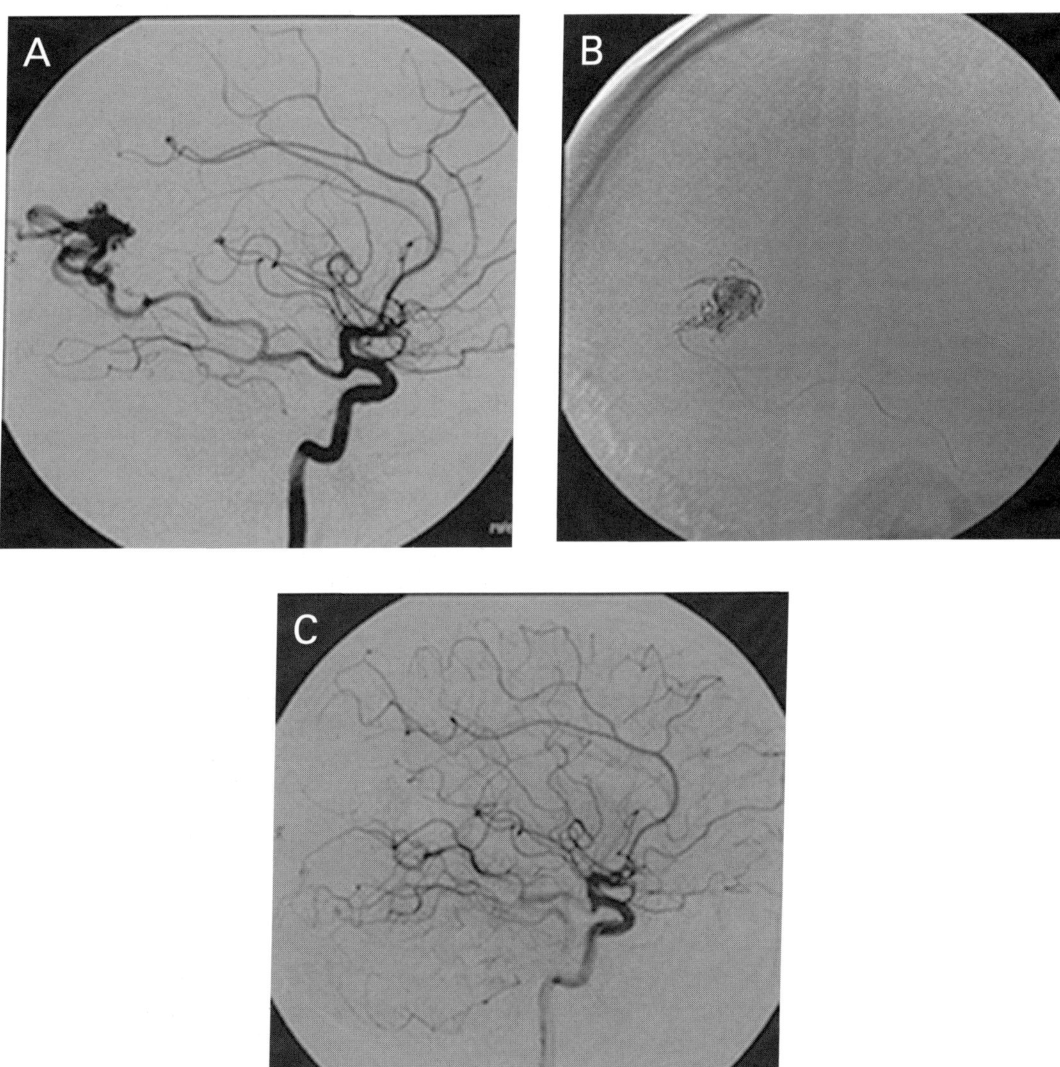

Fig. 9a.5 Embolization of an angioma with onyx. Angiogram of the left ICA shows an occipito-parietal high-flow angioma (A). A microcatheter is navigated into the BAVM nidus and onyx is injected via the MC resulting in a nice cast of the glue (B). Final angiogram demonstrates nearly complete occlusion of the BAVM (C).

complications of therapy. Post-operative mortality was 3.3% with permanent post-operative morbidity of 8.6%, varying from 1.5% to 18.7%. Pre-surgical embolization alone also carried a substantial permanent morbidity varying from 4% to 8.9%. However, clinical outcome after embolization has improved over the last two decades depending on catheter technique, embolization material and knowledge regarding brain AVM anatomy. Persistent neurological deficits have been documented in 9% of patients, with a 2% case fatality [39].

A recent multicenter overview on endovascular AVM therapy (presented at the 2005 World Federation of

Interventional and Therapeutic Neuroradiology meeting) revealed a 10% to 20% frequency of self-reported treatment-related complications in numerous well-established international centers. In a series of patients treated with combined endovascular and surgical intervention, Vinuela *et al.* detected a mild overall long-term morbidity of 6% with an additional moderate to severe morbidity and mortality rate of 13% [40].

To find out the relation between treatment risk and natural risk of BAVM the international, multicenter trial 'A Randomized Trial of Unruptured Brain AVMs' (ARUBA) – is poised to randomize patients with unruptured brain AVMs to medical management versus best interventional therapy, but this has not been completed yet [41].

AV fistulas are classified according to the classification of Cognard *et al.* [42]. Indications for treatment are fistulas classified as dangerous abnormalities (> grade 2A), fistulas which result in neurological deficits (i.e. ophthalmoplegia) or induce unacceptable tinnitus.

Embolization is usually the first treatment of choice. Embolization materials are either coils or Onyx, depending on the fistula size and anatomy (Fig. 9a.6).

Carotis cavernous fistulas (CCF) are differentiated in high-flow and low-flow fistulas. High-flow fistulas are either the result of trauma with dissection of the carotid vessel wall or follow rupture of carotid aneurysm in the sinus part. The cause of low-flow CCFs is often uncertain, these fistulas are supplied by small feeders from the external carotid or from the internal carotid vessel wall. High-flow fistulas are usually treated with coiling via the transcarotidal approach, sometimes with additional stenting. In the case of severe carotid wall disruption a sacrificing of the carotid may be the best treatment option. The permanent carotid occlusion is done with coils (i.e. volume coils) or specific occlusion devices (i.e. amplatzer occluder). Low-flow fistulas are treated primarily using the venous approach either via the inferior petrous sinus or via the orbital vein. Later, a surgical section of the dilated superior ophthalmic vein is sometimes necessary. Additional transarterial embolization of the main arterial feeders may be helpful.

Other fistulas are often the late result of previous cortical vein or sinus thrombosis. The most frequent location for this type of fistula is the lateral transversal sinus fistula.

DAVFs with direct drainage into a cortical vein or with chronic venous reflux require treatment aimed at a complete and definitive fistula closure because they have a high risk of hemorrhage and venous infarction. The treatment may also be indicated for fistulas seen as

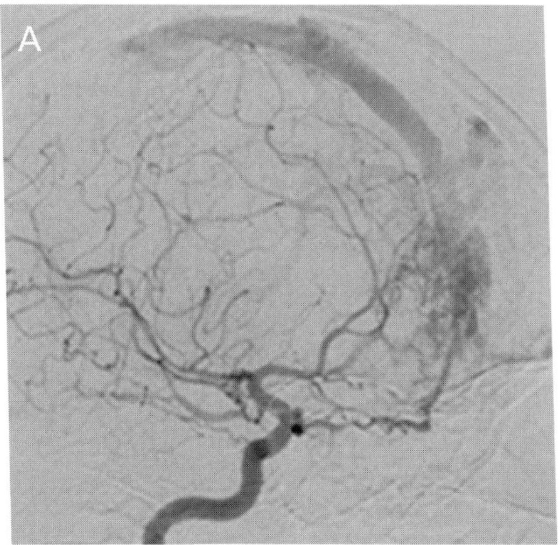

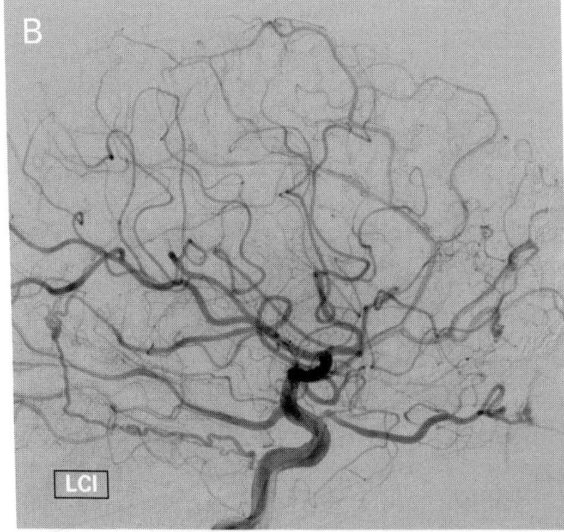

Fig. 9a.6 Embolization of a frontal AV fistula. Angiogram shows a frontal dural high-flow fistula before (A) and after (B) embolization with onyx.

benign (no chronic venous reflux) when the patient cannot tolerate the symptoms, usually pulsatile tinnitus from the high-flow shunt or headache related to intracranial hypertension.

Previously the transvenous approach with coil occlusion of the affected sinus part was the primary treatment option. However, transarterial embolization with Onyx is now the principal recommended therapy [43].

In a recent published series, in 36 of 44 procedures (81%), the authors obtained a cure with just a single procedure. Of the remaining eight fistulas, three resulted in an angiographic cure with a second embolization session and one required a third endovascular treatment. In a minority of lesions (five of 44), both transarterial and transvenous approaches were used to effect a cure. The remaining four patients did require additional open neurosurgical intervention for lesion eradication. Overall, by using a treatment algorithm based on arterial injection of Onyx, complemented by transvenous embolization, the authors embolized and cured 40 of the 44 (91%) fistulas treated. Better anatomic outcome was related to the presence of direct meningeal artery feeders, whereas embolization through transosseous feeders was less effective [44]. The authors concluded that the treatment of DAVFs by using Onyx in an arterial approach is effective and safe and allows the complete occlusion of the arterial venous shunt in a single session in most cases. In the subset of DAVFs with direct drainage into a dural sinus, the arterial approach can be used with Onyx injection and the venous sinus can be preserved.

REFERENCES

1. Shi Z-S, Loh Y, Walker G, Duckwiler GR. Clinical outcomes in middle cerebral artery trunk occlusions versus secondary division occlusions after mechanical thrombectomy: pooled analysis of the Mechanical Embolus Removal in Cerebral Ischemia (MERCI) and Multi MERCI trials. *Stroke.* 2010;**41** (5): 953–60.
2. Nogueira RG, Lutsep HL, Gupta R, *et al.* Trevo versus Merci retrievers for thrombectomy revascularisation of large vessel occlusions in acute ischaemic stroke (TREVO 2): a randomised trial. *Lancet.* 2012;**380**(9849): 1231–40.
3. Pexman JH, Barber PA, Hill MD, *et al.* Use of the Alberta Stroke Program Early CT Score (ASPECTS) for assessing CT scans in patients with acute stroke. *AJNR Am J Neuroradiol.* 2001;**22**(8): 1534–42.
4. Riedel CH, Zimmermann P, Jensen-Kondering U, *et al.* The importance of size: successful recanalization by intravenous thrombolysis in acute anterior stroke depends on thrombus length. *Stroke.* 2011;**42**(6): 1775–7.
5. Schulte-Altedorneburg G, Brückmann H, Hamann GF, *et al.* Ischemic and hemorrhagic complications after intra-arterial fibrinolysis in vertebrobasilar occlusion. *AJNR Am J Neuroradiol.* 2007;**28**(2): 378–81.
6. Saver JL, Jahan R, Levy EI, *et al.* Solitaire flow restoration device versus the Merci Retriever in patients with acute ischaemic stroke (SWIFT): a randomised, parallel-group, non-inferiority trial. *Lancet.* 2012;**380** (9849): 1241–9.
7. Koh JS, Lee SJ, Ryu C-W, Kim HS. Safety and efficacy of mechanical thrombectomy with solitaire stent retrieval for acute ischemic stroke: a systematic review. *Neurointervention.* 2012;**7**(1): 1–9.
8. Almekhlafi MA, Menon BK, Freiheit EA, *et al.* Analysis of observational intra-arterial stroke therapy studies using the Merci device, penumbra system, and retrievable stents. *AJNR Am J Neuroradiol.* 2012;**34**(1): 140–45.
9. Randomised trial of endarterectomy for recently symptomatic carotid stenosis: final results of the MRC European Carotid Surgery Trial (ECST). *Lancet.* 1998;**351**(9113): 1379–87.
10. Kasner SE, Chimowitz MI, Lynn MJ, *et al.* Predictors of ischemic stroke in the territory of a symptomatic intracranial arterial stenosis. *Circulation.* 2006;**113**(4): 555–63.
11. Rothwell PM, Eliasziw M, Gutnikov SA, *et al.* Analysis of pooled data from the randomised controlled trials of endarterectomy for symptomatic carotid stenosis. *Lancet.* 2003;**361**(9352): 107–16.
12. Endovascular versus surgical treatment in patients with carotid stenosis in the Carotid and Vertebral Artery Transluminal Angioplasty Study (CAVATAS): a randomised trial. *Lancet.* 2001;**357**(9270): 1729–37.
13. Brott TG, Hobson RW, Howard G, *et al.* Stenting versus endarterectomy for treatment of carotid-artery stenosis. *N Engl J Med.* 2010;**363**(1): 11–23.
14. Ederle J, Dobson J, Featherstone RL, *et al.* Carotid artery stenting compared with endarterectomy in patients with symptomatic carotid stenosis (International Carotid Stenting Study): an interim analysis of a randomised controlled trial. *Lancet.* 2010;**375**(9719): 985–97.

15. Ringleb PA, Allenberg J, Brückmann H, *et al.* 30 day results from the SPACE trial of stent-protected angioplasty versus carotid endarterectomy in symptomatic patients: a randomised non-inferiority trial. *Lancet.* 2006;**368**(9543): 1239–47.
16. Chimowitz MI, Lynn MJ, Howlett-Smith H, *et al.* Comparison of warfarin and aspirin for symptomatic intracranial arterial stenosis. *N Engl J Med.* 2005;**352**(13): 1305–16.
17. Kurre W, Berkefeld J, Brassel F, *et al.* In-hospital complication rates after stent treatment of 388 symptomatic intracranial stenoses: results from the INTRASTENT multicentric registry. *Stroke.* 2010;**41**(3): 494–8.
18. Chimowitz MI, Lynn MJ, Derdeyn CP, *et al.* Stenting versus aggressive medical therapy for intracranial arterial stenosis. *N Engl J Med.* 2011;**365**(11): 993–1003.
19. Jansen O, Fiehler J, Hartmann M, Brückmann H. Protection or nonprotection in carotid stent angioplasty: the influence of interventional techniques on outcome data from the SPACE Trial. *Stroke.* 2009;**40**(3): 841–6.
20. Tietke MWK, Kerby T, Alfke K, *et al.* Complication rate in unprotected carotid artery stenting with closed-cell stents. *Neuroradiology.* 2010;**52**(7): 611–18.
21. Bonati LH, Jongen LM, Haller S, *et al.* New ischaemic brain lesions on MRI after stenting or endarterectomy for symptomatic carotid stenosis: a substudy of the International Carotid Stenting Study (ICSS). *Lancet Neurol.* 2010;**9**(4): 353–62.
22. Biondi A, Le Jean L, Puybasset L. Clinical experience of selective intra-arterial nimodipine treatment for cerebral vasospasm following subarachnoid hemorrhage. *AJNR Am J Neuroradiol.* 2006;**27**(3): 474; author reply 474.
23. Eddleman CS, Hurley MC, Naidech AM, Batjer HH, Bendok BR. Endovascular options in the treatment of delayed ischemic neurological deficits due to cerebral vasospasm. *Neurosurg Focus.* 2009;**26**(3): E6.
24. Aralasmak A, Akyuz M, Ozkaynak C, Sindel T, Tuncer R. CT angiography and perfusion imaging in patients with subarachnoid hemorrhage: correlation of vasospasm to perfusion abnormality. *Neuroradiology.* 2009;**51**(2): 85–93.
25. Beck J, Raabe A, Lanfermann H, *et al.* Effects of balloon angioplasty on perfusion- and diffusion-weighted magnetic resonance imaging results and outcome in patients with cerebral vasospasm. *J Neurosurg.* 2006;**105**(2): 220–7.
26. Jestaedt L, Pham M, Bartsch AJ, *et al.* The impact of balloon angioplasty on the evolution of vasospasm-related infarction after aneurysmal subarachnoid hemorrhage. *Neurosurgery.* 2008;**62**(3): 610–17.
27. Fiehler J. [Unruptured brain aneurysms: when to screen and when to treat?]. *Rofo.* 2012;**184**(2): 97–104.
28. Clarke M. Systematic review of reviews of risk factors for intracranial aneurysms. *Neuroradiology.* 2008;**50**(8): 653–64.
29. Connolly ES Jr, Rabinstein AA, Carhuapoma JR, *et al.* Guidelines for the management of aneurysmal subarachnoid hemorrhage: a guideline for healthcare professionals from the American Heart Association/American Stroke Association. *Stroke.* 2012;**43**(6): 1711–37.
30. Kotowski M, Naggara O, Darsaut TE, Raymond J. Systematic reviews of the literature on clipping and coiling of unruptured intracranial aneurysms. *Neurochirurgie.* 2012;**58**(2–3): 125–39.
31. Naggara ON, Lecler A, Oppenheim C, Meder J-F, Raymond J. Endovascular treatment of intracranial unruptured aneurysms: a systematic review of the literature on safety with emphasis on subgroup analyses. *Radiology.* 2012; **263**(3): 828–35.
32. Van der Schaaf I, Algra A, Wermer M, *et al.* Endovascular coiling versus neurosurgical clipping for patients with aneurysmal subarachnoid haemorrhage. *Cochrane Database Syst Rev.* 2005;(4): CD003085.
33. Wiebers DO, Whisnant JP, Huston J, *et al.* Unruptured intracranial aneurysms: natural history, clinical outcome, and risks of surgical and endovascular treatment. *Lancet.* 2003;**362**(9378): 103–10.
34. Wermer MJH, Van der Schaaf IC, Algra A, Rinkel GJE. Risk of rupture of unruptured intracranial aneurysms in relation to patient and aneurysm characteristics: an updated meta-analysis. *Stroke.* 2007;**38**(4): 1404–10.
35. Byrne J, Szikora I. Flow diverters in the management of intracranial aneurysms: A review. *EJMINT.* 2012; 1225000057.
36. Hartmann A, Mast H, Choi JH, Stapf C, Mohr JP. Treatment of arteriovenous malformations of the brain. *Curr Neurol Neurosci Rep.* 2007;**7**(1): 28–34.
37. Spetzler RF, Martin NA. A proposed grading system for arteriovenous malformations. *J Neurosurg.* 1986;**65**(4): 476–83.
38. Castel JP, Kantor G. [Postoperative morbidity and mortality after microsurgical exclusion of cerebral arteriovenous malformations. Current data and analysis of recent literature]. *Neurochirurgie.* 2001;**47**(2–3 Pt 2): 369–83.
39. Taylor CL, Dutton K, Rappard G, *et al.* Complications of preoperative embolization of cerebral arteriovenous malformations. *J Neurosurg.* 2004;**100**(5): 810–12.
40. Viñuela F, Dion JE, Duckwiler G, *et al.* Combined endovascular embolization and surgery in the management of

cerebral arteriovenous malformations: experience with 101 cases. *J Neurosurg.* 1991;**75**(6): 856–64.

41. Mohr JP, Moskowitz AJ, Stapf C, *et al.* The ARUBA trial: current status, future hopes. *Stroke.* 2010;**41**(8): e537–540.
42. Cognard C, Gobin YP, Pierot L, *et al.* Cerebral dural arteriovenous fistulas: clinical and angiographic correlation with a revised classification of venous drainage. *Radiology.* 1995;**194**(3): 671–80.
43. De Keukeleire K, Vanlangenhove P, Kalala Okito J-P, *et al.* Transarterial embolization with ONYX for treatment of intracranial non-cavernous dural arteriovenous fistula with or without cortical venous reflux. *J Neurointerv Surg.* 2011;**3**(3): 224–8.
44. Abud TG, Nguyen A, Saint-Maurice JP, *et al.* The use of Onyx in different types of intracranial dural arteriovenous fistula. *AJNR Am J Neuroradiol.* 2011;**32**(11): 2185–91.

9b

Neuroradiological interventions in cerebrovascular disease: intracranial revascularization

Martin Radvany and Philippe Gailloud

Introduction

Intracranial atherosclerotic disease (ICAD), the most common cause of stroke worldwide (1), is characterized by progressive involvement of the major intracranial arteries and is associated with a high risk of new and recurrent strokes (2). In particular, patients with a history of recent transient ischemic attack or stroke and a significant intracranial stenosis (70–99%) have been shown to be prone to recurrent stroke despite treatment with aspirin and management of their vascular risk factors (3). The use of percutaneous angioplasty, with and without stent placement, has been proposed in this patient population as an effort to decrease the incidence of new ischemic events and improve outcomes. Angioplasty alone has a technical success rate of over 80% (4–7). When performed on an elective basis, complication rates as low as 4–6% have been observed (4,8), leading some practitioners to advocate the use of angioplasty only. However, angioplasty followed by stent placement is usually preferred, as it overcomes some of the limitations of angioplasty alone, including immediate elastic recoil, dissection, acute vessel closure, and residual stenosis. Both balloon-expandable and self-expanding stents have been used, with a technical success rate exceeding 90% (9–13).

The Stenting versus Aggressive Medical Therapy for Intracranial Arterial Stenosis (SAMMPRIS) trial (13) was the first randomized, prospective trial to compare endovascular treatment with the Wingspan stent system (Boston Scientific, Natick, MA) with best medical management. Enrollment in the trial was stopped after 451 patients because of a stroke or death rate of 14.7% in the stenting group versus 5.8% in the medical management group. The surprising findings in this study were that the risk of stroke with medical management was lower than expected, while the risk of PTAS with the Wingspan system was higher than expected. The principal message of the SAMMPRIS study is that intracranial stenting cannot be considered as the first line therapy of ICAD at this time. However, two important points must be remembered: 1) the SAMMPRIS study investigated a single device (the Wingspan system), and 2) intracranial stenting remains an important tool for patients with ICAD failing optimal medical therapy.

This chapter provides a practical outline of the technique used for intracranial angioplasty and stenting at our institution.

Patient preparation

Candidates for endovascular treatment of ICAD are patients with a severe stenosis, recent ischemic symptoms, and a score on NIH stroke scale greater than one (14). For acute stroke patients who are stable or improving, the procedure can be delayed 4 to 6 weeks in order to reduce the risk of hemorrhagic transformation of the infarct or of hemorrhage related to perfusion

Critical Care of the Stroke Patient, ed. Stefan Schwab, Daniel Hanley, and A. David Mendelow. Published by Cambridge University Press.

pressure breakthrough phenomenon (15). In view of the SAMMPRIS trial results, angioplasty and stenting is currently limited to patients who became symptomatic under optimal medical therapy.

Anti-platelet therapy

The need for dual antiplatelet therapy is derived from the literature on coronary stenting (16,17). Patients should be pre-treated with a combination of aspirin and a second antiplatelet medication to lower the risk of thromboembolic complications during and after the procedure. Aspirin is usually given as a daily dose of 325 mg orally. Clopidogrel (Plavix, Bristol-Myers Squibb, New York, NY) is the most commonly used and preferred second antiplatelet medication. Pre-treatment should be initiated at least 3 days but preferably 7 days prior to procedure. If optimal preparation is not possible, a loading dose of 300 mg within 24 hours or 600 mg within 6 hours can be used (18). Ticlopidine (Roche Laboratories, Nutley, NJ) at a dose of 250 mg orally twice daily can be used as an alternative for clopidogrel, but patients must be monitored for thrombocytopenia as a side effect of the medication. For emergent procedures, intravenous antiplatelet agents can be given in place of oral antiplatelet agents. Abciximab (Reopro, Eli Lilly, Indianapolis, IN) can be given as a bolus dose of 0.20 mg/kg immediately before the procedure, with a maintenance intravenous drip of 0.125 mcg/kg/min (maximum 10 mcg/min) for 12 hours after the procedure. In this case, adjunctive intraprocedural heparin is typically not administered in order to decrease the risk of hemorrhage (19). Eptifibatide is another intravenous agent that can be given as a bolus dose of 180 mcg/kg/min at the beginning of the procedure (20). While intravenous aspirin is not available in the US, aspirin suppositories (300 mg) can be administered immediately prior to or during an urgent procedure.

Warfarin is usually discontinued 3 to 4 days before stenting in order to allow normalization of the international normalized ratio (INR). For patients depending on systemic anticoagulation (e.g., atrial fibrillation), warfarin can be replaced by heparin prior to the procedure. In emergent situations, fresh frozen plasma can be given to reverse the effects of warfarin.

Procedural considerations

Anesthesia

There is no clear evidence in favor of performing intracranial angioplasty and stenting under conscious sedation rather than general endotracheal anesthesia. General anesthesia has the advantages of maintaining a stable patient position throughout the procedure, allowing for optimal imaging and stenosis measurement, as well as high-quality roadmap imaging for intracranial navigation and accurate device positioning. In addition, pharmacological paralysis prevents patient motion from occurring at critical times, such as during vessel dilation, when a temporary reduction in cerebral perfusion might lead to confusion or agitation. Stopping patient motion also reduces the risk of perforation or vessel rupture. General anesthesia also helps in the management of potentially life-threatening periprocedural complications (e.g., arterial dissection, perforation).

Access

A femoral arterial access is the standard approach for intracranial procedures. In some cases, patient anatomy may dictate a brachial approach due to vessel tortuosity. This is usually more of a concern for stenosis in the posterior circulation. In rare, extreme cases of brachiocephalic tortuosity, a direct carotid approach can be considered (21). In such instances, surgical removal of the arterial sheath with direct repair of the arteriotomy site is preferable to compressing the carotid artery, avoiding the risk of neck hematoma and flow reduction through a freshly placed stent.

Anticoagulation

Systemic anticoagulation is usually initiated once access has been obtained. Intravenous heparin can be administered on a weight-based titration or, preferably, monitored through activated clotting times (ACT). For weight-based heparinization, an intravenous bolus of 50–80 units per kilogram is given, followed by a thousand units hourly. With ACT monitoring, a value of

250–300 seconds is targeted. ACT monitoring also helps adjust the anticoagulation level in patients placed under heparin therapy prior to the procedure.

When glycoprotein IIb/IIIa inhibitors are used, either as a substitute for oral antiplatelet agents or to treat a thromboembolic complication, the heparin dosing is usually adjusted to obtain an ACT value of 200 seconds in order to reduce the risk of a hemorrhagic complication.

Technical details

Baseline angiography

Before treating an intracranial stenosis, it is important to perform a four-vessel diagnostic cerebral angiogram evaluating the cerebrovascular anatomy and potential collateral pathways specific to each patient. The location, length, and morphology of the stenosis must be precisely defined, an accurate vessel diameter proximal and distal to the stenosis determined. The configuration of the distal cerebral branches needs to be carefully evaluated, as this initial study provides the baseline anatomy against which control angiograms will be compared in order to evaluate for distal emboli and/or branch occlusion. The optimal working projections for the angioplasty and stenting should also be determined at that time; rotational angiography with three-dimensional reconstructions can facilitate this step by minimizing the number of injections, the contrast load, and the radiation exposure (in particular when using low-dose protocols). Finally, this baseline angiogram also assesses the presence of incidental lesions, such as an intracranial aneurysm.

Guiding catheters and sheaths

A stable endovascular platform is an essential element for successful internal carotid or intracranial revascularization procedures. Multiple combinations of arterial sheaths and guiding catheters can be employed; the selection of a platform depends upon individual patient anatomy and operator preferences. In a patient with a favorable anatomy, relatively straight vessels, and a stenosis in the intracranial carotid artery or one of its branches, a guiding catheter with good support (e.g., 6-French Envoy, Codman & Shurtleff, Inc., Raynham, MA) is usually adequate. If a stronger platform is required, for example in the case of marked tortuosity of the internal carotid artery, a long sheath advanced into the distal common carotid artery can offer additional support. The Shuttle sheath (6F to 8F, Cook, Bloomington, IN), a long arterial sheath with a Tuohy Borst adapter at its proximal extremity, is a good choice for neurovascular procedures; it is compatible with a range of variously shaped 6.5F coaxial catheters that facilitate navigation in difficult arch configurations. Occasionally, a guidewire carefully parked in the external carotid artery may be needed to offer enough support for the coaxial advancement of the 6.5F catheter and Shuttle sheath. Such maneuver needs to be performed under roadmap guidance in order to avoid vessel damage or perforation by the guidewire tip.

When facing a higher degree of tortuosity, a flexible guiding catheter with an atraumatic tip, such as the Distal Access Catheter (DAC, Codman & Shurtleff, Inc., Raynham, MA) or the Neuron (Penumbra, Inc., Alameda, CA), can be advanced up to the petrous segment of the internal carotid artery, if needed. These catheters carry the disadvantage of increased complexity with a tri-axial configuration (22). These principles of stable platform and distal access apply similarly in the vertebrobasilar circulation.

Balloon angioplasty versus stent-assisted angioplasty

Because it is not possible to predict how an arterial stenosis will respond to balloon angioplasty, all the equipment necessary to deliver a stent should be available in the angiography suite. When angioplasty of a stenosis results in an excellent result, without elastic recoil, the problems associated with stent placement and prolonged dual antiplatelet therapy can be avoided. However, the only intracranial angioplasty system approved by the FDA for use in the US (Wingspan, Boston Scientific, Natick, MA) requires a combination of angioplasty and stenting.

Both self-expanding and balloon-expandable stents (Pharos Vitesse, Codman & Shurtleff, Inc., Raynham,

MA) have been specifically designed for intracranial use. Each system has specific advantages and disadvantages.

The Wingspan system requires a two-step approach, with predilation of the stenosis followed by deployment of the stent. This presents the disadvantage of having to maintain a guidewire in a stable position across the stenosis during the whole procedure, which can be challenging in very tortuous anatomy; distal migration of the guidewire during the exchange between the angioplasty balloon and the stent delivery catheter carries some risks, in particular when the tip advances into small branches that can be perforated. Self-expanding stents do not have the radial force of balloon expandable stents, and may therefore not be as well apposed to the vessel wall, a factor potentially leading to restenosis. At the same time, a lower radial force appears to decrease the risk of in-stent endothelial hyperplasia and delayed restenosis.

Balloon-expandable stents can often be placed in a single step procedure, avoiding the need for exchange maneuvers, though in some cases predilation may be required as well. While having greater radial force, balloon-expandable stents are stiffer and more difficult to deliver to the stenosis site, especially in patients with tortuous anatomy, a problem exacerbated by increasing stent length. Among the disadvantages of balloon-expandable stents is the higher risk of vessel rupture during deployment, and the fact that the stent straightens the artery in which it is delivered, potentially damaging small surrounding perforators. The Pharos Vitesse is currently undergoing clinical trials in the US.

Balloon selection and angioplasty technique

Extreme care must be taken when treating intracranial blood vessels. As opposed to vessels in other locations, which are surrounded by muscle and whose downstream tissues and organs can tolerate distal embolization, intracranial vessels are essentially suspended in fluid and the cerebral parenchyma they supply is highly intolerant to reduced blood flow and emboli. If an intracranial vessel is ruptured or perforated, there is no adjacent tissue able to tamponade the leakage, which can have catastrophic consequences. For this reason, cerebral angioplasty is typically performed by selecting a balloon sized to 70–80% of the diameter of the adjacent, non-diseased vessel.

Angioplasty balloons come in over-the-wire (OTW) or rapid exchange (RX) configurations. OTW systems have two lumens, one for a guidewire, the second for the contrast and saline mixture that expands the balloon. The Gateway balloon (Boston Scientific, Natick, MA) is specifically designed for intracranial use. While dual lumen systems have the disadvantage of a larger crossing profile, their pushability and trackability are superior to RX systems, in particular when addressing tortuous anatomy. A theoretical advantage of RX systems is that they do not require an exchange-length wire. However, the use of an exchange-length wire is recommended even with RX systems, as it facilitates subsequent advancement of a microcatheter towards and across the treated area without losing wire access across the stent. This feature can be critical when facing the need to address acute in-stent thrombosis and/or distal cerebral thromboembolic events.

Situations in which conventional angioplasty balloons cannot be advanced to the target lesion can require the use of more compliant balloon catheters. The Hyperglide balloon (ev3, Irvine, CA), a single lumen OTW balloon designed for the treatment of cerebral vasospasm, is more compliant and trackable than a conventional angioplasty balloon, but generates lower radial forces. As the quality of the angioplasty will be suboptimal, this technique should only be considered when conventional options have failed. The use of newer, more stable guiding catheter platforms, as previously described, should reduce the need to resort to compliant balloon.

Wire selection

The ideal guidewire for intracranial angioplasty should have a soft, atraumatic, and shapeable tip that maintains its shape, has a good torque response and thus a good steerability, and enough body to support stent deployment systems without distorting the fragile intracranial vasculature. Unfortunately, such a wire does not currently exist. Most balloons and stent delivery systems used to treat intracranial atherosclerosis are combined with 0.014 inch guidewires. These wires come in standard (180–90 cm) and exchange (300 cm) lengths. Their respective advantages and disadvantages were mentioned above.

The Transend EX 0.014 inch guidewire (Boston Scientific, Natick, MA) provides a good starting point for many cases. It has a soft, shapeable tip with a medium support. The wire has good torque response and is relatively atraumatic. It comes in both a standard and exchange length version suitable for angioplasty and stent delivery. However, the tip of the Transend wire can easily penetrate small perforating branches, which represents a hazard during exchange maneuvers. The Synchro wire (Boston Scientific, Natick, MA) provides a very soft, atraumatic tip with excellent steerability, but it suffers from poor shape retention and offers less support.

The Luge (Boston Scientific, Natick, MA) is an excellent exchange wire with a very soft and atraumatic tip and a robust body. While the strong support provided by its body may distort the arterial anatomy, the soft tip is unlikely to cause damage, in particular by unwarranted penetration into small branches.

Crossing the stenosis

One may get only one chance at crossing a significant stenosis, as arterial dissection and/or occlusion may follow a failed attempt and prevent endovascular therapy. It is therefore critical to ensure that the initial attempt is successful. Prior to navigating the wire through the stenosis, we like to verify that anticoagulation is adequate (i.e., by obtaining an ACT), and confirm that the patient is fully paralyzed (if under general anesthesia, as it is the case in our practice) and the blood pressure appropriate. A patient waking up and moving during this critical portion of the procedure may lead to catastrophic consequences. If the patient has moved and the roadmap has been degraded, it is worth waiting for the anesthesia to take effect before repeating the roadmap.

Some short, moderate to severe stenoses can be crossed with an angioplasty balloon catheter advanced over a guidewire previously threaded through the narrowing. For very tight, long, or irregular lesions, we prefer to use a low-profile microcatheter (1.7F–1.9F) instead of the balloon catheter. The combination of a low-profile microcatheter with a steerable microwire offers better control over the guidewire advancement through the stenosis under roadmap guidance. Once the wire has passed the stenosis, the microcatheter is advanced until its tip is safely positioned distal to the lesion. The steerable wire (e.g., a Transend 14) is then replaced by an exchange length wire offering more support, but with an atraumatic tip (the Luge wire in our practice). A distal position of the wire increases the stability of the delivery system; however, it is important to keep the wire tip in the fluoroscopic field of view, and ensure that it is freely moving within a distal vessel (i.e., not wedged in a small branch).

Angioplasty technique

Angioplasty balloons to be used in the carotid and vertebrobasilar circulation must be prepped with great care in order to avoid the presence of air within the inflation system. A bursting balloon releasing free air in the cerebral circulation is a catastrophic event. Angioplasty should be performed using an inflation device equipped with a manometer that allows the operator to monitor the pressure, and remain within the values recommended by the manufacturer. An exception to that rule is represented by compliant balloons, for which the degree of inflation is rated in volume rather than pressure.

Rapid dilation with an oversized balloon can lead to vessel dissection and/or rupture. As discussed earlier, it is safer to under-dilate a fragile intracranial vessel. The goal of treating a critical stenosis is to achieve an acceptable and adequate result with the least possible risk. The technique of balloon angioplasty has been well described; the inflation should be performed slowly over the course of 2 to 3 minutes, increasing the pressure by 1–2 atmospheres every 15 seconds. The inflation should be monitored under fluoroscopy to ensure that the balloon remains in the correct location, and that it is not too large for the target vessel (23). Once the desired pressure is reached, the balloon is slowly deflated. It should be withdrawn proximal to the treated segment with the wire maintained across the stenosis so that the balloon can be quickly advanced back into position if needed. A control angiogram is then performed to evaluate the results of the angioplasty.

Stent placement

The role of stenting in ICAD is debated. As previously discussed, some operators believe that stent placement should be reserved for treatment in which angioplasty results in an unsatisfactory result, while other operators think that stents should be used in all cases. Again, the only system currently approved in the US requires the combination of angioplasty and stenting.

The stent size should be chosen so that the vessel is neither stressed by over dilation, nor under dilated, in which case the stent will not be well apposed to the vessel wall, increasing the risk of delayed thromboembolic complications. The stent should be long enough to cover the entire length of the lesion, extending proximally and distally into normal appearing vessel. If primary angioplasty is performed with a balloon-mounted stent, the inflation technique is the same as for balloon angioplasty

Complications

The most serious complication of intracranial angioplasty is arterial rupture leading to life-threatening subarachnoid hemorrhage. Maintaining wire access across the stenosis at all times allows prompt re-advancement and inflation of the balloon across the ruptured segment, in order to gain immediate control of the hemorrhage and tamponade the rupture. Protamine sulfate is administered to reverse the systemic heparinization. Protamine must be readily available in the angiography suite, in the unlikely event that it is needed.

Other significant complications include device-related events, such as arterial dissection and/or occlusion, thrombus formation at the treated site, with or without embolic dissemination, and occlusion of small perforating branches by displaced plaque material. While thromboembolic complications must be carefully looked for and addressed immediately, for example with the superselective and systemic administration of abciximab (Reopro), small perforator occlusion by extruded plaque is unlikely to be detectable.

Non-specific angiographic complications include the risks of groin hematoma, contrast allergy, and kidney impairment.

Post-procedural management

At our institution, patients are transferred to a neurological critical care unit for post-procedural observation. It is important to manage systemic blood pressure to reduce the risk of perfusion pressure breakthrough phenomenon bleeding. Some operators discontinue heparin after the procedure; our preference is to maintain heparin overnight with a target partial thromboplastin time (PTT) of 50–80 seconds. Dual antiplatelet therapy is continued, with clopidogrel (75 mg daily) for 30 days to a year depending upon the clinical situation (ideally 6 months in our practice), and aspirin (81–325 mg daily) for life.

Follow-up

Patients are followed clinically after discharge. CT angiography and MR angiography typically yield sub-optimal results in patients who have undergone stenting due to metal artifacts. If follow-up angiography is needed, it can be performed 3 to 6 months after treatment.

Conclusion

Technical developments in stent, wire, and catheter technology are improving the safety and efficacy of intracranial angioplasty and stenting. Continuing refinements in equipment technology will likely result in better outcomes and a lower risk of recurrent ischemic events in patients with symptomatic ICAD. The precise role and timing of endovascular therapy of ICAD remains to be determined.

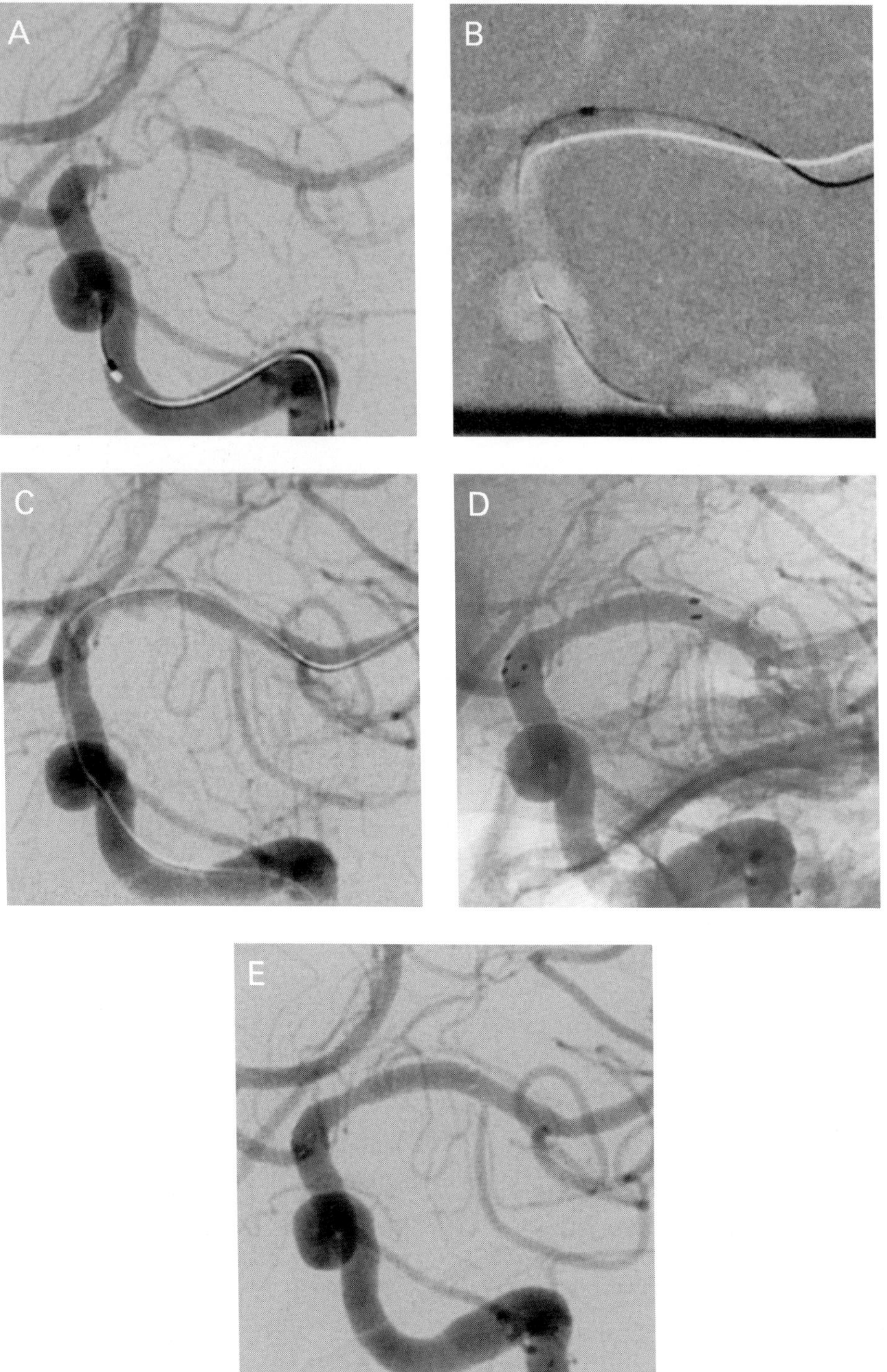

Fig. 9b.1 A 68-year-old man with a past history of strokes, presenting with acute onset aphasia and right hemiparesis, was found to have a left MCA stenosis with a significant perfusion deficit by MRI. He was started on aspirin, clopidogrel, and a statin. During his hospital stay, he was subsequently diagnosed with atrial fibrillation and begun on coumadin. He had recurrent symptoms, with MRI demonstrating progression of white matter ischemic damage. Angioplasty and stenting were recommended in the setting of failed medical therapy. A) DSA, left carotid injection, left anterior oblique projection, prior to endovascular treatment, demonstrating pre-occlusive stenosis of the distal left ICA and left MCA. B) Roadmap image, same projection, showing the angioplasty balloon (1.5 mm × 9 mm) inflated at the stenosis site. C) DSA, same projection, revealing some residual stenosis after angioplasty. D) DSA, same projection, native view post-stent placement, with resolution of the MCA stenosis, showing the proximal and distal markers of the stent. E) DSA, same projection, subtracted view obtained 15 minutes after stent placement to confirm the absence of acute in-stent clot formation.

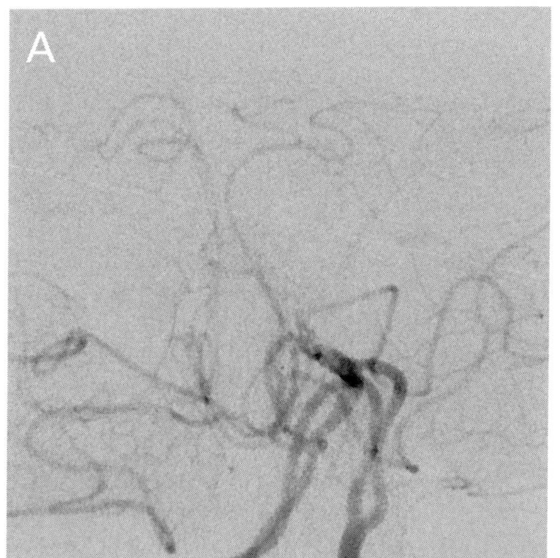

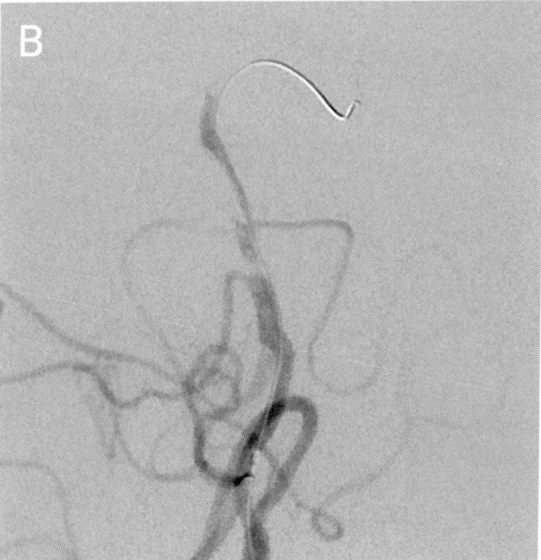

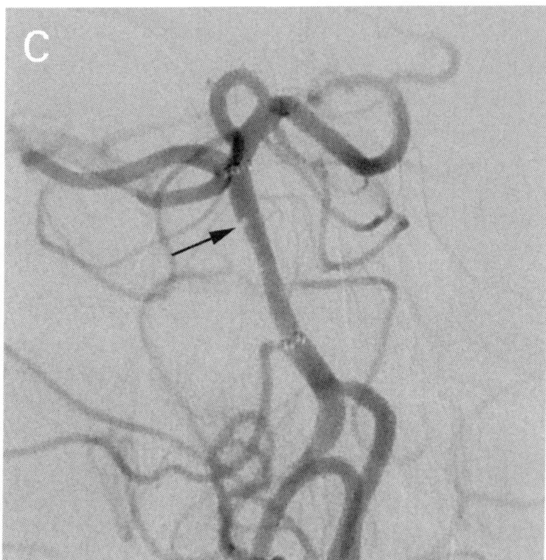

Fig. 9b.2 58-year-old female with history of high blood pressure, diabetes mellitus, and tobacco use, presenting with gait imbalance, right hemiparesis, and dysarthria/dysphagia. MRI showed an acute stroke in the left pons, right cerebellum, and posterior right medulla oblongata. MR angiography was suggestive of severe stenosis of the right vertebral artery and basilar artery. A) DSA, left vertebral artery injection, anteroposterior projection, shows a pre-occlusive stenosis of the basilar artery. B) DSA, same projection, demonstrating residual stenosis in the mid basilar region with poor distal flow after angioplasty. Note that wire access is maintained across the stenosis. C) DSA, same projection, after stent placement, showing resolution of the stenosis. Note a plaque fragment trapped between the stent and the vessel wall (arrow).

REFERENCES

1. Gorelick PB, Wong KS, Bae HJ, Pandey DK. Large artery intracranial occlusive disease: a large worldwide burden but a relatively neglected frontier. *Stroke.* 2008;**39**(8): 2396–9.
2. Chimowitz MI, Lynn MJ, Howlett-Smith H, *et al.* Comparison of warfarin and aspirin for symptomatic intracranial arterial stenosis. *N Engl J Med.* 2005;**352**(13): 1305–16.
3. Kasner SE, Chimowitz MI, Lynn MJ, *et al.* Predictors of ischemic stroke in the territory of a symptomatic intracranial arterial stenosis. *Circulation.* 2006;**113**(4): 555–63.
4. Marks MP, Wojak JC, Al-Ali F, *et al.* Angioplasty for symptomatic intracranial stenosis. *Stroke.* 2006;**37**(4): 1016–20.
5. Higashida RT, Tsai FY, Halbach VV, *et al.* Transluminal angioplasty for atherosclerotic disease of the vertebral and basilar arteries. *J Neurosurg.* 1993;**78**(2): 192–8.
6. Kim JT, Lee SH, Choi SM, *et al.* Long-term durability of percutaneous transluminal angioplasty in patients with symptomatic middle cerebral artery stenosis. *J Clin Neurol.* 2009;**5**(1): 24–8.
7. Yoon W, Seo JJ, Cho KH, *et al.* Symptomatic middle cerebral artery stenosis treated with intracranial angioplasty: Experience in 32 patients. *Radiology.* 2005;**237**(2): 620–6.
8. Alazzaz A, Thornton J, Aletich VA, *et al.* Intracranial percutaneous transluminal angioplasty for arteriosclerotic stenosis. *Arch Neurol.* 2000;**57**(11): 1625–30.
9. du Mesnil de Rochemont R, Turowski B, Buchkremer M, *et al.* Recurrent symptomatic high-grade intracranial stenoses: Safety and efficacy of undersized stents: Initial experience. *Radiology.* 2004;**231**(1): 45–9.
10. Jiang W-J, Wang Y-J, Du B, *et al.* Stenting of symptomatic M1 stenosis of middle cerebral artery. *Stroke.* 2004;**35**(6): 1375–80.
11. Fiorella D, Chow MM, Anderson M, *et al.* A 7-year experience with balloon-mounted coronary stents for the treatment of symptomatic vertebrobasilar intracranial atheromatous disease. *Neurosurgery.* 2007;**61**(2): 236–43.
12. Lylyk P, Vila J, Miranda C, *et al.* Endovascular reconstruction by means of stent placement in symptomatic intracranial atherosclerotic stenosis. *Neurol Res.* 2005;**27**(7): 84–8.
13. Chimowitz MI, Lynn MJ, Derdeyn CP, *et al.* Stenting versus aggressive medical therapy for intracranial arterial stenosis. *N Engl J Med.* 2011;**365**(11): 993–1003.
14. Derdeyn CP, Chimowitz MI. Angioplasty and stenting for atherosclerotic intracranial stenosis: rationale for a randomized clinical trial. *Neuroimaging Clin N Am.* 2007;**17**(3): 355–63.
15. Cross DT, Moran CJ, Derdeyn CP. Technique for intracranial balloon and stent-assisted angioplasty for atherosclerotic stenosis. *Neuroimaging Clin North Am.* 2007;**17**(3): 365–80.
16. King SB, III, Smith SC Jr, Hirshfeld JW Jr, *et al.* 2007 focused update of the ACC/AHA/SCAI 2005 guideline update for percutaneous coronary intervention. *J Am Coll Cardiol.* 2008;**51**(2): 172–209.
17. Wright RS, Anderson JL, Adams CD, *et al.* 2011 ACCF/AHA focused update of the guidelines for the management of patients with unstable angina/non-ST-elevation myocardial infarction (updating the 2007 guideline): A report of the American College of Cardiology Foundation/ American Heart Association Task Force on practice guidelines developed in collaboration with the American College of Emergency Physicians, Society for Cardiovascular Angiography and Interventions, and Society of Thoracic Surgeons. *J Am Coll Cardiol.* 2011;**57**(19): 1920–59.
18. Zaidat OO. Periprocedural management of patients with endovascular treatment of intracranial atherosclerotic disease. *J Neuroimaging.* 2009;**19**(S1): 35S–8S.
19. Eckert B, Koch C, Thomalla G, *et al.* Aggressive therapy with intravenous abciximab and intra-arterial rtPA and additional PTA/stenting improves clinical outcome in acute vertebrobasilar occlusion. *Stroke.* 2005;**36**(6): 1160–5.
20. Levy EI, Ecker RD, Horowitz MB, *et al.* Stent-assisted intracranial recanalization for acute stroke: Early results. *Neurosurgery.* 2006;**58**(3): 458–63.
21. Blanc R, Piotin M, Mounayer C, Spelle L, Moret J. Direct cervical arterial access for intracranial endovascular treatment. *Neuroradiology.* 2006;**48**(12): 925–9.
22. Spiotta AM, Hussain MS, Sivapatham T, *et al.* The versatile distal access catheter: The Cleveland Clinic experience. *Neurosurgery.* 2011;**68**(6): 1677–86.
23. Connors JJ, Wojak JC. Percutaneous transluminal angioplasty for intracranial atherosclerotic lesions: evolution of technique and short-term results. *J Neurosurg.* 1999;**91**(3): 415–23.

The use of hypothermia in cerebrovascular disease

Dan Holmes, Sara Pitoni, Louise Sinclair, and Peter J. D. Andrews

Introduction

Therapeutic hypothermia is the intentional reduction of core body temperature below normal physiological levels and in this chapter we will consider it's efficacy to protect areas of potentially salvageable brain after acute injury. Hypothermia has been recognized as possessing anti-inflammatory and neuroprotective properties since antiquity [1], though the first modern case reports of the effects of induced hypothermia appeared in the 1940s [2]. Thereafter, laboratory work on the effect of hypothermia on physiology has shed light on a number of mechanisms underlying therapeutic hypothermia and neuroprotection [3]. Animal models, in multiple species and injury models, have repeatedly demonstrated attenuation of neuronal injury and improved global functional recovery after ischemic stroke [4].

Early clinical studies of therapeutic hypothermia (TH) were limited by side effects and practical difficulties, and TH was not widely adopted [2,5]. More recently, with randomized controlled trials demonstrating outcome benefit after out of hospital VT/VF cardiac arrest in adults [6,7] and in neonatal birth asphyxia [8], TH has become commonplace in intensive care units. Feasibility studies have also shown that TH has the potential to be delivered safely in stroke patients outside the intensive care environment [9]. Increasing experience by medical and nursing staff of TH, improvements in preventing and treating complications and a substantial body of ongoing research mean that use of TH after stroke and traumatic brain injury is becoming increasingly common.

Mechanisms of action

Therapeutic hypothermia supports metabolic status by slowing ATP breakdown, preserving cerebral glucose and reducing cerebral oxygen consumption by 5% for every 1°C decrease in body temperature. Intracranial pressure is also reduced by hypothermia, due to a reduction in intracranial blood volume secondary to cerebral vasoconstriction. These effects were previously thought to be the most important mechanisms by which hypothermia produced neuroprotection.

More recent evidence suggests that a myriad of other mechanisms are involved. A reduction or cessation of cerebral blood flow triggers an acute cascade of events, causing inflammation, blood-brain barrier (BBB) disruption, protein breakdown and mitochondrial dysfunction [10]. The result is a combination of apoptotic and necrotic neuronal cell death. Whereas pharmacological agents studied for neuroprotection often targeted individual steps in these cascades, hypothermia influences many of the key processes involved [11], though the relative importance of each mechanism in providing neuroprotection remains unclear.

Critical Care of the Stroke Patient, ed. Stefan Schwab, Daniel Hanley, and A. David Mendelow. Published by Cambridge University Press.

Anoxic depolarization

Anoxic depolarization (AD) is a profound depolarization of cortical and subcortical neurones occurring after an ischemic episode and reflects glutamate mediated neuronal calcium influx. AD lasts 3–4 hours and is associated with worsening ischemia and edema in the penumbra (potentially salvageable cerebral tissue). Hypothermia may exert a neuroprotective effect by attenuating neuronal ischemia during the period of AD [12]. Most studies have been performed in models of global ischemia therefore, and the relevance of these effects in focal ischemia are unclear.

Glutamate release

Glutamate is an excitatory neurotransmitter found in high levels in plasma and CSF after acute ischemic stroke. 'Excitotoxic' ischemia may play a role in the pathophysiology of acute stroke, and drugs which antagonize glutamate have been shown to reduce infarct volume in experimental models. Hypothermia reduces post-ischemic glutamate release which may contribute to reduction of ischemic damage during AD [13].

Calcium influx

A rise in intracellular calcium secondary to glutamate mediated N-methyl-D-aspartate (NMDA) receptor activation is an important factor in neuronal death. Hypothermia-induced delay in calcium influx during AD may contribute to its neuroprotective action in global ischemia, although its role in focal damage is unclear. Hypothermia may also have direct inhibitory actions on calcium/calmodulin kinase, which translocate to neuronal synapses after ischemic damage.

Matrix metalloproteinases

Matrix metalloproteinases (MMPs) are zinc-dependent enzymes capable of both producing and degrading extracellular proteins. Activity of certain MMPs such as MMP-9 includes binding to the basal lamina and destruction of collagen, laminin and fibronectin. Elevated levels of MMPs found after stroke are associated with early BBB disruption and hemorrhagic transformation. MMP levels are reduced in animal models of ischemic stroke subjected to moderate hypothermia [14].

Inflammation and free radical formation

The importance of post-ischemic inflammation associated with secondary injury has been increasingly recognized during the past 20 years. Hypothermia reduces inflammation in part by reducing ischemic damage by the mechanisms outlined above. However, these mechanisms alone are unable to account for the neuroprotectant effect of hypothermia.

Leucocyte infiltration after ischemic or traumatic brain injury occurs through binding of signal proteins on the leucocyte surface with intercellular cell adhesion molecule 1 (ICAM-1) on the endothelial wall. ICAM-1 production is upregulated after ischemia. Induction of hypothermia inhibits expression of ICAM-1 and reduces leucocyte infiltration in the acute phase. Microglial and monocyte activation, pro-inflammatory cytokines and nitric oxide synthase are also inhibited by hypothermia [15].

During both the post-ischemic and reperfusion phases, reactive oxygen species (ROS) such as superoxide anion (O_2^-) are produced by a variety of sources, including activated leucocytes, and can result in cellular protein and DNA damage. In addition to reducing ROS release by inhibiting leucocytes, hypothermia directly reduces production of ROS in the penumbra when applied both during ischemia and (of more relevance to stroke patients) during reperfusion [16].

Blood-brain barrier function

Blood-brain barrier disruption is an event common to all types of brain injury, whether caused by trauma, vaso-occlusive disease, cerebral hemorrhage or hypoxia. Crossing of substances normally only found intravascularly occurs into the parenchyma and is associated with worsening inflammation, edema and secondary brain injury. Disruption to the BBB may persist for several days after brain injury and is attenuated by mild to moderate hypothermia in animal models, which may in part be due to its anti-leucocyte actions (see above).

Basic physiology and physics of inducing therapeutic hypothermia

Human thermoregulation

Thermoregulation can be described by considering the human body as two compartments: an inner 'central core' comprising the brain and internal organs, and an outer peripheral compartment including the skin and extremities. Humans maintain core temperature very tightly between 36.2°C and 37°C with peripheral temperature being, under normal circumstances, up to 4°C lower. The anterior hypothalamic nucleus in the preoptic area is responsible for thermoregulation and receives afferent input from core and peripheral temperature sensors, sending efferent projections to the hypothalamus.

The initial response to a core or peripheral temperature decrease includes behavioral changes such as applying extra clothing and seeking warmth. Once core temperature reaches the vasoconstriction threshold at around 36.5°C, vasoconstriction restricts blood exchange between the core and peripheral compartments, reducing heat transfer and maintaining core temperature. Heat loss from the peripheral compartment is also reduced by mechanisms including peripheral vasoconstriction. At approximately 35°C, shivering and brown fat metabolism (in neonates) increase to maintain core temperature. Piloerection is a vestigial reflex in humans with no effect on heat loss. The use of sedative and anesthetic drugs in the intensive care unit decreases arteriolar constriction thereby improving heat exchange between the core and peripheral compartments as well as increasing heat loss from the periphery to the environment. Thus thermoregulation is impaired and central hypothermia facilitated.

Many of these temperature control mechanisms are better preserved in young adults, rendering such patients more resistant to induction of hypothermia. Overcoming these protective mechanisms, in particular shivering, represents one of the key challenges to inducing and maintaining TH (see below).

Physics of temperature and heat transfer

The temperature of a substance in degrees Kelvin is directly proportional to the kinetic energy of the particles within the substance. Temperature is thus distinguished from heat, which is the total energy content of a substance, both kinetic and potential. Transfer of heat to a substance usually increases the kinetic energy (temperature) of the particles in the substance, but may instead increase the potential energy, for example by converting ice to water.

Heat can be transferred to or from a substance by one of four mechanisms – convection, conduction, radiation, and evaporation. The human body loses most of its heat through radiation by infrared electromagnetic waves. Exposure of the skin will increase radiative heat loss, and the application of water and alcohol sprays is used to promote evaporative heat loss. Though these methods are often used as adjuncts, TH is usually induced in humans by controlling the other two processes, conduction and convection.

Conduction is defined as the transfer of heat energy to neighboring molecules in direct contact due to the presence of a thermal gradient. In humans this mechanism accounts for only 5% of heat loss under normal conditions. Nevertheless, most methods currently used for inducing hypothermia increase conductive heat loss, including infusion of cold fluids, surface cooling with ice packing, water mattresses and cooling jackets/heat exchange pads, and placement of intravascular cooling catheters (some also utilize convection).

Convection is the transfer of heat to the surrounding air, and is responsible for 'wind chill'. Convective heat loss is increased both by increasing the movement of air over the body and by reducing the temperature of the surrounding air. Convective air blankets cool by increasing air flow across the entire body. Research is ongoing into the effectiveness of convective head-cooling devices on reducing brain temperature, thus avoiding some of the side effects of systemic hypothermia.

Methods of cooling

Methods of reducing temperature can be categorized in a number of ways. Cooling devices can be non-invasive or invasive, cooling can be applied locally (to the brain) or systemically, and by utilizing each of the four physical mechanisms of heat loss, though most commonly convective and conductive heat loss. Although TH is mostly associated with physical cooling methods, agents which can produce pharmacological hypothermia including neurotensin analogs and hydrogen sulphide are being investigated.

Non-invasive cooling methods

Most non-invasive cooling devices apply whole body surface cooling. The main advantage of such devices is that their use does not require specialist skills and avoids the complications of obtaining central venous access. The simplest and least expensive form involves placement of ice packs directly onto the skin. Particularly when combined with infusion of cold intravenous fluids, this method allows rapid cooling, but fine control is difficult and over- or under-treatment is common. Use of ice packs may be a convenient initial step in the emergency department until more sophisticated cooling devices can be employed.

Used as an adjunct to other techniques, fans can increase convective heat loss and applying alcohol sprays or cold water sponging to exposed areas will increase evaporative heat loss. Adding these simple techniques to maintenance (of hypothermia) cooling methods (see below) can help reduce time to target temperature, which may be associated with reduced parenchymal damage and improved outcome.

A variety of commercial surface-cooling devices are available which utilize cold water circulating through pads or mattresses. These can be placed both underneath and on top of the patient, and target temperature can be reached within as little as 2 hours, particularly if adjunctive measures are used. As with any form of surface cooling, shivering may be difficult to control, particularly if the patient is not adequately prepared for cooling, including administration of anti-pyretic agents, adequate sedation (hypnotic and opiate) and peripheral/focal body warming. Cool forced air blankets, more often associated with surface warming rather than cooling, are an alternative that can be placed over the exposed body surface. Most trials into the effects of TH have used cold water or forced air convective cooling devices.

Other methods which have been assessed include selective brain cooling using convective or conductive helmet devices, and cooling using cold intranasal fluid or air. Such devices are now commercially available (BeneChill International AG, HZW/Alte Winterthurerstrasse 14, CH-8304 Wallisellen, Switzerland) or are the subject of ongoing research (QuickCool, Ideon Science Park, Beta 6, Scheelevägen 17, SE-223 70 Lund).

Invasive cooling methods

Infusion of 20–30 ml/kg 0.9% refrigerated saline solution (~4°C) over 30 minutes has been shown to rapidly and safely induce hypothermia [17]. Target temperature can be reached within 30 minutes, though once temperature has been reached, an alternative method must be used for maintenance.

Intravascular cooling catheters have been the subject of several feasibility trials, and show promising results. These catheters are placed in the inferior vena cava, typically accessed by the femoral route, and consist of a catheter and either a coil or a series of balloons through which warm or cold saline can be circulated. Thus core temperature, as measured by an oesophageal or intravascular thermistor (core temperature measurement is mandatory), can be closely controlled by a closed-loop feedback system [18].

Intravascular cooling devices do not appear to induce thrombus formation, but nevertheless require expertise to insert and come with the procedure-related risks of all central venous access devices. Although induction of hypothermia can be achieved in less than 1 hour once in situ, there is a delay associated with placement. Nevertheless, the main advantage of intravascular heat exchange devices is that shivering is reported to be less problematic, and surface warming may be readily employed. These devices have been successfully used in awake or minimally sedated stroke patients [19].

Other invasive methods which can be used to reduce temperature include peritoneal and bladder lavage and extracorporeal circuits.

Non-invasive and invasive cooling systems with closed-loop feedback permit close control of core temperature, particularly during rewarming.

Clinical application of therapeutic hypothermia in stroke

Acute ischemic stroke

Due to the global impact of stroke, it is critical that treatments are simple, readily available and cost-effective. To date, however, treatments have been slow to progress. Current therapies for acute ischemic stroke are aimed at improving or re-establishing blood supply, principally using antiplatelet or thrombolytic therapy, and secondary prevention with lifestyle measures, antihypertensive, antiplatelet, and cholesterol lowering drugs. Administration of aspirin 160–300 mg within 48 hours of onset of symptoms reduces disability and death by approximately 1% (OR 0.95, 95% CI 0.91 to 0.99) [20]. Thrombolytic therapy such as recombinant tissue-plasminogen activator (rt-PA) has also been shown to reduce death and disability when administered within 3 hours of onset of symptoms (OR 0.71, 95% CI 0.52 to 0.96) [21].

Due to the short time window, however, thrombolytic therapy is only available to a limited number of patients. This calls for new developments for treatment strategies and one such strategy is reduction of body temperature [22], which may provide neuroprotection to prevent further damage in the at-risk area of penumbra surrounding the non-viable ischemic core. Many small clinical studies have been conducted to assess the safety and feasibility of hypothermia as a treatment after acute ischemic stroke, mostly in the intensive care unit (ICU).

The COOLAID trial was the first RCT to assess the effects of endovascular cooling for inducing hypothermia after acute ischemic stroke; it used meperidine, buspirone and surface warming to control shivering and was compared with standard care in the ICU. The trial enrolled 40 patients within 12 hours of stroke onset.

Results showed that endovascular cooling to 33°C for 24 hours is feasible in this patient group and that the complication rate between groups was similar. However, 80% (n = 8) patients in the hypothermia group required intubation during their hospital stay (one during the hypothermia period) compared to one patient in the control group (p = 0.002). This difference may have been as a result of the sedative actions of the drugs used to control shivering [23]. No difference was seen in clinical outcomes; however, the study was not powered to detect this.

Time from onset of ischemic stroke to initiation of treatment

Earlier application of hypothermia during or after acute ischemic stroke is associated with smaller infarct volumes and better outcomes in laboratory studies. The greatest effects occur when hypothermia is induced prior to ischemia, a situation not usually feasible in the clinical setting. However, application of hypothermia after stroke onset has been shown to reduce infarct size and attenuate the damaging biochemical cascade after stroke, particularly if commenced within three hours of ischemia onset. There have been conflicting results from studies reporting on hypothermia initiated after this time, although there are encouraging results from trials with a therapeutic window of 6 hours followed by prolonged treatment [24].

The time from onset of symptoms to initiation of hypothermia has varied across all clinical trials ranging from 3 to 72 hours post onset. There remains no consensus on the maximum length of the time window between onset of stroke and initiation of treatment.

Target temperature

Mild hypothermia is a decrease in core body temperature to between 32°C and 35°C, with moderate hypothermia in the range of 28–32°C. Temperatures lower than this (deep hypothermia) are associated with practical difficulties and significant complications and have never been tested in acute stroke in humans. As well as causing hypokalemia, arrhythmias, and heart failure in stroke patients, deep hypothermia may worsen stroke by further reducing cerebral blood flow.

From animal studies, there appears to be a U-shaped effectiveness curve for hypothermia on ischemic stroke with the optimum target being 33–34°C [25]. The trials of hypothermia for neuroprotection in patients after cardiac arrest and in neonatal asphyxia aimed for moderate hypothermia [6–8] and most ongoing and recently completed trials of hypothermia in acute stroke aimed for a target temperature of 33–35°C. These targets have been shown to be achievable without the need for invasive ventilation (see comments above) and with acceptably low complication rates [9].

Duration of treatment

There is no consensus on the optimal duration of this therapy after an acute stroke. Both brief and prolonged hypothermia have been studied in animal models, showing interdependence between time from ischemia to onset of treatment and duration of treatment. Brief hypothermia of 2–3 hours may be effective if hypothermia is initiated prior to ischemia or very early after onset, but the most impressive effects have been shown with duration of treatment of 22 hours or more [26]. Indeed there may be benefit in even longer treatment albeit at the risk of increasing side effects. Animal data are difficult to extrapolate to humans because of significant inter species and treatment differences. Nevertheless human trials after cardiac arrest used treatment duration of 12–24 hours, and most current human trials in acute stroke stipulate a time at target temperature of between 12 and 48 hours.

Rewarming

Rewarming is potentially hazardous, particularly if raised intracranial pressure or intracranial mass effect is present, such as malignant middle cerebral artery infarction. Whilst hypothermia causes cessation or reduction of the metabolic cascade occurring after stroke (see above), rapid or uncontrolled rewarming may enhance the cascade causing further damage.

Controlled rewarming reduces infarct size, compared with passive rewarming [27]. Passive rewarming is also associated with an increase in ICP and reduction in CPP [28] and the use of passive rewarming may explain the lack of effect of therapeutic hypothermia after stroke in earlier trials. There is no agreed standard to define slow rewarming, but a rate of 0.1–0.25°C per hour is the current standard.

Hypothermia and thrombolysis

Current recommendations for the use of thrombolysis in acute stroke include a treatment window of 3 hours from onset of symptoms to administration of the thrombolytic agent, t-PA. The difficulty in achieving treatment within this time frame is one of the reasons that a relatively small number of stroke patients benefit from t-PA. There is increasing interest in using hypothermia as neuroprotection therapy which may extend the time window during which thrombolysis may be beneficial. Experimental models show a reduction in infarct size if hypothermia is applied during reperfusion [29].

The ICTuS-L trial [30] aimed to assess the feasibility and safety of endovascular hypothermia in patients receiving thrombolytic therapy within 6 hours of symptom onset. This is the largest multi-centre RCT of hypothermia to have been completed in stroke patients, enrolling 58 patients.

Results showed no difference in outcome or event reporting between groups; however, pneumonia rates were significantly higher in patients who received hypothermia ($p < 0.05$). This small trial was not powered to detect differences in outcome, including mortality, and findings showed no affect on 90-day outcome ($p = 0.355$) or mortality ($p = 0.744$) between groups.

Future direction and ongoing trials

The most recent Cochrane review [22] found no significant effect on poor outcome (death and disability) at final follow up (OR 0.9, 95% CI 0.6–1.4); however, a trend towards more reported infections in the intervention groups was found, although this was not significant (OR 1.5, 95% CI 0.8–2.6).

The review concludes that trials to date have been too small to detect intervention effects therefore there is currently not enough evidence to support use of routine temperature reduction strategies in this patient group. Larger randomized controlled trials are required and should focus on proper blinding and treatment allocation procedures along with assessing adverse events [22].

Having assessed the feasibility of endovascular cooling after acute stroke in the ICTuS trial [9] and the safety of endovascular cooling after thrombolytic treatment with t-PA in the ICTuS-L trial [31], a follow-on study by the ICTuS investigators is currently underway. The ICTuS 2/3 trial is a prospective, randomized, single-blind multicentre phase 2/3 trial which aims to determine whether the treatment combination of t-PA and hypothermia leads to improved outcome at 90 days compared to treatment with t-PA alone. Eligible patients will receive an infusion of t-PA within 3 hours of the onset of symptoms and then hypothermia will be initiated in the hypothermia group by a cold saline infusion and maintained using an endovascular catheter to achieve a target temperature of 33°C. Cooling will continue for 24 hours then patients will be re-warmed over a period of 12 hours [32].

This will be the largest trial of hypothermia in stroke patients with 450 patients estimated to be enrolled into the phase two feasibility stage. An interim analysis is then planned and if specific milestones are met, a further 1200 patients will be included in the phase three trial.

Another large, ongoing trial is EuroHYP-1, a European phase three prospective, open randomized controlled trial involving a projected 1500 awake stroke patients. The aim of the trial is to identify whether hypothermia (target temperature 34–35°C) delivered by either surface or endovascular devices within 90 minutes of t-PA infusion or 90 minutes of hospital admission (for patients who are not eligible for t-PA infusion) affects outcome at 90 days [32]. Analysis of this large trial will assess the most appropriate depth of hypothermia and method of cooling along with increasing the understanding of the interaction between hypothermia and t-PA treatments [33].

Recruitment to both trials is ongoing.

Hemorrhagic stroke

Although first investigated in the 1950s, there have been few studies of TH following intracranial hemorrhage. Hemorrhagic stroke can be due to primary intraparenchymal bleeding (intra-axial hemorrhage), subarachnoid hemorrhage, and hemorrhagic transformation into an area of pre-existing ischemic area.

Unlike models of acute ischemic stroke, hypothermia following intracerebral hemorrhage has not shown consistent benefit in terms of reducing the area of damage. Applying hypothermia after intracerebral hemorrhage may reduce associated edema, and can reduce the inflammatory and oxidative factors associated with blood in the brain parenchyma. There may also be benefit in reducing raised intracranial pressure associated with mass lesions. However, there has been no consistent evidence of outcome benefit in either experimental models or human trials. This may be due to adverse blood pressure effects of hypothermia and its effects on the coagulation and thrombolytic pathways [34].

Hypothermia also appears to improve parenchymal metabolic derangement after subarachnoid hemorrhage [34] but there are no studies showing improvement in outcomes. Patients treated with hypothermia for even a prolonged period have shown no significant improvement after subarachnoid hemorrhage, though numbers studied are small [35]. The Intraoperative Hypothermia for Aneurysm Surgery Trial (IHAST) showed no outcome benefit and an increase in bacteremia when mild hypothermia was applied during aneurysm clipping [36].

Combination therapy

The effect of a combination of drugs and hypothermia on stroke patients seems to reduce damage synergistically as they are thought to work through different but complementary neuro-chemical mechanisms. These treatment regimens might be useful for acute stroke management and for prevention of cerebral injury during cerebrovascular surgery. Studies of combination therapy have been conducted with drugs such as Tirilazad, N-acetylcysteine, magnesium, and dexmedetomidine. Tirilazad mesylate is a drug with free radical-scavenging and lipid peroxidation inhibiting properties. N-acetylcysteine has antioxidant properties, inhibiting the production of free radicals. Magnesium is effective in reducing neurological damage in several animal models due to decreased glutamate-related neurotoxicity. Dexmedetomidine is a centrally acting α_2-agonist known to reduce neuronal injury following cerebral ischemia. In experimental models the neuroprotective efficacy of hypothermia is increased by pharmacological interventions, like the antagonism of excitatory amino acids and free radicals. So far, outcome benefit to patients of this strategy has not been shown.

In an attempt to target various stages of the ischemic cascade, Martin-Schild *et al.* [37] conducted a phase I non-randomized study of a combination of three treatments; t-PA therapy, hypothermia, and a caffeinol infusion (incorporating a combination of caffeine and ethanol). The aim of the study was to assess the feasibility and safety of all three treatments in combination. The study enrolled 20 awake, non-intubated patients presenting within 3 hours of onset of symptoms. All patients received a standard dose of t-PA, a 2-hour caffeinol infusion then initiation of hypothermia therapy (target temperature 33–34°C) using both surface and intravascular cooling methods. A similar anti-shivering protocol to the ICTuS and ICTuS-l studies was used with patients receiving a meperidine infusion and regular oral buspirone. Hypothermia was maintained for 24 hours.

The feasibility of administering the combination of t-PA and caffeinol was confirmed in 16 patients who received both interventions. However, therapeutic blood levels of caffeine and ethanol were not reached in all patients with nine (53%) patients reaching target caffeine levels and 12 (67%) reaching target ethanol levels. No explanation is given for this.

Although hypothermia was initiated in 18 patients (eight patients using an endovascular catheter and 10 using surface cooling devices), only 13 reached target temperature and of these eight (62%) remained within the target for at least 12 hours. All of the patients in the surface cooling group reached target temperature (n = 10) compared to only three patients (38%) in the endovascular group.

Similar to previous studies, this study has shown that achieving hypothermia in awake stroke patients is particularly challenging and a fine balance needs to be achieved between temperature reduction and the sedative effects of the anti-shivering regimen. Despite many small feasibility studies being conducted, none has yet developed a robust hypothermia protocol for stroke patients, therefore further studies are required to develop this.

Side effects of hypothermia

Hypothermia treatment causes significant physiological changes including cutaneous vasoconstriction, metabolic upset, shivering, hemodynamic changes, alteration in electrolyte levels, changes to drug handling and obtunds the immune system. Some of these homeostatic consequences are caused by an autonomic or stress-like response which may increase morbidity, negating potential hypothermia related benefits [38].

Metabolic side effects

Shivering

Core body temperature is tightly maintained in a narrow physiological range, with fluctuations outside the range triggering autonomic regulatory responses (see above). Shivering generally develops at a core temperature of around 35.5°C, and reaches its peak intensity over a range of around 1° C. The threshold varies in some physiologic conditions – for example in women the thresholds are 0.3–0.5°C higher than men and can increase further in the luteal phase of menstruation. Age also influences thermoregulation, with vasoconstriction and shivering occurring at a lower temperature in the elderly.

Shivering manifests as uncoordinated and involuntary activity of skeletal muscles, generating heat during contraction. Much of the heat is released to the environment rather than being retained in the core. Thus shivering is relatively inefficient, and is capable of markedly increasing the basal metabolic rate. It can raise oxygen consumption by 120%, which is particularly undesirable in patients with ischemic, hypoxic, and traumatic brain injury. Shivering also results in a rapid respiratory rate, increases perioperative cardiac events and causes patient discomfort. For these reasons, prevention and treatment of shivering is vital to the successful delivery of TH. Aids in assessment such as the Bedside Shivering Assessment Scale (BSAS) [39] have been developed as simple and reliable tools to evaluate and allow protocolised treatment of shivering (Table 10.1).

The only physical method of shivering control available is skin surface warming, though there are several pharmacological options. Many are restricted to use in either intensive care or high-dependency units, as the administration of strong sedatives and opioids by intravenous infusion requires strict monitoring. Protocols combining surface cooling with opioids and sedatives such as meperidine, buspirone, and clonidine have been shown to be safe and feasible outside critical care [9].

Mean skin temperature contributes around 20% of the afferent input to the control of vasoconstriction and shivering. Thus, and perhaps somewhat counter-intuitively, application of skin-surface warming is a useful method for minimizing shivering during core body cooling. Indeed this is one important advantage of invasive cooling, allowing surface warming. Cutaneous warming can be either generalized or localized, though generalized warming is more effective than warming only the extremities [40].

Table 10.1 The Bedside Shivering Assessment Scale [39]

Score	Physical effects	Increase in resting energy expenditure
0	No shivering.	Up to 10%
1	Shivering localized to the neck/thorax. May be seen only as artifact on ECG or felt by palpation.	24%
2	Intermittent involvement of the upper extremities +/− thorax.	65%
3	Generalized shivering or sustained upper/lower extremity shivering.	165%

The sedative drug propofol at a plasma concentration of 2 μg/ml lowers the shivering threshold to 35°C, and at 4 μg/ml to 34°C [41]. Midazolam produces more modest impairment of thermoregulatory control and is thus less effective at controlling shivering, though it has the advantage that it produces less hypotension than propofol. Volatile anesthetics also blunt thermoregulatory autonomic defenses effectively but because of their technical requirements are rarely used outside the operating theatre.

Meperidine (pethidine), a combined μ- and k-agonist opioid, is one of the most frequently used drugs to combat post-operative shivering outside the ICU. Because of its significant k-receptor activity, it markedly decreases the shivering threshold, by twice as much as the vasoconstriction threshold [42]. Opioids such as alfentanil, fentanyl, and morphine are pure μ-receptor agonists and all impair shivering to a lesser degree than meperidine. Alfentanil, administered by continuous infusion, seems to be the most effective pure μ-agonist, lowering the vasoconstriction and shivering thresholds linearly in a dose-dependent manner [43]. Cessation of high-dose opiates may be associated with a rebound increase in shivering due to development of an acute tolerance to μ-receptor activity [44].

Clonidine and dexmedetomidine are centrally acting α_2-agonists shown to be effective for post-operative shivering and pain control, producing a dose-dependent decrease in both vasoconstriction and shivering. Buspirone, a partial serotonin 1a-receptor agonist, slightly reduces the shivering threshold and has the advantage of avoiding respiratory depression. Other treatments to reduce the shivering threshold, including drugs with opioid activity (tramadol and nalbuphine), or other serotonin antagonists (nefopam, ketanserin and ondansetron) have shown less clinical usefulness.

The optimal method for minimizing shivering during therapeutic hypothermia depends on the method of cooling employed, the patient, and disease factors. Nevertheless, a combination of surface warming

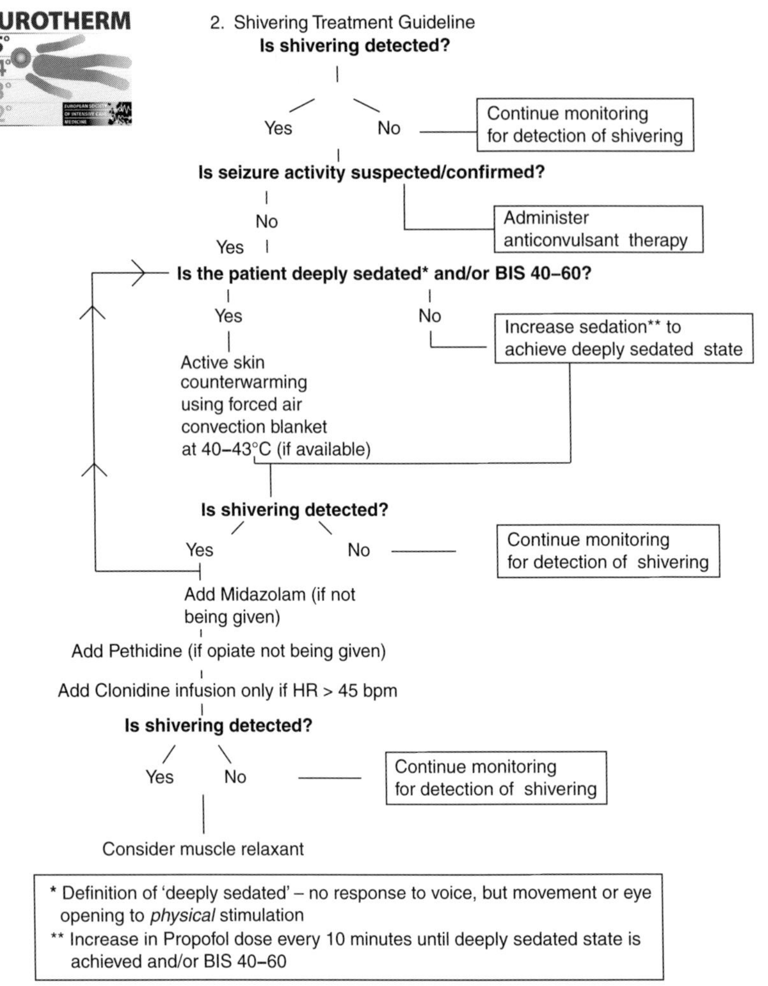

Fig. 10.1 The shivering guideline used in the ongoing Eurotherm3235 trial.

(where possible) with synergistically acting drugs, such as buspirone and meperidine, is a feasible and sensible approach and can be used outside the intensive care unit [9]. In the intensive care environment the optimization of sedation with propofol and opioids and, if necessary, the addition of muscle relaxants, can adequately control shivering. Muscle relaxants such as atracurium should be used as a last resort as, while they decrease metabolic load produced by shivering, they do not reduce the underlying autonomic effects. Figure 10.1 shows the shivering guideline used in the ongoing Eurotherm3235 trial: an ongoing RCT of hypothermia following severe TBI in intubated patients admitted to ICU which will assess the effect of hypothermia on 6-month outcomes.

Glycemic control

Hypothermia alters glucose homeostasis by two mechanisms – a reduction in insulin secretion from pancreatic islet cells and a decrease in peripheral insulin sensitivity. This leads to hyperglycemia, which adversely affects the outcome in critically ill patients and has specific negative effects on patients with neurological injuries by increasing secondary injury. During hypothermia treatment severe hyperglycemic episodes can be avoided by following appropriate protocols on glucose blood level monitoring and IV insulin therapy. The rewarming phase requires particularly strict glucose monitoring in order to avoid rebound of hypoglycemia, due to a combination of a temperature-related reduction in blood glucose level and the effects of multiple doses of insulin required during the maintenance phase [38].

Other metabolic effects

As part of the sympathetic mediated defense against hypothermia, breakdown of fat stores is increased. This leads to an increase in lactate, ketoacids, and a mild metabolic acidosis. Rarely lactate may rise as high as 7 mmol l^{-1}, causing a more significant acidemia. Cortisol levels may also rise, particularly with core temperatures of less than 33°C.

Infection and immunosuppression

Hypothermia inhibits the pro-inflammatory response mechanism, reducing secondary cerebral damage at the cost of an increased risk of infection (see above). Leucocyte count is lowered, neutrophil and macrophage function impaired and pro-inflammatory cytokines are suppressed. There is also a risk of hyperglycemia which if uncontrolled may contribute to immune suppression. Infection risks are generally associated with prolonged hypothermia of 48 hours or more, and may be minimized by meticulous monitoring and management.

Ventilator associated pneumonia

In earlier studies, pneumonia was the most common infectious complication associated with hypothermia treatment. At present the majority of cooled patients are invasively ventilated, with endotracheal intubation and mechanical ventilation already increasing the risk of lower respiratory tract infection (ventilator associated pneumonia, VAP). While short-term hypothermia treatment does not appear to be associated with an increased risk of pneumonia [7]. the risk of intubated patients developing pneumonia with prolonged hypothermia treatment may be as high as 45%. Late-onset VAP (occurring 5 days or more after intubation) is particularly important as it is more likely to be caused by resistant pathogens and is associated with a significant increase in morbidity and mortality.

VAP is diagnosed by a combination of clinical, radiological, laboratory, and microbiological grounds, with initial antibiotic treatment depending on risk factors for resistant pathogens and local antimicrobial policy. A combination of preventative measures ('VAP bundle'), clinical vigilance, and prompt investigation and treatment make any potential increased risk of pneumonia manageable.

Wound infection

Patients undergoing hypothermia treatment are at increased risk of wound infection, probably due to a combination of immune suppression and vasoconstriction affecting vascular supply to the affected area. This applies to ulcers and pressure areas as well as to surgical wounds. Prevention strategies and nursing care of wounds and at-risk areas should be meticulous in patients being cooled.

Alterations in drug pharmacology

Hypothermia alters the pharmacokinetics (PK) of drugs due to changes in metabolism of the drug or alterations to its mechanism of action. Studies conducted on drug PK during hypothermia treatment have shown that drug concentrations in the blood are typically increased with a decrease in volume of distribution and decreased clearance. Reduced clearance is due to a reduction in affinity of the drug for the cytochrome system responsible for its metabolism, and a reduction in hepatic blood flow. This particularly affects drugs with a high hepatic extraction ratio. Drugs which fit a multicompartmental model such as propofol, a commonly used sedative in anesthesia and intensive care, show decreased intercompartmental clearance (Table 10.2).

Table 10.2 Alterations of drug pharmacokinetics during hypothermia

Pharmacokinetic property	Effect of hypothermia
Blood concentration	Decreased
Protein binding	Minimal effect
Volume of distribution	Decreased
Systemic clearance	Decreased
Intercompartmental clearance	Decreased

Whilst plasma levels may be increased, potency and efficacy of drugs can be reduced, producing a global narrowing of the therapeutic index [44]. Decreasing body temperature to 30°C for example reduces morphine potency, related to a reduction in the affinity of morphine for the μ-receptor [45].

Many of the sedative, hypnotic, opioid, antiarrhythmic, anticonvulsant and antimicrobial drugs used in ICUs are metabolized in the liver by the cytochrome P450 system (CYP450). CYP450 comprises a very large and diverse group of enzymes responsible for metabolizing a wide variety of drugs and toxic compounds. Mild to moderate hypothermia decreases the systemic clearance of CYP450-metabolized drugs by between 7% and 22% per degree Celsius below 37°C [46].

Sedatives

The pharmacokinetics of both propofol and midazolam, two sedatives commonly administered by continuous infusion in intensive care units, appears to change markedly during hypothermia. Propofol concentration at steady state increases by approximately 28% during treatment, due to decreased inter-compartmental clearance as well as decreased hepatic clearance secondary to reductions in hepatic blood flow and CYP450 activity [47]. A five-fold increase in blood concentration of midazolam due to a 100-fold decrease in systemic clearance during hypothermia has been reported [48].

Opioids

Hypothermia results in reduced clearance and increased blood concentrations of μ-receptor-agonist opioids such as fentanyl, alfentanil, and remifentanil. Fentanyl blood levels may even remain raised for more than 6 hours after rewarming. Moreover fentanyl may also contribute to secondary brain damage, having been shown to be detrimental in rat models of TBI treated with hypothermia, and can induce seizures in the 'healthy' temporal lobe in partial complex seizure disorder [49].

Other drugs

There are limited data studying specific pharmacokinetic changes in other drugs during treatment with hypothermia, though it seems likely that reduced clearance and increased plasma levels could occur more generally. There is no general rule in terms of drug effect, however, as hypothermia may alter receptor affinity. Clearance of muscle relaxants, propranolol, and phenobarbitone is reduced [50]. Gentamicin shows an increased serum concentration, prolonged elimination half-life and reduced total body clearance, though there are few studies of the effects on antibiotics.

Hemodynamic effects

Hypothermia can influence myocardial performance, affecting heart rhythm, contractility, and coronary perfusion. Mild and moderate hypothermia have been demonstrated to be protective of myocardial tissue, whilst deep hypothermia can be harmful.

Electrocardiographic changes

Variations in heart rhythm can occur during cooling. During induction the heart rate tends to increase until core temperature falls to around 35.5°C. Tachycardia can be further accentuated at this time by hypovolemia, shivering, and inadequate sedation. However, as the temperature decreases further, the heart rate reduces gradually due to a decrease in the rate of spontaneous depolarization of the pacemaker cells.

Hypothermia can be accompanied by other electrocardiograph (ECG) changes. Prolongation of the cardiac action potential and a slight decrease in the speed of myocardial impulse conduction result in prolongation of the PR and QT intervals and widening the QRS complex. Treatment is rarely required for such ECG changes. Globally, mild and moderate hypothermia have been demonstrated to reduce the risk of serious arrhythmias by stabilizing myocardial cell membranes and increasing the likelihood of successful defibrillation. However, deep hypothermia (below 28°C) can decrease the myocardial responsiveness to drugs and defibrillation.

Effects on myocardial performance

Mild and moderate hypothermia improve myocardial contractility in sedated, euvolemic patients. Whilst systolic function is improved, there is a relative bradycardia and a mild impairment in diastolic function resulting in an overall decrease in cardiac output, coupled with a reduction in systemic metabolic requirements. Some studies have reported a successful use of moderate hypothermia as a rescue therapy for refractory cardiac shock.

Effects on ischemic myocardium

Mild to moderate hypothermia has a protective effect on the ischemic myocardium, reducing myocardial oxygen consumption by producing bradycardia and improving oxygen supply through coronary vasodilatation. Animal data indicate that mild induced hypothermia results in improved myocardial salvage, reduced infarct size, left ventricular remodeling, and better long-term left ventricular function. Deep hypothermia, complicated by shivering and tachycardia, increases myocardial damage.

Volume status and hypothermia

Intravascular volume status needs to be carefully monitored and maintained during hypothermia. Hypothermia-induced diuresis may be exacerbated by diabetes insipidus and/or treatment with mannitol and lead to hypovolemia and hypotension, which may worsen outcome. Despite relative hypovolemia, urine output may remain paradoxically high because of the increased activation of atrial natriuretic peptide, decreased levels of antidiuretic hormone, renal tubular dysfunction and increased venous return due to systemic vasoconstriction.

Acid-base balance and electrolytes

During cooling, the extracellular pH level decreases while there is a slight rise in intracellular pH. Hypothermia causes a mild metabolic acidosis due to an increase in fat metabolism causing increased levels of keto-acids, lactic acid, free fatty acids and glycerol. The associated metabolic acidosis usually requires only monitoring, should not be considered evidence of other pathology such as bowel ischemia, and rarely necessitates any treatment.

A reduction in metabolic rate, oxygen consumption and CO_2 production occur together. Therefore, ventilator settings need regular adjustment, particularly during the induction phase. It is necessary to monitor arterial pH and CO_2 levels during treatment. Two different pH and CO_2 measurement methods are available: the alpha-stat system, which measures the CO_2 partial pressure in blood at 37°C and the pH-stat system, in which the $PaCO_2$ tension is corrected to actual body temperature. These systems require different ventilator strategies but, as pH stat is associated with loss of autoregulation and an increase in cerebral blood volume, fi-stat is recommended.

During the different phases of hypothermia application, serum potassium, magnesium, and phosphate are liable to fluctuation. In the induction and maintenance phase, plasma electrolyte levels decrease due to intracellular shift and renal tubular dysfunction leading to electrolyte loss. Monitoring is essential, and in general electrolyte levels should be kept in the high-normal range to avoid arrhythmias, hypotension, and other potential complications. Magnesium depletion should be corrected promptly because its supplementation has been associated with improved neurological outcome and hypomagnesemia is associated with cardiac arrhythmias and worsened cerebral and myocardial injury. During rewarming, plasma electrolyte concentrations tend to rise quickly as they are released from cells. This is particularly true of potassium, though in patients with normal renal function, a slow and controlled rewarming process allows the kidneys to excrete the excess potassium and avoids complications.

Coagulopathy

A moderate reduction in core temperature causes minor impairment of platelet function and mild thrombocytopenia. Once core temperature reaches 33°C the synthesis of clotting enzymes and plasminogen activator inhibitors is inhibited and the kinetics of the coagulation cascade altered. It is important to bear in mind that standard laboratory tests of coagulation will usually demonstrate normal clotting function as they are performed at 37°C. Despite the effects on coagulation, clinically significant bleeding is rare when using hypothermia, even in patients with traumatic brain injury. The use of hypothermia in patients with more widespread traumatic injury is more controversial, and it should not be used where there is major bleeding or cardiovascular instability. If bleeding occurs, or surgical procedures are performed under hypothermic conditions, fresh frozen plasma and platelet transfusion can be used [38].

Conclusion

Therapeutic hypothermia is a theoretically attractive intervention that is already embedded in clinical practice, which could be used after acute brain injury. However, the effects of this intervention are complex and successful delivery requires training and experience. There are considerable endeavors ongoing to increase the evidence base for this intervention (www.EUROTHERM3235Trial.eu and www.eurohyp.org/) and the output from these is eagerly awaited.

REFERENCES

1. Hippocrates (460–375 BC). *De Vetere Medicina.* Jones WHS, Withington ET, trans. Hippocrates. Loeb Classical Library.
2. Fay T. Observations on prolonged human refrigeration. *N Y St J Med* 1940;**40**: 1351–4.
3. Krieger DW, Midori A, Yenari MD. Therapeutic hypothermia for acute ischaemic stroke. What do laboratory studies teach us? *Stroke* 2004;**35**: 1482–9.
4. van der Worp H, Sena ES, Donnan GA *et al.* Hypothermia in animal models of acute ischaemic stroke: a systematic review and meta-analysis. *Brain* 2007;**130**: 3063–74.
5. Williams GR, Spencer F. The clinical use of hypothermia following cardiac arrest. *Ann Surg* 1959;**148**: 462–8.
6. Darby JM, Padosch SA, Kern KB *et al.* Mild therapeutic hypothermia to improve the neurologic outcome after cardiac arrest *NEJM* 2002;**346**: 549–56.
7. Bernard SA, Gray TW, Buist MD *et al.* Treatment of comatose survivors of out-of-hospital cardiac arrest with induced hypothermia. *NEJM* 2002;**346**: 557–63.
8. Gluckman PD, Wyatt JS, Azzopardi D *et al.* Selective head cooling with mild systemic hypothermia after neonatal encephalopathy: multicentre randomised trial. *Lancet* 2005;**365**: 663–70.
9. Lyden PD, Allgren RL, Ng K *et al.* Intravascular Cooling in the Treatment of Stroke (ICTuS): early clinical experience. *J Stroke Cerebrovascular Dis* 2005;**14**(3): 107–14.
10. Zhao H, Steinberg G, Sapolsky RM. General versus specific actions of mild-moderate hypothermia in attenuating cerebral ischemic damage. *J Cereb Blood Flow Metab* 2007;**27**: 1879–94.
11. Krieger DW, Midori A, Yenari MD. Therapeutic hypothermia for acute ischemic stroke. What do laboratory studies teach us? *Stroke* 2004;**35**: 1482–9.
12. Takeda Y, Namba K, Higuchi T. Quantitative evaluation of the neuroprotective effects of hypothermia ranging from 34°C to 31°C on brain ischemia in gerbils and determination of the mechanism of neuroprotection. *Crit Care Med* 2003;**31**: 255–60.
13. Berger C, Schabitz W, Wolf M *et al.* Hypothermia and brain-derived neurotrophic factor reduce glutamate synergistically in acute stroke. *Exp Neurol* 2004;**185**: 305–12.
14. Horstmann S, Kalb P, Koziol J. Profiles of matrix metalloproteinases, their inhibitors, and laminin in stroke patients: Influence of different therapies. *Stroke* 2003;**34**: 2165–72.
15. Wang GJ, Deng HY, Maier CM *et al.* Mild hypothermia reduces ICAM-1 expression, neutrophil infiltration and microglia/monocyte accumulation following experimental stroke. *Neuroscience* 2002; **114**(4): 1081–90.
16. Maier CM, Sun GH, Cheng D. Effects of mild hypothermia on superoxide anion production, superoxide dismutase expression, and activity following transient focal cerebral ischemia. *Neurobiol Dis* 2002;**11**: 28–42.

17. Bernard S, Buist M, Smith K, *et al.* Induced hypothermia using large volume, ice-cold intravenous fluid in comatose survivors of out-of-hospital cardiac arrest: a preliminary report. *Resuscitation* 2003;**56**: 9–13.
18. Hammer MD, Krieger DW. Acute ischaemic stroke: Is there a role for hypothermia? *Cleveland Clinic J Med* 2002;**69**(10): 770–85.
19. Georgiadis D, Schwarz S, Kollmar R, *et al.* Endovascular cooling for moderate hypothermia in patients with acute stroke: first results of a novel approach. *Stroke* 2001;**32**: 2250–3.
20. Sandercock PAG, Counsell C, Gubitz GJ, Tseng MC. Antiplatelet therapy for acute ischaemic stroke. *Cochrane Database of Systematic Reviews* 2009.
21. Wardlaw JM, Murray V, Berge E, del Zoppo, GJ. Thrombolysis for acute ischaemic stroke. *Cochrane Database of Systematic Reviews* 2009.
22. Den Hertog HM, van der Worp HB, Tseng MC, Dippel DWJ. Cooling therapy for acute stroke. *Cochrane Database of Systematic Reviews* 2009.
23. De Georgia MA, Krieger DW, Abou-Chebl A, *et al.* Cooling for acute ischaemic brain damage (COOL AID): a feasibility trial of endovascular cooling. *Neurology* 2004;**63**: 312–17.
24. MacLellan CL, Clark DL, Silasy G *et al.* Use of prolonged hypothermia to treat ischaemic and haemorrhagic stroke. *J Neurotrauma* 2009;**26**: 313–23.
25. Kollmar R, Blank T, Han JL *et al.* Different degrees of hypothermia after experimental stroke. *Stroke* 2007;**38**: 1585–9.
26. Yanamoto H, Nagata I, Nakahara I *et al.* Combination of intraischemic and postischemic hypothermia provides potent and persistent neuroprotection against temporary focal ischemia in rats. *Stroke* 1999;**30**: 2720–6.
27. Berger C, Xia F, Kohrmann M *et al.* Hypothermia in acute stroke. Slow versus fast rewarming: an experimental study in rats. *Exp Neuro* 2007;**204**: 131–7.
28. Steiner T, Friede T, Aschoff A *et al.* Effect and feasibility of controlled rewarming after moderate hypothermia in stroke patients with malignant infarction of the middle cerebral artery. *Stroke* 2001;**32**: 2833–5.
29. Kurasako T, Zhao L, Pulsinelli WA *et al.* Transient cooling during early reperfusion attenuates delayed edema and infarct progression in the spontaneously hypertensive rat. Distribution and time course of regional brain temperature change in a model of postischemic hypothermic protection. *J Cerebral Bloodflow Metab* 2007;**27**: 1919–30.
30. Hemmen TM, Raman R, Guluma KZ, *et al.* Intravenous thrombolysis plus hypothermia for acute treatment of ischaemic stroke (ICTuS-L) final results. *Stroke* 2010;**41**: 2265–70.
31. Hemmen T, Rapp K, Raman R, *et al.* Phase 2/3 study of intravenous thrombolysis and hypothermia for acute treatment of ischaemic stroke (ICTuS 2/3). *Crit Care* 2012;**16** [Suppl 2]: 17–18.
32. Wu TC, Grotta JC. Hypothermia for acute ischaemic stroke. *Lancet Neurol* 2013;**12**: 275–84.
33. van der Worp BH, Macleod MR, Kollmar R. For the European Stroke Research Network for Hypothermia (EuroHYP) Therapeutic hypothermia for acute ischaemic stroke: ready to start large randomised trials? *J Cerebral Blood Flow Metab.* 2010;**30**: 1079–93.
34. Tang XN, Yenari MA. Hypothermia as a cytoprotective strategy in acute tissue injury. *Ageing Res Rev* 2010;**9**: 61–8.
35. Gasser S, Kahn N, Yonekawa Y *et al.* Long-term hypothermia in patients with severe brain edema after poor-grade subarachnoid hemorrhage. *J Neurosurg Anesthesiol* 2003;**15**(3): 240–8.
36. Todd MM, Hindman BJ, Clarke WR *et al.* (IHAST investigators). Mild intraoperative hypothermia during surgery for intracranial aneurysm. *N Engl J Med* 2005;**352**(2); 135–45.
37. Martin-Schild S, Hallevi H, Shaltoni H, *et al.* Combined neuroprotective modalities coupled with thrombolysis in acute ischaemic stroke: a pilot study of caffeinol and mild hypothermia. *J Stroke Cerebrovasc Dis* 2009;**18**[2]: 86–96.
38. Polderman KH, Herold I. Therapeutic hypothermia and controlled normothermia in the intensive care unit: practical considerations, side effects, and cooling methods. *Crit Care Med* 2009;**37**: 1101–20.
39. Badjatia N, Strongilis E, Gordon E, *et al.* Metabolic impact of shivering during therapeutic temperature modulation: the Bedside Shivering Assessment Scale. *Stroke* 2008;**39**: 3242–7.
40. Badjatia N, Strongilis E, Prescutti M, *et al.* Metabolic benefits of surface counter warming during therapeutic temperature modulation. *Crit Care Med* 2009;**37**: 1893–7.
41. Matsukawa T, Kurz A, Sessler DI. Propofol linearly reduces the vasoconstriction and shivering thresholds. *Anesthesiology* 1995;**82**: 1169–80.
42. Kurz A, Go JC, Sessler DI, *et al.* Alfentanil slightly increases the sweating threshold and markedly reduces the vasoconstriction and shivering thresholds. *Anesthesiology* 1995;**83**: 293–9.
43. Nakasuji M, Nakamura M, Imanaka M *et al.* Intraoperative high dose remifentanil increases post-anaesthetic shivering. *Br J Anaesthesia* 2010;**105**(2): 162–7.

44. Polderman KH. Mechanisms of action, physiological effects, and complications of hypothermia. *Crit Care Med* 2009;**37**: S186–202.
45. Puig MM, Warner W, Tang CK *et al.* Effects of temperature on the interaction of morphine with opioid receptors. *Br J Anaesthesia* 1987;**59**: 459–64.
46. Tortorici MA, Kochanek PM, Bies RR *et al.* Therapeutic hypothermia-induced pharmacokinetic alterations on CYP2E1 chlorzoxazone-mediated metabolism in a cardiac arrest rat model. *Crit Care Med* 2006;**34**: 785–91.
47. Leslie K, Sessler DI, Bjorksten AR *et al.* Mild hypothermia alters propofol pharmacokinetics and increases the duration of action of atracurium. *Anesthesia Analgesia* 1995;**80**: 1007–14.
48. Fukuoka N, Aibiki M, Tsukamoto T *et al.* Biphasic concentration change during continuous midazolam administration in brain-injured patients undergoing therapeutic moderate hypothermia. *Resuscitation* 2004;**60**: 225–30.
49. Tempelhoff R, Modica PA, Bernardo KL *et al.* Fentanyl-induced electrocorticographic seizures in patients with complex partial epilepsy. *J Neurosurg* 1992;**77**: 201–8.
50. Polderman KH. Application of therapeutic hypothermia in the intensive care unit: Opportunities and pitfalls of a promising treatment modality – Part 2: Practical aspects and side effects. *Intensive Care Med* 2004;**30**: 757–69.

11

External ventricular drainage in hemorrhagic stroke

Mahua Dey, Jennifer Jaffe, and Issam A. Awad

Introduction

Stroke (cerebrovascular accidents) can be broadly classified into two categories: ischemic, accounting for 85% of all strokes, and hemorrhagic, accounting for about 15% of all strokes. Both pathologies may cause increased intracranial pressure (ICP), one due to brain swelling and edema from infracted brain, and the other by virtue of mass effect from hemorrhage or associated hydrocephalus. Increased ICP in the setting of cerebrovascular accident is usually managed both medically and surgically. Arguably the most common neurosurgical procedure done, usually at the bedside, is the placement of an external ventricular drain (EVD) for monitoring and managing ICP, and assisting with clearance of intraventricular blood.

We review herein the topic of EVD in hemorrhagic stroke, articulating the scope of the problem and prognostic factors, clinical indications, technical aspects, surgical adjuncts and other management issues, and relevant questions for future research. The review is based on a systematic Pubmed literature search of all original publications and previous reviews on this topic with key words of external ventricular drain and intraventricular hemorrhage/placement/insertion/infection/hemorrhage. Specific citations were selected from this reference list for the purpose of illustrating individual aspects of the topic.

Epidemiology of EVDs for hemorrhagic stroke: the scope of the problem

Intracerebral hemorrhage (ICH) and subarachnoid hemorrhage (SAH) account for the majority of hemorrhagic strokes. Although spontaneous ICH with or without intraventricular extension accounts for only 10–15% of all strokes, this devastating disease accounts for disproportionate outcomes, with 30-day mortality rates of 35–52%, and half of those deaths occurring in the first two days (1–6). It has been postulated that rupture of ICH into the ventricles would be beneficial in order to lessen the mass effect from the large ICH on surrounding structures, but in fact the extension of ICH into the ventricles (Fig. 11.1) has been consistently demonstrated as an independent predictor of poor outcome in patients with ICH (7–17). In a series of patients with ICH and intraventricular hemorrhage (IVH), Young *et al.* (18) demonstrated a strong predictor between ventricular blood volume and poor outcome, and determined a 'lethal volume' of blood that predicted poor outcomes. Patients with more than 20 ml blood all had died or were in a persistent vegetative state. However, a study examining patients with large intraventricular hemorrhages found that the etiology of the IVH was more important in predicting outcome than the volume of IVH (19). A careful study by Turhim *et al.* demonstrated a direct correlation between IVH volume and outcome, and this correlation persisted when

Critical Care of the Stroke Patient, ed. Stefan Schwab, Daniel Hanley, and A. David Mendelow. Published by Cambridge University Press.

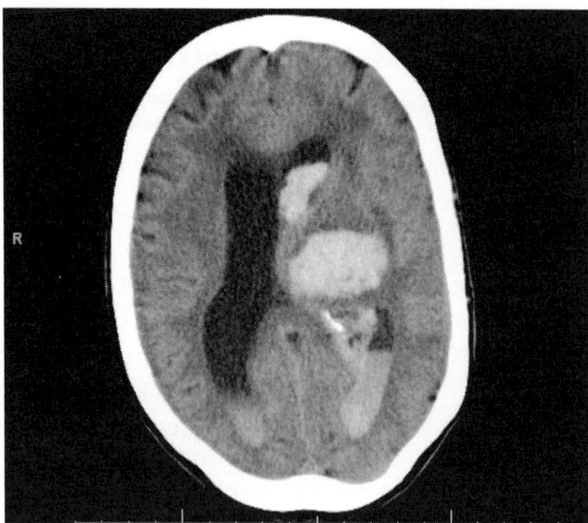

Fig. 11.1 CT scan of a typical intracerebral hemorrhage with extension into the ventricles.

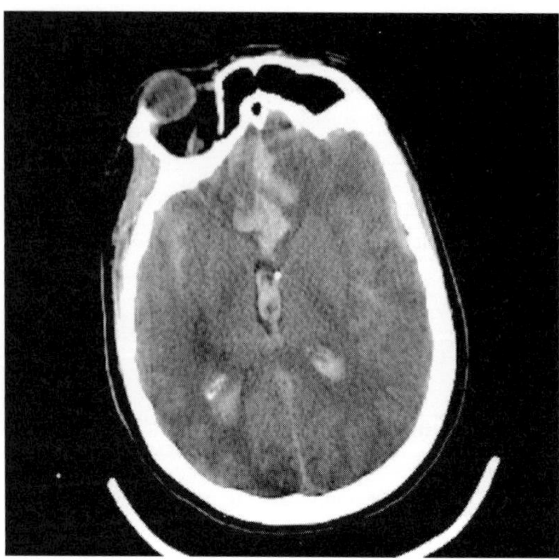

Fig. 11.2 CT scan of a typical subarachnoid hemorrhage with intraventricular hemorrhage.

controlling for the presence or absence of hydrocephalus and size of associated ICH (8).

Subarachnoid hemorrhage (SAH) accounts for approximately 5% of all strokes and affects as many as 30000 Americans each year, with 30-day mortality rates as high as 45% (20), and those who survive often have noteworthy morbidity following the event. Predictors of poor outcome include severity of initial hemorrhage, older age, longer time to treatment, and size and location of aneurysm. The rupture of saccular or berry aneurysms at the circle of Willis is the most common cause of SAH. When aneurysms rupture, the blood often collects in the subarachnoid space causing many devastating effects including blockage of CSF circulation resulting in acute hydrocephalus. The aneurysmal bleeding may also extend into the cerebral ventricles, contributing to obstruction of CSF circulation and acute hydrocephalus (Fig. 11.2). A build-up of CSF can cause the ventricle or subarachnoid space to expand and dilate. Untreated acute hydrocephalus associated with IVH or SAH can increase intracranial pressure (ICP), which causes acute herniation of brain tissue and subsequently death. Several studies have demonstrated the impact of IVH as an independent poor prognostic indicator after aneurysmal SAH (21–23).

Several recent studies have attempted to grade the extent of IVH in relation to patient outcome (8,13,18,19). The 'Graeb score' (Table 11.1) considers the extent of involvement of the respective ventricles and associated ventriculomegaly, and has been extensively validated in outcomes studies (13,24,25).

Indications for EVD in hemorrhagic stroke

Acute obstructive hydrocephalus following IVH and SAH causing high ICP, can lead to significant morbidity and mortality. Even though ICP can be managed medically with sedation and osmotic diuretics, such management is often insufficient to reduce ICP and those settings call for EVD placement (26). An analysis of IVH cohort in a large prospective randomized study of surgery for ICH (27), demonstrated that continuous drainage of CSF contributes to the normalization of ICP. However, the placement of EVD does not eliminate the morbidity and mortality of IVH, perhaps due to underlying damage from the associated stroke, and the toxic effects of ventricular blood on adjacent periventricular brain tissue, including the hippocampus, diencephalon, and brainstem. Catheter occlusions

Table 11.1 Graeb score (modified from Graeb, *et al.* Computed tomographic diagnosis of intraventricular hemorrhage. Etiology and prognosis. *Radiology*. 1982;143:91–6).

Location	Score
Lateral ventricles (each lateral ventricle is scored separately)	
	0= no blood
	1= trace of blood or mild bleeding
	2= less than half of the ventricle is filled with blood
	3= more than half of the ventricle is filled with blood
	4= ventricle is filled with blood and expanded
Third and fourth ventricles	
	0= no blood
	1= blood present, ventricle size normal
	2= ventricle filled with blood and expanded
Total	Range: 0–12

occur frequently in the setting of large IVH volume, with casting and clotting on ventricular blood, and these can result in poor ICP control. Catheter occlusions also require repeated catheter removals and insertions, thus increasing the risks of hemorrhage and infection (28).

EVD and clearance of IVH

The placement of EVD does not immediately clear the IVH. In a study by Naff *et al.* (29), it was shown that blood clot resolution in CSF follows first-order kinetics, and it has been suggested that EVD could even potentially slow the rate of IVH clearance by removing the tissue plasminogen activator (tPA) released from the clot into the CSF. Conversely, the injection of thrombolytic agents into the ventricular space would increase the rate of clot resolution. Thrombolytic therapy for IVH has evolved in response to the problems of catheter obstruction and slow IVH clearance, and has been shown to be safe and effective in animal studies (16,30,31), and in small clinical case series (32–36). The safety and feasibility of intraventricular thrombolysis was recently tested in Phase II clinical trials (29), and the dose of intraventricular thrombolysis has been optimized, with 1 mg every 8 hours achieving the most enhanced clearance without increasing hemorrhage risk. The effect of intraventricular thrombolysis on survival and functional outcome in comparison to EVD alone with placebo irrigation is being tested in ongoing Phase III clinical trials (www.cleariii.org).

Techniques of EVD insertion

In the setting of hemorrhagic stroke, where timely ICP management is critical, the EVD is usually inserted at the bedside in the emergency room or intensive care unit (ICU). Keen in 1890 first reportedly used skull landmarks to cannulate the lateral ventricle (37) and in 1918 Dandy published a technique involving anterior and occipital ventricular horn punctures for air ventriculography (38). The standard neurosurgical technique for bedside EVD insertion has gradually evolved in subsequent decades using preassembled kits, and ultimately the introduction of disposable instruments and drills and tunneling of the catheter (39). Ghajar introduced the principle of cannulating the cerebral ventricle by precise perpendicular trajectory to the skull surface, and he developed a tool to facilitate this approach (40). Roitberg *et al.* reported minimal complications and successful EVD placement and maintenance for the duration of required drainage, in a retrospective series of 103 consecutive cases of bedside EVD placement in the ICU, with sterile technique and short subcutaneous tunneling of the catheter (41). Kakarla *et al.* confirmed the safety and accuracy of EVD placement by neurosurgical trainees by bedside ventriculostomy for ICP monitoring and CSF drainage (42).

Due to occasional complications associated with bedside EVD placement some have recommended placement of the EVD in the operating room, with a rationale of better sterile technique, and more optimal visualization and hemostatasis of burr hole exposure and brain surface cannulation (41). However, the added time involved with operating room access and patient transport have continued to favor the emergent use of bedside technique.

Standard technique of EVD insertion

The typical technique for bedside placement of EVD is illustrated in Figure 11.3. Usually the right, non-dominant side is preferred for EVD insertion unless specific contra-indications are present like right lateral ventricle hematoma, AVM/lesion in the trajectory of the EVD, etc. Kocher's point is frequently used for placement of frontal EVD. Kocher's point is located at 2–3 cm lateral to the midline (approximately the mid-pupillary line with forward gaze) avoiding the sagittal sinus, and 1 cm anterior to the coronal suture (about 10.5 cm behind the nasion) avoiding the motor cortex (43). Once Kocher's point is identified, the hair around the planned insertion site and EVD exit site is clipped and the area is prepped with sterile prepping technique. A short incision is planned, typically 1–2 cm long, parallel to the midline. After the incision is made, the periostium is elevated, a self-retaining retractor is placed, and the burr hole is drilled with a twist drill. Durotomy is accomplished using a needle or probe, and the EVD catheter is advanced with an internal stylet, perpendicular to the surface of the brain aiming towards the medial canthus of the ipsilateral eye in the coronal plane and towards the tragus of the ear in the sagittal plane. Once CSF is obtained, which is usually at a depth of about 4–5 cm, the stylet is removed and the catheter is advanced another 1 cm or so. This technique of EVD insertion places the catheter in the anterior horn of the lateral ventricle, with its tip at or near the foramen of Munro.

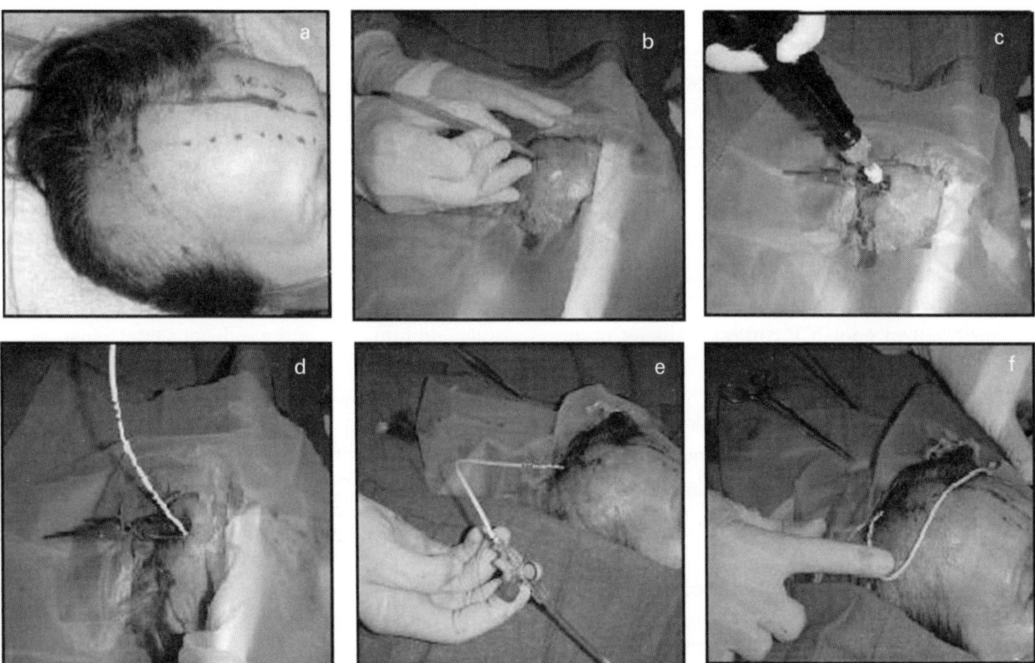

Fig. 11.3 EVD entry point is marked 10.5 cm behind the nasion and 2.5 cm from the midline (a) and a short (approximately 2 cm) incision is made down to the pericranium (b). Twist drill hole is made through both tables of the skull using a manual drill with guard adjusted to avoid plunging (c). The stylet is removed with catheter depth at 5.5 cm to 6 cm from the outer table of the skull (d) and the EVD catheter is connected to the closed bag drainage system incorporating a three-way stopcock. Secure the catheter with suture to the skin at a second point, insuring that the catheter is not kinked or obstructed (f).

Insertion of EVD is a technical procedure and thus is operator dependent. Very few studies have been done to assess the precision of EVD placement, and these have not used standardized or adjudicated criteria (42,44–51). Successful cannulation of the ventricle (subjective, and series dependent), number of catheter passes, and inadvertent EVD placement in brain tissue or subarachnoid space varied vastly depending on the study (and what was assessed and reported). For example, misplacement rate was observed to be 50% by Toma *et al.* (44), 22.4% by Huyette *et al.* (45), 20% by Khanna *et al.* (46), 13% by Kakarla *et al.* (42), 11% by Bogdahn *et al.* (47) etc.

Technical adjuncts

Given that the body of the lateral ventricle lies in the midpupillary line and the curve of the superior aspect of the anterior horn parallels the curve of the overlying cranium, thus a catheter directed at a right angle to the cranial surface in the midpupillary line will enter the ventricle. Based on this principle, Ghajar designed a device that, when placed over a burr hole at Kocher's point, guides a catheter perpendicular to the skull surface. The efficacy of the guide was studied in 17 patients who required ventriculostomy. Cerebrospinal fluid was obtained in all patients on the first pass of the catheter at an approximate intracranial distance of 5 cm. Eleven patients had confirmation of correct catheter placement in the ipsilateral anterior horn of the lateral ventricle by intraoperative fluoroscopy or post-operative computerized tomography (40). However, this technique is useful only when a mass lesion has not distorted the patient's brain anatomy. A study comparing the freehand technique of catheter placement using external landmarks with the use of the Ghajar guide showed that successful cannulation was achieved using either technique; however, the catheters placed using the Ghajar guide were closer to the target (51).

Lollis and Roberts proposed the use of robotic technique, and reported a small prospective series with safe, highly accurate, and reliable EVD placement with robot guided trajectory even in patients with very small ventricles (52). Image-guided frameless stereotaxy is increasingly being used for ventricular catheter placement in shunt procedures for hydrocephalus, demonstrating greater accuracy and better placement of the catheter in even difficult cases like slit ventricles, and shift due to mass lesion or cysts, etc. (53). While this practice has not translated into routine use for emergent EVD placement because of time constraints and the life-threatening nature of acute hydrocephalus, it may be most appropriate for catheter replacements after initial poor placement, or for second catheters targeted at trapped or casted ventricles (Fig. 11.4). In selected situations, EVD placement may be accomplished with real-time image guidance in the CT scanner under sterile technique, as per procedures of real-time CT-guided biopsy (Fig. 11.5).

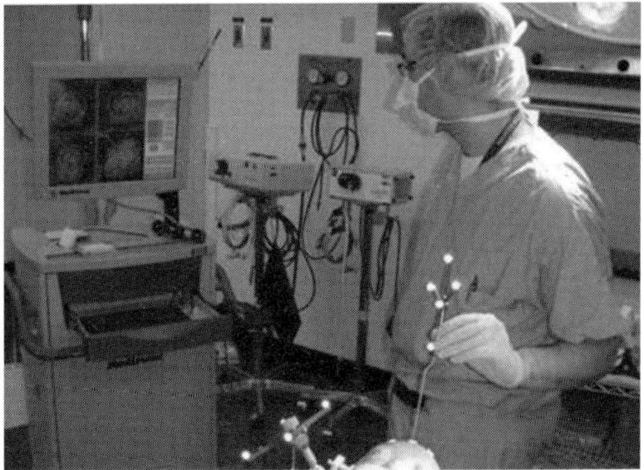

Fig. 11.4 Image-guided EVD placement using frameless stereotaxy.

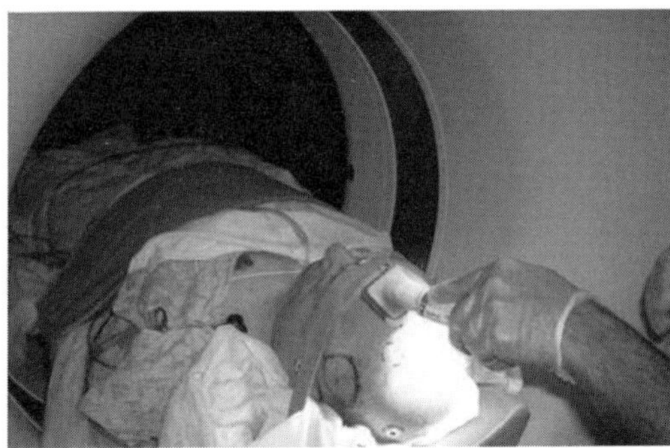

Fig. 11.5 Image-guided placement of EVD in CT scanner.

Special surgical considerations

Despite the technical ease of their placement, misplacement of the ventricular catheter can lead to a range of complications including hemorrhage and infection (54). In a meta-analysis performed by Binz *et al.*, they reported new bleeding on CT scan after 5.7% of EVD placements, with less than 1% risk of clinically significant hemorrhage (3). Even though hemorrhage associated with ventriculostomy placement is a known risk, it is very poorly studied and quantified. Complication rate may be influenced by many factors like the institutional and individual practitioner's practice patterns, timing of the CT scan, the thresholds on coagulation studies to indicate safety, use of platelet infusion for patients treated with antiplatelet agents, access site, drill bit size and thread distance, aggressive drilling, use of saline to irrigate the twist drill hole, removal of all bone fragments prior to dural opening, sharp or blunt dural penetration, sharp or blunt pial opening, slow or quick access of the frontal horn, removal of the stylet at ventricular entry or after advancement to the foramen of Monro, or even tightness of scalp closure (3). Gardner *et al.* noted a possible trend, but no statistically significant reduction of hemorrhage risks when EVDs are placed in the operating room as compared to the ICU (55). Other authors have reported modified techniques in an attempt to lower the risk of EVD-associated hemorrhage. In a retrospective study of 50 patients using a modified spinal needle for ventricular access Hassler and Zentner demonstrated a 0% 'symptomatic' hemorrhage rate (56). Using a stainless steel, blunt-tip needle for percutaneous ventriculostomy, Meyer *et al.* reported an intracranial hemorrhage rate of 1% with only 0.5% caused by the actual ventricular puncture in 200 patients (57). Careful, well-designed studies are needed to objectively define and estimate the risk of EVD-associated hemorrhage. Adjudicated data in this regard will emerge from ongoing trials of thrombolysis versus placebo in EVD for IVH (29,58–60).

Management of EVD

Measuring opening pressure

One of the most important pieces of information obtained from EVD is the opening ICP measurement. This value has significant prognostic implications, and it influences the subsequent strategy and threshold of CSF drainage through the EVD. In all but cases of impending cerebral herniation, special attention is paid so as not to allow significant CSF escape from the EVD before documenting pressure, and this can be accomplished with a manometer or transducer. Once the pressure is measured, the EVD catheter is secured and connected with the drainage bag system and pressure transducer.

Opening level, intermittent versus continuous drainage

There are several options of managing EVD drainage, depending on the opening pressure and the underlying pathology. In the setting of SAH and untreated aneurysm, the conventional wisdom is to not lower the ICP too drastically. The rationale is to avoid changing the transmural pressure across the wall of recently ruptured aneurysm, predisposing to rebleeding (61). While some studies did not confirm an increased risk of rebleeding with EVD after aneurysmal SAH (62), current best practice aims not to drain too much CSF too fast. There has been no comparison of intermittent drainage strategies (regularly scheduled intermittent volume, or as needed in response to ICP elevations), versus continuous drainage with the drip chamber set a particular level (drainage as needed when ICP exceeds that level). Continuous drainage may allow more rapid clearance of ventricular blood, and presumably spasmogenic and irritative contents of bloody CSF, but may also be vulnerable to overdrainage during patient suctioning and mobilization (experienced units protocolize temporary clamping of the EVD during those maneuvers). Others have cautioned that overdrainage of CSF could predispose to cerebral vasospasm as well as hydrocephalus (63).

Infection prophylaxis

Incidence of ventriculostomy-related infections have been reported from 0% to 22% (64–68). This frequently necessitates replacement of EVD, prolonged hospital stay, antibiotics-associated cost and morbidities, and occasionally life-threatening sequelae. Risk factors that have been suggested in association with EVD-related infections include previous craniotomy, systemic infection, depressed cranial fracture, lack of tunneling of the catheter, intraventricular hemorrhage, duration of EVD, catheter irrigation, site leaks, and frequency of CSF sampling (69). Yet many of these factors have not been carefully adjudicated in controlled studies, or even in multivariate analyses. Factors suggested to reduce infectious complications include strict sterile insertion technique with tunneling of the EVD catheter, wound care, closed system devices, and minimum interruption of the closed systems (70). Most of these suggestions have attributed particular interventions to a low infection rate, or have compared sequential periods or different series with various protocols, but there have not been careful controlled studies addressing these adjuncts. Some studies showed an associated risk of infection if the catheter is left more than five days (71), and a linear correlation between infection rates and the duration of the catheter and CSF leakage (72). Other studies have shown that length of EVD duration has no effect on the rate of infection (73).

Antibiotic use

To reduce infections associated with EVD, a common practice is to administer intravenous antibiotics to cover common skin flora (71). However, antibiotics prophylaxis may contribute to the development of resistant organisms, or much more morbid gram negative ventriculitis (74). Protocols of antibiotic use have varied widely, including peri-operative use at and for short periods after EVD insertion, or continued for the duration of drainage (71, 75). A meta-analysis of randomized clinical trials and observational studies concluded that the use of prophylactic systemic antibiotics throughout the duration of EVD and use of antibiotic-coated EVD appears beneficial in preventing ventriculostomy-related infection (75–79); however, the absolute and relative risk reduction of EVD infections, if any, with antibiotic use has not been carefully assessed and requires further carefully controlled trials. In the setting CSF infection with indwelling EVD, it is commonly advised to remove the presumably colonized EVD, and replace it with a clean EVD, preferentially at a different 'clean' site. The new EVD allows resumption of CSF drainage, may enhance clearance of ventriculitis, allows CSF sampling to monitor response to treatment, and provides a route for intraventricular antibiotics administration. The latter may be lifesaving in fulminant ventriculitis. In addition to changing the EVD, intravenous antibiotics should be started or adjusted in response to the specific offending agent, and intraventricular antibiotic instillation should be considered for more fulminant or recalcitrant infections. Protocols of managing bacterial ventriculitis in association with EVD have varied widely, with a number of protocols resulting in successful eradication of infection (78,80,81).

CSF surveillance

To proactively monitor development of infection in the setting of EVD, regular CSF samples may be collected under sterile conditions and examined for organisms, cells, glucose, and protein, and sent for microbiological culture. Infection may be gleaned from CSF WBC pleocytosis, relative CSF hypoglycemia, positive gram stain or positive PCR for bacterial DNA, but positive CSF culture is the ultimate proof of infection (82). There is wide variation in current practices regarding CSF surveillance, ranging from routine CSF monitoring on a daily basis or other regular intervals, to CSF sampling only when there is clinical concern for infection, and in documenting clearance of infection. Gram stain and newer PCR techniques may allow rapid identification of colonization or early infections, and the initiation of treatment before the serious sequelae of intraventricular purulence.

Antibiotic impregnated catheters

Drawing from the success of antibiotic-impregnated central venous catheters in decreasing central line associated sepsis, antibiotic-impregnated EVD catheters have been developed with the aim of decreasing infection risk. One prospective randomized study found that catheters impregnated with minocycline and rifampin were one half as likely to become colonized as the control catheters and positive CSF cultures were seven times less frequent in patients with antibiotic-impregnated catheters compared with those in the control group (83). However, another similar study found no reduction of infection using the hydrogel-coated catheters when presoaked in low-concentration bacitracin solution when compared with regular catheters (84). One of the biggest concerns for using antibiotic-impregnated catheters is that surveillance specimens obtained from them may be less likely to demonstrate bacterial growth and thus potentially delay the detection of infection until more advanced ventriculitis. A recent study confirms that the risk of a false-negative culture result may be increased when a CSF sample is drawn through an antibiotic-impregnated catheter (85).

Removal of EVD

With IVH and SAH, there is often obstruction of arachnoid villi and the ventricular and cisternal drainage pathways causing acute hydrocephalus and hence the need for EVD. However, CSF flow dynamics may recover in some cases after clearance of ventricular blood, allowing the EVD to be discontinued. In other cases, chronic hydrocephalus develops requiring the need for long-term CSF diversion by shunt placement. The decision of EVD removal or conversion to shunt is based on EVD weaning and clamping trials.

Weaning and clamping trials

Extrapolating from other medical devices like chest or endotracheal tubes, the conventional way of EVD removal is a multiday stepwise weaning by progressive height elevation of the drainage system leading to clamping of the EVD. During this multiday process the size of the ventricles is usually monitored with serial imaging, along with the patient's neurologic condition and the volume of CSF drained at various thresholds. If the size of the ventricles increases during this process, or significant ICP elevations of persistent need of drainage are otherwise documented, those patients are deemed to be in need of a permanent CSF diversion strategy like a shunt. However, a study looking at the gradual versus rapid weaning of the EVD in the setting of SAH found that multistep gradual EVD weaning may have provided no definite advantage, only delaying the ultimate shunt procedure, and contributed to more prolonged ICU and hospital stays (86). However, it is clear that different patients recover from EVD dependency at varying rates, and many would not require a shunt after longer periods of EVD drainage, which could best be gauged through repeated clamping trials, if not gradual weaning.

Indication and timing of VP shunt placement

In the setting of aneurysmal subarachnoid hemorrhage older studies have shown many factors loosely associated with increased risk for needing a VP shunt like advanced age (87–89), more extensive SAH with higher Fisher grade (87,90,91), poorer neurological condition with higher Hunt and Hess grade (87,91–93), presence of acute hydrocephalus (90,92,94), increased CSF drainage time (94, 95), continuous CSF drainage (63), and female sex (87,91,92). Chan *et al.* studied the clinical factors predisposing a patient to long-term shunt dependency and tried to formulate a Failure Risk Index (FRI) that strongly and linearly correlated with the risk of EVD challenge failure (96). They also found that CSF protein level at the time of challenge was the single most predictive factor. However, this index has not been validated with prospective study. A very recent study suggests that permanent CSF diversion after aneurysmal SAH may be independently predicted by hyperglycemia at admission, findings on the admission CT scan (Fisher Grade 4, fourth ventricle intraventricular hemorrhage, and bicaudate index ≥ 0.20), and development of nosocomial meningitis (97).

Special consideration

EVD and thromboprophylaxis

EVD is associated with 0–33% risk of hemorrhagic complications (3) and many patients requiring EVD are coagulopathic due to their underlying brain illness or previous therapies. Coagulation parameters are measured before starting the procedure, and in all but life-threatening impending herniation, the conventional practice is to measure coagulation parameters and platelet counts, and to correct the coagulopathy (if INR > 1.2–1.4) or administer platelets (if platelet counts are <100000) before or during insertion of EVD. In the case of previous antiplatelet therapies, it is common to administer platelets for emergent EVD placement, or to document normal platelet aggregation assays if time permits. While most practitioners advocate platelet transfusion for clopidogrel (Plavix) effect, there is controversy whether aspirin use alone should preclude safe EVD placement. Exact thresholds of coagulopathy for safe EVD placement have largely been derived from empiric experience, rather than carefully controlled studies. Similarly, normal coagulation parameters must be insured for any catheter manipulations, catheter removal, or during thrombolytic administration through the EVD.

Most patients with stroke, including those requiring EVD, are unconscious or immobile, with demonstrated higher risk of developing deep venous thrombosis. Sequential stockings should be used from the time of patient admission, and there is no rationale for delaying administration of mini dose anticoagulation for thromboprophylaxis after placement of EVD, as long as the hemorrhagic stroke has stabilized and the underlying aneurysm or vascular malformation has been secured. Patients are closely monitored clinically and if needed radiographically after removal of EVD.

Future directions

Much controversy persists regarding various facets of EVD management, and these should be clarified in controlled studies. There is much variability in EVD placement, including whether anatomical landmarks should be used, placing the EVD in a freehand manner, or using image guidance to place the catheter. Suboptimal placement is more likely when using anatomical landmarks for insertion, but this is often the most efficient technique in emergent situations, and image guidance is not always readily available. Other variability exists in terms of target placement, whether to place the catheter through the lateral ventricle with greater or lesser blood, or how far from the foramen of Monro the catheter should be placed. Analyses of ICP control, catheter obstructions, and clot resolution rates in relation to various catheter placement strategies should be performed in order to enhance the efficacy of EVD in hemorrhagic stroke.

REFERENCES

1. Chiewvit P, Danchaivijitr N, Nilanont Y, Poungvarin N. Computed tomographic findings in non-traumatic hemorrhagic stroke. *J Med Assoc Thai.* 2009;**92**(1):73–86.
2. Badjatia N, Rosand J. Intracerebral hemorrhage. *Neurologist.* 2005;**11**(6):311–24.
3. Binz DD, Toussaint LG, 3rd, Friedman JA. Hemorrhagic complications of ventriculostomy placement: a meta-analysis. *Neurocrit Care.* 2009;**10**(2):253–6.
4. Ehtisham A, Taylor S, Bayless L, Klein MW, Janzen JM. Placement of external ventricular drains and intracranial pressure monitors by neurointensivists. *Neurocrit Care.* 2009;**10**(2):241–7.
5. Murry KR, Rhoney DH, Coplin WM. Urokinase in the treatment of intraventricular hemorrhage. *Ann Pharmacother.* 1998;**32**(2):256–8.
6. Sudlow CL, Warlow CP. Comparable studies of the incidence of stroke and its pathological types: results from an international collaboration. International Stroke Incidence Collaboration. *Stroke.* 1997;**28**(3):491–9.
7. Jakovljevic D, Sarti C, Sivenius J, *et al.* Socioeconomic differences in the incidence, mortality and prognosis of intracerebral hemorrhage in Finnish Adult Population. The FINMONICA Stroke Register. *Neuroepidemiology.* 2001;**20**(2):85–90.
8. Tuhrim S, Horowitz DR, Sacher M, Godbold JH. Volume of ventricular blood is an important determinant of outcome in supratentorial intracerebral hemorrhage. *Crit Care Med.* 1999;**27**(3):617–21.
9. St Louis EK, Wijdicks EF, Li H, Atkinson JD. Predictors of poor outcome in patients with a spontaneous cerebellar hematoma. *Can J Neurol Sci.* 2000;**27**(1):32–6.
10. Holloway RG, Benesch CG, Burgin WS, Zentner JB. Prognosis and decision making in severe stroke. *JAMA.* 2005;**294**(6):725–33.
11. Bhattathiri PS, Gregson B, Prasad KS, Mendelow AD. Intraventricular hemorrhage and hydrocephalus after spontaneous intracerebral hemorrhage: results from the STICH trial. *Acta Neurochir Suppl.* 2006;**96**:65–8.

12. Ozdemir O, Calisaneller T, Hasturk A, *et al.* Prognostic significance of third ventricle dilation in spontaneous intracerebral hemorrhage: a preliminary clinical study. *Neurol Res.* 2008;**30**(4):406–10.
13. Hanley DF. Intraventricular hemorrhage: severity factor and treatment target in spontaneous intracerebral hemorrhage. *Stroke.* 2009;**40**(4):1533–8.
14. Goh KY, Poon WS. Recombinant tissue plasminogen activator for the treatment of spontaneous adult intraventricular hemorrhage. *Surg Neurol.* 1998;**50**(6):526–31; discussion 31–2.
15. Ohwaki K, Yano E, Nagashima H, *et al.* Blood pressure management in acute intracerebral hemorrhage: relationship between elevated blood pressure and hematoma enlargement. *Stroke.* 2004;**35**(6):1364–7.
16. Pang D, Sclabassi RJ, Horton JA. Lysis of intraventricular blood clot with urokinase in a canine model: Part 2. In vivo safety study of intraventricular urokinase. *Neurosurgery.* 1986;**19**(4):547–52.
17. Passero S, Ciacci G, Reale F. Potential triggering factors of intracerebral hemorrhage. *Cerebrovasc Dis.* 2001;**12** (3):220–7.
18. Young WB, Lee KP, Pessin MS, *et al.* Prognostic significance of ventricular blood in supratentorial hemorrhage: a volumetric study. *Neurology.* 1990;**40**(4):616–9.
19. Roos YB, Hasan D, Vermeulen M. Outcome in patients with large intraventricular haemorrhages: a volumetric study. *J Neurol Neurosurg Psychiatry.* 1995;**58**(5):622–4.
20. Broderick JP, Brott TG, Duldner JE, Tomsick T, Leach A. Initial and recurrent bleeding are the major causes of death following subarachnoid hemorrhage. *Stroke.* 1994;**25**(7):1342–7.
21. Rosen DS, Macdonald RL, Huo D, *et al.* Intraventricular hemorrhage from ruptured aneurysm: clinical characteristics, complications, and outcomes in a large, prospective, multicenter study population. *J Neurosurg.* 2007;**107** (2):261–5.
22. Mayfrank L, Hutter BO, Kohorst Y, *et al.* Influence of intraventricular hemorrhage on outcome after rupture of intracranial aneurysm. *Neurosurg Rev.* 2001;**24**(4):185–91.
23. Mohr G, Ferguson G, Khan M, *et al.* Intraventricular hemorrhage from ruptured aneurysm. Retrospective analysis of 91 cases. *J Neurosurg.*1983;**58**(4):482–7.
24. Graeb DA, Robertson WD, Lapointe JS, Nugent RA, Harrison PB. Computed tomographic diagnosis of intraventricular hemorrhage. Etiology and prognosis. *Radiology.* 1982;**143**(1):91–6.
25. Hallevi H, Dar NS, Barreto AD, *et al.* The IVH score: a novel tool for estimating intraventricular hemorrhage volume: clinical and research implications. *Crit Care Med.* 2009;**37** (3):969–74, e1.
26. Ronning P, Sorteberg W, Nakstad P, Russell D, Helseth E. Aspects of intracerebral hematomas – an update. *Acta Neurol Scand.* 2008;**118**(6):347–61.
27. Ziai WC, Torbey MT, Naff NJ, *et al.* Frequency of sustained intracranial pressure elevation during treatment of severe intraventricular hemorrhage. *Cerebrovasc Dis.* 2009;**27** (4):403–10.
28. Carhuapoma JR. Thrombolytic therapy after intraventricular hemorrhage: do we know enough? *J Neurol Sci.* 2002;**202**(1–2):1–3.
29. Naff NJ, Hanley DF, Keyl PM, *et al.* Intraventricular thrombolysis speeds blood clot resolution: results of a pilot, prospective, randomized, double-blind, controlled trial. *Neurosurgery.* 2004;**54**(3):577–83; discussion 83–4.
30. Pang D, Sclabassi RJ, Horton JA. Lysis of intraventricular blood clot with urokinase in a canine model: Part 3. Effects of intraventricular urokinase on clot lysis and post-hemorrhagic hydrocephalus. *Neurosurgery.* 1986;**19** (4):553–72.
31. Pang D, Sclabassi RJ, Horton JA. Lysis of intraventricular blood clot with urokinase in a canine model: Part 1. Canine intraventricular blood cast model. *Neurosurgery.* 1986;**19** (4):540–6.
32. Shen PH, Matsuoka Y, Kawajiri K, *et al.* Treatment of intraventricular hemorrhage using urokinase. *Neurol Med Chir (Tokyo).* 1990;**30**(5):329–33.
33. Huttner HB, Tognoni E, Bardutzky J, *et al.* Influence of intraventricular fibrinolytic therapy with rt-PA on the long-term outcome of treated patients with spontaneous basal ganglia hemorrhage: a case-control study. *Eur J Neurol.* 2008;**15**(4):342–9.
34. Vereecken KK, Van Havenbergh T, De Beuckelaar W, Parizel PM, Jorens PG. Treatment of intraventricular hemorrhage with intraventricular administration of recombinant tissue plasminogen activator: A clinical study of 18 cases. *Clin Neurol Neurosurg.* 2006;**108** (5):451–5.
35. Kumar K, Demeria DD, Verma A. Recombinant tissue plasminogen activator in the treatment of intraventricular hemorrhage secondary to periventricular arteriovenous malformation before surgery: case report. *Neurosurgery.* 2003;**52**(4):964–8; discussion 8–9.
36. Findlay JM, Weir BK, Stollery DE. Lysis of intraventricular hematoma with tissue plasminogen activator. Case report. *J Neurosurg.* 1991;**74**(5):803–7.
37. Keen W. Surgery of the lateral ventricles of the brain. *Lancet.* 1890;**136**(3498):553–5.

38. Dandy WE. Ventriculography following the injection of air into the cerebral ventricles. *Ann Surg.* 1918;**68**(1):5–11.
39. Friedman WA, Vries JK. Percutaneous tunnel ventriculostomy. Summary of 100 procedures. *J Neurosurg.* 1980;**53**(5):662–5.
40. Ghajar JB. A guide for ventricular catheter placement. Technical note. *J Neurosurg.* 1985;**63**(6):985–6.
41. Roitberg BZ, Khan N, Alp MS, *et al.* Bedside external ventricular drain placement for the treatment of acute hydrocephalus. *Br J Neurosurg.* 2001;**15**(4):324–7.
42. Kakarla UK, Kim LJ, Chang SW, Theodore N, Spetzler RF. Safety and accuracy of bedside external ventricular drain placement. *Neurosurgery.* 2008;**63**(1 Suppl 1):ONS162–6; discussion ONS6–7.
43. Greenberg M. *Handbook of Neurosurgery.* 7th ed: Thieme; 2010.
44. Toma AK, Camp S, Watkins LD, Grieve J, Kitchen ND. External ventricular drain insertion accuracy: is there a need for change in practice? *Neurosurgery.* 2009;**65**(6):1197–1200; discussion 1200–1.
45. Huyette DR, Turnbow BJ, Kaufman C, *et al.* Accuracy of the freehand pass technique for ventriculostomy catheter placement: retrospective assessment using computed tomography scans. *J Neurosurg.* 2008;**108**(1):88–91.
46. Khanna RK, Rosenblum ML, Rock JP, Malik GM. Prolonged external ventricular drainage with percutaneous long-tunnel ventriculostomies. *J Neurosurg.* 1995;**83**(5):791–4.
47. Bogdahn U, Lau W, Hassel W, *et al.* Continuous-pressure controlled, external ventricular drainage for treatment of acute hydrocephalus – evaluation of risk factors. *Neurosurgery.* 1992;**31**(5):898–903; discussion, 904.
48. Anderson RC, Kan P, Klimo P, *et al.* Complications of intracranial pressure monitoring in children with head trauma. *J Neurosurg.* 2004;**101**(1 Suppl):53–8.
49. Stangl AP, Meyer B, Zentner J, Schramm J. Continuous external CSF drainage – a perpetual problem in neurosurgery. *Surg Neurol.* 1998;**50**(1):77–82.
50. Khan SH, Kureshi IU, Mulgrew T, Ho SY, Onyiuke HC. Comparison of percutaneous ventriculostomies and intraparenchymal monitor: a retrospective evaluation of 156 patients. *Acta Neurochir Suppl.* 1998;**71**: 50–2.
51. O'Leary ST, Kole MK, Hoover DA, *et al.* Efficacy of the Ghajar Guide revisited: a prospective study. *J Neurosurg.* 2000;**92**(5):801–3.
52. Lollis SS, Roberts DW. Robotic catheter ventriculostomy: feasibility, efficacy, and implications. *J Neurosurg.* 2008;**108**(2):269–74.
53. Azeem SS, Origitano TC. Ventricular catheter placement with a frameless neuronavigational system: a 1-year experience. *Neurosurgery.* 2007;**60**(4 Suppl 2):243–7; discussion 247–8.
54. Saladino A, White JB, Wijdicks EF, Lanzino G. Malplacement of ventricular catheters by neurosurgeons: a single institution experience. *Neurocrit Care.* 2009;**10**(2):248–52.
55. Gardner PA, Engh J, Atteberry D, Moossy JJ. Hemorrhage rates after external ventricular drain placement. *J Neurosurg.* 2009;**110**(5):1021–5.
56. Hassler W, Zentner J. Ventricle puncture for external CSF drainage and pressure measurement using a modified puncture needle. *Acta Neurochir (Wien).* 1988;**94**(1–2):93–5.
57. Meyer B, Schaller K, Rohde V, Hassler W. Percutaneous needle trephination. Experience in 200 cases. *Acta Neurochir (Wien).* 1994;**127**(3–4):232–5.
58. Dunatov S, Antoncic I, Bralic M, Jurjevic A. Intraventricular thrombolysis with rt-PA in patients with intraventricular hemorrhage. *Acta Neurol Scand.* Feb 8.
59. Staykov D, Bardutzky J, Huttner HB, Schwab S. Intraventricular fibrinolysis for intracerebral hemorrhage with severe ventricular involvement. *Neurocrit Care.* Jun 4.
60. Morgan T, Awad I, Keyl P, Lane K, Hanley D. Preliminary report of the clot lysis evaluating accelerated resolution of intraventricular hemorrhage (CLEAR-IVH) clinical trial. *Acta Neurochir Suppl.* 2008;**105**: 217–20.
61. Hasan D, Lindsay KW, Vermeulen M. Treatment of acute hydrocephalus after subarachnoid hemorrhage with serial lumbar puncture. *Stroke.* 1991;**22**(2):190–4.
62. Hellingman CA, van den Bergh WM, Beijer IS, *et al.* Risk of rebleeding after treatment of acute hydrocephalus in patients with aneurysmal subarachnoid hemorrhage. *Stroke.* 2007;**38**(1):96–9.
63. Kasuya H, Shimizu T, Kagawa M. The effect of continuous drainage of cerebrospinal fluid in patients with subarachnoid hemorrhage: a retrospective analysis of 108 patients. *Neurosurgery.* 1991;**28**(1):56–9.
64. Holloway KL, Barnes T, Choi S, *et al.* Ventriculostomy infections: the effect of monitoring duration and catheter exchange in 584 patients. *J Neurosurg.* 1996;**85**(3):419–24.
65. Chan KH, Mann KS. Prolonged therapeutic external ventricular drainage: a prospective study. *Neurosurgery.* 1988;**23**(4):436–8.
66. Kanter RK, Weiner LB. Ventriculostomy-related infections. *N Engl J Med.* 1984;**311**(15):987.
67. Park P, Garton HJ, Kocan MJ, Thompson BG. Risk of infection with prolonged ventricular catheterization. *Neurosurgery.* 2004;**55**(3):594–9; discussion 599–601.

68. Dasic D, Hanna SJ, Bojanic S, Kerr RS. External ventricular drain infection: the effect of a strict protocol on infection rates and a review of the literature. *Br J Neurosurg.* 2006;**20**(5):296–300.
69. Hoefnagel D, Dammers R, Ter Laak-Poort MP, Avezaat CJ. Risk factors for infections related to external ventricular drainage. *Acta Neurochir (Wien).* 2008;**150**(3):209–14; discussion 214.
70. Schade RP, Schinkel J, Visser LG, *et al.* Bacterial meningitis caused by the use of ventricular or lumbar cerebrospinal fluid catheters. *J Neurosurg.* 2005;**102**(2):229–34.
71. Beer R, Lackner P, Pfausler B, Schmutzhard E. Nosocomial ventriculitis and meningitis in neurocritical care patients. *J Neurol.* 2008;**255**(11):1617–24.
72. Lyke KE, Obasanjo OO, Williams MA, *et al.* Ventriculitis complicating use of intraventricular catheters in adult neurosurgical patients. *Clin Infect Dis.* 2001;**33**(12): 2028–33.
73. Korinek AM, Reina M, Boch AL, *et al.* Prevention of external ventricular drain-related ventriculitis. *Acta Neurochir (Wien).* 2005;**147**(1):39–45; discussion 46.
74. Ortiz R, Lee K. Nosocomial infections in neurocritical care. *Curr Neurol Neurosci Rep.* 2006;**6**(6):525–30.
75. Lucey MA, Myburgh JA. Antibiotic prophylaxis for external ventricular drains in neurosurgical patients: an audit of compliance with a clinical management protocol. *Crit Care Resusc.* 2003;**5**(3):182–5.
76. Wong GK, Poon WS, Lyon D, Wai S. Cefepime vs. Ampicillin/Sulbactam and Aztreonam as antibiotic prophylaxis in neurosurgical patients with external ventricular drain: result of a prospective randomized controlled clinical trial. *J Clin Pharm Ther.* 2006;**31**(3):231–5.
77. Sonabend AM, Korenfeld Y, Crisman C, *et al.* Prevention of ventriculostomy-related infections with prophylactic antibiotics and antibiotic-coated external ventricular drains: A systematic review. *Neurosurgery.* Jan 6.
78. Pfausler B, Spiss H, Beer R, *et al.* Treatment of staphylococcal ventriculitis associated with external cerebrospinal fluid drains: a prospective randomized trial of intravenous compared with intraventricular vancomycin therapy. *J Neurosurg.* 2003;**98**(5):1040–4.
79. Pons VG, Denlinger SL, Guglielmo BJ, *et al.* Ceftizoxime versus vancomycin and gentamicin in neurosurgical prophylaxis: a randomized, prospective, blinded clinical study. *Neurosurgery.* 1993;**33**(3):416–22; discussion 422–3.
80. Beer R, Pfausler B, Schmutzhard E. Management of nosocomial external ventricular drain-related ventriculomeningitis. *Neurocrit Care.* 2009;**10**(3):363–7.
81. Elvy J, Porter D, Brown E. Treatment of external ventricular drain-associated ventriculitis caused by *Enterococcus faecalis* with intraventricular daptomycin. *J Antimicrob Chemother.* 2008;**61**(2):461–2.
82. Pfisterer W, Muhlbauer M, Czech T, Reinprecht A. Early diagnosis of external ventricular drainage infection: results of a prospective study. *J Neurol Neurosurg Psychiatry.* 2003;**74**(7):929–32.
83. Zabramski JM, Whiting D, Darouiche RO, *et al.* Efficacy of antimicrobial-impregnated external ventricular drain catheters: a prospective, randomized, controlled trial. *J Neurosurg.* 2003;**98**(4):725–30.
84. Kaufmann AM, Lye T, Redekop G, *et al.* Infection rates in standard vs. hydrogel coated ventricular catheters. *Can J Neurol Sci.* 2004;**31**(4):506–10.
85. Stevens EA, Palavecino E, Sherertz RJ, Shihabi Z, Couture DE. Effects of antibiotic-impregnated external ventricular drains on bacterial culture results: an in vitro analysis. *J Neurosurg.* 2010;**113**(1):86–92.
86. Klopfenstein JD, Kim LJ, Feiz-Erfan I, *et al.* Comparison of rapid and gradual weaning from external ventricular drainage in patients with aneurysmal subarachnoid hemorrhage: a prospective randomized trial. *J Neurosurg.* 2004;**100**(2):225–9.
87. Graff-Radford NR, Torner J, Adams HP Jr, Kassell NF. Factors associated with hydrocephalus after subarachnoid hemorrhage. A report of the Cooperative Aneurysm Study. *Arch Neurol.* 1989;**46**(7):744–52.
88. Lanzino G, Kassell NF, Germanson TP, *et al.* Age and outcome after aneurysmal subarachnoid hemorrhage: why do older patients fare worse? *J Neurosurg.* 1996;**85**(3):410–18.
89. Lin CL, Kwan AL, Howng SL. Acute hydrocephalus and chronic hydrocephalus with the need of postoperative shunting after aneurysmal subarachnoid hemorrhage. *Kaohsiung J Med Sci.* 1999;**15**(3):137–45.
90. Schmieder K, Koch R, Lucke S, Harders A. Factors influencing shunt dependency after aneurysmal subarachnoid haemorrhage. *Zentralbl Neurochir.* 1999;**60**(3):133–40.
91. Vale FL, Bradley EL, Fisher WS, 3rd. The relationship of subarachnoid hemorrhage and the need for postoperative shunting. *J Neurosurg.* 1997;**86**(3):462–6.
92. Sheehan JP, Polin RS, Sheehan JM, Baskaya MK, Kassell NF. Factors associated with hydrocephalus after aneurysmal subarachnoid hemorrhage. *Neurosurgery.* 1999;**45**(5):1120–7; discussion 1127–8.
93. van Gijn J, Hijdra A, Wijdicks EF, Vermeulen M, van Crevel H. Acute hydrocephalus after aneurysmal subarachnoid hemorrhage. *J Neurosurg.* 1985;**63**(3):355–62.

94. Widenka DC, Wolf S, Schurer L, Plev DV, Lumenta CB. Factors leading to hydrocephalus after aneurysmal subarachnoid hemorrhage. *Neurol Neurochir Pol.* 2000;**34** (6 Suppl):56–60.
95. Ohwaki K, Yano E, Nakagomi T, Tamura A. Relationship between shunt-dependent hydrocephalus after subarachnoid haemorrhage and duration of cerebrospinal fluid drainage. *Br J Neurosurg.* 2004;**18**(2):130–4.
96. Chan M, Alaraj A, Calderon M, *et al.* Prediction of ventriculoperitoneal shunt dependency in patients with aneurysmal subarachnoid hemorrhage. *J Neurosurg.* 2009; **110**(1):44–9.
97. Rincon F, Gordon E, Starke RM, *et al.* Predictors of long-term shunt-dependent hydrocephalus after aneurysmal subarachnoid hemorrhage. Clinical article. *J Neurosurg.* **113**(4):774–80.

12

Management of lumbar drains in cerebrovascular disease

Dimitre Staykov and Hagen B. Huttner

Introduction

Post-hemorrhagic hydrocephalus and drainage of cerebrospinal fluid

Post-hemorrhagic hydrocephalus is a common complication occurring after subarachnoid or intraventricular hemorrhage (IVH). IVH may lead to casting of the third and fourth ventricles, causing acute obstruction of the cerebrospinal fluid (CSF) outflow from the ventricular system into the subarachnoid space [1]. Another pathomechanism is the impairment of CSF resorption in the Pacchioni granulations of the arachnoidea leading to a communicating (aresorptive) hydrocephalus [1]. This form of hydrocephalus is either caused directly by blood in the subarachnoid space after subarachnoid hemorrhage (SAH), or occurs with a delay after IVH, mediated by circulating blood breakdown products [1,2]. Irrespective of its underlying mechanism, hydrocephalus leads to a gradual increase in intracranial pressure (ICP), supported by the ongoing production of CSF in the choroid plexus, mainly in the lateral ventricles. This is accompanied by clinical deterioration, beginning with headache, nausea, and vomiting, and leading to a gradual decline of consciousness from somnolence to deep coma [1,2].

In such patients, extracorporal diversion of CSF represents an essential therapeutic intervention usually becoming necessary at an early stage during the course of treatment [3]. Both obstructive and communicating hydrocephalus can be treated with external ventricular drainage (EVD), a catheter placed uni- or bilaterally in the frontal horn of the lateral ventricle. Although a life-saving procedure and the only treatment option in acute obstructive hydrocephalus, EVD is highly invasive and may lead to secondary complications such as e.g. catheter tract bleeding [4,5] during or after placement, catheter-associated infection with increasing duration of CSF drainage, or symptomatic seizures [6]. Furthermore, every exchange of an EVD because of catheter malfunction, obstruction or infection causes additional parenchymal brain injury.

In the past decade, another treatment alternative has emerged for patients with communicating post-hemorrhagic hydrocephalus. Lumbar drainage (LD), a simple and less invasive bedside technique, has been increasingly used to replace EVD, reduce EVD duration, and avoid EVD exchange procedures in such patients [1,2,7]. Moreover, an additional therapeutic effect of LD mediated by removal of blood and its breakdown products from the subarachnoid space has been suggested, because of reduction of vasospasm after SAH [8,9], or reduction of the incidence of permanent hydrocephalus after ICH with severe ventricular involvement [1,7]. Communication between the ventricular and the subarachnoid CSF space is essentially necessary for the usage of LD in such patients.

Critical Care of the Stroke Patient, ed. Stefan Schwab, Daniel Hanley, and A. David Mendelow. Published by Cambridge University Press.

ruptured intracranial aneurysms. *Neurosurgery*, 1999. **44** (3):503–9; discussion 509–12.

15. Pare, L., R. Delfino, R. Leblanc, The relationship of ventricular drainage to aneurysmal rebleeding. *J Neurosurg*, 1992;**76**(3):422–7.
16. McIver, J. I., *et al.*, Preoperative ventriculostomy and rebleeding after aneurysmal subarachnoid hemorrhage. *J Neurosurg*, 2002;**97**(5):1042–4.
17. Ruijs, A. C., *et al.*, The risk of rebleeding after external lumbar drainage in patients with untreated ruptured cerebral aneurysms. *Acta Neurochir (Wien)*, 2005;**147** (11):1157–61; discussion 1161–2.
18. Ochiai, H., Y. Yamakawa, Continuous lumbar drainage for the preoperative management of patients with aneurysmal subarachnoid hemorrhage. *Neurol Med Chir (Tokyo)*, 2001;**41**(12):576–80; discussion 581.
19. Hellingman, C. A., *et al.*, Risk of rebleeding after treatment of acute hydrocephalus in patients with aneurysmal subarachnoid hemorrhage. *Stroke*, 2007;**38**(1):96–9.
20. Connolly, E. S., Jr., *et al.*, The safety of intraoperative lumbar subarachnoid drainage for acutely ruptured intracranial aneurysm: technical note. *Surg Neurol*, 1997;**48** (4):338–42; discussion 342–4.
21. Crowley, R. W., *et al.*, New insights into the causes and therapy of cerebral vasospasm following subarachnoid hemorrhage. *Drug Discov Today*, 2008;**13**(5–6):254–60.
22. Weir, B., R. L. Macdonald, M. Stoodley, Etiology of cerebral vasospasm. *Acta Neurochir Suppl*, 1999;**72**:27–46.
23. Friedman, J. A., *et al.*, Volumetric quantification of Fisher Grade 3 aneurysmal subarachnoid hemorrhage: a novel method to predict symptomatic vasospasm on admission computerized tomography scans. *J Neurosurg*, 2002;**97** (2):401–7.
24. Al-Tamimi, Y. Z., *et al.*, Lumbar drainage of cerebrospinal fluid after aneurysmal subarachnoid hemorrhage: a prospective, randomized, controlled trial (LUMAS). *Stroke*, 2012;**43**(3):677–82.
25. Bardutzky, J., *et al.*, EARLYDRAIN-outcome after early lumbar CSF-drainage in aneurysmal subarachnoid hemorrhage: study protocol for a randomized controlled trial. *Trials*, 2011;**12**:203.
26. Tuettenberg, J., *et al.*, Clinical evaluation of the safety and efficacy of lumbar cerebrospinal fluid drainage for the treatment of refractory increased intracranial pressure. *J Neurosurg*, 2009;**110**(6):1200–8.
27. Munch, E. C., *et al.*, Therapy of malignant intracranial hypertension by controlled lumbar cerebrospinal fluid drainage. *Crit Care Med*, 2001;**29**(5):976–81.
28. Grady, M. S., Editorial. Lumbar drainage for increased intracranial pressure. *J Neurosurg*, 2009;**110**(6):1198–9.
29. Abadal, J. M., *et al.*, Lumbar drainage for intracranial pressure. *J Neurosurg*, 2009;**111**(6):1295; author reply 1295–6.
30. Bhattathiri, P. S., *et al.*, Intraventricular hemorrhage and hydrocephalus after spontaneous intracerebral hemorrhage: results from the STICH trial. *Acta Neurochir Suppl*, 2006;**96**:65–8.
31. Steiner, T., *et al.*, Dynamics of intraventricular hemorrhage in patients with spontaneous intracerebral hemorrhage: risk factors, clinical impact, and effect of hemostatic therapy with recombinant activated factor VII. *Neurosurgery*, 2006;**59**(4):767–73; discussion 773–4.
32. Tuhrim, S., *et al.*, Volume of ventricular blood is an important determinant of outcome in supratentorial intracerebral hemorrhage. *Crit Care Med*, 1999;**27**(3):617–21.
33. Diringer, M. N., D. F. Edwards, A. R. Zazulia, Hydrocephalus: a previously unrecognized predictor of poor outcome from supratentorial intracerebral hemorrhage. *Stroke*, 1998;**29**(7):1352–7.
34. Adams, R. E., M. N. Diringer, Response to external ventricular drainage in spontaneous intracerebral hemorrhage with hydrocephalus. *Neurology*, 1998;**50**(2):519–23.
35. Staykov, D., *et al.*, Intraventricular fibrinolysis for intracerebral hemorrhage with severe ventricular involvement. *Neurocrit Care*, 2010;**15**(1):194–209.
36. Naff, N. J., *et al.*, Intraventricular thrombolysis speeds blood clot resolution: results of a pilot, prospective, randomized, double-blind, controlled trial. *Neurosurgery*, 2004;**54**(3):577–83; discussion 583–4.
37. Huttner, H. B., *et al.*, Influence of intraventricular fibrinolytic therapy with rt-PA on the long-term outcome of treated patients with spontaneous basal ganglia hemorrhage: a case-control study. *Eur J Neurol*, 2008;**15**(4):342–9.
38. Staykov, D., *et al.*, Single versus bilateral external ventricular drainage for intraventricular fibrinolysis in severe ventricular haemorrhage. *J Neurol Neurosurg Psychiatry*, 2010;**81**(1):105–8.
39. Tung, M. Y., *et al.*, A study on the efficacy of intraventricular urokinase in the treatment of intraventricular haemorrhage. *Br J Neurosurg*, 1998;**12**(3):234–9.
40. O'Kelly, C. J., *et al.*, Shunt-dependent hydrocephalus after aneurysmal subarachnoid hemorrhage: incidence, predictors, and revision rates. Clinical article. *J Neurosurg*, 2009;**111**(5):1029–35.
41. Speck, V., *et al.*, Lumbar catheter for monitoring of intracranial pressure in patients with post-hemorrhagic

communicating hydrocephalus. *Neurocrit Care*, 2010;**14**(2):208–15.

42. Dagnew, E., H. R. van Loveren, J. M. Tew, Jr., Acute foramen magnum syndrome caused by an acquired Chiari malformation after lumbar drainage of cerebrospinal fluid: report of three cases. *Neurosurgery*, 2002;**51**(3):823–8; discussion 828–9.
43. Bloch, J., L. Regli, Brain stem and cerebellar dysfunction after lumbar spinal fluid drainage: case report. *J Neurol Neurosurg Psychiatry*, 2003;**74**(7):992–4.
44. Manley, G. T., W. Dillon, Acute posterior fossa syndrome following lumbar drainage for treatment of suboccipital pseudomeningocele. Report of three cases. *J Neurosurg*, 2000;**92**(3):469–74.
45. Snow, R. B., W. Kuhel, S. B. Martin, Prolonged lumbar spinal drainage after the resection of tumors of the skull base: a cautionary note. *Neurosurgery*, 1991;**28**(6):880–2; discussion 882–3.
46. Acikbas, S. C., *et al.*, Complications of closed continuous lumbar drainage of cerebrospinal fluid. *Acta Neurochir (Wien)*, 2002;**144**(5):475–80.
47. Staykov, D., *et al.*, Early recognition of lumbar overdrainage by lumboventricular pressure gradient. *Neurosurgery*, 2011;**68**(5):1187–91; discussion 1191.
48. Shapiro, S. A., T. Scully, Closed continuous drainage of cerebrospinal fluid via a lumbar subarachnoid catheter for treatment or prevention of cranial/spinal cerebrospinal fluid fistula. *Neurosurgery*, 1992;**30**(2):241–5.
49. Scheithauer, S., *et al.*, Prospective surveillance of drain associated meningitis/ventriculitis in a neurosurgery and neurological intensive care unit. *J Neurol Neurosurg Psychiatry*, 2009;**80**(12):1381–5.
50. Puzzilli, F., *et al.*, Cytochemical and microbiological testing of CSF and catheter in patients with closed continuous drainage via a lumbar subarachnoid catheter for treatment or prevention of CSF fistula. *Neurosurg Rev*, 1998;**21**(4):237–42.
51. Governale, L. S., *et al.*, Techniques and complications of external lumbar drainage for normal pressure hydrocephalus. *Neurosurgery*, 2008;**63**(4 Suppl 2):379–84; discussion 384.
52. Olivar, H., *et al.*, Subarachnoid lumbar drains: a case series of fractured catheters and a near miss. *Can J Anaesth*, 2007;**54**(10):829–34.
53. Ruiz-Sandoval, J. L., *et al.*, Multiple simultaneous intracerebral hemorrhages following accidental massive lumbar cerebrospinal fluid drainage: case report and literature review. *Neurol India*, 2006;**54**(4):421–4.
54. Settepani, F., *et al.*, Intracerebellar hematoma following thoracoabdominal aortic repair: an unreported complication of cerebrospinal fluid drainage. *Eur J Cardiothorac Surg*, 2003;**24**(4):659–61.

SECTION 3

Critical Care of Ischemic Stroke

Intravenous and intra-arterial thrombolysis for acute ischemic stroke

Martin Köhrmann and Stefan Schwab

Introduction

Occlusion of a brain vessel leads to a critical reduction in cerebral perfusion and, within minutes, to ischemic infarction with a central infarct core of irreversibly damaged brain tissue and a more or less large area of hypoperfused but still vital brain tissue (the ischemic penumbra), which can be salvaged by rapid restoration of blood flow. Therefore, the underlying rationale for thrombolytic agents is the lysis of the occluding thrombus, re-establishment of cerebral blood flow with subsequent reperfusion, and salvage of the ischemic penumbra. After introduction of thrombolytic therapy for the treatment of acute myocardial infarction in the early 1990s, major trials for the evaluation of this new therapeutic approach to ischemic stroke were initiated.

There are, in general, two strategies in thrombolytic therapy, a local (intra-arterial) approach and a systemic (intravenous) application of the thrombolytic agent. Only the latter has been proven to be effective in larger randomized trials and is a Class 1/Level A recommendation in national or international guidelines. This chapter summarizes the evidence for thrombolytic therapy of acute ischemic stroke with emphasis on progress regarding the approved intravenous treatment. Finally intra-arterial approaches as well as combined systemic and interventional therapies are discussed.

Intravenous thrombolysis

The early rt-PA trials

In 1995 the first two large randomized trials on thrombolytic treatment using recombinant tissue plasminogen activator (Alteplase; rt-PA) – the NINDS and the ECASS I trial – were published (1,2). These were followed by ECASS II in 1998 (3) and ATLANTIS in 1999 and 2000 (4,5). Overall a total of 2657 patients were randomized to treatment with placebo (n = 1316 patients) or intravenous rt-PA (n = 1341 patients) within 0–3 hours (NINDS), 3–5 hours (ATLANTIS), or 0–6 hours (ECASS I and II) after symptom onset. All four studies treated patients mainly based on exclusion of intracerebral hemorrhage using a baseline non-contrast CT. In addition, all studies except for the NINDS study also established CT exclusion criteria such as major early signs of infarction. All trials used a 0.9 mg/kg bodyweight dose up to a maximum of 90 mg rt-PA, except ECASS I, in which 1.1 mg/kg up to a maximum dose of 100 mg was given (2). Since ECASS I showed increased bleeding complications using the slightly higher dose, the present standard dosing of 0.9 mg/kg bodyweight was established. Ten percent of the total dose is given as a bolus; the rest is infused over 1 hour. Only the NINDS trial showed a significant benefit of rt-PA treatment over placebo with respect to the chosen primary endpoint. However, it has to be noticed that, even though ECASS I

Critical Care of the Stroke Patient, ed. Stefan Schwab, Daniel Hanley, and A. David Mendelow. Published by Cambridge University Press.

formally failed, there was a clear efficacy signal and it would have succeeded if the combined endpoint of the NINDS trial had been applied (6).

Mainly based on the positive results of the NINDS study, the American Food and Drug Administration (FDA) approved rt-PA in 1996 for the treatment of acute ischemic stroke within the 3-hour time window. The European Medicines Agency (EMEA) gave conditional approval in 2000.

Meta- and pooled analyses

Several meta-analyses of the early randomized Alteplase trials have been performed (7–9). The overall number needed to treat (NNT) in favor of rt-PA for all doses and time windows is 11; within 3 hours it is seven. The OR for death and dependence was 0.79 (CI 0.68–0.92, p = 0.001) for all time windows and doses. For the approved 3-hour time window the OR was 0.58 (CI 0.46 to 0.74, p = 0.00001).

In 2004, a combined analysis of the data from the NINDS, ECASS I and II, and ATLANTIS studies aimed to confirm the importance of rapid treatment and influence of time was published (10). Common data elements from the trials were pooled and re-analysed using multi-variable logistic regression to assess the relation of the interval from stroke onset to start of treatment on favorable 3-month outcome and on the occurrence of clinically relevant parenchymal ICH. 2775 patients from these trials were included in the analysis. Odds of a favorable 3-month outcome decreased as onset to treatment time increased (p = 0.005). Odds were 2.8 (95% CI 1.8–4.5) for 0–90 min, 1.6 (1.1–2.2) for 91–180 min, 1.4 (1.1–1.9) for 181–270 min, and 1.2 (0.9–1.5) for 271–360 min in favor of the rt-PA group. The hazard ratio for death adjusted for baseline NIHSS was not different from 1.0 for the 0–90 min, 91–180 min, and 181–270 min intervals; for 271–360 min it was 1.45 (1.02–2.07). ICH was seen in 82 (5.9%) rt-PA patients and 15 (1.1%) controls (p < 0.0001). In contrast to the efficacy analysis ICH was not associated with OTT but was with rt-PA treatment (p = 0.0001) and age (p = 0.0002). In 2010 data from ECASS-3 (821 patients) and EPITHET (100 patients) were added to the dataset (9). The analysis confirmed the results of the first calculation and yielded almost identical numbers. In both papers the authors concluded that the sooner rt-PA is given to stroke patients, the greater the benefit, especially if treatment is started within 90 min. This is of major importance since it has been previously reported in large cohorts that in IVT for stroke a so-called '3-hour effect' exists (11–13). The earlier a patient is admitted, the longer the treating physician takes to initiate thrombolysis. This reverse correlation is mainly attributed to a psychological effect of the physician feeling that there is no rush to make the 3-hour time window in which IVT is approved (11–13). The phenomenon was first reported for the population in the 'Standard Treatment with Alteplase to Reverse Stroke' study (STARS) in which every 30-min delay between stroke onset and ED arrival was associated with a 15-min decrease in the time between arrival and initiation of rt-PA therapy (regression coefficient, − 0.56; p < .001) (11). The same effect was recently shown in more than 10 000 thrombolysis patients from the 'Get with the Guidelines-Stroke Database'. OTD and DTN were again reversely correlated (r = −0.3) and treatment was significantly delayed in patients arriving within 1 hour after symptom onset compared to patients arriving later (13). However, neither the pre-hospital emergency caregivers nor the emergency and stroke physicians in the hospital have more time. Not only based on pathophysiological considerations but also as shown in both pooled analyses thrombolysis is more effective the earlier it is applied. Thus especially in very early time windows every single minute counts and logistics should be optimized wherever possible ('Lost time is lost brain'; 'Time is brain').

Ecass III

In 2000 the European Medicines Agency (EMEA) gave only conditional approval to rt-PA, imposing the implementation of a Phase IV registry monitoring the use of rt-PA in clinical practice as well as the evaluation of the treatment in an extended time window beyond 3 hours in a randomized trial, ECASS III (14). The original protocol was designed to include patients up to 4 hours. This was changed in early 2005, in adaptation to low recruitment rates and the detection of the effectiveness of the 4.5-hour time window in the above-mentioned pooled analysis from 2004. ECASS III was a double-blind, randomized, placebo-controlled trial of standard dose rt-PA in the 3-4.5 hour time window with 400 patients per study arm (rt-PA vs. placebo). Inclusion criteria were matched to the current European label of rt-PA, treatment was based on non-contrast CT as in the previous studies. The primary endpoint was a mRS score of 0–1 at day 90, the secondary endpoint was a global outcome analysis comparable to the one used in the NINDS trials (mRS 0–1, BI 95–100, GOS 0–1, NIHSS 0–1). Safety end points included death and symptomatic ICH. A total of 821 patients were enrolled into the study, 418 received rt-PA and 403 a placebo. The median time for the administration of medication was 3 hours 59 min. More patients had a favorable outcome according to the primary endpoint with rt-PA than with placebo (52.4% versus 45.2%; OR = 1.34; 95% CI 1.02–1.76; $p = 0.04$). In the global analysis, the outcome was also improved by active treatment (OR = 1.28; 95% CI 1.00–1.65; $p < 0.05$). Both OR were even more in favor of rt-PA in the per protocol analysis. Interestingly the achieved OR of 1.4 almost exactly replicated the base on the first pooled analysis of the early trials calculated results. This demonstrated the robustness of the treatment effect. Although the incidence of sICH was higher with rt-PA than with placebo, hemorrhagic complications were rare (2.4% versus 0.2%; $p = 0.008$), mortality did not differ between the two groups (7.7% and 8.4%)(14).

ECASS III is clearly a positive study not only opening the door to treatment in the extended 4.5 hour time window but also strengthening the confidence in thrombolytic therapy overall. An extension of the labeling in Europe is underway and even though treatment outside the 3 hour window is still off label – albeit one which is based on CLASS 1 evidence – several national and international guidelines already recommend treatment up to 4.5 hours.

Phase IV studies and registries for intravenous thrombolysis

After initial approval of rt-PA, several Phase IV studies and registries were undertaken to monitor the implementation of Alteplase into clinical routine practice. The largest such registry was the European Safe Implementation of Thrombolysis in Stroke – Monitoring Study (SITS-MOST) which was initially started as mandated in the conditional approval by the EMEA (15). SITS-MOST was a web-based registry embedded into the pre-existing larger SITS-ISTR database. 6483 patients were recruited from 285 centers between 2002 and 2006. Primary outcomes were the modified Rankin Score at 90 days as well as symptomatic ICH and mortality. Results were compared to the pooled randomized controlled trials. While the rate of symptomatic ICH with 1.7% (SITS-MOST definition) and 7.3% using the NINDS/Cochrane definition was comparable, the mortality rate was significantly lower (11.3% vs. 17.3%). Independent outcomes were in the upper percent range of the randomized trials. Further analysis, however, demonstrated that the slightly improved results regarding mortality and outcome were grounded on slightly more favorable baseline characteristics (16). Thus SITS-MOST confirmed that intravenous thrombolysis with rt-PA in clinical routine is at least as safe and effective as in the randomized trials (15). Table 13.1 summarizes the main inclusion and exclusion criteria for intravenous thrombolysis.

In another analysis SITS-ISTR (Safe Implementation of Thrombolysis in Stroke – international stroke treatment registry), the 'over-registry' of SITS-MOST compared outcome in patients treated between 3 hours and 4.5 hours versus those treated within 3 hours (from SITS-MOST and SITS-ISTR) (16). 664 patients with ischemic stroke and IVT between 3 hours and 4.5 hours were compared with 11 865 patients receiving treatment within 3 hours. Outcome measures were symptomatic ICH within 24 hours, mortality and independence (mRS score 0–2) at 3 months. The 3–4.5 hour cohort had a symptom start to treatment time of 195 min (IQR 187–210 min) versus 140 min (IQR 115–165 min); $p < 0.0001$. Median age was younger and stroke severity was lower (NIHSS score 11 versus 12 points, $p < 0.0001$) in the cohort treated in the extended time window. There were no significant differences between both cohorts for any safety of efficacy outcome measure. Consistent with the findings of ECASS III, IVT with rt-PA remains safe when given in between 3–4.5 hours and does not significantly differ from standard treatment within 3 hours in efficacy (16).

Table 13.1 Main inclusion and exclusion criteria for intravenous thrombolysis

Inclusion criteria	Exclusion criteria
- Acute focal neurological syndrome consistent with the diagnosis ischemic stroke	- Stroke or serious head trauma within 3 months
- Age 18–80 years (European license)	- Oral anticoagulation
- Symptom onset < 3 hours (< 4.5 hours for ECASS-3 patient cohort **but still 'off-label'**)	- History of significant bleeding (i.e. gastrointestinal)
	- Symptoms suggestive of subarachnoid hemorrhage
- Exclusion of ICH (e.g. non-contrast CT)	- Seizure at stroke onset
- Monitoring on an ICU or Stroke Unit	- Arteriovenous malformation or untreated cerebral aneurysm
	- Intramuscular or arterial puncture at a non-compressible site
	- Uncontrollable arterial hypertension
	- Significant surgery within the last 3 months
	- Severe liver disease or other disease with elevated bleeding risk
	- Intracranial neoplasm

Intravenous thrombolysis based on advanced MRI

Two MRI techniques have received much attention for acute stroke treatment over the past 15 years: diffusion-weighted-sequences (DWI) and perfusion-imaging (PI). In the classical model the DWI lesion represents the irreversibly damaged core of the infarct. Recent research has to a certain extent refined this approach. Now that more patients have been evaluated with stroke MRI and at early time points, partial reversal of the initial DWI lesion has been reported, suggesting that the DWI lesion might be included in the therapeutic target (17). DWI lesion reversal is associated with ultra-early and permanent reperfusion and this per se is a far stronger predictor of clinical and imaging outcome (18). In most instances, especially in later time windows, the DWI lesion may adequately reflect permanently damaged brain tissue. Also, PI does not measure quantitative perfusion. Most authors agree that time-based parameters such as mean transit time (MTT) or time to peak (TTP) give the best prognostic information. Thus, while hypoperfusion remains a key pathophysiological mechanism in stroke, more practically, the 'ischemic penumbra' may be operationally defined as those brain regions which are at risk of infarction but remain salvageable (19).

The volume difference of DWI and PI – also termed PI/DWI-mismatch – gives an approximate measure of this tissue at risk of infarction (20). While its non-quantitative approach suffers from, in part, inaccurate PI measurements and the fact that DWI abnormalities may reverse (17), they serve their purpose of easy clinical application. In fact, most experts agree that from a practical standpoint this simple model of PI/DWI-mismatch is sufficiently accurate in most acute stroke patients, and furthermore stroke MRI findings are consistent with our understanding of the pathophysiology of acute ischemia (21).

Applying the mismatch concept in addition to other parameters such as vessel occlusion may identify the individual time window for the patient and thus allow therapeutic decision making based on an individual vascular and hemodynamic situation, rather than the elapsed time. Additional MR findings not captured by CT, such as early blood–brain barrier disruption (22) and old microbleeds (23) may predict a poor outcome after thrombolysis and therefore can be used to improve patient selection. However, the presence of microbleeds currently should not influence our treatment practice, but in the face of doubt may be used as an exclusion criterion in reperfusion studies to increase safety (Fig. 13.1).

DEFUSE and EPITHET

The mismatch concept has recently been validated in the DEFUSE study (24). DEFUSE was a seven-centers trial, which recruited 74 patients treated with rt-PA

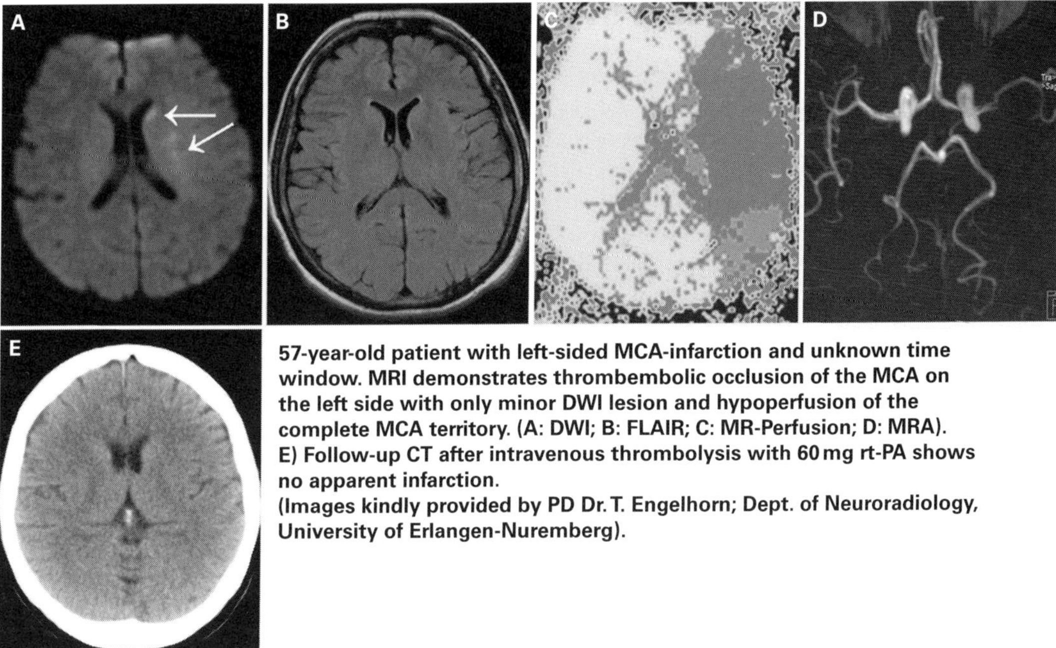

Fig. 13.1 Case presentation MRI-based thrombolysis. (See plate section for color version).

within 3–6 hours after symptom onset. Treatment was based on CT findings but an MRI was obtained immediately prior to and after rt-PA. Early reperfusion was associated with significantly better chance of a favorable clinical response to thrombolysis in patients with a PI/DWI-mismatch. Patients without a mismatch did not benefit from early reperfusion. Large infarctions already seen on baseline DWI experienced fatal sICH upon reperfusion, while small (lacunar) infarcts did reasonably well with or without a mismatch (24). The EPITHET trial, also recently published, was a placebo-controlled randomized study design, which tested the effect of rt-PA versus placebo within the 3–6 hour time window (25). Patients were again selected by CT and received MRI before the study drug was given, i.e. MRI was **not** used to select patients. Inasmuch, EPITHET was similar to DEFUSE, but randomized. The primary endpoint was reduction of stroke lesion volume growth (geometric mean) at day 90; secondary endpoints included various volume and clinically-based outcomes, as well as reperfusion at day 3–5. 101 patients were recruited (52 rt-PA and 49 placebo); of these, 85 had mismatch. While EPITHET failed the primary outcome, trends and significant results were seen for secondary outcomes such as reperfusion – which occurred more often with rt-PA (56% vs. 26%), and was associated with reduced infarct growth, and with improved neurological as well as functional outcomes (25). The recently started Australian EXTEND study now randomizes in a larger phase III design patients in a 3–9 hour time window selected based on MRI-mismatch to receive either rt-PA or placebo. With a primary clinical endpoint it will shed more light onto the role of imaging-based thrombolysis.

Non-randomized observational studies

After earlier smaller studies, three large observational studies using stroke MRI in an extended time window in clinical practice have been published (23,26,27). Thomalla *et al.* compared outcome and symptomatic bleeding complications of intravenous rt-PA within 6 hours of symptom onset in MRI-selected patients with acute MCA infarction with the pooled data of the large stroke rt-PA trials (26). Favorable outcome was more frequent in MRI-selected rt-PA patients compared with pooled placebo and pooled rt-PA patients. Interestingly the rate of sICH in MRI-selected rt-PA patients was lower than in the pooled rt-PA group and comparable to the pooled placebo group. Another single-center study compared patients who were treated with rt-PA based on CT findings within 3 hours with patients treated MRI based within and beyond 3 hours (27). Clinical outcome and occurrence of sICH were prospectively assessed in 382 consecutive patients. Patients were divided into three groups: (1) CT-based < 3 hours (n = 209 patients), (2) MRI-based < 3 hours (n = 103 patients), and (3) MRI-based > 3 hours (n = 70 patients). The rate of independent outcomes in groups 1–3 was 47.8%, 50.5% and 55.7%. Mortality was trendwise reduced, and sICH were significantly reduced in the MRI-based groups. MRI-selected patients overall had a significantly lower risk for sICH and mortality. In multi-variate analysis only age and treating MRI-based were significant predictors of sICH, whereas for independent outcome and mortality age, NIHSS score and sICH were predictive. Time to treatment proved to be irrelevant for all outcomes in uni-variate and multi-variate analyses (27). A similar analysis in a multi-center dataset on 1210 patients yielded similar but stronger results (23). The predefined primary 'efficacy' outcome was favorable outcome (mRS 0–1), safety endpoints were sICH and mortality. The overall use of MRI significantly reduced symptomatic intracranial hemorrhage (OR: 0.520, 95% CI: 0.270 to 0.999, p = 0.05). Use of stroke MRI beyond 3 hours (compared to CT or MRI within 3 hours), the use of MRI significantly predicted a favorable outcome (OR: 1.467; 95% CI: 1.017 to 2.117, p = 0.040). Within 3 hours and for all secondary endpoints, there was a trend in favor of MRI-based selection over standard < 3-hour CT-based treatment (23).

The desmoteplase trial program

Two parallel phase II trials (DIAS, DEDAS) with a 3–9 hour time window using desmoteplase and another thrombolytic drug were completed (28, 29). In DIAS reperfusion rates up to 71.4% were observed compared with 19.2% with placebo (28). Favourable 90-day clinical outcome was found in 22.2% of placebo-treated patients and between 13.3% (62.5 μg/kg; p = 0.757) and 60.0% (125 μg/kg; p = 0.009) of desmoteplase-treated patients. Early reperfusion correlated favorably with clinical outcome (p = 0.0028). Favorable outcome occurred in 52.5% of patients experiencing reperfusion versus 24.6% of patients without reperfusion (28). The DEDAS study yielded confirmatory results (29). Interestingly in both studies, imaging parameters paralleled the clinical outcome proving that the MRI parameters function as adequate surrogate parameters.

After these promising results a follow-up phase III study – DIAS-2 – was undertaken but yielded negative results (30). 193 patients were again randomized to receive desmoteplase (90 or 125 μg/kg) or placebo. In contrast to the previous studies treatment based on CT imaging was allowed. The primary endpoint was clinical response rates at 90 days, defined as a composite of improvement in NIHSS score of at least 8 points, a mRS of 0–2 points, and a Barthel Index of 75–100. Forty-seven percent in the lower and 36% of patients in the higher desmoteplase dose tier showed clinical response. This, however, compared to a placebo response rate of 46%. Intracranial hemorrhage rates were again acceptable. Mortality was increased in the higher desmoteplase group. The reasons for these disappointing results are not fully understood yet. However, overall stroke severity was milder, median lesion volume small, and the placebo response rate of 46% was very high (30). Currently two parallel phase III trials (DIAS 3/4) are underway using slightly modified inclusion criteria allowing only patients with proximal vessel occlusion to be randomized.

Intra-arterial thrombolysis and combined treatment approaches

The delivery of thrombolytic agents locally, at or within the occluding thrombus, has the advantage of providing a higher concentration of the particular thrombolytic agent where it is needed while minimizing the systemic concentration. Hence, local intra-arterial thrombolysis has the potential for greater efficacy with regard to arterial recanalization rates and greater safety with regard to lower risk of hemorrhage. The technique involves performing a cerebral arteriogram, localizing the occluding clot, navigating a microcatheter to the site of the clot, and administering the lytic agent at or inside the clot with or without mechanical dissolution of the thrombus. The potential advantages of the intra-arterial approach are contrasted by several specific drawbacks, mainly the high technical needs and the considerable time delay to angiography, and from initiation of angiography to clot lysis.

Over the past decade multiple mainly smaller studies using different techniques have been published. In contrast to intravenous treatment there is not a standard intra-arterial procedure derived from these studies. Many different thrombolytic agents as well as different interventional devices were used in these studies. This may have hampered further clinical evaluation of the treatment approach and even though the interventional approach is nowadays often used in dedicated centers for the treatment of strokes caused by proximal vessel occlusion, larger clinical trials with clinical endpoints are mostly missing.

PROACT I and II

The PROACT I trial was published in 1998 and compared intra-arterial recombinant pro-urokinase (rpro-UK) versus placebo in patients with angiographically documented proximal middle cerebral artery occlusion (31). Among the 40 treated patients, 26 received rpro-UK and 14 placebo at a median of 5.5 hours from symptom onset. Recanalization was significantly associated with rpro-UK but outcome was unchanged (31). PROACT II randomized 180 patients to rpro-UK and heparin or heparin alone. Both regarding the primary outcome endpoint (mRS 0–2) as well as regarding recanalization of the target vessel, a significant benefit of active treatment was shown (32). Mortality was not significantly different. Despite these positive results the FDA did not approve the therapy and another study (PROACT III) of intra-arterial pro-urokinase for acute stroke within 6 hours had been intended but currently is not planned due to lack of funding.

Combined intravenous and interventional treatment: the 'bridging concept'

One way to combine the potential benefits of the local intra-arterial approach with the advantage of the easy-to-use and early intravenous thrombolysis is the so-called 'bridging concept' in which immediate intravenous thrombolysis 'bridges' the time gap until intra-arterial therapy is initiated (Fig. 13.2).

Interventional management of stroke (IMS) and the penumbra trial

In a first study, the IMS group investigated the safety of a combined IV/IA approach to recanalization in patients with ischemic stroke (33). Patients aged 18–80 with an NIHSS >/= 10 at baseline had IV rt-PA started (0.6 mg/kg, 60 mg maximum over 30 minutes) within 3 hours of onset. Additional rt-PA was then administered via a microcatheter at the site of the thrombus up to a total dose of 22 mg over 2 hours of infusion or until thrombolysis. Primary comparisons were made with historical controls (rt-PA-treated subjects from the NINDS rt-PA stroke trial). 80 patients with a median baseline NIHSS score of 18 were included in a median time to initiation of IV rt-PA of 140 min. The 3-month mortality in IMS patients (16%) was non-significantly lower than the mortality of placebo (24%) and rt-PA-treated subjects (21%) in the NINDS rt-PA stroke trial. The rate of sICH (6.3%) in IMS subjects was similar to that of rt-PA-treated subjects (6.4%) but higher than the rate in placebo-treated subjects (1.0%, $p = 0.018$) in the NINDS rt-PA stroke trial. Despite the higher baseline severity, IMS subjects had a significantly better outcome at 3 months than NINDS placebo-treated subjects for all outcome measures (33).

The IMS-2 study used the same protocol as in the IMS study (34). One of the main goals of the study was to gain data on the use of another interventional device, the EKOS ultrasound device. Here the catheter tip emanates low-frequency ultrasound waves that aid in thrombus fragmentation. The median NIHSS was 19, a recanalization was achieved in 57.7%, mortality was 16%, sICH rate was 11%, favorable and independent outcomes were seen in 33% (mRS 0–1) and 45% (mRS 0–2), respectively (34).

Another trial examined the use of another interventional device, the 'Penumbra-System, a thrombus

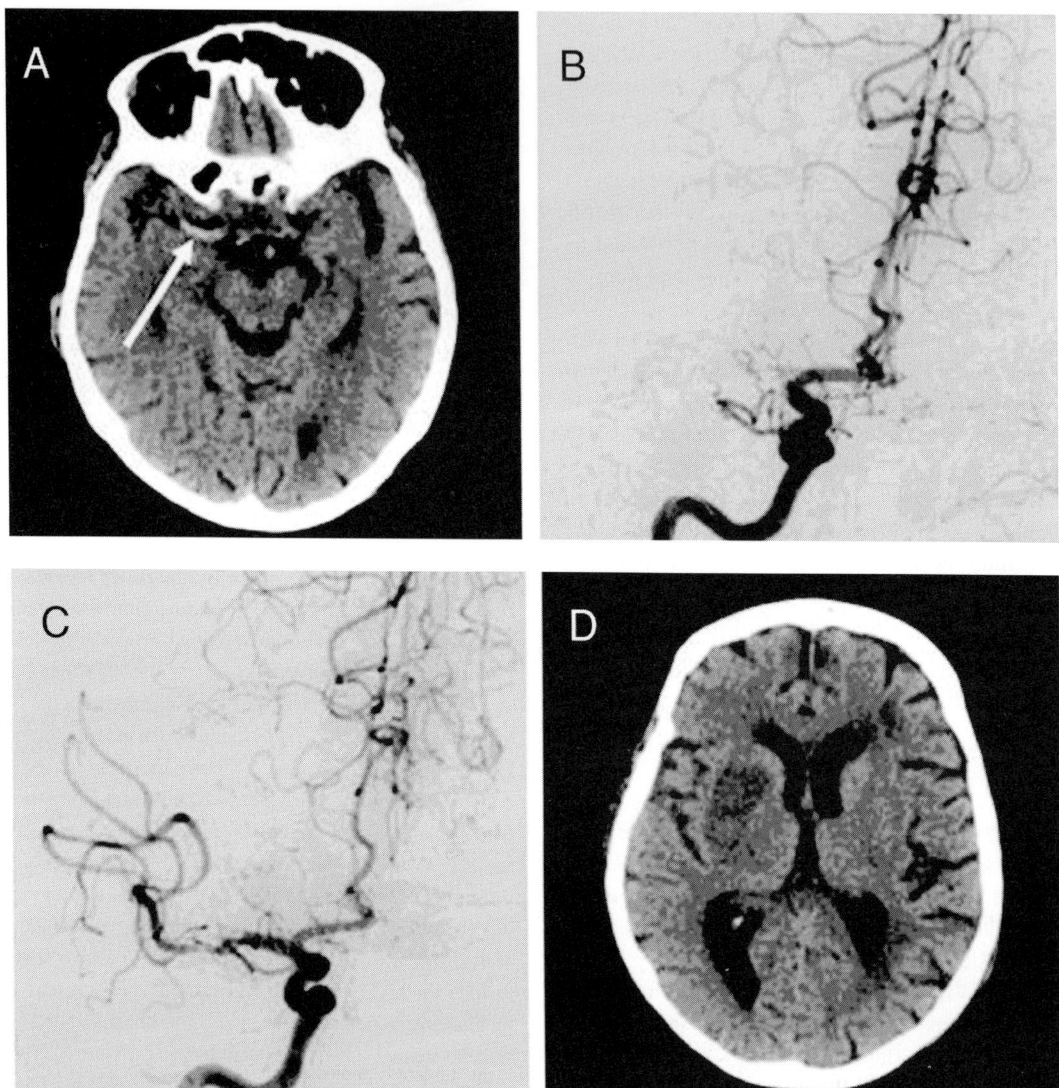

Fig. 13.2 'Bridging lysis'
58-year-old patient with severe right-sided MCA syndrome presenting 2 hours after symptom onset. A) Non-contrast CT on admission shows a dense MCA sign (arrow) but no early ischemic changes. B) Angiogram after full dose 'bridging lysis' (rt-PA) with persisting MCA occlusion. C) Successful recanalizaion using the Penumbra-System. D) Follow-up CT demonstrates only minor infarction on the right side. (Images kindly provided by Dr. T. Struffert; Dept. of Neuroradiology; University of Erlange-Nuremberg).

debulking and aspiration device specifically designed for embolectomy in acute stroke' (35). The study also allowed rt-PA therapy with a majority of the 125 patients included into this single arm study receiving primary thrombolysis. Recanalization of the 'target vessel' was achieved in 81.6%; however, mortality was 33% and only 25% of patients achieved a favorable clinical outcome (mRS 0–2). The discrepancy between a very high recanalization rate and the disappointing clinical outcome may at least be explained by the definition of recanalization of the target vessel used in the trial (35).

A large randomized, open label phase III trial – the IMS-3 trial – is now being conducted as a follow-up trial to the first IMS studies (36). It will include 900 patients within 3 hours and randomizes patients to receive either intravenous standard rt-PA therapy alone or a bridging lysis of 0.6 mg/kg over 40 min followed by angiography in the IV/IA arm. If an occlusion is seen then the patient will be treated with either of the approved devices (i.e. EKOS, Merci retriever, Penumbra-System or conventional microcatheter). This trial will yield first conclusive data on the combination of IV and IA treatment and the clinical value of interventional therapies in general (36).

Conclusion and summary

Intravenous thrombolysis is a highly effective and safe therapy of acute ischemic stroke which is still underused. Recent studies and registries strengthen the confidence in this valuable treatment and demonstrate safe implementation into clinical routine practice. In addition, the randomized placebo controlled ECASS-3 trial yields robust evidence of a treatment effect up to 4.5 hours. However, time is brain and thrombolysis is the more effective the earlier it is applied. Thus it is the responsibility of all medical personal to keep pre- and intrahospital delays to an absolute minimum. In the future, MRI-based treatment may even further extend the time window for treatment. The clinical value of intra-arterial therapy alone or in combination with systemic thrombolysis is not clear to date. Future studies are needed to evaluate interventional therapies for acute ischemic stroke.

CONFLICT OF INTEREST

MK received travel grants from Boehringer Ingelheim the manufacturer of rt–PA. PDS and SS are members of the advisory board and the speakers bureau of Boehringer Ingelheim the manufacturer of rt–PA

REFERENCES

1. Tissue plasminogen activator for acute ischemic stroke. The National Institute of Neurological Disorders and Stroke rt-PA Stroke Study Group. *N Engl J Med.* 1995;**333**(24):1581–7.
2. Hacke W, Kaste M, Fieschi C, *et al.* Intravenous thrombolysis with recombinant tissue plasminogen activator for acute hemispheric stroke. The European Cooperative Acute Stroke Study. *JAMA.* 1995;**274**:1017–25.
3. Hacke W, Kaste M, Fieschi C, *et al.* Randomised double-blind placebo-controlled trial of thrombolytic therapy with intravenous alteplase in acute ischaemic stroke (ECASS II). *Lancet.* 1998;**352**:1245–51.
4. Clark WM, Wissman S, Albers GW, *et al.* Recombinant tissue-type plasminogen activator (Alteplase) for ischemic stroke 3 to 5 hours after symptom onset. The ATLANTIS Study: a randomized controlled trial. *Alteplase Thrombolysis for Acute Noninterventional Therapy in Ischemic Stroke. JAMA.* 1999;**282**(21):2019–26.
5. Clark WM, Albers GW, Madden KP, Hamilton S. The rtPA (alteplase) 0 to 6-hour acute stroke trial, part A (A0276g): results of a double-blind, placebo-controlled, multicenter study. Thrombolytic therapy in acute ischemic stroke study investigators. *Stroke.* 2000;**31**(4):811–16.
6. Hacke W, Bluhmki E, Steiner T, *et al.* Dichotomized efficacy end points and global end-point analysis applied to the ECASS intention-to-treat data set. *Post Hoc Analysis of ECASS 1. Stroke.* 1998;**29**:2073–5.
7. Hacke W, Brott T, Caplan L, *et al.* Thrombolysis in acute ischemic stroke: controlled trials and clinical experience. *Neurology.* 1999;**53**(7):S3–14.
8. Wardlaw JM, del Zoppo G, Yamaguchi T. Thrombolysis for acute ischaemic stroke (Cochrane Review). *The Cochrane Library*; 2002.
9. Lees KR, Bluhmki E, von Kummer R, *et al.* Time to treatment with intravenous alteplase and outcome in stroke: an updated pooled analysis of ECASS, ATLANTIS, NINDS, and EPITHET trials. *Lancet.* 2010;**375**(9727):1695–703.
10. Hacke W, Donnan G, Fieschi C, *et al.* Association of outcome with early stroke treatment: pooled analysis of ATLANTIS, ECASS, and NINDS rt-PA stroke trials. *Lancet.* 2004;**363**(9411):768–74.
11. Albers GW, Bates VE, Clark WM, *et al.* Intravenous tissue-type plasminogen activator for treatment of acute stroke: the Standard Treatment with Alteplase to Reverse Stroke (STARS) study. *JAMA.* 2000;**283**(9):1145–50.

12. Sattin JA, Olson SE, Liu L, Raman R, Lyden PD. An expedited code stroke protocol is feasible and safe. *Stroke.* 2006;**37**(12):2935–9.
13. Saver JL, Smith EE, Fonarow GC, *et al.* The 'golden hour' and acute brain ischemia: presenting features and lytic therapy in > 30,000 patients arriving within 60 minutes of stroke onset. *Stroke.* 2010;**41**(7):1431–9.
14. Hacke W, Kaste M, Bluhmki E, *et al.* Thrombolysis with alteplase 3 to 4.5 hours after acute ischemic stroke. *N Engl J Med.* 2008;**359**(13):1317–29.
15. Wahlgren N, Ahmed N, Davalos A, *et al.* Thrombolysis with alteplase for acute ischaemic stroke in the Safe Implementation of Thrombolysis in Stroke-Monitoring Study (SITS-MOST): an observational study. *Lancet.* 2007;**369**(9558):275–82.
16. Wahlgren N, Ahmed N, Eriksson N, *et al.* Multivariable analysis of outcome predictors and adjustment of main outcome results to baseline data profile in randomized controlled trials: Safe Implementation of Thrombolysis in Stroke-MOnitoring STudy (SITS-MOST). *Stroke.* 2008;**39**(12):3316–22.
17. Kidwell CS, Alger JR, Saver JL. Beyond mismatch: evolving paradigms in imaging the ischemic penumbra with multimodal magnetic resonance imaging. *Stroke.* 2003;**34**(11):2729–35.
18. Chalela JA, Kang DW, Luby M, *et al.* Early magnetic resonance imaging findings in patients receiving tissue plasminogen activator predict outcome: Insights into the pathophysiology of acute stroke in the thrombolysis era. *Ann Neurol.* 2004;**55**(1):105–12.
19. Schlaug G, Siewert B, Benfield A, Edelman RR, Warach S. Time course of the apparent diffusion coefficient (ADC) abnormality in human stroke. *Neurology.* 1997;**49**(1):113–19.
20. Warach S. Tissue viability thresholds in acute stroke: The 4-factor model. *Stroke.* 2001;**32**(11):2460–1.
21. Schellinger PD, Fiebach JB, Hacke W. Imaging-based decision making in thrombolytic therapy for ischemic stroke: present status. *Stroke.* 2003;**34**(2):575–83.
22. Latour LL, Kang DW, Ezzeddine MA, Chalela JA, Warach S. Early blood-brain barrier disruption in human focal brain ischemia. *Ann Neurol.* 2004;**56**(4):468–77.
23. Fiehler J, Albers GW, Boulanger JM, *et al.* Bleeding risk analysis in stroke imaging before thrombolysis (BRASIL): pooled analysis of T2*-weighted magnetic resonance imaging data from 570 patients. *Stroke.* 2007;**38**(10):2738–44.
24. Albers GW, Thijs V, Wechsler L, *et al.* Results of the Diffusion-Weighted Imaging Evaluation for Understanding Stroke Evolution (DEFUSE) Study. *Stroke.* 2006;**37**(2):635–6.
25. Davis SM, Donnan GA, Parsons MW, *et al.* Effects of alteplase beyond 3 h after stroke in the Echoplanar Imaging Thrombolytic Evaluation Trial (EPITHET): a placebo-controlled randomised trial. *Lancet Neurol.* 2008;**7**(4):299–309.
26. Thomalla G, Schwark C, Sobesky J, *et al.* Outcome and aymptomatic bleeding complications of intravenous thrombolysis within 6 hours in MRI-selected stroke patients: Comparison of a German multicenter study with the pooled data of ATLANTIS, ECASS, and NINDS rtPA trials. *Stroke.* 2006;**37**(3):852–8.
27. Köhrmann M, Jüttler E, Schwark C, et al. MRI-based thrombolysis within and beyond the 3 hour time window is as safe and effective as standard CT-based treatment. *Lancet Neurology.* 2006: submitted for publication.
28. Hacke W, Albers G, Al-Rawi Y, *et al.* The Desmoteplase in Acute Ischemic Stroke Trial (DIAS): a phase II MRI-based 9-hour window acute stroke thrombolysis trial with intravenous desmoteplase. *Stroke.* 2005;**36**(1):66–73.
29. Furlan AJ, Eyding D, Albers GW, *et al.* Dose Escalation of Desmoteplase for Acute Ischemic Stroke (DEDAS): evidence of safety and efficacy 3 to 9 hours after stroke onset. *Stroke.* 2006;**37**(5):1227–31.
30. Hacke W, Furlan AJ, Al-Rawi Y, *et al.* Intravenous desmoteplase in patients with acute ischaemic stroke selected by MRI perfusion-diffusion weighted imaging or perfusion CT (DIAS-2): a prospective, randomised, double-blind, placebo-controlled study. *Lancet Neurol.* 2009;**8**(2):141–50.
31. del Zoppo GJ, Higashida RT, Furlan AJ, *et al.* PROACT: A Phase II randomized trial of recombinant pro-urokinase by direct arterial delivery in acute middle cerebral artery stroke. *Stroke.* 1998;**29**:4–11.
32. Furlan A, Higashida R, Wechsler L, *et al.* Intra-arterial prourokinase for acute ischemic stroke. The PROACT II study: a randomized controlled trial. *Prolyse in Acute Cerebral Thromboembolism. JAMA.* 1999;**282**(21):2003–11.
33. The IMS Study Investigators. Combined intravenous and intra-arterial recanalization for acute ischemic stroke: the Interventional Management of Stroke Study. *Stroke.* 2004;**35**(4):904–11.
34. Gruber A. The Interventional Management of Stroke (IMS) II Study. *Stroke.* 2007;**38**(7):2127–35.
35. American Heart Association. The penumbra pivotal stroke trial: safety and effectiveness of a new generation of mechanical devices for clot removal in intracranial large vessel occlusive disease. *Stroke.* 2009;**40**(8):2761–8.
36. Khatri P, Hill MD, Palesch YY, *et al.* Methodology of the interventional management of stroke III trial. *Int J Stroke.* 2008;**3**(2):130–7.

Decompressive surgery and hypothermia

Rainer Kollmar, Patrick Lyden, and Thomas M. Hemmen

Large ischemic stroke often requires critical care treatment, because of mass effects leading to life-threatening situations. Basically, there are two major options for treatment: giving space for the injured brain and/or reducing mass effects by medical or physical methods to prevent and treat herniation. This chapter gives a detailed overview about decompressive surgery as the surgical option and therapeutic hypothermia as the physical method for neuroprotection and edema treatment.

Decompressive surgery for the treatment of space-occupying ischemic stroke

Large ischemic stroke leads to ischemic brain edema which may cause life-threatening complications such as severe midline shift, brain herniation, increased intracranial pressure (ICP), and occlusion hydrocephalus (1). Decompressive surgery has been investigated for two major types of ischemic stroke over the last 15 years: large infarction in the territory of middle cerebral artery (MCA) and large cerebellar infarction (2,3).

Space-occupying or 'malignant' MCA infarction

Subtotal or complete MCA infarctions are found in up to 10% of patients with supratentorial ischemia (4). The yearly incidence of a malignant acute ischemic stroke ranges between 10 and 20 per 100 000 people (4). The etiology of malignant MCA infarctions is mostly due to thrombosis or embolic occlusion of either the internal carotid artery or the proximal MCA. Depending on anatomical variances, the anterior and/or posterior cerebral artery territories might be involved concomitantly. Anatomical variances and pathological findings that predispose an individual to a malignant MCA infarction include abnormalities of parts of the ipsilateral circle of Willis (mainly a hypoplasia or an atresia) and an insufficient number and caliber of leptomeningeal collateral vessels that are available for collateralization (5).

The clinical picture is characterized by severe hemiparesis, severe sensory deficits, head and eye deviation, hemi-inattention, and, if the dominant hemisphere is involved, global aphasia (2,4). Over the first days, patients with malignant MCA infarctions show a progressive deterioration of consciousness which is mainly caused by ischemic brain edema, which again leads to a reduced ventilatory drive, requiring mechanical ventilation (4). The resulting increased ICP and tissue shifts lead to further destruction of formerly healthy brain tissue, giving rise to the term malignant MCA infarction. These large cerebral infarctions often result in severe shifting of midline structures with subsequent uncal or even transtentorial herniation, and thus have been associated with a poor prognosis in more than 80% of cases (4).

Critical Care of the Stroke Patient, ed. Stefan Schwab, Daniel Hanley, and A. David Mendelow. Published by Cambridge University Press.

While the success of conservative treatment for ischemic brain edema and increased ICP is limited (6), decompressive surgery offers a powerful therapeutic option. There are three compartments in the incompressible skull: brain tissue, cerebrospinal fluid (CSF), and blood. According to the thesis of Monroe and Kellie, the cranium and its constituents create a state of volume equilibrium, such that any increase in volume of one of the cranial constituents must be compensated by a decrease in volume of another. If the compensatory mechanisms are depleted, ICP increases in an exponential manner (1). Removing a part of the cranium by decompressive surgery enables the outward swelling of ischemic brain tissue without compromising healthy brain areas by midline shift and ventricular compression. The normalizing of increased intracranial pressure levels results in raised cerebral blood flow and improved cerebral perfusion pressure, which leads to better oxygenation of brain tissue that is still healthy (7). In rodent studies, especially early decompressive surgery increased the survival rate and decreased the final infarct volume. In patients, decompressive surgery is done by hemicraniectomy in combination with a duraplasty (2). After incision of the skin in the shape of a question mark, a bone flap that has a diameter of at least 12 cm is removed, including parts of the frontal, parietal, temporal, and occipital squama. The removed bone flap must be of a sufficient size to prevent additional ischemic lesions (8). After the opening of the dura, a dural patch is inserted, which usually consists of homologous periosteum or a temporal fascia. Ischemic brain tissue is not resected. From 6 weeks up to 6 months after removal, the stored bone flap, or an artificial replacement, is used for reconstituting cranioplasty (1).

Early case series, observational studies and non-randomized trials of decompressive surgery indicated beneficial effects in patients with malignant MCA stroke. In 2004, a review of 12 clinical studies including 129 patients with large MCA stroke was published (9). In contrast to the high historical mortality rate following conservative medical therapy, decompressive surgery led to only 24%. Seven percent of the patients reached an mRS of 0 or 1, 35% an mRS of 2 or 3, and 58% an mRS between 4 and 6. These studies were followed by so far six controlled-randomized clinical trials:

1. **DESTINY** (Decompressive Surgery for the Treatment of Malignant Infarction) (10).
2. **DESTINY II** (Decompressive Surgery for the Treatment of Malignant Infarction in over 60-year-old patients).
3. **DECIMAL** (Decompressive Craniectomy in Malignant Middle Cerebral Artery Infarcts) (11).
4. **HAMLET** (Hemicraniectomy after Middle Cerebral Artery Infarction with Life-Threatening Oedema) (12).
5. **HeADDFIRST** (Hemicraniectomy and Durotomy upon Deterioration from Infarction Related Swelling Trial).
6. **HeMMI** (Hemicraniectomy for Malignant Middle Cerebral Artery Infarcts).

While official data from the American HeADDFIRST study and the Philippine HeMMI trial are awaited, there are robust data from European studies which show increased survival and indicate less disability after decompressive surgery. Details of the studies are shown in Table 14.1.

After discontinuation of DECIMAL and DESTINY, data were analyzed including the preliminary results of

Table 14.1 Characteristics of European randomized trials for decompressive surgery in large MCA stroke

	DECIMAL	DESTINY	HAMLET
Age	18–55	18–60	18–60
NIHSS dominant	> 15	> 20	> 20
NIHSS non-dominant	> 15	> 18	> 15
Consciousness	LOC ≥ 1	LOC ≥ 1	GCS ≤ 13
Dominant included	Yes	Yes	Yes
CT	½ MCA (< 6 hours) +total MCA (> 6 hours)	2/3 MCA, edema	2/3 MCA, edema
MRI	DWI ≥ 145 ml	–	–
Time window (hours)	0–30	12–36	0–99
Time to operation	6 hours	6 hours	3 hours

LOC: level of consciousness; NIHSS: National Institutes of Health Stroke Scale

Table 14.2 Inclusion and exclusion criteria for pooled analysis. Reproduced (12) with permission

Inclusion criteria

- Age 18–60 years
- Clinical deficits suggestive of infarction in the territory of the MCA with a score on the NIHSS > 15
- Decrease in the level of consciousness to a score of 1 or greater on item 1a on the NIHSS
- Signs on CT of an infarct of at least 50% of the MCA territory, with or without additional infarction in the territory of the anterior or posterior cerebral artery on the same side, or infarct volume of > 145 mm^3 as shown on diffusion-weighted MRU
- Inclusion within 45 hours after onset of symptoms
- Written informed consent by the patient or a legal representative

Exclusion criteria

- Pre-stroke score on the mRS ≥ 2
- Two fixed dilated pupils
- Contralateral ischemia or other brain lesion that could affect outcome
- Space-occupying hemorrhagic transformation of the infarct (≥ parenchymal hemorrhage grade 2)
- Life expectancy < 3 years
- Other serious illness that could affect outcome
- Known coagulopathy or systemic bleeding disorder
- Contraindication for anesthesia
- Pregnancy

HAMLET (13). Inclusion and exclusion criteria for the pooled analysis are shown in Table 14.2. A total of 93 patients were evaluated (DECIMAL, n = 38; DESTINY, n = 32; HAMLET, n = 28) (13). The primary endpoint was the outcome after 1 year dichotomized for mRS ≤ 4 versus mRS ≤ 3. Secondary outcome parameters were mortality after 1 year and outcome dichotomized by mRS ≤ 3 versus mRS 4–6. All of these outcome parameters showed a significant difference.

Mortality: The mortality after decompressive surgery was 29% in contrast to 79% for conservative treatment. Therefore, the absolute risk reduction for the primary endpoint accounted to 51% and transferred into a number needed to treat of two for survival. The NNT for survival with an mRS of ≤ 3 was **functional outcome.** The usual scores were used for description of the functional outcome and degree of disability; Glasgow Outcome Score (GOS), Barthel Index (BI), and modified Rankin Scale (mRS). In addition, functional outcome is divided into favorable and poor outcome. Mostly, favorable outcome is defined by a GOS of 4 and a BI of over 60 or an mRS of 0–3. In the pooled analysis, even an mRS of 0–4 is defined as a favorable outcome. However, these rather simple scales which do not sufficiently consider neuropsychological or cognitive deficits and certainly cannot represent the individual evaluation of quality of life are an important matter for discussion. The pooled analysis showed that 43% of patients with decompressive surgery and only 21% of the conservatively treated patients had a favorable outcome after 1 year as defined by an mRS of ≥ 3. Another result was of great importance for justifying surgery after large ischemic stroke. The number of patients with an mRS of 5 which is defined as a vegetative state did not increase by decompressive surgery. However, the total number of patients with meaningful disability defined by an mRS of 4 increased by factor 10. As the three studies did not include patients aged over 60 years, their data cannot be transferred to older people. However, effects of decompressive surgery in over-60-year-olds are currently being investigated in the DESTINY II study.

Quality of life: Scales such as mRS, GOS, and BI do not measure the patient`s quality of life (QOL). In patients with large ischemic stroke, severe impairment such as cognitive deficits, aphasia or depressive disorders complicate assessment of QOL. However, small case series indicate that QOL is only moderately affected in the majority of patients. When being asked after therapy, the vast majority of patients and relatives would again choose treatment despite the sometimes severe disability. However, the range is between 100% in DESTINY and 41% in a previously published study in 2004 (for an overview, see 1,7).

Prognostic factors and open questions

- Age: As in most acute neurological diseases, age is a major outcome factor in large ischemic stroke. However, the available data of randomized studies do not address this question sufficiently. As other results for older people come from non-randomized

trials and case series, it cannot be stated that decompressive surgery is superior to medical treatment. Since results in younger patients clearly show the superiority of surgery and there is an acceptable explanation for these results, withdrawal of the best treatment (decompressive surgery) leads to the question of whether to treat these patients at all.
- Site of infarction: At first glance, maximal treatment including decompressive surgery in patients with infarction in the speech-dominant hemisphere appears not to be reasonable because of potential severely disabling deficits. However, to date, available data do not support this impression. Randomized studies do not show a significant difference for functional outcome in patients with stroke in the dominant or non-dominant hemisphere. Small studies indicate that patients with infarcts in the dominant hemisphere recover very well. A study in eight patients with large left-sided stroke and initially severe aphasia showed that only a single patient had a persistent global aphasia and was severely disabled with a mean observation study time of 14 months (for overview see 1,7). All other patients had only a mild to moderate aphasia.
- Time to surgery: Animal experiments indicate that early surgery is superior to delayed treatment for survival, functional outcome, and infarct size. While there are publications that favor early treatment, the pooled analysis of DECIMAL, DESTINY, and HAMLET showed no difference in outcome for patients being operated before and after 24 hours (12).

Complications

The rate of complications due to decompressive surgery accounts for up to 25%. In up to 10%, surgery has to be done again (1). Complications include: hemorrhagic transformation or intraparenchymal hemorrhage in the infarcted brain area; additional ipsi- and/or contralateral infarcts; hygroma; meningitis; cerebral abscess; subdural hematoma; wound infections; and epidural, subdural hemorrhages after re-implantation of the bone, etc. A dramatic and life-threatening complication is the sinking skin flap syndrome which is shown in Figure 14.1. While most of the other complications do not contribute to a higher mortality rate, they prolong the in-hospital stay and delay rehabilitation (1).

Imaging and prediction of a malignant course

Cranial CT is widely used for the diagnosis and monitoring of patients with malignant MCA infarction (Fig. 14.2) (1,14). Repeated CT imaging during the first 3 days might be possible to reliably determine the extent of infarction. Generally, a neuroradiological definition of a malignant MCA infarction assumes that at least two-thirds of the MCA territory is affected. Other authors predict a malignant course with development of severe edema if more than 50% of the rostral MCA territory and the basal ganglia show ischemic alterations (1,7,14). Additionally, infarctions of the ipsilateral anterior or posterior cerebral arteries can occur concomitantly with MCA infarctions. The definite infarction volume visualized on MRI is evident as hyperintense lesions on FLAIR (fluid-attenuated inversion recovery) sequences; however, in the hyperacute stages, even diffusion-weighted sequences can be used to reliably predict a malignant MCA infarction if the lesion volume is more than 145 cm^3 (1,7,15).

Decompressive surgery in cerebellar infarction

Patients with infarcts in the posterior cerebral fossa rarely require intensive care management and surgical treatment. However, the swelling of a large space-occupying cerebellar infarct might lead to compression of the brain stem and midbrain or cause a hydrocephalus. Patients with a subtotal or total cerebellar infarct in CT or MR imaging should be monitored in an intensive care unit. A decrease of consciousness indicates compression of the brainstem or hydrocephalus. Because of the potential compression of healthy brain regions and hydrocephalus, these patients should be treated with

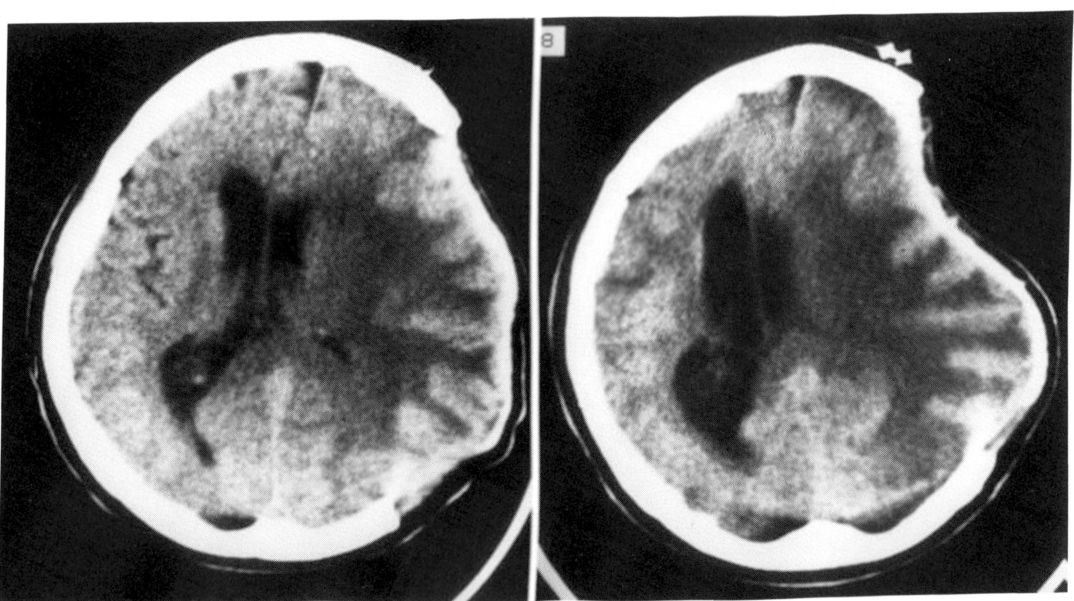

Fig. 14.1 Sinking skin flap syndrome. The left CT shows a moderate midline shift after decompressive surgery. In the right CT, the brain collapses and leads to severe midline shift. (Schwab *et al.*, Nervenarzt (1998);69:896–900).

external ventricular drainage (EVD) and decompressive surgery, providing only extraventricular drainage of the CSF does not reduce local compression of the brainstem or midbrain.

Clinical data on decompressive surgery after cerebellar infarction is limited. The German Austrian Cerebellar Infarct Study observed prospectively 84 patients who were treated with decompressive surgery and EVD (n = 34), only EVD (n = 14), or conservative treatment (n = 36) (3). Patients were followed from 21 days up to 3 months. The treatment groups differed regarding the level of consciousness, signs of mass effect in CT imaging, and signs of brainstem involvement. A major result was that the overall risk for poor outcome depended on the level of consciousness after clinical deterioration. While there was no significant overall treatment effect for awake/drowsy or somnolent/stupor patients, half of the patients deteriorating to coma treated with EVD or decompressive surgery had a good outcome defined by an mRS of ≤ 2. Since none of the deteriorating patients was only medically treated, there was no control group.

Two recent retrospective clinical studies investigated the outcome of patients treated by decompressive surgery after cerebellar infarction (16,17). In one study, 40% (n = 21) had a good outcome as defined by an mRS of ≤ 2 over a mean follow-up period of 4.7 years (16). An additional brainstem infarction was associated with poor outcome.

Because of the small investigated patient number, there are still many open questions. It is not clear whether decompressive surgery and EVD is superior to decompressive surgery or EVD. However, not every medical therapy can be investigated in a randomized manner. Combination of decompressive surgery and EVD is in our opinion the treatment of choice in patients with a deteriorating, decreased state of consciousness because of space-occupying cerebellar infarction. In addition, it is not clear whether additional resection of infarcted cerebellar tissue is superior to only decompression. Moreover, open questions include optimal timing for surgical treatment, therapeutic decision in patients with additional brainstem infarcts, and influence of presurgical state of consciousness.

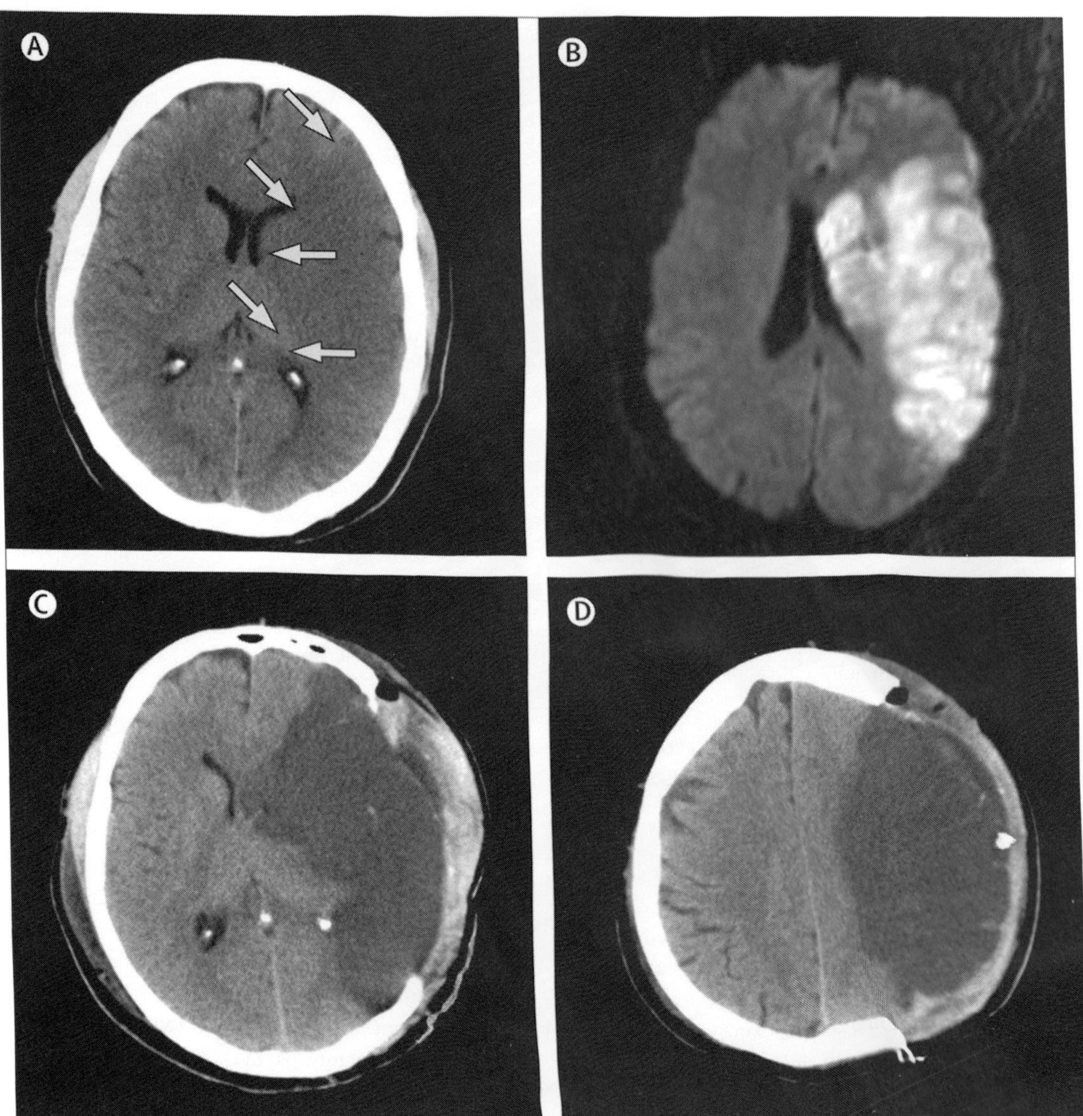

Fig. 14.2 Brain imaging findings before and after hemicraniectomy in malignant MCA infarction. (A) Axial cranial CT 7 h after stroke onset. Arrows indicate the margins of the infarction. (B) Axial diffusion-weighted MRI in the acute phase of malignant MCA infarction. (C) and (D) Axial CT on day 2 after symptom onset after hemicraniectomy. Note that despite decompressive surgery, a compression of the ventricular system with slight midline shifting (C; axial CT at the level of the basal ganglia) and a beginning outward swelling (D; axial CT at the supraventricular level) of the ischemic brain tissue is evident. MCA = middle cerebral artery. From Huttner and Schwab (7) with permission.

Induced hypothermia

Background

Hypothermia (HY) is the most powerful neuroprotective therapy in pre-clinical models and the only proven clinical therapy for patients with global cerebral ischemia. In experimental and early phase human trials, HY was rated as one of the most active modes of neuroprotection (18,19). HY improves neurological outcome in survivors of cardiac arrest (20,21) and in infants with hypoxic-ischemic encephalopathy (22).

The neuroprotective potential of HY after ischemic stroke and traumatic brain injury remains under investigation. Studies in acute ischemic stroke that target the acute phase and aim to reduce neurological injury from ischemia are ongoing and early reports of its feasibility and safety are promising (23). The use of HY showed promise in the reduction of mortality after stroke that causes a space-occupying lesion (24).

In patients with space-occupying ischemic stroke, HY can be neuroprotective and reduce cerebral edema and may therefore be complementary to decompressive surgery. Decompressive surgery does not reduce edema formation, but prevents death and severe neurological impairment by prevention of intracranial herniation. The prevention and therapy of cerebral edema with induced hypothermia has long been used as a potent strategy in the treatment of space-occupying stroke (25).

Mechanism of action

HY induces neuroprotection after ischemia utilizing many modes of action, including induction of ischemic tolerance by affecting the expression of early genes including c-fos and the release of excitatory neurotransmitters, such as glutamate; a reduced cerebral metabolic rate; prevention of cell death by apoptosis and necrosis; reduced inflammatory response and matrix metalloproteinases activity; and stabilization of the blood–brain barrier (26–28). It is not known if HY, through these mechanisms, prevents neuronal death or only delays ischemic injury (6).

Reduction of edema after ischemia is better understood (29–31), making its use in patients who develop irreversible neuronal injury that leads to swelling of the ischemic stroke with space-occupying effect and cerebral herniation reasonable.

Clinical efficacy

Induced HY reduces mortality after malignant middle cerebral artery (MCA) stroke to 44%, compared to 78% in historical controls (4). In early clinical trials, however, the risk of pneumonia was increased in patients treated with HY (24) and rebound edema after HY caused mortality in 30% (25). These safety concerns and other challenges regarding feasibility and safety have limited the clinical efficacy of HY in the treatment of space-occupying stroke. Georgiadis *et al.* have shown that decompressive surgery is superior to HY in the reduction of mortality after larger MCA stroke. Patients treated with HY had 47% mortality compared to 12% in the surgical group (32). The combination of decompressive surgery and HY may be compelling, but concerns of increased bleeding and infection when using hypothermia in the peri-surgical time have to be addressed.

Mode of cooling

In general, two methods of induced cooling are used in the application of HY after stroke, surface or endovascular hypothermia. Surface cooling methods include convective air blankets, water mattresses, alcohol bathing, cooling jackets, and ice packing. These have been used for many years in the treatment of fever. Most studies of HY in patients after massive stroke, cardiac arrest, and the neonatal asphyxia studies used surface cooling. Patients with these conditions are usually comatose, endotracheally intubated, and ventilated (33,34).

The advantages of surface cooling are that it does not require advanced equipment or expertise in catheter placement and avoids the risks associated with central venous catheter placement. External cooling, however, is slower and for temperatures below 35°C the use of sedatives and paralytics to prevent discomfort and shivering in most cases is required. Paralytics render neurological assessments and detection of neuro-worsening during the cooling period virtually impossible (34). Cooling of the skin surface induces vasoconstriction and reduces heat exchange in cooled patients. This reduces temperature control and may lead to target temperature overshoot and lack of control during rewarming (35). The latter was associated with rebound edema and death.

Newer surface-cooling systems, such as energy transferring skin pads (36), may demonstrate a reduction in the time to target temperature and allow better temperature control, but this has not been confirmed in controlled clinical trials (37).

Endovascular cooling using catheters with antithrombotic coatings is feasible and safe (23). The catheter attached to a cooling unit comprise an in-dwelling heat transfer system without requiring cold fluid infusion or extra corporal heat transfer (38).

Endovascular cooling allows rapid heat exchange and faster cooling towards target temperature. Shivering is in part driven through skin receptors; endovascular cooling allows concurrent skin warming, which reduces shivering to make heat exchange more efficient and temperature control tighter. This control avoids target temperature overshoot and incidental rewarming, which can lead to increase in brain edema and intracranial pressure (39).

Temperature control and shivering

The human thermoregulatory system tightly controls core body temperature near 37°C. Protective mechanisms against hypothermia include muscle shivering and cutaneous vasoconstriction. Cutaneous vasoconstriction reduces heat conduction through the skin; shivering produces energy and heat through repetitive muscle contractions (40).

Shivering in the conscious patient creates great discomfort and reduces the effectiveness of cooling. Most patients with large ischemic stroke have a reduced state of consciousness but are not comatose. To assure comfort of patients with space-occupying stroke and to cool effectively, shivering must be reduced with centrally active substances. These alter hypothalamic thermoregulatory centers and avoid cooling to moderate HY without induction of shivering (41). In patients who receive endovascular HY, skin warming, which reduces the trigger of shivering through skin temperature sensors, can be added.

The best studied field of shivering treatment is in the postoperative period. Over 20 clinical trials have shown that meperidine (pethidine), clonidine, and doxapram are the most effective without significant respiratory depression and effective dosages (42). More recent studies have shown that propofol, buspirone, magnesium, tramadol, and dexmedetomidine are effective therapies as well (43). Because of the significant respiratory depression in propafol and dexmedetomidine, these are usually restricted to endotracheally intubated patients.

In addition to substances that alter the hypothalamic temperature control, neuromuscular blocking agents (NMBA) are effective against shivering. Proper sedation is required in conjunction with NMBA and monitoring of the neurological exam is limited during their use. In the clinical trials of hypothermia in patients after cardiac arrest NMBAs were used to prevent and treat shivering (21).

Optimal cooling temperature

Most preclinical models of hypothermia after brain injury and stroke have used temperatures from 24°C to 35°C (29,44). While infarct size and edema were reduced in most models, animals with hypothermia between 28°C and 34°C experienced greater recovery than those with temperatures below 28°C (45). No previously reported study of induced hypothermia after space-occupying stroke has used target temperatures below 33°C.

Onset and duration of cooling

HY is more effective early after ischemia. The diagnosis of a space-occupying stroke, however, may be delayed and the prophylactic use of HY to prevent the development of space-occupying stroke is not established. CT- and MRI-based surrogate markers may aid in the early diagnosis of a space-occupying lesion after stroke (46–48). Hypothermia should be induced as early as possible to achieve maximum neuroprotection and edema blocking effect (49). From preclinical studies we know that HY can abolish ischemia when induced during the onset of ischemia and that HY within 3 hours after ischemia onset significantly reduced infarct size (50,51). Some reports found that delaying hypothermia for more than 3 hours after ischemia showed no significant neuroprotection (52), while Colbourne *et al.* have shown that cooling over 24 hours has neuroprotective effects, even when the treatment was delayed by 6 hours (53).

The optimum duration of cooling after stroke is not known. Yamamoto *et al.* compared cooling for 22 and 3 hours after transient middle cerebral artery occlusion (tMCAo). Animals in the longer treatment group had better neuroprotection (54). In the gerbil two vessel occlusion (2-VO) model, intra-ischemic hypothermia completely prevented cell damage in the hippocampus when continued for 4–6 hours, cooling for 2 hours showed less and 0.5–1 hour showed no protective effect (52). In addition, shorter periods of cooling may lead to only transient neuroprotection. The studies with best long-term outcome treated for 24 hours with hypothermia (55).

Longer periods of cooling in the treatment of brain edema have been used clinically in observational studies. These have targeted the HY by intracranial pressure monitoring and cerebral microdialysis (56).

Conclusion

Induced HY alone or in combination with decompressive surgery in patients with space-occupying stroke holds great promise at reducing cerebral edema and death. If HY can lead to clinically effective neuroprotection and prevention of neuronal cell death after ischemic stroke remains to be seen in future clinical studies.

REFERENCES

1. Uhl E. Decompressive hemicraniectomy for space-occupying cerebral infarction. *Cen Eur Neurosurg.* 2009;**70**(4):195–206.
2. Schwab S, Steiner T, Aschoff A, *et al.* Early hemicraniectomy in patients with complete middle cerebral artery infarction. *Stroke* 1998;**29**:1888–93.
3. Jauss M, Krieger D, Hornig C *et al*: Surgical and medical management of patients with massive cerebellar infarctions: results of the German-Austrian Cerebellar Infarction Study. *J Neurol* 1999;**246**:257–64.
4. Hacke W, Schwab S, Horn M, *et al.* 'Malignant' middle cerebral artery territory infarction: clinical course and prognostic signs. *Arch Neurol* 1996;**53**:309–15.
5. Jaramillo A, Gongora-Rivera F, Labreuche J, Hauw JJ, Amarenco P. Predictors for malignant middle cerebral artery infarctions: a postmortem analysis. *Neurology* 2006;**66**:815–20.
6. Bardutzky J, Schwab S. Antiedema therapy in ischemic stroke. *Stroke* 2007;**38**:3084–94.
7. Huttner HB, Schwab S. Malignant middle cerebral artery infarction: clinical characteristics, treatment strategies, and future perspectives. *Lancet Neurol.* 2009;**8**(10):949–58.
8. Wagner S, Schnippering H, Aschoff A, *et al.* Suboptimum hemicraniectomy as a cause of additional cerebral lesions in patients with malignant infarction of the middle cerebral artery. *J Neurosurg* 2001;**94**:693–6.
9. Gupta R, Connolly ES, Mayer S, Elkind MS. Hemicraniectomy for massive middle cerebral artery territory infarction: a systematic review. *Stroke* 2004;**35**:539–43.
10. Jüttler E, Schwab S, Schmiedek P, *et al.* Decompressive Surgery for the Treatment of Malignant Infarction of the Middle Cerebral Artery (DESTINY): a randomized, controlled trial. *Stroke* 2007;**38**:2518–25.
11. Vahedi K, Vicaut E, Mateo J, *et al.* Sequential-Design, Multicenter, Randomized, Controlled Trial of Early Decompressive Craniectomy in Malignant Middle Cerebral Artery Infarction (DECIMAL trial). *Stroke* 2007;**38**:2506–17.
12. Hofmeijer J, Kappelle LJ, Algra A, *et al.* Surgical decompression for space-occupying cerebral infarction (the Hemicraniectomy After Middle Cerebral Artery Infarction with Life-threatening Edema Trial [HAMLET]): a multicentre, open, randomised trial. *Lancet Neurol* 2009;**8**:326–33.
13. Vahedi K, Hofmeijer J, Juettler E, *et al.* Early decompressive surgery in malignant infarction of the middle cerebral artery: a pooled analysis of three randomised controlled trials. *Lancet Neurol* 2007;**6**:215–22.
14. Sarov M, Guichard JP, Chibarro S, *et al.* Sinking skin flap syndrome and paradoxical herniation after hemicraniectomy for malignant hemispheric infarction. *Stroke.* 2010;**41**(3):560–2.
15. Barber PA, Demchuk AM, Zhang J, *et al.* Computed tomographic parameters predicting fatal outcome in large middle cerebral artery infarction. *Cerebrovasc Dis* 2003;**16**:230–5.
16. Thomalla GJ, Kucinski T, Schoder V, *et al.* Prediction of malignant middle cerebral artery infarction by early

perfusion- and diffusion-weighted magnetic resonance imaging. *Stroke* 2003;**34**:1892–9.

17. Pfefferkorn T, Eppinger U, Linn J, *et al.* Long-term outcome after suboccipital decompressive craniectomy for malignant cerebellar infarction. *Stroke.* 2009;**40**(9):3045–50.
18. Popovic R, Liniger R, *et al.* Anesthetics and mild hypothermia similarly prevent hippocampal neuron death in an in vitro model of cerebral ischemia. *Anesthesiology* 2000;**92**(5):1343–9.
19. O'Collins VE, Macleod MR, *et al.* 1,026 experimental treatments in acute stroke. *Ann Neurol* 2006;**59**(3):467–77.
20. The Hypothermia After Cardiac Arrest Study Group. Mild therapeutic hypothermia to improve the neurologic outcome after cardiac arrest. *N Engl J Med* 2002;**346** (8):549–56.
21. Bernard SA, Gray TW, *et al.* Treatment of comatose survivors of out-of-hospital cardiac arrest with induced hypothermia. *N Engl J Med* 2002;**346**(8):557–63.
22. Shankaran S, Laptook AR, *et al.* Whole-body hypothermia for neonates with hypoxic-ischemic encephalopathy. *N Engl J Med* 2005;**353**(15):1574–84.
23. Hemmen TM, Raman R, *et al.* Intravenous Thrombolysis Plus Hypothermia for Acute Treatment of Ischemic Stroke (ICTuS-L). Final results. *Stroke.* 2010;**41**:2265–70.
24. Schwab S, Schwarz S, *et al.* Moderate hypothermia in the treatment of patients with severe middle cerebral artery infarction. *Stroke* 1998;**29**(12):2461–6.
25. Rosomoff HL. Protective effects of hypothermia against pathological processes of the nervous system. *Ann N Y Acad Sci* 1959;**80**:475–86.
26. Karibe H, Zarow GJ, *et al.* Mild intra-ischemic hypothermia reduces postischemic hyperperfusion, delayed postischemic hypoperfusion, blood-brain barrier disruption, brain edema, and neuronal damage volume after temporary focal cerebral ischemia in rats. *J Cereb Blood Flow Metab* 1994;**14**(4):620–7.
27. Xu L, Yenari MA, *et al.* Mild hypothermia reduces apoptosis of mouse neurons in vitro early in the cascade. *J Cereb Blood Flow Metab* 2002;**22**(1):21–8.
28. Thornhill J, Corbett D. Therapeutic implications of hypothermic and hyperthermic temperature conditions in stroke patients. *Can J Physiol Pharmacol* 2001;**79**(3):254–61.
29. Kawai N, Kawanishi M, *et al.* Effects of hypothermia on thrombin-induced brain edema formation. *Brain Res* 2001;**895**(1–2):50–8.
30. Guluma KZ, Oh H, *et al.* Effect of endovascular hypothermia on acute ischemic edema: morphometric analysis of the ICTuS trial. *Neurocrit Care* 2008;**8**(1):42–7.
31. Kawanishi M, Kawai N, *et al.* Effect of delayed mild brain hypothermia on edema formation after intracerebral hemorrhage in rats. *J Stroke Cerebrovasc Dis* 2008;**17**(4):187–95.
32. Georgiadis D, Schwarz S, *et al.* Hemicraniectomy and moderate hypothermia in patients with severe ischemic stroke. *Stroke* 2002;**33**(6):1584–8.
33. Schwab S, Georgiadis D, *et al.* Feasibility and safety of moderate hypothermia after massive hemispheric infarction. *Stroke* 2001;**32**(9):2033–5.
34. Krieger DW, De Georgia MA, *et al.* Cooling for acute ischemic brain damage (cool aid): an open pilot study of induced hypothermia in acute ischemic stroke. *Stroke* 2001;**32**(8):1847–54.
35. Gillies MA, Pratt R, *et al.* Therapeutic hypothermia after cardiac arrest: A retrospective comparison of surface and endovascular cooling techniques. *Resuscitation* **81** (9):1117–22.
36. Mayer SA, Kowalski RG, *et al.* Clinical trial of a novel surface cooling system for fever control in neurocritical care patients. *Crit Care Med* 2004;**32**(12):2508–15.
37. Zweifler RM, Mahmood MA, Alday DD. Induction and maintenance of mild hypothermia by surface cooling in nonintubated subjects. *J Stroke Cerebrovasc Dis* 2003;**12**:237–43.
38. Mack WJ, Huang J, *et al.* Ultra-rapid, convection-enhanced intravascular hypothermia: a feasibility study in nonhuman primate stroke. *Stroke* 2003;**34**(8):1994–9.
39. Flint AC, Hemphill JC, *et al.* Therapeutic hypothermia after cardiac arrest: performance characteristics and safety of surface cooling with or without endovascular cooling. *Neurocrit Care* 2007;**7**(2):109–18.
40. Jessen, K. An assessment of human regulatory nonshivering thermogenesis. *Acta Anaesthesiol Scand* 1980;**24**(2):138–43.
41. Doufas AG, Lin CM, *et al.* Dexmedetomidine and meperidine additively reduce the shivering threshold in humans. *Stroke* 2003;**34**(5):1218–23.
42 Kranke P, Eberhart LH, *et al.* Pharmacological treatment of postoperative shivering: a quantitative systematic review of randomized controlled trials. *Anesth Analg* 2002;**94** (2):453–60.
43. Weant KA, Martin JE, *et al.* Pharmacologic options for reducing the shivering response to therapeutic hypothermia. *Pharmacotherapy* 2012;**30**(8):830–41.
44. Krieger DW, Yenari MA. Therapeutic hypothermia for acute ischemic stroke: what do laboratory studies teach us? *Stroke* 2004;**35**(6):1482–9.
45. Maier CM, Ahern K, *et al.* Optimal depth and duration of mild hypothermia in a focal model of transient cerebral

ischemia: effects on neurologic outcome, infarct size, apoptosis, and inflammation. *Stroke* 1998;**29**(10):2171–80.

46. Krieger DW, Demchuk AM, *et al.* Early clinical and radiological predictors of fatal brain swelling in ischemic stroke. *Stroke* 1999;**30**(2):287–92.
47. Barber PA, Demchuk AM, *et al.* Computed tomographic parameters predicting fatal outcome in large middle cerebral artery infarction. *Cerebrovasc Dis* 2003;**16**(3):230–5.
48. Jaramillo A, Gongora-Rivera F, *et al.* Predictors for malignant middle cerebral artery infarctions: a postmortem analysis. *Neurology* 2006;**66**(6):815–20.
49. Delgado P, Sahuquillo J, *et al.* Neuroprotection in malignant MCA infarction. *Cerebrovasc Dis* 2006;**21** Suppl 2:99–105.
50. Chen H, Chopp M, *et al.* Effect of mild hyperthermia on the ischemic infarct volume after middle cerebral artery occlusion in the rat. *Neurology* 1991;**41**(7):1133–5.
51. Zhang RL, Chopp M, *et al.* Postischemic (1 hour) hypothermia significantly reduces ischemic cell damage in rats subjected to 2 hours of middle cerebral artery occlusion. *Stroke* 1993;**24**(8):1235–40.
52. Dietrich WD, Busto R, *et al.* Intra-ischemic but not post-ischemic brain hypothermia protects chronically following global forebrain ischemia in rats. *J Cereb Blood Flow Metab* 1993;**13**(4):541–9.
53. Colbourne F, Corbett D. Delayed postischemic hypothermia: a six month survival study using behavioral and histological assessments of neuroprotection. *J Neurosci* 1995;**15**(11):7250–60.
54. Yamamoto H, Nagata I, *et al.* Combination of intra-ischemic and postischemic hypothermia provides potent and persistent neuroprotection against temporary focal ischemia in rats. *Stroke* 1999;**30**(12):2720–6; discussion 2726.
55. Colbourne F, Li H, *et al.* Indefatigable CA1 sector neuroprotection with mild hypothermia induced 6 hours after severe forebrain ischemia in rats. *J Cereb Blood Flow Metab* 1999;**19**(7):742–9.
56. Polderman KH. Induced hypothermia and fever control for prevention and treatment of neurological injuries. *Lancet* 2008;**371**(9628):1955–69.

15

Space-occupying hemispheric infarction: clinical course, prediction, and prognosis

H. Bart van der Worp and Stefan Schwab

Acknowledgment

H. Bart van der Worp is supported by a grant from the Dutch Heart Foundation (2010T075).

In the first days to weeks after symptom onset, large infarcts in the flow territory of the middle cerebral artery (MCA) are commonly associated with brain edema. In severe cases, this may lead to herniation. Life-threatening, space-occupying MCA infarcts are often referred to as 'malignant' (1,2). There is no generally accepted definition of space-occupying or malignant MCA infarction, but for therapeutic and prognostic purposes, the joint inclusion criteria used in recent randomized trials have proven helpful (Table 15.1) (3). Case fatality was 71% in patients aged between 18 and 60 years who fulfilled these criteria in the first 48 hours of stroke onset, and were treated conservatively (4).

The exact proportion of patients with ischemic stroke who develop malignant MCA infarction is unknown. Most authors cite a frequency of between 1% and 10% of all ischemic strokes (2–4), but the referred studies were performed in selected patient populations, and the actual frequency is likely to be at the lower end of this range. Younger patients with MCA infarction appear to have a higher risk of herniation than elderly patients.

Clinical features and prognosis

Malignant hemispheric infarction is most often caused by acute occlusion of the internal carotid artery or the proximal MCA (2). Concomitant infarction in the territories of the anterior or posterior cerebral artery increases the risk of life-threatening edema formation. Involvement of the anterior choroidal artery and an incomplete ipsilateral part of the circle of Willis have also been associated with a higher risk of herniation (5).

Patients who ultimately develop life-threatening edema usually present with the syndrome of large cortical MCA infarction, including aphasia or neglect, partial or complete conjugate eye deviation, hemianopia, and a severe hemiparesis. Most often, there is a gradual decrease in consciousness over the first 1–3 days, together with the development of pupillary asymmetry. Usually, the ipsilateral pupil first becomes dilated and fixed due to compression of the third nerve, followed by involvement of the contralateral pupil. In an observational intensive-care-based study of 55 patients with complete MCA infarction, pupils became dilated and fixed between 24 hours and 7 days after stroke onset (1). Brain tissue shifts rather than a globally increased intracranial pressure are the most important cause of the initial neurological deterioration (6), but intracranial pressure values higher than 30 mmHg have been found in all patients with pupillary asymmetry (1). In the abovementioned observational study, 49 of the 55 patients (89%) required mechanical ventilation during the first days, and 43 (78%) died, despite anti-edema therapy. All deaths occurred within 7 days after stroke onset, and most on days 2 to 4 (1). Other observational studies have reported case fatality rates of 55% to79% on con-

Critical Care of the Stroke Patient, ed. Stefan Schwab, Daniel Hanley, and A. David Mendelow. Published by Cambridge University Press.

Table 15.1 Early symptoms and signs suggestive of malignant middle cerebral artery (MCA) infarction

- Clinical deficits suggestive of infarction in the territory of the MCA with a score on the National Institutes of Health stroke scale (NIHSS) > 15;
- Decrease in the level of consciousness to a score of 1 or greater on item 1a of the NIHSS;
- Signs on CT of an infarct of at least 50% of the MCA territory, with or without additional infarction in the territory of the anterior or posterior cerebral artery on the same side, or
- Infarct volume > 145 cm^3 as shown on diffusion-weighted MRI.

Adapted from (3).

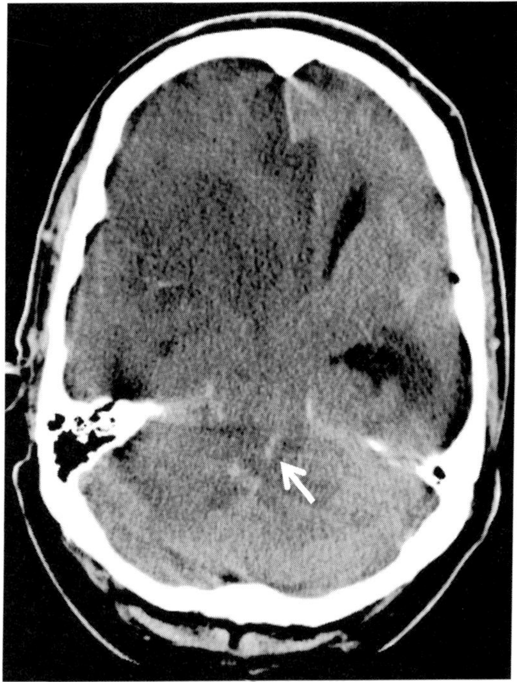

Fig. 15.1 Duret hemorrhages in a patient with space-occupying infarction of the right anterior and middle cerebral artery.

servative treatment (7,8). In the conservatively treated patients included in randomized trials of decompressive surgery within 48 hours of symptom onset, case fatality at 1 year was 71%, with the large majority of deaths occurring in the first week after stroke onset (4). With or without surgery, just a minority of the survivors become independent in their activities of daily life (3,4,9), and most have long-term global cognitive impairment (10).

Herniation

The most common cause of death in patients with space-occupying infarction is cerebral herniation. Cingulate herniation occurs when brain tissue shifts across the midline, forcing the cingulate gyrus under the falx cerebri, thereby compressing and displacing the internal cerebral vein and the anterior cerebral artery (ACA). This commonly precedes downward shift and transtentorial herniation, which may cause compression of the great cerebral vein. Uncal herniation occurs when the swollen tissue in the temporal lobe shifts the inner, basal edge of the uncus and hippocampal gyrus toward the midline so that these bulge over the incisural edge of the tentorium. The resultant crowding at the notch flattens the adjacent midbrain, pushing it against the opposite incisural edge. The ipsilateral third nerve and posterior cerebral artery are often caught between the overhanging swollen uncus and the free edge of the tentorium (11).

Compression of the ACA may lead to additional infarction in its flow territory, most commonly in the ipsilateral paracentral lobule or superior frontal gyrus (12,13). Involvement of the PCA may result in ipsilateral, contralateral, or bilateral occipital lobe infarction (14). Compression of the large cerebral veins reduces venous outflow and increases hydrostatic pressure in the territories they drain. Both uncal and transtentorial herniation can compress the aquaduct and lead to an obstructive hydrocephalus, which further increases intracranial pressure. Transtentorial herniation displaces the midbrain and pons downward, stretching the perforating branches of the basilar artery and thereby causing brainstem ischemia. This is commonly associated with small hemorrhages in the midbrain and pons, the so-called Duret hemorrhages (Fig. 15.1) (11).

Predicting fatal edema formation

In patients with space-occupying infarction, decompressive surgery is only of proven benefit if initiated within 48 hours of stroke onset (see Chapter 8). For this reason, patients at risk of developing fatal edema should be identified as early as possible. Several early predictors of space-occupying edema formation have been described, ranging from the presence of vomiting to a variety of infarct sizes. In a systematic review that included articles published up to 2007, the major determinants for developing fatal edema after MCA infarction were infarct size larger than 50% and a perfusion deficit larger than 66% of the MCA territory. Other associated determinants were early mass effect, involvement of other vascular territories, higher body temperature, internal carotid artery occlusion, and need for mechanical ventilation. However, positive and negative predictive values were too low to be useful in the clinic (15).

Paradoxically, MCA occlusion was associated with a lower risk of life-threatening edema. This is probably a result of selection bias within the studies included in the meta-analysis, because the group of patients with an MCA occlusion consisted mainly of patients with distal MCA occlusions, whereas occlusions of the MCA trunk have been associated with poor outcome. The presence of a hyperdense MCA sign is usually indicative of MCA trunk occlusion, and in the meta-analysis a hyperdense MCA sign on CT appeared associated with an increased risk. Unfortunately, the meta-analysis was limited by the large variety of inclusion criteria and methods of analysis among the included studies (15).

At the time of the systematic review, early lesion volume on diffusion-weighted imaging could not be subjected to meta-analysis, because this had not been tested in a sufficient number of studies. In two retrospective studies, lesion volume of more than 145 ml on diffusion-weighted imaging (DWI) within 14 hours after the onset of symptoms (16) and more than 82 ml on apparent diffusion coefficient maps in the first 6 hours (17) predicted the development of life-threatening brain edema with positive predictive values of 91% and 82%, and negative predictive values of 100% and 92%, respectively. The value of DWI lesion volume for the prediction of space-occupying infarction was recently confirmed in a prospective, multi-center, observational cohort study of patients with acute ischemic stroke and MCA main stem occlusion, in which a DWI lesion volume greater than 82 ml in the first 6 hours of stroke had a positive predictive value of 88% and a negative predictive value of 90%. However, sensitivity was low (52%), indicating that a substantial proportion of the patients who ultimately developed space-occupying edema would have been missed if treatment decisions would be based on DWI lesion volume alone (18). In this study, the definition of malignant MCA infarction was based on the inclusion criteria of the aforementioned randomized trials of surgical decompression. Because measurement of infarct volume with DWI is simple and reliable, this appears to be the method of choice for predicting edema formation both in the clinic and in clinical trials.

Medical treatment of space-occupying infarction

Several conservative treatment strategies have been proposed to limit brain tissue shifts and reduce intracranial pressure, such as sedation with barbiturates or propofol, hyperventilation, and osmotic therapy with glycerol, mannitol, or hypertonic saline hydroxyethyl starch (HES). However, no trials have addressed the efficacy of these therapies to improve clinical outcome, and several reports suggest that these are ineffective or even detrimental (19). Still, the use of osmotherapy with glycerol or mannitol may be considered as a bridging therapy prior to decompressive surgery (20). The value of ICP monitoring has also not been established. ICP monitoring may reduce iatrogenic errors, but is probably not helpful in guiding long-term treatment (21).

Two non-randomized studies in patients with severe space-occupying edema after MCA infarction suggested that moderate hypothermia (32–34°C) on an ICU could help to control critically elevated ICP values and improve clinical outcome. Hypothermia was associated with several side effects, of which thrombocytopenia, bradycardia, and pneumonia were most frequently encountered. Most deaths occurred during rewarming as a result of excessive ICP rise and herniation (22,23). A shorter rewarming period was associated with a more pronounced rise of ICP (23). Rebound ICP rise may be prevented by slow and controlled, instead of passive, rewarming (24). Randomized trials of cooling for space-occupying edema formation have not been performed (19). The only therapy of proven benefit is decompressive surgery, as discussed in Chapter 14.

REFERENCES

(1) Hacke W, Schwab S, Horn M, *et al.* 'Malignant' middle cerebral artery infarction. Clinical course and prognostic signs. *Arch Neurol* 1996;**53**:309–15.

(2) Huttner HB, Schwab S. Malignant middle cerebral artery infarction: clinical characteristics, treatment strategies, and future perspectives. *Lancet Neurol* 2009;**8**:949–58.

(3) Vahedi K, Hofmeijer J, Juettler E, *et al.* Early decompressive surgery in malignant infarction of the middle cerebral artery: a pooled analysis of three randomised controlled trials. *Lancet Neurol* 2007;**6**:215–22.

(4) Hofmeijer J, Kappelle LJ, Algra A, *et al.* Surgical decompression for space-occupying cerebral infarction (the Hemicraniectomy After Middle Cerebral Artery Infarction with Life-threatening Edema Trial [HAMLET]): a multicentre, open, randomised trial. *Lancet Neurol* 2009;**8**:326–33.

(5) Jaramillo A, Gongora-Rivera F, Labreuche J, Hauw JJ, Amarenco P. Predictors for malignant middle cerebral artery infarctions: a postmortem analysis. *Neurology* 2006;**66**:815–20.

(6) Frank JI. Large hemispheric infarction, deterioration, and intracranial pressure. *Neurology* 1995;**45**:1286–90.

(7) Wijdicks EFM, Diringer MN. Middle cerebral artery territory infarction and early brain swelling: progression and effect of age on outcome. *Mayo Clin Proc* 1998;**73**:829–36.

(8) Berrouschot J, Sterker M, Bettin S, Köster J, Schneider D. Mortality of space-occupying ('malignant') middle cerebral artery infarction under conservative intensive care. *Intensive Care Med* 1998;**24**:620–3.

(9) Zhao J, Su YY, Zhang Y, *et al.* Decompressive hemicraniectomy in malignant middle cerebral artery infarct: a randomized controlled trial enrolling patients up to 80 years old. *Neurocrit Care* 2012;**17**:161–71.

(10) Hofmeijer J, Van der Worp HB, Kappelle LJ, *et al.* Cognitive outcome of survivors of space-occupying hemispheric infarction. *J Neurol* 2013;**260**:1396–403.

(11) Plum F, Posner JB. *The diagnosis of stupor and coma.* 3 ed. Philadelphia: F.A. Davis Company; 1982.

(12) Sohn D, Levine S. Frontal lobe infarcts caused by brain herniation. Compression of anterior cerebral artery branches. *Arch Pathol* 1967;**84**:509–12.

(13) Rothfus WE, Goldberg AL, Tabas JH, Deeb ZL. Callosomarginal infarction secondary to transfalcial herniation. *AJNR Am J Neuroradiol* 1987;**8**:1073–6.

(14) Sato M, Tanaka S, Kohama A, Fujii C. Occipital lobe infarction caused by tentorial herniation. *Neurosurgery* 1986;**18**:300–5.

(15) Hofmeijer J, Algra A, Kappelle LJ, Van der Worp HB. Predictors of life-threatening brain edema in middle cerebral artery infarction. *Cerebrovasc Dis* 2008;**25**:176–84.

(16) Oppenheim C, Samson Y, Manai R, *et al.* Prediction of malignant middle cerebral artery infarction by diffusion-weighted imaging. *Stroke* 2000;**31**:2175–81.

(17) Thomalla GJ, Kucinski T, Schoder V, *et al.* Prediction of malignant middle cerebral artery infarction by early perfusion- and diffusion-weighted magnetic resonance imaging. *Stroke* 2003;**34**:1892–9.

(18) Thomalla G, Hartmann F, Juettler E, *et al.* Prediction of malignant middle cerebral artery infarction by magnetic resonance imaging within 6 hours of symptom onset: A prospective multicenter observational study. *Ann Neurol* 2010;**68**:435–45.

(19) Hofmeijer J, Van der Worp HB, Kappelle LJ. Treatment of space-occupying hemispheric infarction. *Crit Care Med* 2003;**31**:617–25.

(20) Guidelines for management of ischaemic stroke and transient ischaemic attack 2008. *Cerebrovasc Dis* 2008;**25**:457–507.

(21) Schwab S, Aschoff A, Spranger M, Albert F, Hacke W. The value of intracranial pressure monitoring in acute hemispheric stroke. *Neurology* 1996;**47**:393–8.

(22) Schwab S, Schwarz S, Spranger M, *et al.* Moderate hypothermia in the treatment of patients with severe middle cerebral artery infarction. *Stroke* 1998;**29**:2461–6.

(23) Schwab S, Georgiadis D, Berrouschot J, *et al.* Feasibility and safety of moderate hypothermia after massive hemispheric infarction. *Stroke* 2001;**32**:2033–5.

(24) Steiner T, Friede T, Aschoff A, *et al.* Effect and feasibility of controlled rewarming after moderate hypothermia in stroke patients with malignant infarction of the middle cerebral artery. *Stroke* 2001;**32**:2833–5.

16

Critical care of basilar artery occlusion

Perttu J. Lindsberg, Tiina Sairanen, and Heinrich P. Mattle

Characterization of the syndrome

Historical note

In 1946 Kubik and Adams published a landmark paper on 18 patients who died from basilar artery occlusions (BAO) and four patients who survived [1]. This was the first detailed report delineating clinical and pathologic features of embolic and thrombotic BAO. Another landmark study by Lou Caplan appeared in 1980. He described the 'top of the basilar syndrome', usually resulting from a distal embolic occlusion of the basilar artery (BA) and characterized by a variable combination of a midbrain stroke with thalamic, temporomedial or temporobasal and occipital lobar strokes [2].

Vascular anatomy dictates neurological deficits

Roughly one fifth of cerebral infarctions occur in the posterior circulation territory, and a small portion of these are BAOs. The BA is located on the ventral aspect of the brainstem and feeds blood to the pons, cerebellum, mesencephalon, thalamus and, with a variable degree, to the territory of the posterior cerebral artery. The location and length of the vascular occlusion dominates the clinical picture resulting from BAO. BA and its branches subserve three main territories: the anteromedial, anterolateral, and dorsolateral territories [3]. Anterolateral lesions commonly produce somewhat mild motor deficits, whereas in anteromedial lesions pyramidal tract interruption and tetraplegia is the rule. Cranial nerve palsies and ophthalmoplegia result usually from dorsolateral lesions. However, a complete occlusion of the BA characteristically results in massive neurological deficits with tetraplegia, ophtalmoplegia, and reduced consciousness [4].

Etiology

The most common etiological mechanism is atherothrombosis, including local thrombosis and artery-to-artery embolism, originating usually from atherosclerotic vertebrobasilar arteries. This etiology has been reported in some large series in 35% to 44% of BAO cases [5,6]. Vertebral artery lesions are found roughly in half of BAO patients, most often in the intracranial segments [7]. Other common causes are cardioembolism (32% to 36%) and vertebral artery dissection (5% to 14%). Occasionally the syndrome is caused by dolichoectasy of the vertebral or basilar arteries. Distal BAO tends to be more frequently of embolic origin, whereas midbasilar and proximal occlusions tend to result from local thrombosis building on atherosclerotic lesions of the vertebrobasilar arteries [8].

Clinical phenotypes

The mode of symptom onset can be quite variable. The most common clinical presentation is a stepwise progressive course of neurological symptoms such as vertigo, gaze palsy, double vision, dysarthria,

Critical Care of the Stroke Patient, ed. Stefan Schwab, Daniel Hanley, and A. David Mendelow. Published by Cambridge University Press.

paresthesia, and hemiparesis. Up to 60% of the patients experience prodromal symptoms, which are mostly rather non-specific such as nausea, headache, tinnitus, hearing loss, and vertigo [7,9]. These transient symptoms can precede the onset of the monophasic, progressive deficits by days, but typically by several weeks [7]. In these patients the etiology is usually atherothrombosis of the vertebral arteries. Another phenotype of BAO presents with rapid onset of severe, often bilateral motor weakness, variable forms of ophthalmoplegia and gaze palsy and reduced consciousness or coma. Occasionally the muscle tone is elevated and even seizure-like jerking and forceful incomprehensible vocalizations can occur, making the differential diagnosis with epileptic convulsions sometimes a subject of consideration. In cases of very severe symptoms with tetraplegia, ophthalmoplegia, and coma, a gloomy clinical picture is on the horizon. If the condition cannot be reversed quickly, death or devastating outcomes such as locked-in syndrome will result. The locked-in syndrome is characterized by retained consciousness and cognition but loss of active motor functions except for vertical gaze movements. A person becomes a prisoner in his or her own body.

To illustrate the breadth of salient features and their neuroanatomical correlation in BAO in settings of critical care, the characteristic symptoms and the involved brain structures are summarized in Table 16.1.

Table 16.1 Cardinal symptoms of BAO and the respective brain structures

Symptom	Brain structure
Reduced consciousness or coma	Ascending reticular activating system
Disturbance of respiration and autonomic nervous system	Nuclei of the medulla oblongata
Dysarthria and bulbar symptoms	Cerebellum and cranial nerve nuclei of the medulla oblongata and lower brainstem
Ophthalmoplegia, double vision, nystagmus	Cerebellum and the oculomotor nuclei of the brainstem
Ptosis, non-reactive dilated pupillae, disorientation	Mesencephalon, thalamus
Dysequilibrium, falling	Cerebellum and the brainstem cranial nerve nuclei regulating balance
Blindness	Occipital lobes
Ataxia, loss of coordination of limbs and posture	Cerebellum and linked proprioceptive and motor tracts
Bilateral motor and sensory paresis	Pontine pyramidal tract, medial lemniscus and spinothalamic tract
Extension rigidity and jerking	Pontine pyramidal tract

Diagnostics and imaging procedures

Differential diagnosis

The clinical diagnosis of BAO can often be tricky if one compares to the common presentations of hemispheric stroke. Especially when presented with rapid onset of tetraplegia and coma, many other disorders affecting cerebral function are relevant in the differential diagnosis on admission. In many instances the patient is found unconscious with non-witnessed symptom onset. Often a number of ancillary investigations are necessary to rule out other disorders. The non-contrast head CT is typically unremarkable at the early stage. Occasionally a dense BA sign is present and directs to the correct diagnosis. The most common differential diagnostic conditions are summarized in Table 16.2.

Diagnostic imaging procedures

The quickest way to the correct diagnosis is CT angiography (CTA), MR angiography (MRA) or digital subtraction angiography (DSA) once the suspicion of BAO has been raised. Occasionally the clot that caused the clinical syndrome has already dislodged or dissolved. This is often the case in the 'top of the basilar' syndrome (Fig. 16.1), and then the actual exact vascular

Table 16.2 Common differential diagnostic disorders and relevant ancillary investigations

Disorder	Ancillary investigation
Subarachnoidal hemorrhage	Head CT, CT or MR angiography
Non-convulsive status epilepticus or postictal state	Clinical picture, history, EEG
Hypoglycemic or other metabolic coma, intoxication	Clinical picture, history, blood chemistry, EEG
Hypoxic-ischemic encephalopathy	Clinical picture, history, ECG, EEG
CNS infection (meningitis, encephalitis)	Clinical picture, cerebrospinal fluid
Bilateral hemispheric stroke	Head CT or MRI, carotid ultrasound, cardio-ECHO
Cardiogenic or hemorrhagic circulatory shock	Hemodynamics, ECG, chest x-ray, cardio-ECHO
Guillain–Barré syndrome or cranial neuritis, Miller–Fisher syndrome, botulism, myasthenic crisis	Clinical picture (reflexes), cerebrospinal fluid, ENMG

diagnosis may be obscured. Patients are often restless and uncooperative, and imaging results are likely to be compromised by movement artifacts, so short-acting sedative agents are advisable. Occasionally it is necessary to intubate and ventilate the patients and use anesthesia for diagnostic and subsequent therapeutic procedures.

Prognostic imaging studies

Using quite variable algorithms to score the signs of early ischemic lesions, correlation of imaging findings have been reported both for diffusion-weighted (DWI) MR and CT and BAO outcome after varying treatments [10]. Puetz *et al.* modified the Acute Stroke Prognosis Early CT score (ASPECTS) for posterior circulation from CTA source images (CTASI) and described a score range for the extent of hypoattenuation that sorts out patients likely to have a poor outcome and in whom the dismal disease course would probably not be reversed even in the case of recanalization [11]. This scoring was also predictive for the final infarct size [12]. Ostrem *et al.* demonstrated that mismatch in diffusion and perfusion MRI can identify a potentially salvageable brain area at risk, also in the posterior circulation and brainstem, and that thrombolytic therapy could diminish this mismatch area and presumably rescue some tissue at risk [13]. Later studies have confirmed the association of DWI lesions with outcome and refined prognostic algorithms for imaging of BAO, which take into account strategic brain regions important for survival such as the brainstem, rather than lesion volume alone [14,15].

Recent data are interpreted so that the clinician should respect the extent of the ischemic changes on the admission scan when making the treatment decision, and not rigidly the clock [16,17]. When a clot lodges suddenly in the BA, there is a drop in the downstream perfusion pressure of the artery, which can lead to reversed flow from the posterior communicating arteries. While preventing the clot from advancing more distally, this reflux may also augment residual blood flow in the branches located distally to the clot. Indeed, a case series (n = 20) has supported that strong collateral flow to the BA may increase the duration of BAO tolerated by the brain tissue at risk, and may even promote favorable outcome [18]. Of patients with collateral filling of the distal BA, five (83%) had a good neurologic outcome and one did not. Of those without collateral flow, one (17%) had a good neurologic outcome and five did not.

Imaging studies such as those described above may assist in determining whether an individual patient might benefit from recanalization therapies in BAO [16,17]. This is important since the time window for recanalization therapies such as thrombolysis is not well established [16]. Repeated investigations may help in deciding whether to continue intensive care or to discontinue it.

Recanalization therapies

Conventional therapy

Available evidence on the efficacy of different treatment protocols is predominantly based on retrospective or prospective patient cohorts and case series from centers

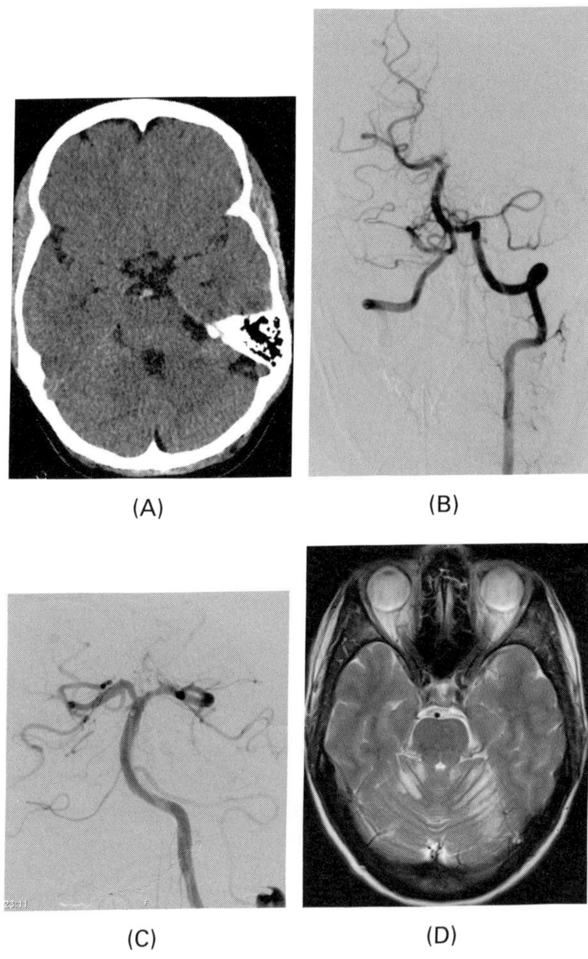

Fig. 16.1 'Top of the basilar syndrome'. This 31-year-old woman experienced sudden severe headache, tinnitus, nausea, double vision, and soon became drowsy. When she arrived at the emergency room 2.5 hours later there was bilateral ptosis, vertical gaze palsy, bilateral internal rectus paresis, and her left pupil was dilated and barely reactive to light. The CT scan showed a dense basilar artery at its top (A). It was decided to start i.v. thrombolysis with rt-PA followed by endovascular treatment. Arteriography showed thrombotic material at the top of the basilar artery occluding both superior cerebellar arteries, the thalamic arteries and the left posterior cerebral artery (B). With mechanical fragmentation of the thrombus and urokinase, recanalization of the thalamic arteries and the left posterior cerebral artery was achieved, but not the superior cerebellar arteries (C). As a result MRI after 1 day showed infarcts in both superior cerebellar artery territories (D). Three months later the neurological examination was normal. (Images courtesy of G. Schroth, Institute of Diagnostic and Interventional Neuroradiology, University Hospital, Bern).

using a variety of recanalization therapy protocols, which have evolved rapidly over time. Most case series report single center experiences of using intra-arterial thrombolysis rather than intravenous thrombolysis or conventional therapy with antithrombotics. Even antithrombotic therapy, which probably has been used most commonly for treating BAO patients in the past, has been reported scarcely as consecutive case series. In the conventional therapy (antiplatelet agents and/or anticoagulation) mortality has ranged from 23% to

86% [16,19,20]. The likelihood of favorable outcome defined as modified Rankin Scale (mRS) score 0 to 3 has been 13% to 21%. Of note, BAO was confirmed radiologically only in 30% of the 82 patients in the study by Schonewille *et al.* [19]. Similar lack of angiographic proof of BAO is evident for other studies with conservative treatment as well [16]. A more benign outcome without recanalization therapies has been reported mainly in cases with short segment occlusion of atherothrombotic origin and good collaterals. Without recanalization, the likelihood of good outcome (mRS 0 to 2) is roughly 2% across a wide range of case series studies even when thrombolytic therapy has been used either i.v. (IVT) or i.a. (IAT) [21].

Thrombolytic therapy

Zeumer and colleagues were the first to report a successful fibrinolytic therapy of a BAO in a young woman [22]. However, still today therapy decisions in BAO are hampered by the lack of randomized controlled trials (RCT) using anticoagulants or antiplatelet agents in a face-to-face comparison with thrombolysis. There is only one small RCT that compared intra-arterial urokinase against anticoagulation in 16 patients, which suggested that intra-arterial urokinase was associated with a better outcome [23]. However, the study was discontinued prematurely for logistical reasons and is much too small to support general guidelines for management.

The lack of RCTs in the therapy of BAO is a continuing subject of controversy also for selecting the therapeutic approach (IVT or IAT) in experienced stroke centers using thrombolysis routinely for treating ischemic stroke both in anterior and posterior circulation [4,24–26]. On the practical side, there are advantages and disadvantages in both IVT and IAT. IVT can in most hospitals be initiated faster, it is less straining for the patient and theoretically the thrombolytic agent will reach the clot from both distal and proximal aspects. IVT is accessible much more widely, not only in highly specialized academic stroke centers. IAT, on the other hand, offers a possibility to reach higher local concentration of fibrinolytics, to disintegrate and otherwise maneuver the clot, and also enables monitoring of vessel patency during the procedure. Furthermore mechanical devices have been developed that enhance the recanalization rates and shorten the time to recanalization compared to pharmacological thrombolysis. However, it requires a skilled interventive neuroradiologist (or other intervention specialist) and rapid access to an angiography suite equipped with a dedicated team including an anesthesiologist. Emerging clinical experience supports the prioritization of adequate analgosedation without anesthesia to avoid time delay and hypotension, but the choice of anesthesia or sedation has to be taken individually by the interventional team.

Preparations for thrombolysis include placement of urinary catheter, monitoring of cardiac rhythm and blood pressure. BAO patients may develop hypotension and cardiorespiratory failure very rapidly, so an anesthesiologist should be at hand with short notice especially during prolonged imaging studies.

Case series using IAT and IVT

Representative consecutive patient series of BAO treated with either IVT or IAT have been published [4]. The drawbacks in comparing different series include gross variability in the definitions of outcome and follow-up time. Quite variable therapeutic protocols have been used with variable degrees of neurological deficits on admission and disparate treatment delays.

Most of the published case series have applied IAT. The largest series was reported by Eckert *et al.* [27], which included 83 patients treated within 18 hours of symptom onset. Forty-three percent of them were treated within 6 hours. The cohort included a minor proportion of patients with bilateral vertebral artery occlusion. Forty percent of the patients survived, recanalization was achieved in 66% and a favorable outcome (Barthel index 90–100) in 23%. More favorable results have been reported when treatment commenced within a more narrow time window. Arnold *et al.* treated 40 patients with IAT within 12 hours of symptom onset, 42% of which within 6 hours. Fifty-eight percent of the patients survived and 65% of the occlusions recanalized [28]. Good outcome (mRS 0 to 2) was reached in 35%.

An earlier consecutive series of patients treated with IVT (alteplase) comprised 50 patients treated per protocol within 48 hours after symptom onset in the progressive BAO phenotype and within 12 hours in the sudden onset phenotype [5]. Heparin was used as an adjuvant. Sixty percent of the patients survived and the recanalization rate (time-of-flight MRA) was reported to be 52%. Good outcome (functional independence, Barthel index 95–100) was achieved in 24% of the patients. The proportion of good outcome was similar in this continued single-center consecutive BAO cohort when increased to 116 patients, which included the previous 50 patients [29]. Importantly, among 184 patients registered by February 2012 recanalization of BAO up to 48 hours was seldom futile and produced good outcomes in 50% of patients when there was absence of extensive ischemia on admission scan [17].

One systematic analysis has been published consisting of reported case series of at least 10 patients that comprised altogether 420 BAO patients [21]. Patients treated with IVT (76) and IAT (344) had equal odds of death or dependency: 78% after IVT and 76% after IAT (p = 0.82) (Fig. 16.2). A total of 24% of patients treated with IAT and 22% treated with IVT reached favorable outcome (p = 0.82). Recanalization was noted more frequently after IAT (65%) than after IVT (53%; p = 0.05), but surprisingly this did not translate into better clinical outcome. If recanalization was not achieved, there was hardly any chance of a good outcome (2%), but when at least some patency of BA could be gained, the odds of favorable outcome increased substantially to 38% (Fig. 16.3).

In this analysis, hemorrhagic changes were slightly but not significantly more frequent after IVT (11%) than after IAT (8%; p = 0.59). Furthermore, the symptomatic hemorrhages after IVT were observed only after failed recanalization in patients destined to poor prognosis. Overall, the risk of symptomatic hemorrhages after IAT or IVT for BAO is quite similar to the bleeding risk of thrombolysis for anterior circulation strokes. Therefore, although the presence of hemorrhagic lesions is always a contraindication for thrombolysis, one should not fear for it more than in the thrombolytic therapy of anterior circulation strokes despite longer symptom durations, keeping in mind the devastating prognosis of BAO without recanalization.

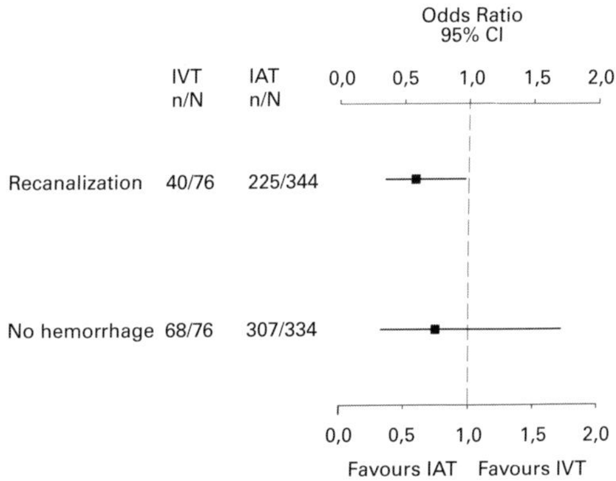

Fig. 16.2 The ORs and 95% CIs for death, dependence, and death/dependence. Reprinted from Lindsberg and Mattle. *Stroke* (2006);**37**:922–8.

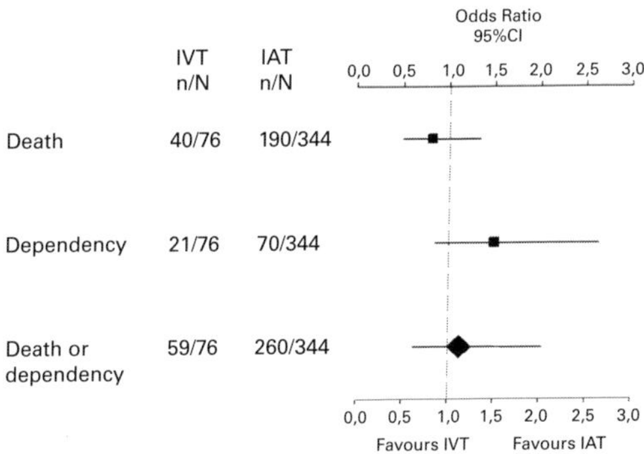

Fig. 16.3 The ORs and 95% CIs for post-thrombolytic signs of recanalization and the likelihood of avoiding symptomatic hemorrhage or parenchymal hematoma. Reprinted from Lindsberg and Mattle. *Stroke* (2006);**37**:922–8.

The main results of the largest prospective multicenter observational registry (BASICS) of 592 BAO patients treated between 2002 and 2007 were reported in 2009 [6]. The patients received either conventional therapy (antiplatelet drugs or anticoagulation, n = 183), IVT (n = 121, some patients treated with on-demand IAT) or intra-arterial approaches (n = 288, IAT, mechanical thrombectomy, stenting, or their combinations). Compared with conventional therapy, patients with a severe deficit (coma, tetraplegia or locked-in state; n = 347) had a lower risk of unfavorable outcome (mRS 4 to 6) at 1 month after IVT (adjusted RR 0.88, 0.76–1.01) or intra-arterial therapy (adjusted RR 0.94, 0.86–1.02), whereas outcomes were similar after treatment with IAT or IVT (adjusted RR 1.06, 0.91–1.22). Interestingly, patients with a mild-to-moderate deficit (n = 245) had less favorable outcome after intra-arterial therapies compared with IVT (adjusted RR 1.49, 1.00–2.23). Similarly to the aforementioned systematic analysis [16], intra-arterial therapy was not unequivocally superior to IVT in leading to good outcome, although vessel recanalization was achieved slightly more frequently with intra-arterial therapies (72%) than with IVT (67%). The conclusion of these investigators was that patients with mild-to-moderate symptoms should be treated with IVT as soon as possible, and that those with severe deficits should be treated with either IVT or IAT. Finally, it was concluded that an RCT should be conducted. Whether the benefit of IVT over IAT in milder strokes is due to shorter treatment delay remains to be further tested as well.

Indications for recanalization therapies

Indications and contraindications for recanalization therapies for BAO have not been well established and different centers follow empirically or intuitively evolved variable protocols. Some argue that coma and bilateral motor symptoms on presentation predict poor or desperate prognosis that makes recanalization therapies futile. To this end, studies summarized by Levy *et al.* revealed coma at the time of treatment to portend decreased survival rates [30]. Generally, roughly half of BAO patients present with coma at the time of treatment [21]. In the IVT series from Helsinki, out of 71 patients who presented with coma, 16 (22.5%) eventually reached a moderate outcome (mRS up to 3) and eight additional patients reached mRS 4 [29]. This is in line with the BASICS registry, where in thrombolysed patients with coma, tetraplegia or locked-in state, good outcome at 1 month was noted in 17% (34 out of 196, IAT) to 26% (19 out of 72, IVT) [6]. Therefore, while coma on presentation is a negative prognostic variable, recanalization therapies should not be refused from acutely comatose patients with BAO. However, absent brainstem reflexes and spontaneous respiration, widespread brainstem infarction or hemorrhagic transformation are generally held as contraindications for recanalization therapies. Furthermore, previous independence in daily activities and lack of serious comorbidities that limit the life expectancy are regarded as additional criteria to select patients for recanalization therapy. Naturally, angiographic proof of total or near total BAO is a prerequisite for the treatment. The most important contraindications for thrombolytic therapy to be considered on an individual basis are summarized in Table 16.3.

Time window for thrombolysis

In posterior circulation strokes the time window for recanalization therapies has not been established. Almost all case series have included patients with considerably longer durations from symptom onset than what is accepted for the anterior circulation, up to 4.5 to 6 hours for IVT or IAT and 8 hours for mechanical thrombectomy. It has been speculated that different collateral flow patterns, and relatively low hemorrhage rates due to smaller infarct volumes

Table 16.3 Suggested contraindications for thrombolytic therapy in BAO

Most important exclusion criteria
Absent brainstem refexes and/or lack of spontaneous respiration
Extensive brainstem infarction in brain imaging
Hemorrhage in brain imaging or serious bleeding or trauma elsewhere in the body*
Serious failure of hemostasis or current bleeding or diathesis*
Previous lack of independence in daily activities
Multiple comorbidities with limited life expectancy
Duration of massive BAO symptoms longer than 12 hours or longer than 48 hours in the phenotype where gradually progressing symptoms reach a severe degree
Persistently elevated blood pressure (> 185/110 mmHg) despite adequate antihypertensive medication

*Endovascular treatment may still be considered

may render brain tissue in the territory of BA more tolerant to ischemia. [13]

In a systematic analysis of case series that included altogether 420 BAO patients treated with either IVT or IAT, the time window for treatment varied from 7 to 48 hours after symptom onset [21]. In the IVT protocols the fraction of patients treated within 12 hours was 77% and 29% within 6 hours. In the IAT protocols the corresponding fractions were 76% and 42%, respectively. In the BASICS registry cohort (n = 619), longer time to treatment predicted poor outcome among other admission characteristics [31], but in a large single-center cohort (n = 184) outcome was independent of time to treatment [17]. Clearly, the severity of neurological deficits and the presence and length of coma have an influence on the duration of BAO after which thrombolysis is still deemed a viable option. However, a general consensus on the time window has so far not been formed and decisions will have to be made on an individual basis.

Factors influencing recanalization and outcome

Several factors have been described to affect or predict the likelihood of recanalization of BAO. In the series of Arnold *et al.*, for those patients treated within 6 hours, recanalization was more likely to occur than in those treated between 6 and 12 hours (90% vs. 55%, $p = 0.011$), and therefore time is probably a significant factor [28]. A similar finding was not noted in the series of Ezaki *et al.* (n = 26) and Brandt *et al.* (n = 51) [32,33]. In the latter series occlusions of embolic origin were more likely to be recanalized than those of atherothrombotic origin. There is no evidence of the superiority of urokinase, pro-urokinase or alteplase in achieving recanalization of the BA or survival of the patient [32,34]. Some centers have used glycoprotein IIb/IIIa inhibitors abciximab or tirofiban in an attempt to enhance recanalization [35,36]. Most protocols also apply IV heparin or IV acetylosalicylic acid to ensure patency of BA after recanalization.

The location of the clot also plays a role. Some evidence supports the idea that distal clot location is associated with more favorable clinical outcome. In the series of Cross *et al.* (n = 22) only 15% of the patients with proximal or midbasilar location survived while 71% of those with distal clot survived [37]. According to Levy *et al.* distal BAO is nearly one-half as likely to result in a fatal outcome than BAO that is placed more proximally [30]. In line, in the series of Sliwka *et al.* the top of the basilar occlusions were most likely to be recanalized [34], a finding repeated by Sairanen *et al.* [29]. In the top of the basilar cases branches penetrating into the brainstem and cerebellum are likely to remain patent (Fig. 16.1), which usually is not the case in midbasilar or proximal occlusions where the circulatory failure of penetrating arteries may not be reversed even after successful recanalization of the BA.

Percutaneous transluminal angioplasty (PTA) has also been used as accessory therapy following thrombolysis in patients with stenosing atherosclerotic lesions in the basilar or vertebral arteries [27,32,35]. Stenting a stenosed (> 50%) BA in patients with TIA or stroke without complete BAO has been reported to yield a recurrent stroke rate of 12% and a complication rate of 15% [38,39]. While recanalization rates and eventual vessel patency are improved in artery remodeling procedures, periprocedural complications and recurrences may bear on clinical outcomes. More research is needed in these therapeutic protocols where vessel remodeling is associated with thrombolysis.

Mechanical thrombectomy

Since recanalization is by far the most significant factor influencing the clinical outcome in BAO, more aggressive and invasive approaches have been inspired. These include devices with a catheter placed intra-arterially and mechanical clot removal. Most devices are used in cerebral vessels that are 2–5 mm in diameter. The MERCI-retriever device™ deploys screw-like wire, engages the thrombus, and pulls it backwards to the tip of the catheter, through which the clot is aspirated away from the vasculature. Another device using fragmentation and aspiration of the thrombus is the Penumbra System™. Other devices are based as well on rheolytic clot fragmentation and suction (Angiojet™) or on delivering either photoacoustic energy (EPAR™) or acoustic ultrasound pressure gradient applied transcranially (transcranial Doppler) or intra-arterially (EKOS™). However, the development of Angiojet and EPAR has been discontinued, while EKOS™ is still investigated in clinical stroke trials and aims to disrupt the clot by ultrasound in the presence of thrombolytic agents and thereby enhance the penetration of the fibrinolytic drug into the clot. The most recent development for mechanical recanalization techniques are self-expanding, retrievable stents. One example is the Solitaire® stent. The stent is advanced into the clot, released, left for approximately 5 min and then retrieved with the clot. Self-expanding, retrievable stents are promising, mainly for two reasons: first, they achieve recanalization rates of more than 90%, and second, they are easier to handle than other recanalization devices [4,40].

The published patient series with basilar artery occlusions treated with endovascular mechanical devices comprise 10 to 76 patients [6,41]. The benefit of endovascular therapy options in addition to IVT is investigated in the ongoing BASICS Trial.

The rates of good outcome and survival at 3 months (28% and 66%, respectively, n = 25) with mechanical thrombectomy in BAO are not necessarily more favorable than with IVT or IAT based on the MERCI Multi-MERCI results, even though recanalization was achieved in 76% (19 out of 25 BAO patients) [42]. In these patients treated within 8 hours of symptom onset, symptomatic hemorrhages or procedural complications occurred in 20% and 13% of the patients, respectively. Using the photoacoustic recanalization device (EPAR), successful recanalization rate of 73% was achieved in a series of 11 BAO patients, of whom 27% reached good outcome (mRS score 0–3) while 55% died [43]. It should be noted that in these series the patients were mostly ineligible for IVT and presented with somewhat more severe neurological deficits than those treated with thrombolytic therapy in other studies. This will likely be a weak point in clinical trials yet to come.

More recent approaches to recanalize the BA have deployed a combination of treatments performed as 'bridging therapies', in which the patient is initially evaluated and treated with IVT in a community hospital and then transferred to a fully equipped stroke center for on-demand IAT or endovascular thrombectomy [36]. This type of drip, ship, and retrieve protocols are expected to increase if interventionists are available [40,44]. Telemedical video consultation can be used in these protocols to decide on the initial therapy in the primary community hospital.

Taken together, the acute treatment of verified basilar occlusion differs between centers and it may include only IV thrombolysis (IVT), or bridging IV therapy with intra-arterial therapy, which nowadays most often involves endovascular mechanical thrombectomy (EMT) despite lack of randomized, controlled studies. Also, the adjunctive therapy with antithrombotics and heparinoids differs strongly. Each center uses mainly one of the aforementioned treatment options and the choice is based on the resources including the availability of emergency angiography, interventionist, and anesthesiologist.

Intensive care

After recanalization therapy patients should be monitored in the ICU until their condition is stable. Following complete or partial recanalization heparin or acetylsalicylic acid should be continued in the intensive care unit with frequent blood coagulation and platelet count measurements. Especially in BAO of atherothrombotic origin and associated atherosclerotic stenosis reocclusion is a major peril and therefore neurological function should be monitored frequently by ICU staff. A low-flow state may persist in the BA especially in a patient with limited collaterals and the danger of reocclusion is considerable. In patients with imminent or already occurred reocclusion administration of glycoprotein IIb/IIIa inhibitors and mechanical thrombectomy are foremost treatment options. The possibility of internal bleedings and heparin-induced thrombocytopenia (HIT) should be kept in mind. Warfarin should be started when the patient's condition has been stabilized. Acetosalicylic acid or clopidogrel can be used as adjuvants when more efficient antithrombotic control is deemed necessary to maintain vessel patency.

Thorough cardiac investigations including ECG, cardio-ECHO, and long-term monitoring of cardiac rhythm should be carried out in patients with no stenosing vertebrobasilar or atherosclerotic aortic lesions, or in whom cardioembolic origin is otherwise suspected. Since BAO can cause brainstem and medullary lesions that encompass nuclei regulating vital functions, respiration, cardiac rhythm, and other autonomic hemodynamic functions should be closely monitored in the ICU.

Patients with intracranial occlusive disease are very sensitive to changes in brain perfusion upon hypotension or volume depletion. In the New England Posterior Circulation Registry (n = 430) 36% of the patients with vertebrobasilar occlusive disease had their symptoms worsen by prone position or antihypertensives, so optimizing of the hemodynamic state and adequate hydration are mandatory to maintain sufficient brain perfusion [45].

Brain imaging (CTA, MRA, DSA or transcranial Doppler) should be repeated at 12 to 24 hours and again later on as necessary to exclude potential hemorrhagic transformations and reocclusion especially upon worsening of the patient's neurological condition. Reduction of consciousness can also result from hydrocephalus after extensive cerebellar infarction, in which case ventriculostomy, shunt placement or decompressive craniectomy may become necessary after consultation with a neurosurgeon. There is no evidence that would support the use of hypothermia or putative neuroprotectants in the ICU treatment of BAO.

Large space-occupying infarcts can result from BAO. In such patients, especially when there is no extensive destruction of the brainstem, decompressive surgery should be considered. This is recommended by both the European and American (ESO and AHA) guidelines for stroke treatment, though no randomized controlled trial supports this recommendation to date. To date, only large patient series have been reported [46].

For elderly patients presenting very late in coma, or those with evidence of extensive posterior fossa infarction, the treatment of choice is likely to be palliative care outside the ICU. In patients with persisting BAO after recanalization therapies and prolonged coma, or extensive brainstem and cerebellar infarctions, continuation of ICU treatment is futile. The same is true for patients with absent brainstem reflexes and/or lack of spontaneous respiration.

On the other hand, every effort should be placed on rescuing those with prognostic markers of meaningful recovery, but not denying recanalization therapies from acutely comatose or tetraplegic patients. In survivors after recanalized BAO, those who score 5 on mRS at 3 months tend to die long-term, whereas those who score with 4 or better tend to improve [5]. Even despite substantial disability, long-term survivors rate their quality of life on average 7 on a 10-point scale consisting of 10 different components of quality of life (unpublished data from [5]). Survival with unimpaired cognition can be meaningful for the patient and close family members, even when physical capabilities are limited and continuous care needs to be given.

Conclusion

Clearly, we need more effective diagnostic and treatment strategies to improve the very poor outcomes in BAO. Using either noninvasive or invasive treatment approaches the fraction of patients who achieve favorable outcome is still below 35% in most centers and a considerable portion still die or remain dependent and need continuous care and assistance in daily activities. At present, the therapeutic protocols are quite variable in different stroke centers, which makes face-to-face comparisons demanding. Furthermore, technical advances in devising intravascular mechanical tools evolve rapidly. New techniques are invented frequently while some existing ones are withdrawn. For each new instrument, there is a learning curve for operators. These factors also present challenges in designing study protocols that could recruit enough patients in each intended protocol arm for a powered, systematic RCT in this relatively infrequent disease. Consecutive patient registries have limited power against RCTs of officially approved thrombolytic treatment protocols.

The current wisdom is that IVT should not be delayed while waiting for preparations necessary for conducting IAT or alternative invasive procedures. In hospitals not equipped with invasive neuroradiological services, immediate IVT should be the treatment of choice rather than conventional antithrombotic therapy. These hospitals should consider setting up telemedical service with the nearest fully equipped stroke center and perhaps consider adopting 'bridging therapies'. Advanced imaging modalities should be used to improve patient selection for individualized therapy. It is quite likely that pharmacological therapies alone have a ceiling effect and that the invasive approaches should be investigated more intensively and systematically, and compared with IVT protocols to document their potential superiority in the future.

REFERENCES

[1] Kubik CS, Adams RD. Occlusion of the basilar artery. *Brain* 1946;**69**:73–121.

[2] Caplan LR. 'Top of the basilar' syndrome. *Neurology* 1980;**30**:72–9.

[3] Tatu L, Moulin T, Bogousslavsky J, Duvernoy H. Arterial territories of the human brain: cerebral hemispheres. *Neurology* 1998;**50**:1699–708.

[4] Mattle HP, Arnold M, Lindsberg PJ, Schonewille WJ, Schroth G. Basilar artery occlusion. *Lancet Neurol* 2011;**10**:1002–14.

[5] Lindsberg PJ, Soinne L, Tatlisumak T, *et al.* Long-term outcome after intravenous thrombolysis of basilar artery occlusion. *J Am Med Assoc* 2004;**292**:1862–6.

[6] Schonewille WJ, Wijman CA, Michel P, *et al.* Treatment and outcomes of acute basilar artery occlusion in the Basilar Artery International Cooperation Study (BASICS): a prospective registry study. *Lancet Neurol* 2009;**8**:724–30.

[7] Ferbert A, Brückmann H, Drummen R. Clinical features of proven basilar artery occlusion. *Stroke* 1990;**21**:1135–42.

[8] Caplan LR. Vertebrobasilar embolism. *Clin Exp Neurol* 1991;**28**:1–22.

[9] Baird TA, Muir KW, Bone I. Basilar artery occlusion. *Neurocritical Care* 2004;**3**:319–30.

[10] Mortimer AM, Saunders T, Cook JL. Cross-sectional imaging for diagnosis and clinical outcome prediction of acute basilar artery thrombosis. *Clin Radiol* 2011;**66**:551–8.

[11] Puetz V, Sylaja PN, Coutts SB, *et al.* Extent of hypoattenuation on CT angiography source images predicts functional outcome in patients with basilar artery occlusion. *Stroke* 2008;**39**:2485–90.

[12] Puetz V, Sylaja PN, Hill MD, *et al.* CT angiography source images predict final infarct extent in patients with basilar artery occlusion. *Am J Neuroradiol* 2009;**30**:1877–83.

[13] Ostrem JL, Saver JL, Alger JR, *et al.* Acute basilar artery occlusion: diffusion-perfusion MRI characterization of tissue salvage in patients receiving intra-arterial stroke therapies. *Stroke* 2004;**35**:e30–4.

[14] Cho TH, Nighoghossian N, Tahon F, *et al.* Brain stem diffusion-weighted imaging lesion score: a potential marker of outcome in acute basilar artery occlusion. *Am J Neuroradiol* 2009;**30**:194–8.

[15] Nagel S, Herweh C, Köhrmann M, *et al.* MRI in patients with acute basilar artery occlusion – DWI lesion scoring is an independent predictor of outcome. *Int J Stroke* 2012;**7**:282–8.

[16] Mortimer AM, Bradley M, Renowden SA. Endovascular therapy for acute basilar artery occlusion: a review of the literature. *J Neurointervent Surg* 2012;**4**:266–73.

[17] Strbian D, Sairanen T, Silvennoinen H, *et al.* Thrombolysis of basilar artery occlusion: Impact of baseline ischemia and time. *Ann Neurol* 2013: Mar 28. doi:10.1002/ana.23904 [Epub].

[18] Cross DT 3rd, Moran CJ, Akins PT, *et al.* Collateral circulation and outcome after basilar artery thrombolysis. *Am J Neuroradiol* 1998;**19**:1557–63.

[19] Schonewille WJ, Algra A, Serena J, Molina CA, Kappelle LJ. Outcome in patients with basilar artery occlusion treated conventionally. *J Neurol Neurosurg Psychiatry* 2005;**76**:1238–41.

[20] Hacke W, Zeumer H, Ferbert A, Bruckmann H, del Zoppo GJ. Intra-arterial thrombolytic therapy improves outcome in patients with acute vertebrobasilar occlusive disease. *Stroke* 1988;**19**:1216–22.

[21] Lindsberg PJ, Mattle HP. Therapy of basilar artery occlusion: A systematic analysis comparing intra-arterial and intravenous thrombolysis. *Stroke* 2006;**37**:922–8.

[22] Zeumer H, Hacke W, Kolman HL, Poeck K. Fibrniolysetherapie bei Basilaristhrombose. *Dtsch Med Wschr* 1982;**107**:728–31.

[23] Macleod MR, Davis SM, Mitchell PJ, *et al.* Results of a multicentre, randomised controlled trial of intra-arterial urokinase in the treatment of acute posterior circulation ischaemic stroke. *Cerebrovasc Dis* 2005;**20**:12–17.

[24] Donnan GA, Davis SM, Schellinger PD, Hacke W. Intra-arterial thrombolysis is the treatment of choice for basilar thrombosis: pro. *Stroke* 2006;**37**:2436–7.

[25] Davis SM, Donnan GA. Basilar artery thrombosis: Recanalization is the key. *Stroke* 2006;**37**:2440.

[26] Ford GA. Intra-arterial thrombolysis is the treatment of choice for basilar thrombosis: con. *Stroke* 2006;**37**:2438–9.

[27] Eckert B, Kucinski T, Pfeiffer G, Groden C, Zeumer H. Endovascular therapy of acute vertebrobasilar occlusion: early treatment onset as the most important factor. *Cerebrovasc Dis* 2002;**14**:42–50.

[28] Arnold M, Nedeltchev K, Schroth G, *et al.* Clinical and radiological predictors of recanalisation and outcome of 40 patients with acute basilar artery occlusion treated with intra-arterial thrombolysis. *J Neurol Neurosurg Psychiatry* 2004;**75**:857–62.

[29] Sairanen T, Strbian D, Soinne L, *et al.* Intravenous thrombolysis of basilar artery occlusion: predictors of recanalization and outcome. *Stroke* 2011;**42**:2175–9.

[30] Levy EI, Firlik AD, Wisniewski S, *et al.* Factors affecting survival rates for acute vertebrobasilar artery occlusions treated with intra-arterial thrombolytic therapy: a meta-analytical approach. *Neurosurgery* 1999;**45**:539–45.

[31] Greving JP, Schonewille WJ, Wijman CAC, *et al.* Predicting outcome after acute basilar artery occlusion based on admission characteristics. *Neurology* 2012;**78**:1058–63.

[32] Ezaki Y, Tsutsumi K, Onizuka M, *et al.* Retrospective analysis of neurological outcome after intra-arterial thrombolysis in basilar artery occlusion. *Surg Neurol* 2003;**60**:423–9.

[33] Brandt T, von Kummer R, Müller-Küppers M, Hacke W. Thrombolytic therapy of acute basilar artery occlusion. Variables affecting recanalization and outcome. *Stroke* 1996;**27**:875–81.

[34] Sliwka U, Mull M, Stelzer A, Diehl R, Noth J. Long-term follow-up of patients after intra-arterial thrombolytic therapy of acute vertebrobasilar artery occlusion. *Cerebrovasc Dis* 2001;**12**:214–19.

[35] Eckert B, Koch C, Thomalla G, *et al.* Aggressive therapy with intravenous abciximab and intra-arterial rtPA and additional PTA/stenting improves clinical outcome in acute vertebrobasilar occlusion: combined local fibrinolysis and intravenous abciximab in acute vertebrobasilar stroke treatment (FAST): results of a multicenter study. *Stroke* 2005;**36**:1160–5.

[36] Pfefferkorn T, Holtmannspötter M, Schmidt C, *et al.* Drip, ship, and retrieve: cooperative recanalization therapy in acute basilar artery occlusion. *Stroke* 2010;**41**:722–6.

[37] Cross DT 3rd, Moran CJ, Akins PT, Angtuaco EE, Diringer MN. Relationship between clot location and outcome after basilar artery thrombolysis. *Am J Neuroradiol* 1997;**18**:1221–8.

[38] The SSYLVIA Study Investigators. Stenting of symptomatic atherosclerotic lesions in the vertebral or intracranial arteries (SSYLVIA). Study results. *Stroke* 2004;**35**:1388–92.

[39] Fields JD, Liu KC, Barnwell SL, Clark WM, Lutsep HL. Indications and applications of arterial stents for stroke prevention in atherosclerotic intracranial stenosis. *Curr Cardiol Rep* 2010;**12**:20–8.

[40] Gralla J, Brekenfeld C, Mordasini P, Schroth G. Mechanical thrombolysis and stenting in acute ischemic stroke. *Stroke* 2012;**43**:280–5.

[41] Broussalis E, Hitzl W, McCoy M, Trinka E, Killer M. Comparison of endovascular treatment versus conservative medical treatment in patients with acute basilar artery occlusion. *Vasc Endovasc Surg* 2013 May 19. [Epub]

[42] Shi ZS, Loh Y, Walker G, Duckwiler GR. MERCI and Multi MERCI Investigators. Endovascular thrombectomy for acute ischemic stroke in failed intravenous tissue plasminogen activator versus non-intravenous tissue plasminogen activator patients: revascularization and outcomes stratified by the site of arterial occlusions. *Stroke* 2010;**41**:1185–92.

[43] Lutsep HL, Rymer MM, Nesbit GM. Vertebrobasilar revascularization rates and outcomes in the MERCI and Multi MERCI trials. *J Stroke Cerebrovasc Dis* 2008;**17**:55–7.

[44] Pfefferkorn T, Holtmannspötter M, Schmidt C, *et al.* Drip, ship, and retrieve: cooperative recanalization therapy in acute basilar artery occlusion. *Stroke* 2010;**41**:722–6.

[45] Shin H-K, Yoo K-M, Chang HM, Caplan LR. Bilateral intracranial vertebral artery disease in the New England Medical Center Posterior Circulation Registry. *Arch Neurol* 1999;**56**:1353–8.

[46] Jüttler E, Schweickert S, Ringleb PA, *et al.* Long-term outcome after surgical treatment for space-occupying cerebellar infarction: experience in 56 patients. *Stroke* 2009;**40**:3060–6.

17

Critical care of cerebellar stroke

Tim Nowe and Eric Jüttler

Summary

Space-occupying edema is a frequent complication in cerebellar infarction and occurs in up to 50% of these patients. General treatment of ischemic cerebellar infarction does not differ from other ischemic strokes. The clinician should be aware of life-threatening complications and patients should therefore be closely monitored and treated on an experienced stroke unit or (neuro)intensive care unit (ICU) in the early stage of the disease. However, it is important to keep in mind that deterioration occurs even in late stages and must not be overlooked. If space-occupying edema occurs potential treatments include pharmacological anti-edema and intracranial pressure (ICP)-lowering therapies, ventricular drainage either by EVD or ventriculostomy, suboccipital decompressive surgery with or without resection of necrotic tissue, or a combination of these strategies, depending on the underlying cause of clinical deterioration. Timing of treatment escalation is crucial and should be guided by clinical and neuroradiological measures. There is some evidence in the literature that early and prophylactic treatment might be beneficial. In addition, initially comatose patients due to hydrocephalus and/or local brainstem involvement may also profit from surgical therapy, as long as these conditions are reversible and as long as no irreversible brain injury has occurred. As old age and additional brain stem infarction most strongly predict poor outcome in these patients, this has to be kept in mind for decision-making, which should always be done in close cooperation of neurointensive care physicians, neurologists, and neurosurgeons.

Introduction

Severe ischemic cerebellar infarction and its life threatening complications represent both a diagnostic and therapeutic challenge. After description of the relevant anatomy, including blood supply, specific pathophysiological aspects, and symptomatology, highlighting signs and symptoms of space-occupying infarcts, the emphasis of this chapter will be on diagnostic and treatment strategies relevant for the ICU. General treatment of ischemic stroke, anti-edema therapy, and technical aspects of neurosurgical interventions, especially decompressive surgery, are only mentioned briefly, since these are described in more detail in chapters 7 and 8, respectively. The focus will rather be on a comparison of different treatment strategies including an extensive review of all available retrospective and prospective cohort studies as well as case series of severe cerebellar infarction.

Anatomy and blood supply of the cerebellum

The cerebellum mounts the medulla oblongata and the pons and consists of the two lateral hemispheres and

Critical Care of the Stroke Patient, ed. Stefan Schwab, Daniel Hanley, and A. David Mendelow. Published by Cambridge University Press.

the midline vermis. The cerebellum has various connections with other cerebral nervous system (CNS) structures through the three cerebellar peduncles.

The cerebellum is located in the posterior fossa where it fills it nearly completely. Rigid dural folds, known as the tentorium cerebelli, form the upper boundary; below the cerebellum is embedded in the base of the skull. The cerebellar peduncles form the roof of the fourth ventricle and are located over the aqueduct of Sylvius. This anatomical situation is important to understand the serious complications of space-occupying edema formation after cerebellar stroke, which may rapidly lead to direct brainstem compression and obstructive hydrocephalus by obstruction of the aqueduct and/or the fourth ventricle. As soon as compensating space is consumed subsequent herniation, transforaminal herniation (downward herniation, through the foramen magnum), or transtentorial (upward herniation, through the tentorium) may occur.

The cerebellum receives its blood supply from the posterior circulation also known as the vertebrobasilar system. The extracranial vertebral arteries originate from the subclavian arteries and ascend in the neck through the transverse processes of the cervical spine. They exit at C2 to penetrate the dura and enter the cranium and the confluence to form the unpaired basilar artery. Three main paired arteries feed the cerebellum: the posterior inferior cerebellar arteries (PICA), which usually derive from the distal vertebral artery, the anterior inferior cerebellar arteries (AICA), usually branches from the proximal or mid-basilar artery, and the superior cerebellar arteries (SUCA) usually stems from the distal basilar artery. Shorter, proximal branches from all three of the cerebellar arteries also supply portions of the brainstem, which is mainly supplied by the basilar artery. This organization of the blood supply in the posterior circulation and the physiology of the cerebellum lead to the large variations of symptoms and their severity in cerebellar stroke, which are described below [1].

Epidemiology and risk factors

Acute ischemic cerebellar infarction has an incidence of 1.1% to 4.2% in clinicopathological studies, and constitutes 1.5% to 10.5% of all acute ischemic strokes in stroke registries and larger case series [2–5]. However, these data might underestimate the frequency of cerebellar infarcts because of often unspecific symptoms.

Modifiable risk factors such as hypertension, diabetes, cigarette smoking, and hyperlidemia, and nonmodifiable risk factors such as age, atrial fibrillation, and history of stroke or transient ischemic attack also apply for cerebellar stroke.

The average age of patients with cerebellar infarcts is 60–65 years and seems to be a little lower than in other ischemic stroke populations [6–11]. This could be an effect of a higher proportion of younger patients, however, it is more likely due to selectional bias, because numbers derive from treatment, and retrospective cohorts.

Pathogenesis

The most frequent causes of ischemic cerebellar strokes are cardio embolism and large vessel atherosclerosis. Small artery disease and artery-to-artery embolism are less frequent. Vertebral artery dissection is a relevant cause, especially in younger patients with a peak in the fifth decade; however, it may occur at every age and is not necessarily related to recent trauma, which is reported in only half of the cases [12,13]. Infarcts of the PICA territory are most common, followed by infarcts of the SUCA territory, while infarcts of the AICA are less common. In up to 44% of the patients more than one vessel territory is involved [14].

Space-occupying edema is a common complication in cerebellar infarcts and occurs in 17% up to 54% of the patients, mainly due to cytotoxic and to a minor degree vasogenic and interstitial brain tissue edema [6,7,15–25]. It is more common in infarcts of the PICA, the SUCA, or of multiple territories and uncommon in infarcts of the AICA territory. Beside the coincidence of additional brainstem infarction, it is the most dreaded complication of acute cerebellar infarct. So far it is not clear which factors promote the evolvement of brain edema after stroke. Clinical experience indicates that there is a wide inter-individual range. Sometimes infarcts with large volumes can be accompanied by only small edema, while on the other hand comparably small infarcts can develop extensive swelling. Timing of edema formation is very variable as well. Although data from neuroimaging studies show that in most of the patients the maximum of swelling is present between days two and four, which closely correlates with the clinical picture of most deeply impaired consciousness between day two and day three, again the inter-individual variability is extremely wide and ranges from day one to day nine [15,17,22].

Clinical manifestations of cerebellar infarcts and space-occupying cerebellar edema

The cerebellum is crucial for control and modulation of movement as well as motor learning and adaption. Damage to the cerebellum generally leads to inaccurate, erratic, or uncoordinated movements. Although many of these functions are regionally specified, localization of the anatomical region of a lesion is often difficult in clinical practice. The superior parts of the cerebellum are primarily involved in limb (lateral hemispheres) and trunk (midline vermis) movements and speech articulation (paravermal area). The inferior areas are primarily involved in oculomotor control and vestibular adaptation. Projections between the limbs and cerebellum are either uncrossed or doubly crossed, so that motor deficits after unilateral cerebellar lesion are usually more severe in the ipsilateral limbs. Many deficits, however, are bilateral or of only weak lateralization because of bilateral and partially redundant projections that control coordination of midline muscles of the head, neck, and trunk.

Patients with cerebellar infarcts often show unspecific symptoms such as dizziness, nausea, vomiting, unsteady gait, and headache. More specific neurological signs such as dysarthria, ataxia, and nystagmus are often either only slight or may even be absent [2].

Unfortunately, in the early stage these signs and symptoms are not different from those patients with small cerebellar infarcts and those with large and potentially space-occupying infarcts. The only clinical signs of space-occupying cerebellar infarcts include progressive deterioration of consciousness, brainstem signs, and finally signs of herniation. However, brainstem compression due to increasing edema formation and additional brainstem infarct might present clinically identically, and cannot be clearly differentiated by clinical means only [7,9,10,22].

Vertigo and dizziness

Vertigo or dizziness occurs in about 75% of patients with cerebellar infarcts and in up to 10% of patients dizziness is the main or only complaint. On the other hand, dizziness is also a common symptom of various other neurologic, cardiologic, and psychiatric diseases, head trauma, infections, electrolyte disturbances, dehydration, as well as a side effect of many medications and other conditions and is frequently seen in general practice and emergency departments. The likelihood of ischemic stroke or TIA in patients who report dizziness as the main or even only complaint is very low (about 3% when presenting with other symptoms and even lower (1%) when patients complain about dizziness alone) [26]. The same is true for vertigo, which in most cases is either phobic or due to peripheral vestibular conditions. However, small prospective studies in patients with acute vertigo, especially when vestibular symptoms were present, suggest that in patients with increasing age and the presence of vascular risk factors the frequency of a central nervous cause is considerably high and therefore should be excluded [27]. The key questions in the case of dizziness or vertigo are about timing, duration, trigger factors, medication, cardiac diseases, and accompanying symptoms.

Although dizziness seems to be more common in patients with space-occupying stroke it is not useful for monitoring or timing of treatment.

Nausea and vomiting

About half of the patients with cerebellar infarcts suffer from nausea and vomiting [6–8]. It can even be the dominant symptom and disproportionate to vertigo or dizziness. Again, this symptom is unspecific and its differential diagnostic value in the absence of other signs and symptoms is low. Even though nausea is almost as common as dizziness, a central cause should be considered if associated medical symptoms such as abdominal or chest pain, diarrhea, fever or a context such as recent changes in medication are missing.

Nausea and vomiting also seem to be more frequent in patients with large or space-occupying infarcts. However, it is unclear whether this is due to increased intracranial pressure.

Gait instability

About half of the patients with cerebellar infarcts suffer from gait instability. Unilateral strokes usually lead to unidirectional falls. Although acute peripheral vestibulopathies cause gait instability and directional falling as well, the inability to sit, stand or walk suggest a central cause of the symptoms [6–8]. It is, again, not useful for monitoring of patients with severe cerebellar infarcts or at risk of developing hydrocephalus or brainstem compression.

Headache

As the other symptoms reported so far, headache is an extremely common symptom reported in the patient's history and may be due to at least as many causes as dizziness or nausea. Headache is not a leading symptom of ischemic stroke, but is more commonly reported in posterior than in anterior circulation infarcts, in particular in cerebellar infarcts where nearly 40% of patients complain about headache [28]. It might be due to local swelling or a sign of vertebral arterial dissection, which should always be taken into consideration and prompt further investigation, especially in younger patients, after trauma, when it is unilateral, cervical, or accompanied by focal neurological signs [6].

Level of consciousness

The level of consciousness should be monitored very closely in patients with cerebellar infarction. Progressive deterioration of consciousness is a clinical warning sign of severe edema formation and/or brainstem involvement and may occur at any time in the acute and subacute phase, sometimes late, when the patient is already regarded as stable. Level of consciousness according to GCS scores shows close interaction with neurological status measured on the NIHSS score and other neurological findings such as involvement of cranial nerves [9]. Some authors believe that deterioration of consciousness is the strongest predictor for dangerous space occupation and should be used for decision-making. However, it is a common finding in about 34% of patients with cerebellar infarction and may have various causes other than mass effect [7]. In addition, if it occurs because of mass effect, it usually rapidly progresses to coma, most often within less than 24 hours [15]. It must also be kept in mind that changes in the level of consciousness are unspecific and therefore sometimes misinterpreted in these patients. For example, it is difficult to distinguish clinical signs of brainstem compression, which may be reversible, from irreversible brainstem infarction. Therefore altered level of consciousness should always be accompanied by neuroimaging, if possible MRI, before it should be used for therapy guidance.

Other signs

The most common other signs in patients with cerebellar infarction are dysarthria, ataxia, and nystagmus. If dysarthria occurs together with dizziness it is almost always central, but is not unique to the posterior circulation and therefore should always prompt imaging.

Less than 40% of patients with cerebellar infarcts show limb ataxia in the physical examination. It may be absent even in extensive infarcts [1].

Nystagmus is a common finding in both central and peripheral vestibular syndromes. A standardized examination might help to classify the type of nystagmus. Whenever there is a vertical nystagmus or the type of nystagmus cannot be allocated to definite peripheral syndrome, one should always take a central nervous cause into consideration.

In the cases of cerebellar edema progress, there is often direct compression of the brainstem, which initially affects the posterior part of the pons, leading first to a paresis of the sixth cranial nerve and soon to a complete loss of ipsilateral gaze (due to compression of the nucleus of VI and the lateral gaze center) as well as peripheral facial paresis (due to compression of the facial colliculus).

Diagnosis

Neurological examination

Typical and frequent clinical signs and symptoms have been described above. Neurological examination of the critically ill should, in addition, be accompanied by a standardized protocol. Despite the weakness of single neurological or emergency scales to cover the variability of the disease, they might be helpful to add measurable or pseudo-objective information, especially when different investigators are involved and the patient is investigated repeatedly. It has, however, to be kept in mind that clinical scales alone are insufficient for clinical monitoring and must always be combined with individual patient examination and evaluation as well as appropriate neuroimaging.

Scales

The National Institute of Health Stroke Scale (NIHSS) was originally invented for studies in thrombolysis [29]. It is practical for a detailed documentation of stroke severity, but was primarily invented to estimate the severity of supratentorial infarcts. However, the signs and symptoms of cortical, supratentorial infarcts differ largely from cerebellar infarcts. The previously discussed signs and symptoms of cerebellar infarcts, such as ataxia, vertigo, dysarthria, and others are clearly underrepresented compared to limb and facial paresis, aphasia, or inattention. However, increased NIHSS scores correlate with poor outcome due to the fact that patients that suffer from an additional brainstem infarct score much higher in the NIHSS.

The Glasgow Coma Scale (GCS) is widely used in emergency and intensive care medicine [30]. GCS alone is not a sufficient prognostic scale for patients with cerebellar infarction but seems to be superior as compared with the NIHSS. Monitoring using the GCS is especially helpful to decide if the patient needs intubation and the course of GCS together with neuroimaging findings is very helpful for interdisciplinary decisions on therapy escalation.

Neuroimaging

Non-contrast CT is currently the most widely available and most widely used imaging technique of first choice in patients with clinically suspected cerebellar stroke [31]. Especially clinically unstable or ventilated patients can be monitored adequately in the scanner and benefit from the short scanning time. Multimodal CT imaging, together with CT angiography and CT perfusion provide relevant additional information on the vessel status, especially pathologies of the vertebral arteries or basilar artery. However, non-contrast CT in the acute phase has a very low sensitivity for ischemic changes in the posterior fossa and brainstem due to artifacts from bones and the base of the skull and partial volume effects in that anatomical region (see Fig. 17.1) [32]. Furthermore, hypodense lesions in the lateral structures next to the corticospinal tract are difficult to detect and the angle of the sectional plane in conventional CT might lead to wrong anatomical attribution and misinterpretation of the findings. Moreover, additional saggital imaging is usually impossible and may also lead to misinterpretation. Even imminent complications such as local brain swelling and circulatory disturbance of the cerebrospinal fluid (CSF) might be overlooked in initial CT scans [33,34]. As a result, although the quality of head CT scans has improved tremendously in the last decade, both technical aspects and the anatomy of the posterior fossa are still the same and CT can therefore neither adequately confirm nor exclude cerebellar ischemic infarcts, especially in the early phase (see Fig. 17.1) [35].

On the other hand, in most cases of space-occupying cerebellar infarcts, repeated CT is sufficient for monitoring of tissue shifts, width of basal cisterns, and the ventricular system indicating occlusive hydrocephalus. Jauss and colleagues suggested a numerical score to assess mass effect of cerebellar infarction using a three-item CT score (Table 17.1, Fig. 17.2) including the width of the fourth ventricle, compression of the quadrigeminal cistern, and the width of the lateral ventricles [36].

The score correlates with clinical findings of the levels of consciousness and is of high inter-rater and retest

Table 17.1 Three-item CT score to assess mass effect of space-occupying cerebellar infarcts according to Jauss *et al.* A value of 4 is suggested as cut-off to strongly consider decompressive surgery [36].

Anatomical region/ rated item on CT	Severity (0 = no space-occupying effect; 9 = maximum space-occupying effect)			
Compression of the fourth ventricle	0 = no compression	1 = unilateral compression	2 = shifted midline	3 = not visible
Compression of the quadrigeminal cistern	0 = no compression	1 = mild, with asymmetric compression ipsilateral to the infarction	2 = moderate, with evidence of bilateral compression	3 = severe, bilateral compression with invisible quadrigeminal cistern
Dilatation of the inferior horn of the lateral ventricle	0 = no dilatation	1 = mild	2 = moderate	3 = severe

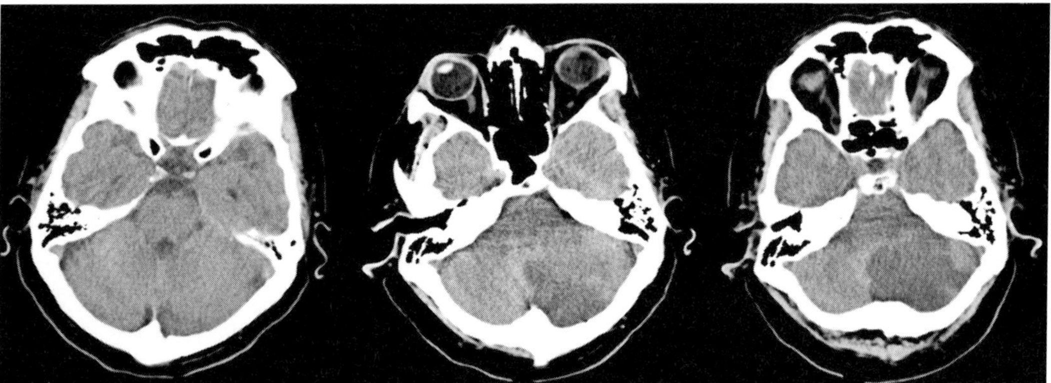

Fig. 17.1 CT imaging of a patient with left-hemispheric space-occupying cerebellar infarct. From left to right: day of symptom onset, 24, and 48 hours after symptom onset.

reliability. It may be used as a supplement to descriptive neuroimaging findings, especially in repeated imaging, and the clinical assessment of the patient, and is also valuable in monitoring the effect of medical and surgical interventions, but its value for predicting survival or long-term outcome is questionable [9].

Magnetic resonance imaging (MRI) is far more sensitive than CT in diagnosis of acute ischemic changes of the brain tissue, with study results indicating an 80% to 95% sensitivity in the first 24 hours when diffusion-weighted imaging (DWI) is used [33,34]. Stroke-MRI protocol consists at least of a DWI-, a T2*- (gradient echo) and a FLAIR (fluid-attenuated-inversion-recovery) sequence with or without perfusion imaging and contrast-enhanced or flow-based vessel imaging such as the time of flight (TOF) angiography. These sequences provide almost all important information in the acute phase.

Especially in the posterior circulation imaging, quality of MRI and sensitivity to detect ischemic changes is far better than non-contrast CT (see Fig. 17.3 and Fig. 17.4). Additional brainstem lesions are detected far more accurately compared with non-contrast CT imaging. However, even DWI sequences can be falsely negative in some cases. The main disadvantage of MRI

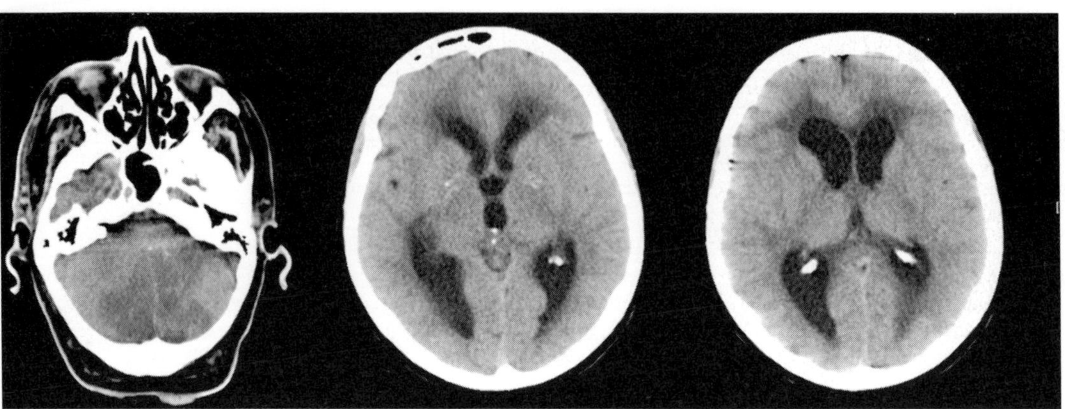

Fig. 17.2 CT imaging of a patient with bilateral cerebellar infarct, compression of the fourth ventricle and subsequent occlusive hydrocephalus with enlargement of the third and the lateral ventricles.

is that it is often not accessible in the acute phase. In particular, imaging of ventilated patients needs specific equipment and experience, even then a close continuous monitoring is difficult to establish in the MRI scanner and emergency interventions are difficult in this setting. In addition, scanning time is considerably longer than for CT [37].

Vascular imaging

Vascular imaging is crucial in ischemic stroke, especially in the posterior circulation. Several techniques can be used, either alone or in combination, including Doppler ultrasound, CT angiography (CTA), MR angiography (MRA), and conventional catheter angiography. Each modality has its advantages and disadvantages, with respect to availability, timing, duration, and accuracy. There are four main objectives of neurovascular imaging in patients with ischemic stroke in the posterior circulation including cerebellar infarcts. 1) To detect or exclude life-threatening or dangerous artery occlusion such as basilar artery occlusion or occlusion of the vertebral arteries. 2) To detect or exclude a potential target of therapy in patients with unknown onset. 3) To find the underlying pathology of stroke and confirm or exclude artery dissection. 4) To directly treat the patient (e.g. intra-arterial thrombolysis, vascular intervention). The advantages of Doppler ultrasound including transcranial Doppler are rapid assessment, portability, and low cost. It is also minimally invasive and can easily be used repeatedly to monitor vascular changes on the ICU bedside. However, this technique is highly operator dependent [38]. This is especially true for vascular flow in the posterior circulation, which is especially subject to misinterpretation.

Although conventional catheter angiography is still the gold standard for cerebrovascular imaging, CTA or MRA are more and more used as alternatives [33]. CTA seems to be more accurate than Doppler ultrasound in patients with vertebral artery pathologies and also more accurate than MRA [39,40] Despite CTA being widely available and extremely quick to do, a potentially toxic dye load and ionizing radiation is required. Although non-contrast MRA avoids the problems of the toxic dye and ionizing radiation, the above-mentioned disadvantages of investigating the critically ill patient in the MRI scanner make it less attractive for vascular imaging compared to CTA. Compared to catheter angiography, CTA and MRI can easily be combined with tissue imaging thereby obtaining structural images of the brain simultaneously with vascular images. On the contrary, catheter angiography enables immediate intervention (i.e. intra-arterial thrombolysis, stenting, etc.) in the same session.

Evoked potentials

Motor evoked potentials (MEPs), somatosensory evoked potentials (SEPs), and brainstem auditory evoked

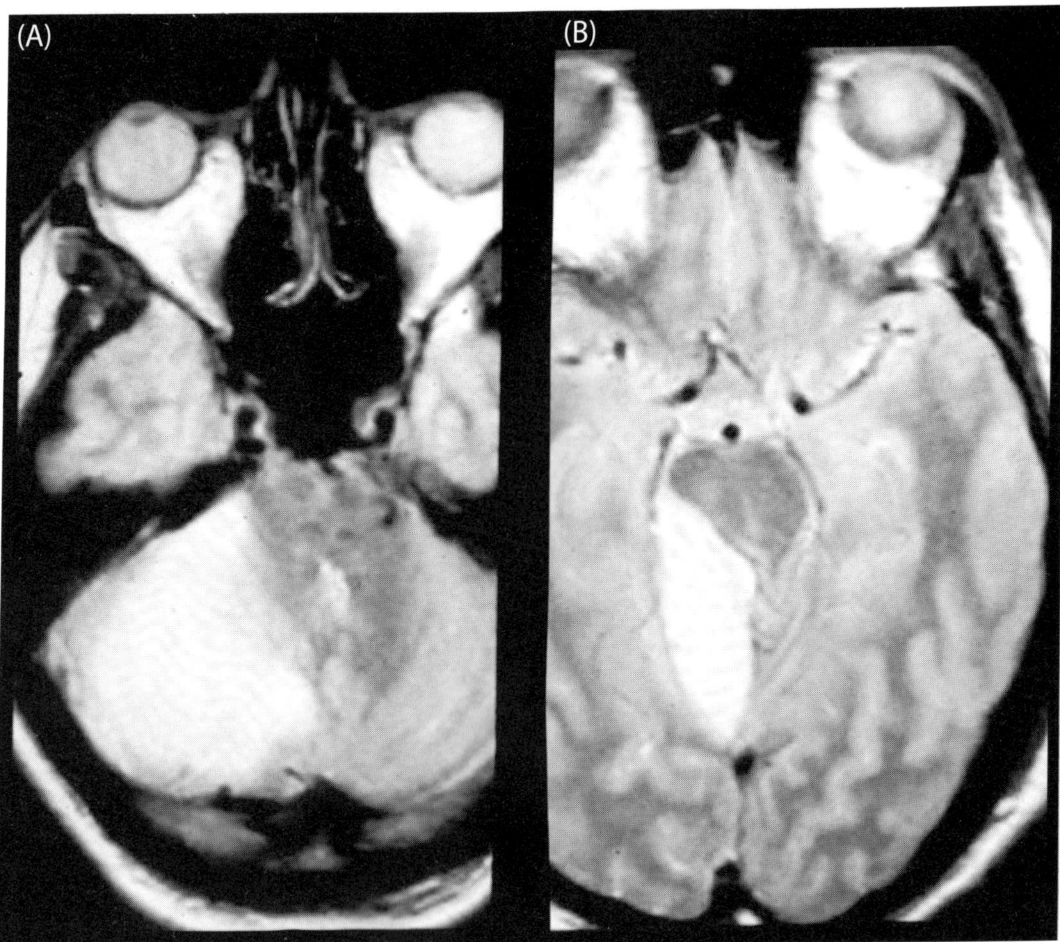

Fig. 17.3 MRI imaging of a patient with space-occupying right-hemispheric cerebellar infarction. (A) T2-imaging showing the extent of the infarct; (B) FLAIR-imaging, demonstrating compression of the pons.

potentials (BAEPs) are widely used in various neurological diseases. They might be helpful to detect additional brainstem lesions when combined. In patients with acute brainstem lesions, MEPs correlate with radiological findings, predict a persisting motor deficit more accurately than clinical findings, and are a reliable diagnostic tool for assessing motor function in otherwise unresponsive patients. In patients with basilar artery thrombosis and/or BAEP and SEP they are mostly abnormal and can indicate the location of the lesion, but may be normal in infarctions of the basis pontis. Furthermore, they have a prognostic value, providing information that cannot be obtained by neurological examination of the patient under sedative drugs [41,42].

Clinical course and outcome in space-occupying cerebellar stroke

It is unclear how many patients with cerebellar infarcts suffer from space-occupying edema. Data from the literature report space-occupying edema in

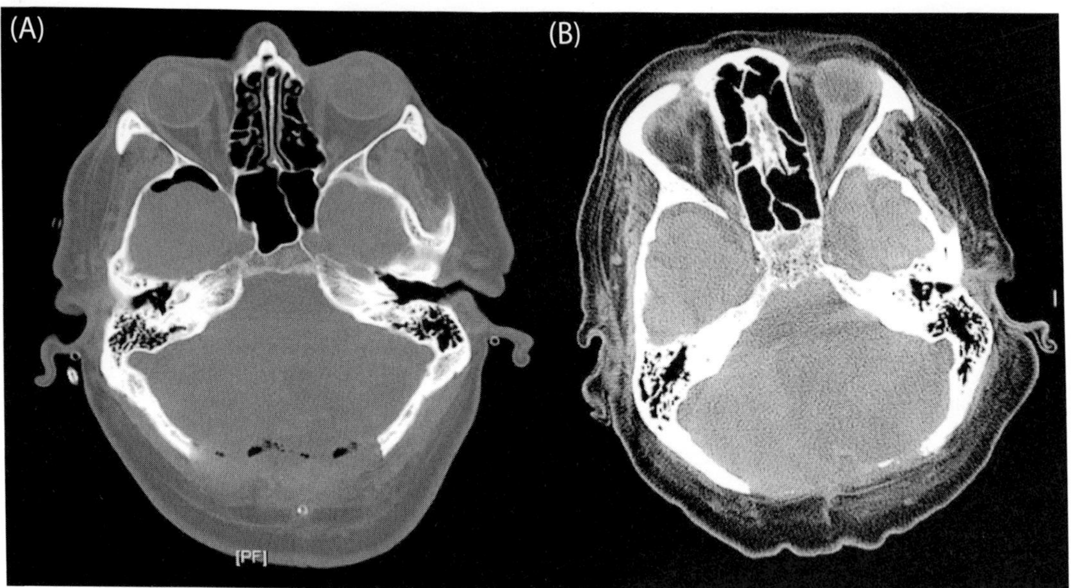

Fig. 17.4 CT imaging of a patient with right-hemispheric space-occupying cerebellar infarct after suboccipital decompressive craniectomy. (A) bone imaging; (B) parenchymal imaging.

17–54% of these patients. It is also unclear how many of those infarcts lead to brainstem compression or hydrocephalus and may thereby be life threatening.

The problem in space-occupying infarcts of the posterior fossa is not increased intracranial pressure, but tissue local shift leading to:

(1) Obstructive hydrocephalus due to the blockage of the fourth ventricle;
(2) Direct compression and damage of vital structures of the pons and midbrain;
(3) Restriction of local blood flow by compression of arterial vessels leading to or worsening blood supply and thereby causing or worsening brainstem and/or cerebellar ischemia.

All of this may eventually lead to:

(4) Upward herniation of the superior vermis cerebelli through the tentorial notch (rarely) and/or;
(5) Downward herniation of the cerebellar tonsils through the foramen magnum (frequently). [6–8,21,24,25].

Table 17.2 shows the typical clinical signs and symptoms of these complications and imaging features in space-occupying cerebellar stroke.

Even though neuroradiological examinations are widely available and serial CT or MRI scans can detect these complications, the course of the disease in individual patients is hard to predict because of large interindividual differences.

Conservative treatment

Alert and clinically stable patients should initially be treated conservatively and monitored closely [44]. However, there are currently no evidence-based conservative treatment options that are specific for cerebellar infarction. Guidelines for general conservative treatment are therefore derived from acute ischemic stroke in general. Baseline standard therapy including airway protection, adequate oxygenation, blood pressure management, management of blood glucose, body temperature, and prevention of deep venous thrombosis (DVT) and pulmonary embolism are at least as important as in an anterior circulation stroke and may even become more important in the subacute

Table 17.2 Typical clinical and radiological findings in space-occupying cerebellar stroke [15,17,42,43].

Common symptoms	Common focal signs	Common CT findings
Early stage (starting after 2 to 4, but up to 9 days after symptom onset)		
Headache	Ataxia	Cerebellar infarction
Vertigo	Dysarthria	+/– Early signs of hydrocephalus
Nausea	Nystagmus	+/– Narrowing of fourth ventricle
Vomiting	Blurred vision	
	Double vision	
Subacute stage (variable)		
Somnolence	Additional	Cerebellar infarction
Irritability	Cranial nerve palsies, including gaze palsy	Clear signs of hydrocephalus with widening of the third ventricle and lateral ventricles
Disorientation	Horner's syndrome	Compression of the fourth ventricle +/– brainstem compression
	Signs of the corticospinal tract	Narrowing of basal cisterns
Late stage (variable)		
Stupor	Additional	Cerebellar infarction
Coma	Tetra paresis	Pronounced hydrocephalus
Cardiovascular instability	Signs of decerebration with opisthotonus	Fourth ventricle not visible
	Pathological breathing patterns or apnea	Basal cisterns not visible
		Brainstem distortion

and late course of cerebellar stroke because of the comparatively high frequency of dysphagia and cardiorespiratory failure due to brainstem affection. Furthermore, an impaired level of consciousness is more frequent in the posterior circulation stroke and should be monitored very closely in these patients. Early neurological deterioration and decreased level of consciousness should always immediately prompt further vascular imaging and neuroimaging as described above.

Escalation of general conservative treatment includes mainly sedation and mechanical ventilation, intensive care of cardiac and circulatory function, and medical treatment of increased intracranial pressure. These treatment concepts are summarized in Table 17.3 [45–47].

It has to be kept in mind that all these conservative treatment concepts are based on a fairly low level of evidence. Randomized trials investigating conservative treatment options on space-occupying stroke are largely lacking, and trials on space-occupying cerebellar stroke as a specific stroke subtype do not exist [48,49]. Therefore, all these treatment concepts always have the character of recommendations rather than guidelines and need to be adapted to national guidelines, local clinical standards, and local circumstances.

Sedation and analgesia

In particular, ICU patients are exposed to various stress factors. Inadequate sedation can lead to increases in ICP and augmented metabolic rate and oxygen consumption. Of importance, sedation is never a substitute for adequate analgesia. Sedation and analgesia are the basis therapy in patients with elevated ICP and space-occupying infarcts.

Table 17.3 Medical therapy and conservative treatment strategies [45–47].

Elevation of head	Positioning of the head 15–30° guided by ICP (< 20 mmHg) and CPP (> 70 mmHg)
Sedation and analgesia	Sedation and analgesia is the basis of intracranial pressure-lowering therapy.
Intubation and ventilation	Intubation and mechanical ventilation is performed at a GCS of 8 or lower or respiratory insufficiency. It is used to prevent aspiration in case of altered consciousness or dysphagia. Early extubation is recommended.
ICP monitoring	ICP monitoring is essential to guide therapy. Intraventricular measurement via a ventricular drain is the gold standard. Intraparenchymal probes should be chosen over extraventricular drainage because of lower complication rates. Epidural problems have lowest complications rates, but at the same time measurement is subject to many artifacts.
Osmotherapy	Osmotherapy is the first choice conservative treatment of increased ICP. Mannitol (20 %), glycerol (10 %), hydroxyethylstarch (HES) (6%) and/or in addition hypertonic saline are available. No drug has proven superiority in randomized controlled trials. Regardless of the therapeutic regimen, it is vital to monitor serum electrolyte levels and osmolality closely while osmotic agents are used.
Hyperventilation	Not recommended generally, only if ICP cannot be controlled otherwise and more effective therapy (i.e. surgical intervention) is planned. Target $PaCO_2$ 30–35 mmHg, target venous PO_2 > 50%.
Buffer solutions	Not recommended generally, only if ICP cannot be controlled otherwise and more effective therapy (i.e. surgical intervention) is planned. Continuous TRIS infusion should be initiated only if the first application leads to significant ICP reduction.
Barbiturates	Should only be used as a therapy of last choice. Thiopental is recommended. Treatment effects must be monitored via EEG on the basis of the appearance of a burst-suppression pattern. Serum drug levels are not useful.

Pulmonary function and mechanical ventilation

Recommendations of airway management and ventilation do not differ from those in ischemic stroke in general. However, dysphagia and respiratory failure are especially frequent in patients with posterior circulation stroke. As soon as there are signs of aspiration pneumonia due to decreased level of consciousness or impaired central respiratory drive, neurogenic pulmonary edema, or in the case of impaired gag reflex, airway protection becomes mandatory and the indication for ventilation should be generous.

Conservative treatment of increased intracranial pressure

The main goal of increased ICP treatment is to minimize secondary ischemic insults and mechanical damage caused by tissue shifts and local compression of healthy brain tissue. Over the past years the focus has changed from a regimen that was purely ICP-oriented to one that aims to maintain CPP. In order to treat increased ICP adequately, it should also be monitored adequately by using an ICP probe. Treating increased ICP on the basis of clinical signs only is inadequate. Treatment options include osmotherapy, buffers, barbiturates, and hyperventilation.

Osmotherapy: Mannitol is currently the most commonly used osmotherapeutic agent for various causes of increased ICP. Available data suggest that mannitol can be effective in acute ICP crisis and thereby possibly bridge the time until further interventions can be initiated.

Glycerol is another frequently used osmotic agent. Theoretically, the risk of a rebound phenomenon is lower compared to mannitol, since glycerol can be metabolized by the brain. Although both agents are effective at lowering ICP, the duration of this effect is usually longer for glycerol. Therefore, it was often used as a basic regimen, whereas mannitol was rather used to counteract sudden increases in ICP. Most centers, however, have left this regimen of continuous or prophylactic application of osmotic substances because of the fear of accumulation in the necrotic tissue.

The effect of hypertonic saline solutions in the treatment of intracranial hypertension has mainly been documented after head trauma. The optimum concentration remains controversial. Multiple concentrations ranging from 3% to 23.4% have been used with different application schedules. Theoretically a combination of mannitol and hypertonic saline is reasonable, because mannitol may lead to hyponatremia, especially after repeated application. Side effects of hypertonic saline include severe hypernatremia, congestive heart failure, and pulmonary edema.

Regardless of the therapeutic regimen, it is vital to monitor serum electrolyte levels and osmolarity closely while osmotic agents are used.

Buffers: Trimethamine (TRIS buffer) leads to a reduction of ICP via vasoconstriction, subsequent decrease in intracranial blood volume, and thereby to a decrease in ICP. Continuous TRIS infusion should be initiated only if the first application leads to significant ICP reduction.

Barbiturates: The main effect of barbiturates is based on a decrease in cerebral metabolism and subsequent vasoconstriction. Because of several potential side effects including severe arterial hypotension, myocardial failure, electrolyte disturbances, impairment of liver function, and predisposition to infection, this treatment should only be used as a therapy of last choice or as a salvage maneuver when an abrupt increase in ICP requires immediate control until further measures can be undertaken. Application of barbiturates should be accompanied by invasive monitoring of MAP and frequent evaluations of serum electrolyte and liver enzyme levels. In neurocritical care units thiopental is mostly used. Barbiturate effects should be monitored via EEG on the basis of the appearance of a burst-suppression pattern. Serum drug levels are not useful.

Hyperventilation: Hyperventilation leads to reduction of arterial CO_2 which, again, causes vasoconstriction. This effect usually occurs within minutes of initiation of hyperventilation. Importantly, autoregulation is not intact in ischemic brain regions where brain arterioles are maximally dilated. Vasoconstriction is therefore limited to vessels supplying intact brain tissue, a feature that could theoretically lead to redistribution of blood (reverse steal phenomenon). It may therefore only be an option for short interventions to counteract sudden ICP increases.

Surgical treatment

In contrast to complex pathophysiological concepts of conservative and medical treatment, surgical therapy is based on mere mechanical reasoning. This includes suboccipital craniectomy or suboccipital decompressive surgery, with or without resection of necrotic tissue, or ventriculostomy, either by extraventricular drainage or by endoscopic third ventriculostomy.

Suboccipital decompressive craniectomy: The idea of external decompressive surgery (in case of space-occupying cerebellar infarction suboccipital decompressive craniectomy, SOD) is to give space for the swelling tissue to expand outside the bone gap and thereby avoid life-threatening compression of neighboring brain structures. There are many different surgical approaches: unilateral versus bilateral craniectomy, with versus without opening of the foramen magnum, with versus without resection of the atlantic arch, with versus without duraplasty, including different techniques of duraplasty. Some neurosurgeons also perform internal decompressive surgery, i.e. surgical removal of necrotic tissue – so-called strokeectomy – to create space within posterior fossa. Strokeectomy provides about 20 milliliters of additional space, depending on size of infarcted tissue. External and internal decompressive surgery are often combined. For further technical details see chapter 8.

Ventriculostomy: Insertion of an extraventricular drain (EVD) is a standard neurosurgical procedure that can be performed bedside. It allows continuous drainage of cerebrospinal fluid (CSF) and is usually indicated when signs of obstructive hydrocephalus are present, in the case of space-occupying cerebellar stroke due to compression of the fourth ventricle and the aqueduct. An alternative option for treating a non-communicating, obstructive hydrocephalus caused by cerebellar mass effect is endoscopic third ventriculostomy (ETV). In this procedure an opening is created in the floor of the third ventricle using an endoscope placed within the ventricular system through a burr hole. The endoscope is navigated through the foramen of Monro into the third ventricle. The floor of the third ventricle is bluntly perforated and the perforation may be enlarged by a balloon catheter to achieve an adequate fenestration size. This allows the CSF to flow directly to the basal cisterns, thereby shortcutting the obstruction [17,50]. It is performed far less frequently than insertion of an EVD. An advantage of ETV may be a lower infection rate as compared with EVD.

Treatment concepts

It is widely accepted among neurosurgeons and neurologists that surgical treatment is the treatment of choice and is superior to conservative measures in patients with space-occupying cerebellar infarcts. In contrast to surgical treatment in space-occupying supratentorial infarcts, surgical intervention in large cerebellar stroke is far less controversial. Most neurosurgeons and neurologists agree that when the procedure is life-saving, clinical outcomes are usually good, which is also reflected by current guidelines and recommendations [16,18,22,24,44,48,49,51]. However, when clinical and neuroimaging factors indicate a neurosurgical approach, which of these approaches should be chosen, whether they should be combined, the exact time point to start surgical treatment, or which factors should trigger which intervention remain unclear. Data on the clinical course and on long-term outcome are very limited. This lack of evidence for standardized, validated, and evidence-based treatment decisions based on reliable prognostic factors, both clinical and neuroradiological, which could guide decision-making is in contrast to the huge and long-standing clinical experience in the treatment of these patients. Major reasons for this are 1) that clinical signs indicating space-occupying mass effect are unspecific [7,15,22] and signs of brainstem involvement are seen in up to 74% of patients [14]. Differentiation between irreversible brainstem infarct and reversible brainstem compression cannot be made clinically. 2) Deterioration of level of consciousness, which is widely used to guide therapy, is not reliable either. It is extremely common in patients with cerebellar infarcts, with or without mass effect, but may have many different reasons, including brainstem compression, brainstem infarct, hydrocephalus, but also other complications such as infection, or side effects of medication [52–54]. This is why even comatose patients may have a chance of good recovery if the cause of deteriorating level of consciousness is reversible [15]. 3) None of the available treatment concepts and procedures has been adequately tested in larger controlled or randomized trials, including conservative treatment, ventriculostomy (either by EVD or EVT), suboccipital decompressive surgery, with or without strokeectomy, or various combinations of these.

Prognosis

First case reports of patients with space-occupying cerebellar infarcts have been published at the end of the 19th century. First reports on decompressive sugery in these patients have been published almost simultaneously by Lindgren and Fairburn and Oliver in 1956 [55,56]. Meanwhile more than 100 original publications are available, including more than 800 patients (see Table 17.4 and Table 17.5, and the reference list at the end of this chapter).

The German–Austrian Space-Occupying Cerebellar Infarction Study (GASCIS) published by Jauss *et al.* and the Tohoku Cerebellar Infarction Study Group are the only available prospective multicenter cohort studies [22,57]. In GASCIS, level of consciousness after clinical deterioration was the strongest predictor of poor outcome. Those patients who were awake/drowsy or somnolent/stuporous had a good functional outcome (mRS 0–2) in 86% or 76%, respectively, but also 47% of patients who were comatose before surgery. The study was not randomized and there was clear selection bias indicated by remarkable imbalances between the treatment groups. Mass effect on CT, lower cranial nerve

Table 17.4 Mortality in space-occupying cerebellar stroke according to treatment.

	All patients with space-occupying cerebellar infarcts (n, (%))		Conservative treatment (n, (%))		Suboccipital decompressive surgery (SOD) without EVD (n, (%))		SOD + EVD (n, (%))		EVD alone (n, (%))	
Survival	dead	survived	dead	survived	dead	survived	dead	survived	dead	survived
Total n = 673	195 (29.0)	478 (71.0)	84 (44.4)	105 (55.6)	27 (23.7)	87 (76.3)	26 (21.1)	97 (78.9)	27 (19.0)	115 (81.0)

involvement, and decreased level of consciousness were far more common in surgically- than in medically-treated patients. In addition, 22.2% of patients initially treated by ventriculostomy required decompressive surgery due to further deterioration.

The only available studies on long-term outcome including a considerable number of patients with a follow-up of at least 1 year were published simultaneously in 2009, including a total of 108 patients [9,10]. In these studies mean time to follow-up was 56.4 and 98.5 months, respectively. Long-term survival rate was 60%. Forty-five percent of survivors showed a favorable outcome (mRS score 0–1), 63% showed an independent outcome (mRS score 0–2). In contrast to the wide belief that prognosis in survivors of space-occupying cerebellar infarcts is usually good with the majority being independent, even in patients with very large cerebellar infarcts, initially comatose patients or those who show severe clinical brainstem signs and signs of herniation, these studies indicate that more than 3 years after the event less than one-third of patients show a favorable outcome, with about 40% being dead. In addition, a considerable number of patients show moderate or severe neurological deficits. Age and especially the presence of brainstem infarction could be identified as the most important independent prognostic factors (see Fig. 17.5). [9,10,14,15] Interestingly, insertion of an EVD, either alone or in combination with decompressive craniectomy, seemed to have no effect on survival or outcome [9,10].

Treatment algorithm

According to these data from the literature, decision-making in space-occupying cerebellar infarcts is much more difficult and controversial than current guidelines suggest. Most clinicians agree that alert and clinically stable patients should be treated conservatively and monitored closely [22,58]. Some believe that deterioration of consciousness is the strongest predictor for dangerous space-occupation and should be used for decision-making [53]. If it occurs due to mass effect, it usually rapidly progresses to coma, most often within less than 24 hours [15]. However, it is a common finding in about 34% of patients with cerebellar infarction and may have various causes others than mass effect [7]. Especially brainstem infarction is a common differential diagnosis, which would even be an argument against therapeutic escalation [10]. Again others believe that it is highly dangerous to base the decision to proceed to surgical intervention on clinical signs only, because they may occur too late to initiate intervention in time and recommend repeated neuroimaging to detect hydrocephalus and brainstem compression early enough, or even recommend preventive intervention, before these signs are present clinically or visible on CT or MRI [44,51,53,54]. They argue that the risk of EVD or craniectomy is fairly small and patients undergoing surgical intervention as an approach preceding hydrocephalus or brainstem compression tend to recover better than those undergoing emergency treatment after deterioration [22]. However, CT signs predicting deterioration and therefore triggering timely surgical treatment are controversial [51]. Although hydrocephalus, brainstem deformity, and basal cistern compression on CT or MRI seem to correlate with clinical deterioration, infarct volume and territorial distribution of infarcts are not different in patients who deteriorate and those who remain stable [59].

Table 17.5 Outcome in survivors of space-occupying cerebellar stroke according to treatment. No or mild disability: modified Rankin Scale (mRS) score 0 or 1, Glasgow Outcome Scale (GOS) score 5, or Barthel-Index (BI) score 90–100; moderate disability: mRS score 2 or 3, GOS score 4, BI score 65–85; severe disability: mRS score 4 or 5; GOS score 2 or 3; BI score ≤ 60.

	All patients with space-occupying cerebellar infarcts (n, (%))			Conservative treatment (n, (%))			Suboccipital decompressive surgery (SOD) without EVD (n, (%))			SOD + EVD (n, (%))			EVD alone (n, (%))		
Disability	no or mild	moderate	severe	no or mild	moderate	severe	no or mild	moderate	severe	no or mild	moderate	severe	no or mild	moderate	severe
Total	136	42	37	33	0	1	11 (44.0)	8	6	26	12	14	28	8	9
n=215	(63.3)	(19.5)	(17.2)	(97.1)	(0.0)	(2.9)		(32.0)	(24.0)	(50.0)	(23.1)	(26.9)	(62.2)	(17.8)	(20.0)

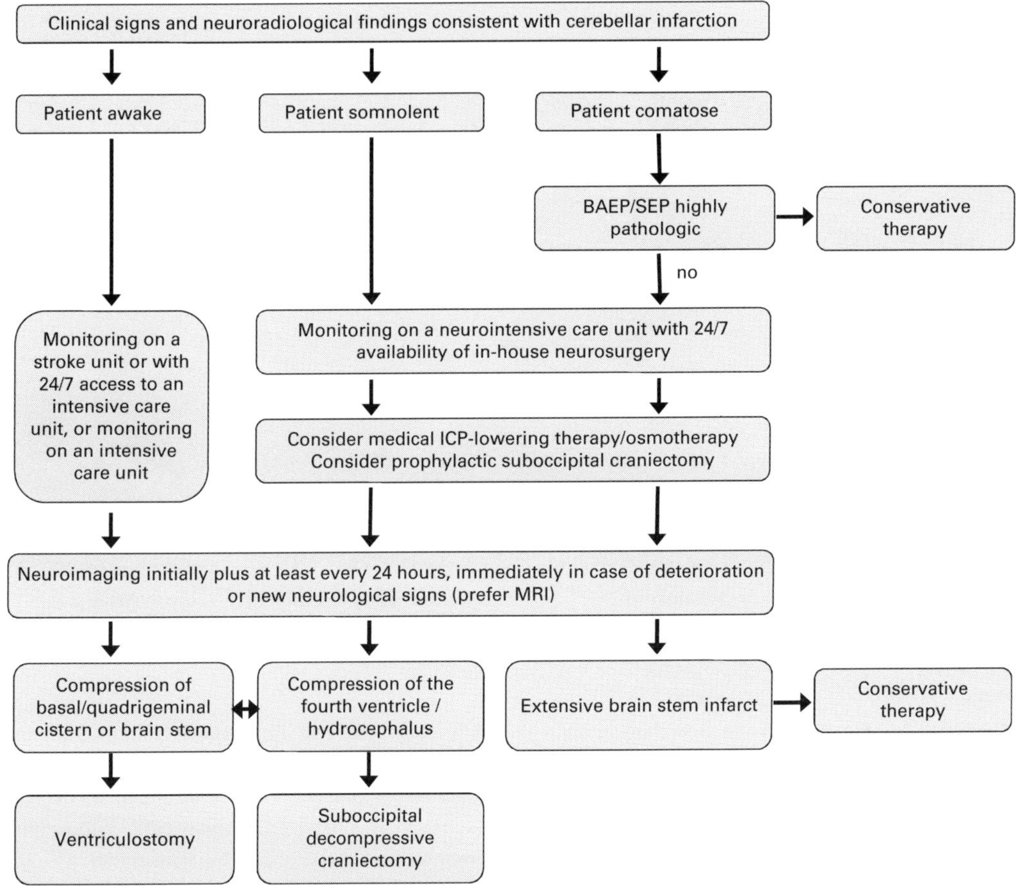

Fig. 17.5 Algorithm for decision-making in cerebellar infarct.

As for the treatment of choice, some authors recommend ventriculostomy as first choice and consider decompressive surgery only when there is further clinical deterioration [24,60]. The rationale is that deterioration of consciousness in most patients with space-occupying cerebellar stroke is primarily due to obstructive hydrocephalus [14,24]. Other authors, however, consider ventriculostomy alone as dangerous in these patients, firstly due to the risk of inducing upward herniation (whereas others consider this risk as overestimated) and secondly, because it does not undo brainstem compression, especially when mass effect is still increasing [43,61,62]. These authors favor suboccipital decompression as first choice treatment, some with additional resection of infarcted tissue [24]. Some of these authors consider suboccipital decompression alone as sufficient in most cases to resolve mass effect and all its complications, including hydrocephalus, while others recommend additional ventriculostomy is necessary when occlusive hydrocephalus is present [63].

In times of evidence-based treatment decisions the value of preventive SDC/EVD versus a 'wait and see strategy' should be evaluated in a randomized trial design.

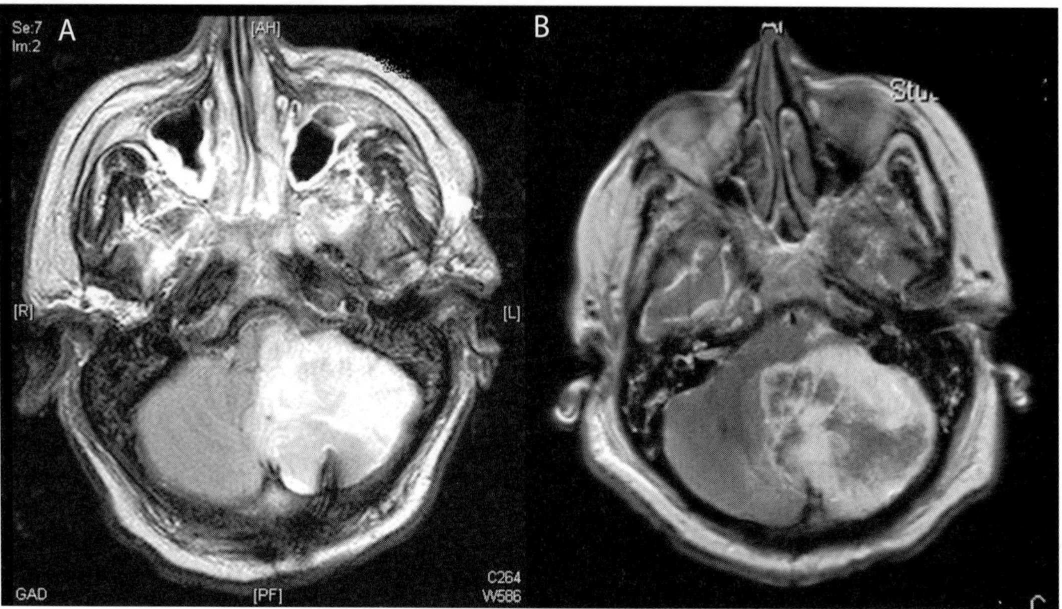

Fig. 17.6 MRI of a patient with left-hemispheric cerebellar infarct and extensive left brainstem infarct. A: FLAIR imaging; B: T2-weighted imaging.

Since these data are not available the flow chart in Fig. 17.5 may be useful for decision-making in everyday clinical practice.

Alert and clinically stable patients should be treated conservatively and monitored closely using GCS and NIHSS, always keeping in mind that they are limited in their predictive value and do not substitute experienced clinical neurological evaluation [24]. Initial monitoring on a stroke unit is possible if there is immediate access to intensive care facilities and neurosurgery. Otherwise transfer and monitoring on a neurointensive care unit is recommended. Because clinical signs of deterioration are unspecific and neuroradiological parameters are uncertain or may be detected too late, a multimodal monitoring approach is recommended, including neuroimaging at least every 24 hours and immediate imaging in case of neurological deterioration or new neurological deficits [22,44,51]. If available, MRI should be preferred over CT to detect the underlying pathology and verify or rule out co-existing brainstem infarction as well as whether other vessel territories are affected. Prophylactic osmotherapy can be considered if there is radiological evidence of edema, but is not generally recommended, because its efficacy is unproven. Prophylactic suboccipital decompressive surgery can be considered as early intervention, if 24/7 emergency intervention cannot be provided, but is also not generally recommended, because its efficacy is unproven and it may cause complications without being necessary.

In patients with impaired consciousness or those who deteriorate, if available and clinically practicable, MRI should be performed to detect brainstem infarction. In patients with extensive brainstem infarction cautious and rather conservative treatment is recommended (see Fig. 17.5). In patients without brainstem infarction further intervention is based on other neuroimaging findings. 1) If there is compression of the fourth ventricle and hydrocephalus is present, a ventriculostomy by extraventrciular drainage should be performed immediately. Additional suboccipital decompressive surgery should be considered in patients who do not improve or worsen after ventriculostomy. 2) In patients with signs of quadrigeminal cistern compression and/or compression of the brainstem immediate suboccipital decompressive surgery is recommended. If there are additional signs of hydrocephalus additional EVD is recommended.

In comatose patients MRI and BAEP/SEP should be performed to detect severe brainstem affection and rule out other pathologic findings. In those with extensive brainstem infarction or highly pathologic BAEP/SEP conservative treatment is recommended. If neither MRI nor BAEP is available, no general recommendation can be given. In patients without brainstem infarction and normal BAEP/SEP, decompressive surgery plus EVD should be performed immediately.

In all patients age and co-morbidities and previous patient wishes should guide the decision. Conservative treatment alone is associated with a high mortality rate of up to 80%. It should always be kept in mind that EVD has an infection rate of 1–2% per day, increasing beyond day four. Removal as early as possible is recommended. ETV may be an alternative.

REFERENCES

1. Kumral E, Kisabay A, Ataç C. Lesion patterns and etiology of ischemia in superior cerebellar artery territory infarcts. *Cerebrovasc Dis.* 2005;**19**:283–90.
2. Edlow JA, Newman-Toker DE, Savitz SI. Diagnosis and initial management of cerebellar infarction. *Lancet Neurol.* 2008;**7**:951–64.
3. Amarenco P, Lévy C, Cohen A, *et al.* Causes and mechanisms of territorial and nonterritorial cerebellar infarcts in 115 consecutive patients. *Stroke.* 1994;**25**:105–12.
4. Bogousslavsky J, Van Melle G, Regli F. The Lausanne stroke registry: Analysis of 1,000 consecutive patients with first stroke. *Stroke.* 1988;**19**:1083–92.
5. Caplan L, Chung C-S, Wityk R, *et al.* New England medical center posterior circulation stroke registry: I. Methods, data base, distribution of brain lesions, stroke mechanisms, and outcomes. *J Clin Neurol.* 2005;**1**:14–30.
6. Kase CS, Norrving B, Levine SR, *et al.* Cerebellar infarction. Clinical and anatomic observations in 66 cases. *Stroke.* 1993;**24**:76–83.
7. Tohgi H, Takahashi S, Chiba K, Hirata Y. Cerebellar infarction. Clinical and neuroimaging analysis in 293 patients. The Tohoku cerebellar infarction study group. *Stroke.* 1993;**24**:1697–701.
8. Macdonell RA, Kalnins RM, Donnan GA. Cerebellar infarction: Natural history, prognosis, and pathology. *Stroke.* 1987;**18**:849–55.
9. Juttler E, Schweickert S, Ringleb PA, *et al.* Long-term outcome after surgical treatment for space-occupying cerebellar infarction: Experience in 56 patients. *Stroke.* 2009;**40**:3060–6.
10. Pfefferkorn T, Eppinger U, Linn J, *et al.* Long-term outcome after suboccipital decompressive craniectomy for malignant cerebellar infarction. *Stroke.* 2009;**40**:3045–50.
11. Heuschmann PU, Di Carlo A, Bejot Y, *et al.* Incidence of stroke in Europe at the beginning of the 21st century. *Stroke.* 2009;**40**:1557–63.
12. Schievink WI. Spontaneous dissection of the carotid and vertebral arteries. *N Engl J Med.* 2001;**344**:898–906.
13. de Bray JM, Penisson-Besnier I, Dubas F, Emile J. Extracranial and intracranial vertebrobasilar dissections: Diagnosis and prognosis. *J Neurol Neurosurg Psychiatry.* 1997;**63**:46–51.
14. Mohsenipour I, Gabl M, Schutzhard E, Twerdy K. Suboccipital decompressive surgery in cerebellar infarction. *Zentralbl Neurochir.* 1999;**60**:68–73.
15. Hornig CR, Rust DS, Busse O, Jauss M, Laun A. Space-occupying cerebellar infarction. Clinical course and prognosis. *Stroke.* 1994;**25**:372–4.
16. Auer LM, Auer T, Sayama I. Indications for surgical treatment of cerebellar haemorrhage and infarction. *Acta Neurochir (Wien).* 1986;**79**:74–9.
17. Baldauf J, Oertel J, Gaab MR, Schroeder HWS. Endoscopic third ventriculostomy for occlusive hydrocephalus caused by cerebellar infarction. *Neurosurgery.* 2006;**59**:539–44.
18. Busse O. Therapie des raumfordernden kleinhirninfarktes. *Aktuelle Neurologie.* 1988;**15**:6–8.
19. Chen HJ, Lee TC, Wei CP. Treatment of cerebellar infarction by decompressive suboccipital craniectomy. *Stroke.* 1992;**23**:957–61.
20. Cuneo RA, Caronna JJ, Pitts L, Townsend J, Winestock DP. Upward transtentorial herniation: Seven cases and a literature review. *Arch Neurol.* 1979;**36**:618–23.
21. Heros RC. Surgical treatment of cerebellar infarction. *Stroke.* 1992;**23**:937–8.
22. Jauss M, Krieger D, Hornig C, Schramm J, Busse O. Surgical and medical management of patients with massive cerebellar infarctions: Results of the German-Austrian cerebellar infarction study. *J Neurol.* 1999;**246**:257–64.

23. Krieger D, Busse O, Schramm J, Ferbert A. German-Austrian space occupying cerebellar infarction study (GASCIS): Study design, methods, patient characteristics. The steering and protocol commission. *J Neurol.* 1992;**239**:183–5.
24. Raco A, Caroli E, Isidori A, Salvati M. Management of acute cerebellar infarction: One institution's experience. *Neurosurgery.* 2003;**53**:1061–5.
25. Shenkin HA, Zavala M. Cerebellar strokes: Mortality, surgical indications, and results of ventricular drainage. *Lancet.* 1982;**2**:429–32.
26. Kerber KA, Brown DL, Lisabeth LD, Smith MA, Morgenstern LB. Stroke among patients with dizziness, vertigo, and imbalance in the emergency department: A population-based study. *Stroke.* 2006;**37**:2484–7.
27. Norrving B, Magnusson M, Holtas S. Isolated acute vertigo in the elderly; vestibular or vascular disease? *Acta Neurol Scand.* 1995;**91**:43–8.
28. Kumral E, Bogousslavsky J, Van Melle G, Regli F, Pierre P. Headache at stroke onset: The Lausanne stroke registry. *J Neurol Neurosurg Psychiatry.* 1995;**58**:490–2.
29. Brott T, Adams HP, Olinger CP, *et al.* Measurements of acute cerebral infarction: A clinical examination scale. *Stroke.* 1989;**20**:864–70.
30. Teasdale G, Jennett B. Assessment of coma and impaired consciousness. A practical scale. *Lancet.* 1974;**2**:81–4.
31. Masdeu JC, Irimia P, Asenbaum S, *et al.* EFNS guideline on neuroimaging in acute stroke. Report of an EFNS task force. *Eur J Neurol.* 2006;**13**:1271–83.
32. Simmons Z, Biller J, Adams HP, Jr., Dunn V, Jacoby CG. Cerebellar infarction: Comparison of computed tomography and magnetic resonance imaging. *Ann Neurol.* 1986;**19**:291–3.
33. Mullins ME, Schaefer PW, Sorensen AG, *et al.* CT and conventional and diffusion-weighted MR imaging in acute stroke: Study in 691 patients at presentation to the emergency department. *Radiology.* 2002;**224**:353–60.
34. Chalela JA, Kidwell CS, Nentwich LM, *et al.* Magnetic resonance imaging and computed tomography in emergency assessment of patients with suspected acute stroke: A prospective comparison. *Lancet.* 2007;**369**:293–8.
35. Weisberg LA. Acute cerebellar hemorrhage and CT evidence of tight posterior fossa. *Neurology.* 1986;**36**:858–60.
36. Jauss M, Müffelmann B, Krieger D, Zeumer H, Busse O. A computed tomography score for assessment of mass effect in space-occupying cerebellar infarction. *J Neuroimaging.* 2001;**11**:268–71.
37. Fiebach JB, Schlamann M, Schellinger PD. [Diffusion and perfusion MR imaging in stroke]. *Radiologe.* 2005;**45**:412–14.
38. Cloud GC, Markus HS. Diagnosis and management of vertebral artery stenosis. *QJM.* 2003;**96**:27–54.
39. Puchner S, Haumer M, Rand T, *et al.* CTA in the detection and quantification of vertebral artery pathologies: A correlation with color Doppler sonography. *Neuroradiology.* 2007;**49**:645–50.
40. Bash S, Villablanca JP, Jahan R, *et al.* Intracranial vascular stenosis and occlusive disease: Evaluation with CT angiography, MR angiography, and digital subtraction angiography. *AJNR Am J Neuroradiol.* 2005;**26**:1012–21.
41. Krieger D, Adams HP, Rieke K, Hacke W. Monitoring therapeutic efficacy of decompressive craniotomy in space-occupying cerebellar infarcts using brain-stem auditory evoked potentials. *Electroencephalogr Clin Neurophysiol.* 1993;**88**:261–70.
42. Krieger D, Aschoff A. Evoked potentials before and following decompression craniotomy in space-occupying cerebellar infarct. *Nervenarzt.* 1989;**60**:36–9.
43. Kase CS, Wolf PA. Cerebellar infarction: Upward transtentorial herniation after ventriculostomy. *Stroke.* 1993;**24**:1096–8.
44. Busse O, Laun A, Agnoli AL. Obstructive hydrocephalus in cerebellar infarcts. *Fortschr Neurol Psychiatr.* 1984;**52**:164–71.
45. Jüttler E, Schellinger PD, Aschoff A, *et al.* Clinical review: Therapy for refractory intracranial hypertension in ischaemic stroke. *Critical care (London, England).* 2007;**11**:231.
46. Hofmeijer J, van der Worp HB, Kappelle LJ. Treatment of space-occupying cerebral infarction. *Crit Care Med.* 2003;**31**:617–25.
47. Bardutzky J, Schwab S. Antiedema therapy in ischemic stroke. *Stroke.* 2007;**38**:3084–94.
48. European Stroke Organisation (ESO) Executive Committee. Guidelines for management of ischaemic stroke and transient ischaemic attack. *Cerebrovasc Dis.* 2008;**25**:457–507.
49. Adams HP, Jr., del Zoppo G, Alberts MJ, *et al.* Guidelines for the early management of adults with ischemic stroke: A guideline from the American Heart Association/American Stroke Association Stroke Council, Clinical Cardiology Council, Cardiovascular Radiology and Intervention Council, and the atherosclerotic peripheral vascular disease and quality of care outcomes in research interdisciplinary working groups. *Circulation.* 2007;**115**: e478–534.

50. Yoshimura K, Kubo S, Nagashima M, *et al.* Occlusive hydrocephalus associated with cerebellar infarction treated with endoscopic third ventriculostomy: Report of 5 cases. *Minim Invasive Neurosurg.* 2007;**50**:270–2.
51. Mathew P, Teasdale G, Bannan A, Oluoch-Olunya D. Neurosurgical management of cerebellar haematoma and infarct. *J Neurol, Neurosurg Psychiatry.* 1995;**59**:287–92.
52. Hojer C, Beil C, Neveling M, Szelies B, Haupt WF. Diagnosis and prognosis of acute cerebellar infarcts. A retrospective study. *Nervenarzt.* 1990;**61**:482–90.
53. Langmayr JJ, Buchberger W, Reindl H. Cerebellar hemorrhage and cerebellar infarct: Retrospective study of 125 cases. *Wien Med Wochenschr.* 1993;**143**:131–3.
54. Kanis KB, Ropper AH, Adelman LS. Homolateral hemiparesis as an early sign of cerebellar mass effect. *Neurology.* 1994;**44**:2194–7.
55. Fairburn B, Oliver LC. Cerebellar softening; a surgical emergency. *Br Med J.* 1956;**1**:1335–6.
56. Lindgren SO. Infarctions simulating brain tumours in the posterior fossa. *J Neurosurg.* 1956;**13**:575–81.
57. Caplan LR, Wityk RJ, Glass TA, *et al.* New England medical center posterior circulation registry. *Ann Neurol.* 2004;**56**:389–98.
58. Jones HR, Millikan CH, Sandok BA. Temporal profile (clinical course) of acute vertebrobasilar system cerebral infarction. *Stroke.* 1980;**11**:173–7.
59. Koh MG, Phan TG, Atkinson JL, Wijdicks EF. Neuroimaging in deteriorating patients with cerebellar infarcts and mass effect. *Stroke.* 2000;**31**:2062–7.
60. Cioffi FA, Bernini FP, Punzo A, D'Avanzo R. Surgical management of acute cerebellar infarction. *Acta Neurochir (Wien).* 1985;**74**:105–12.
61. Tulyapronchote R, Malkoff MD, Selhorst JB, Gomez CR. Treatment of cerebellar infarction by decompression suboccipital craniectomy. *Stroke.* 1993;**24**:478–80.
62. Kudo H, Kawaguchi T, Minami H, *et al.* Controversy of surgical treatment for severe cerebellar infarction. *J Stroke Cerebrovasc Dis.* 2007;**16**:259–62.
63. Ho SU, Kim KS, Berenberg RA, Ho HT. Cerebellar infarction: A clinical and CT study. *Surgical Neurol.* 1981;**16**:350–2.

18

Rare specific causes of stroke

Alexander Beck, Philipp Gölitz, and Peter D. Schellinger

Introduction

The following chapter deals with rare causes of ischemic stroke. We present a selection of 'rare' causes of stroke that is obviously limited by the given size of this chapter. The authors chose therefore some diseases while leaving out others based on their own perception of potential clinical relevance in daily neuro-ICU business.

Stroke due to arterial vessel disease

Cervical artery dissections (CAD)

Dissections within the cervical region can be subdivided into vertebral artery dissections (VAD) and carotid artery dissections (CAD). Most dissections have been reported to occur in the internal carotid artery (ICAD).

The incidence of CAD is estimated at 2.6/100000/year (USA) and appears to be low, but in 25% of ischemic strokes in adults younger than 50 years old CAD is the underlying cause (1–3). ICAD occurs more frequently than VAD (1.7 versus 1.0/100000/year), multiple CADs are seen in 13–16% of cases (3–5). Depending on the reference the gender distribution is about 1:1 with a marginal trend towards men (53–57%) (5–8).

A dissection is a rupture in the vessel wall with blood accumulation in the intima, media or underneath the adventitia or a rupture of the vasa vasorum. Mostly, emboli, which have been formed at the torn site of the intima, cause a cerebral ischemia (4). The exact pathophysiology is still a matter of research; however, a relation between a vasculopathy and a concomitant artery abnormality is described in literature such as fibromuscular dysplasia (9), aortic root dilation (10), hyper-distensibility, and increased arterial stiffness (4,11,12). Monogenetic connective tissue disorders such as Ehlers-Danlos syndrome and Marfan's disease are reported but very rare (13); however, mild connective tissue changes have been shown in skin biopsies in a larger fraction of patients with dissections.

Environmental factors and trauma are also associated with dissections (14). Common causes are chiropractic manipulation (15), sport activities such as golf (16), whiplash injury, sudden neck movements, and severe coughing. These traumas are characterized by hyper-extension, rotation, extension or lateroversion of the neck (4,17). Furthermore non-penetrating and penetrating injuries cause ruptures of the arterial vessel wall (18).

Clinical features include Horner's syndrome, abnormal neck pain, headache, (caudal) cranial nerve palsy (19), and tinnitus may be present alone or in combination as local symptoms. CAD may induce ipsilateral cerebral ischemia with the typical focal neurological deficits. Isolated neck pain also has to be recognized as possibly the only symptom, preferentially in VAD but also in ICAD (4,20).

There are different tools to diagnose CAD. Firstly, T1-weighted axial cervical magnetic resonance images (MRI) with a fat-saturation technique show an excentric hypointense lumen with a semilunar mural hematoma.

Critical Care of the Stroke Patient, ed. Stefan Schwab, Daniel Hanley, and A. David Mendelow. Published by Cambridge University Press.

Additional signs such as flame-shaped occlusion or the string sign visualized on magnetic resonance angiography (MR-A) are typical findings in ICAD. However, in some patients a conventional digital subtraction angiography (DSA) may still be the diagnostic modality of choice (4,8). Secondly, computerized tomography (CT) and angiography (CT-A) provide an equivalent amount of information about CAD, while exposure to radiation has to be considered. In case of a contraindication or absence of an MRI a CT scan is recommended. In general, DSA as a diagnostic tool for ICAD is not the primary imaging modality, because of its invasiveness and difficulty to display the mural hematoma (4,21). Thirdly, color coded duplex and Doppler ultrasound can be used to detect CAD. This non-invasive technique, however, should be applied as a screening tool because of its interpersonal variance and possible difficulties assessing certain locations (skull base and transverse foramina) (22).

Ischemic stroke due to ICAD can be considered for intravenous thrombolysis within the 3-hour time window and considering the usual contraindications (23,24). In case of critical cerebral perfusion pressure (CPP) without embolic occlusions induced hypertension may be indicated at the ICU.

In the acute phase for CAD anticoagulation (2–3 times of base line prothrombin time) or antiplatelets are recommended whereas no high-quality data about superiority by randomized controlled trails (RCT) are available (25,26). The rate of intracranial hemorrhage (ICH) and recurrent ischemic stroke under anticoagulation or antiplatelet therapy is low (0.3–2%) (27). Subsequent oral anticoagulation (OAC) (INR 2–3) is recommended for 3–24 months. In case of full vessel recanalization the OAC can be discontinued. Recanalization (of stenosis and occlusion) rate after 6 months amounted up to 60%, whereas occlusions were less likely to recanalize. Beyond half a year the recanalization rate decreases (28).

Vasculitis/angitis

Vasculitis is responsible in 3–5% of strokes in adults younger than 50 years, therefore extensive laboratory screening for vasculitis in every stroke patient is not cost effective (29,30). The following immune mediated diseases affecting the vessels have an impact on the central nerve system in particular. An inflammatory vessel affecting the nervous system is called primary vasculitis (Table 18.1). If the vasculitis is part of a systemic disease and attacks amongst others the nerve system, it is called secondary (29). Depending on the affected vessel size the vasculitis is subdivided according to the Chapel-Hill criteria (31) (see Table 18.1). Note that syndromes may frequently overlap in symptoms and cause. A vessel lumen reduction can subsequently lead to hemodynamic and embolic strokes, arterial aneurysms may occur. In general, the consequence is a reduction and occlusion of the vessel lumen with a subsequent ischemic stroke. Currently therapeutic strategies have changed towards a steroid saving immunsuppressive medication with methotrexate, cyclophosphamide, or azathioprine in addition to as low dose as possible corticoids. The indication has to be checked individually and carefully but overall

Table 18.1 Selection of primary and secondary vasculitis.

Primary vasculitis	Secondary vasculitis
Primary angiitis of the CNS (PACNS)	Infectious vasculitis Virus, bacteria, fungi Malignancy Lymphoma Solid tumor Collagen vascular disorder SLE Sjögren syndrome Sclerodermia *Large vessel disease* i.e. Takayasu disease (TA)*, giant cell disease (GCA)* *Medium-sized vessel disease* i.e. polyarteritis nodosa (PAN), Kawasaki disease *Small vessel disease* i.e. Churg-Strauss*, Wegener's granulomatosis*

*granulomatous vasculitis

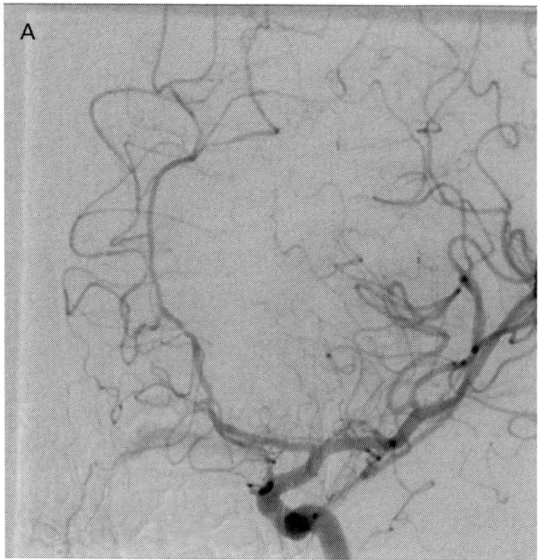

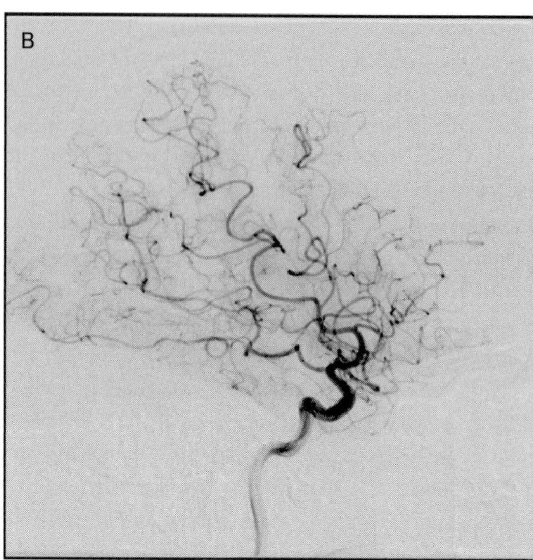

Fig. 18.1 Vasculitis: digital subtraction angiography. Visualization of left ICA after injection of contrast agent. Characteristic irregularities of vessel size of the ACA. Reticular collaterals due to distal vessel occlusion.

immunsuppressive therapy may reduce the demand of steroids (Fig. 18.1).

Primary vasculitis

Primary angiitis of the CNS (PACNS) is characterized by an affection of medium- and small-sized vessels preferentially leptomeningeal and parenchymatous arteries and veins (32). Middle-aged men of about 50 years old are twice as often affected as women (M:F = 2:1) (33). The clinical spectrum includes a subacute onset headache, cognitive and mnestic dysfunction, focal neurological deficits due to ischemic and hemorrhagic strokes, and epileptic seizures (29). Strokes and TIA occur in about 30–50% of patients, however, in less than 20% of patients at onset of disease or in absence of headache or encephalopathy (33,34). Multifocal and widespread ischemic formations with co-existing ischemic and hemorrhagic strokes in neuro-imaging may be indicative (35). In over 80%, imaging demonstrates unspecific alterations. Angiography may show sausage-like arteries and other characteristics of a vasculitis; however, it may be normal in up to 50% of cases (36). Laboratory work-up may show an increase of inflammatory parameters, cerebral spinal fluid (CSF) analysis may reveal a lymphomonocytic pleocytosis and an elevation of the CSF protein. Meningeal biopsy may be necessary for definite diagnosis. After that, therapy consists of either alone or in combination intravenous corticoid pulse therapy (e.g. 1 g/d methylprednisolone over 3 days) and oral methylprednisolone 1 mg/kg/d with or without cyclophosphamide 1 mg/kg/d (36).

Secondary vasculitis

Infectious diseases. A current retrospective study showed that 8.8% of their cohort suffered from ischemic stroke due to community-acquired bacterial meningitis (37). Known pathogens that cause brain infarction are: *Streptococcus pneumoniae* (38), *Neisseria meningitidis* (39), *Haemophilus influenzae* (40), and *Streptococcus aureus* (41). In good agreement with several studies *S. pneumoniae* is most frequently associated with ischemic stroke (37,42,43). Symptom onset with focal neurological deficits (compromised alertness, hemiparesis, cranial nerve paresis) is delayed in the second week of the course of disease. Adjunctive treatment with dexamethasone (before or with the first dose of antibiotics and for four consecutive days) reduced the unfavorable outcome from 25% to 15% in adults with meningitis without serious adverse effects, even with a borderline neurological benefit. Every patient with suspected or proven bacterial meningitis should receive 10 mg Dexamethasone four times a day for 4 days (44,45).

Neuro-tuberculosis presents as basal meningitis with headache, fever, basal cranial nerve palsy, and other possible neurological deficits. Pathogenetically there is a direct invasion of mycobacteria into small and medium-sized arterial walls at the skull base. Tubercle and inflammatory cells cumulate in the adventitia with proliferation of subendothelial cells. TIA or ischemic strokes are caused by subsequent stenosis.

The Herpes simplex virus 1 and 2 (HSV 1/2) and the Varizella-zoster-virus (VZV) belong to the family of herpesviridae with double-stranded DNA genome. After a primary infection the virus persists in the ganglia. A secondary reactivation is well known as Herpes zoster caused by an endogenous prior VZV infection. In the USA, about one million cases per year of Herpes zoster with an estimated lifetime attack rate of 30% has been reported (46). VZV vasculopathy induces ischemic strokes secondary to VZV infection without necessarily having a history of rash (47). The correct diagnosis is sometimes hard to distinguish because often arteriosclerotic pathologies and not virus induced damage is ostensible. Large vessel infarctions, with or without delay, are usually associated with zoster infections whereas VZV infection may trigger multifocal large and mainly small vessel infarctions, and affects both immune-competent and immune-incompetent patients (48). Signs of encephalopathy with headache (before, during or after stroke), eruptable vesicles and focal deficits may be present at clinical examination. CSF analysis shows mild lymphocytic pleocytosis, increased protein and the PCR is positive for virus (HSV or VZV) nucleic acid. Intravenous acyclovir in a dosage of 8 mg/kg every 8 hours is administered. Duration of acyclovir administration follows different protocols and ranges between 7 and 21 days. The use of corticosteroids as an adjunct treatment for HSE is controversial. However, when encephalitis is complicated by severe, vasogenic cerebral edema with neuroimaging evidence of midline shift, high-dose steroids (dexamethasone) may have a role in therapy (49). Seventy-five percent of patients treated with steroids and acyclovir compared to 66% with acyclovir alone improved or stabilized so that the combination might be a therapeutic option (47). This is currently evaluated in a German multicenter study (GACHE). Antiplatelets may be indicated.

CNS mycosis (aspergillosis, candidosis, coccidiomycosis, cryptococcosis, histoplasmosis, mukomycosis) are very rare causes of vasculitis with consecutive stroke.

Giant cell arteritis (GCA) or temporal arteritis is a necrotizing, granulomatous vasculitis affecting the aorta and its main branches (large vessel disease), in particular the temporal artery. The prevalence is 3–9% per 100000 patients, the incidence is estimated to be 20/100000 patients with a female:male ratio of 3:1 (29, 50). The average symptom onset is about 70 years, rarely before 50 years; almost exclusively the white race is affected, increasingly in the north rather than in the south of Europe and America (51). Headache, particularly, not only the affected side, but diffuse or otherwise localized, is the most frequent and initial symptom. Focal symptoms such as vision disturbance with amaurosis or diplopia are further serious signs due to retina or optic nerve ischemia. The American college of Rheumatology (ACR) also includes claudication of jaw or tongue, tenderness of temporal artery, ESR > 50 mm/h and temporal artery biopsy (performance < 48 h of first steroid treatment, low sensitivity) among the diagnostic criteria (52). Doppler sonography shows the affection of ACE and its branches (halo sign). Immediate and intravenous steroids in patients with severe ischemic symptoms (amaurosis) and corresponding diagnostic findings are indicated with 500–1000 mg/d i.v. for 5 days followed by a switch to oral dose of 1 mg/kg (53).

Takayasu arteritis (TA) is a granulomatous giant cell panarteritis that involves the aorta and its main branches preferring the proximal sections (large vessel disease). Predominately young females in their third and fourth decade are affected (54). The incidence in Asia is about 2.6 per million whereas in Europe and USA, TA is very rare (55). Characteristic symptoms and diagnostic findings are missing/different pulse or blood pressure differences, claudication, dizziness after lifting an upper extremity (subclavian steel syndrome), occlusion/stenosis of the aorta and its major branches, in particular the brain feeding arteries. Subsequent neurologic symptoms are syncope, vision disturbance, and other focal neurological deficits due to TIA or ischemic stroke. TIA or strokes, however, are rare (29). Diagnostic work-up includes the detection of angiographic and inflammatory (erythrocyte sedimentation rate, C-reactive protein and fever) abnormalities. Auto-antibodies are missing. The first therapeutic step is the use of steroids. Then, immunsuppressive medication, i.e. azathioprine, cyclophosphamide, and antiplatelet therapy are recommended.

Panarteritis nodosa is a necrotizing, non-granulomatous vasculitis, which is in 70% associated with HBsAg-positive hepatitis (56) (small vessel disease). The annual incidence is 1.6/1000000, the mean age of onset is 51 years (57). Only 40% of the symptoms are caused by an affection of the CNS. Besides headache, cognitive, mnestic, and visual (retinopathy) impairments, ischemic stroke with focal deficits occurs but is very rare. The diagnosis is secured by muscle-nerve biopsy or kidney biopsy. Treatment involves a high dose of steroids and immunsuppressive drugs (cyclophosphamide) (29).

Behcet's disease (BD) is named after a Turkish dermatologist Hulusi Behcet, who published his clinical triad of recurrent oral and genital ulcers and uveitis in 1937. The prevalence in Europe and the United States has been reported to be less than 1/100000 inhabitants and increases to 2.5/100000 in the north-western Mediterranean region. In Turkey the prevalence rates between 4 and 420/100000 (58,59). In general, BD is more present in the Middle East, in the basin and the Far East. Men are twice more often affected than women, age of manifestation is between 20 and 40 years. The pooled average of neurological involvement of BD was 9.4% (60), whereas symptom onset is delayed about 5 years after dermatologic manifestation. Clinical signs are those of cerebral venous thrombosis, meningoencephalitis with affection of brainstem or basal ganglia, headache, cognitive deficits, cranial nerve palsy, and hemiparesis. Ischemic stroke with according focal deficit is rare and is reported in only 1.5% of BD patients (60). Perivascular necrosis and meningeal infiltration may cause 'stroke-like episodes'. These parenchymatous lesions can be recognized in the MRI which is superior to CT scan (61). Laboratory work-up is unspecific. The typical history and clinical presentation make a histological back-up dispensable. Treatment consists of a combination of methylpredisolone (500–1000 mg for 5–7 days) and immunsuppressive medication (i.e. azathioprine).

Mechanisms of secondary vasculitis on the basis of an infectious disease remain complex (62). Different pathogenic agents may induce cerebral vasculitis and are considerable for ischemic stroke.

Moya Moya syndrome

Moya Moya syndrome (MMS) is characterized by progressive bilateral distal ICA and/or proximal intracranial stenosis or occlusion and a typical abnormal vasculature mainly at the brain basis (63). The typical angiographic appearance of the collateral vascular network is called 'puff of smoke' or in Japanese 'moya-moya' (64). In Europe MMS is very uncommon but in Asia, especially in Japan, the disorder predominately occurs in the first and the fourth decade of life. In childhood, patients mostly present with clinical symptoms of cerebral ischemic infarcts due to an occlusion of the cerebral vasculature. In adulthood the clinical manifestation of MMS is found by initial subarachnoidal hemorrhage due to a decompensation of a collateralization of the pathological vessel architecture. Either the MMS is idiopathic or is associated with trisomy 21, neurofibromatosis, arteriosclerosis or cranial irradiation (65). Nowadays the diagnosis can be made by MR-A showing diagnostic findings (66) or angiography. The conservative treatment comprises a daily medication with antiplatelets or the consideration of a neurosurgical revascularization procedure by bypassing the superficial temporal artery to the middle cerebral artery (65) (Fig. 18.2).

Fibromuscular dysplasia (FMD)

FMD is a non-inflammatory, non-artherosclerotic vasculopathy of the small- and medium-sized arteries. The second most common affection after the renal

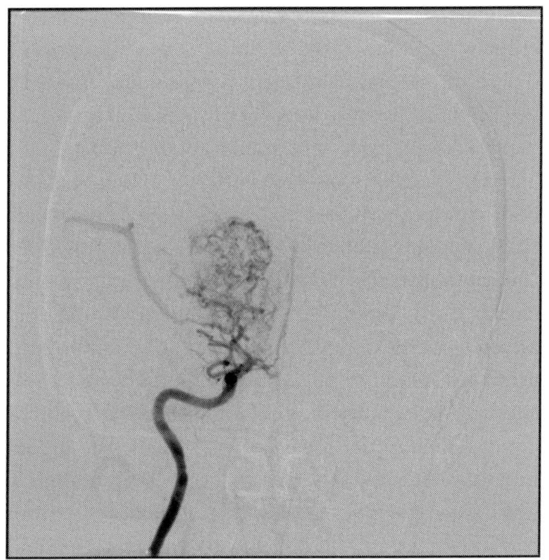

Fig. 18.2 Moya Moya disease: digital subtraction angiography. Visualization of left ICA after injection of contrast agent. Distal right ICA occlusion with characteristic appearance of the collateral vascular network.

arteries are the cervico-cranial vertebral artery and the internal carotid artery (1,67). The cause of the disease is currently not known. FMD is a risk factor for stenosis, dissections, aneurysms, and vessel ruptures. Diagnosis is secured by visualizing the 'string of beads' due to alternating section of stenosis and aneurysms in angiography (gold-standard) (68). Ischemic stroke is a frequent consequence of FMD. Antiplatelet medication is adequate for patients with cervico-cranial affection without symptoms. Patients with strokes may be considered for interventional procedures (69) (Fig. 18.3).

Vasospasm, vasoconstriction (primary, secondary)

Cerebral artery vasospasm occurs primarily in the *Call-Fleming syndrome* or in association with headache. Secondary vasospasms are due to SAH, unruptured intracranial aneurysm, traumatic brain injury and neurosurgery. Furthermore some medication and illicit drugs, malignancy, hypercalcemia, porphyria or eclampsia may cause arterial muscle contraction with subsequent ischemic strokes. Vasospasm is a diagnosis

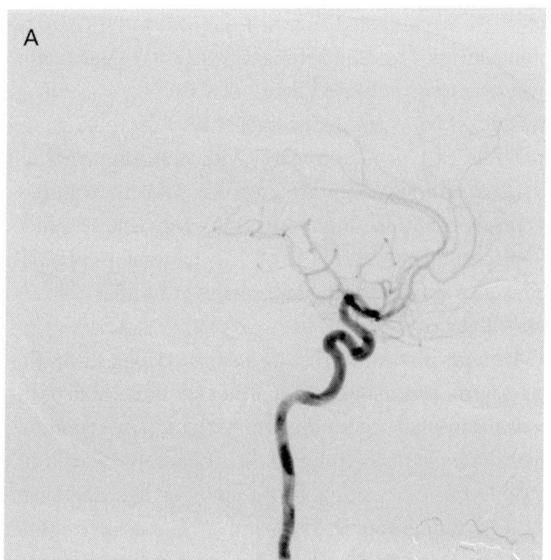

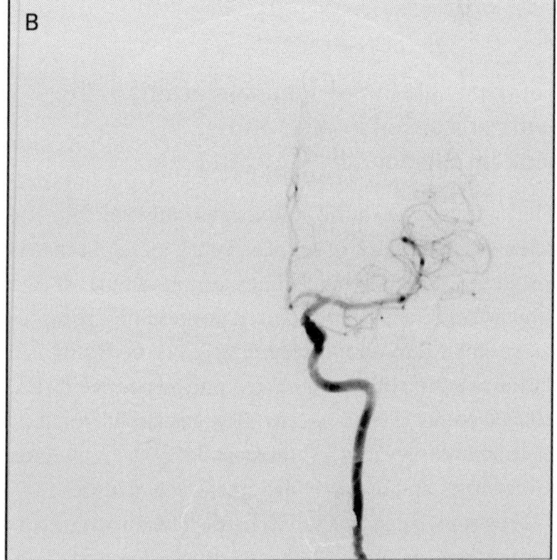

Fig. 18.3 Fibromuscular dysplasia: digital subtraction angiography. Visualization of left ICA after injection of contrast agent. Characteristic 'string of beads' at the distal part of left ICA.

of exclusion. Above all, a cerebrovascular disease such as embolism has to be excluded.

The Call-Fleming syndrome affects young women under labor or postpartum with peracute headache and nausea. Some days later patients may suffer from cortical blindness, Balint syndrome, flicker scotoma, disorientation, aphasia, apraxia, dysarthria, hemiparesis, deafness, and ataxia. Laboratory and CSF analysis are normal besides an elevated CSF protein. Cerebral neuro-imaging shows multiple ischemic infarcts predominately in the posterior vessels. Angiography shows at the brain base several vessel constrictions and dilations. Neurological deficits decline within days and weeks (70).

Vasospasms with headache (thunderclap headache, migraine with/without aura, exposure-induced headache) show many parallels in symptoms, clinical features, and course compared to the Call-Fleming syndrome. Currently it remains unclear if both diseases have the same entity or not; both clinical pictures are diagnosis by exclusion.

Secondary vasospasms occur in subarachnoid hemorrhage, bacterial meningitis, neurosurgical procedures, non-ruptured aneurysms, and pharmaceutical drugs (bromocrytine, ergotamine, lisurid, nasally applied ephedrine, phenyl-propanolamine, sumatriptane, intravenous immunoglobuline).

Cerebral autosomal dominant arteriopathy with subcortical infarcts and leukencephalopathy (CADASIL)

The acronym CADASIL was first introduced into the scientific literature in 1993. The small vessel disease is an autosomal-dominant inherited mutation of the Notch-3 gene on chromosome 19 expressing a receptor on vascular smooth muscle cells (71,72). CADASIL is a rare syndrome with an estimated prevalence of 1.98 per 100000 adults in Scotland (73). The exact epidemiology is unknown because of missing data, the emerging knowledge, and the variable screening of exons.

Frequent symptoms are ischemic subcortical recurrent strokes or TIAs (84%), subcortical dementia with cognitive impairment (progressive or stepwise, 31%), migraine with aura (22%), and mood disorders with depressions (20%). At a mean age of 49 years, ischemic events occur with pure motor or sensory syndrome, dysarthria, clumsy hand or atactic hemiparesis (74), yet the onset of migraine was at a mean age of 38 years. The mean age at death was 65 years (75).

Neuro-imaging, particularly MRI, reveals besides brain atrophy, lacunar, ischemic insults in the pons, basal ganglia, the anterior temporal lobe, and the subcortical (periventricular and deep white matter) parenchyma (74). Lumbar puncture and cerebral vessel screening show normal results. The diagnosis is confirmed by a skin biopsy to detect the mutation of the Notch-3 gene. Furthermore, immunostaining identifies the small affected arterioles with restriction of the lumen, vessel-wall thickening, abnormal muscle cells, and eosinophilia. A specific treatment has not been established yet. Apart from that, handling the common vascular risk factors (serum glucose, blood pressure, and nicotine) seems to improve the clinical course (74,76).

Fabry disease

Fabry disease or Fabry-Andersson disease is an X-linked lysosomal storage disorder caused by mutations in the α-galactosidase-A (α-GAL-A) gene, which encodes the α-galactosidase-A enzyme with according deficiencies. Prevalence ranges from 9 to 14 per 100000 whereas many cases of Fabry disease remain undiagnosed. Stroke prevalence in Fabry disease in young patients has been reported, with 4.9% in men and 2.4% in women. This accounts for 4% in a cohort of cryptogenic stroke in young adults between 18 and 55 years of age. About 1% of the general population presents with cryptogenic cerebrovascular disease showing a GAL-A deficiency (77–79).

Patients present with early onset ischemic stroke due to micro- and macroangiopathies, in particular in the vertebrobasilar artery system with the corresponding symptoms of nausea, dizziness, nystagmus, ataxia, and dysarthria. Correlating vessel changes like dolichoectatic pathology have been found (77). Another frequent diagnostic finding in patients with Fabry disease is proteinuria. Patients with the classic phenotype of Fabry disease usually present in childhood with pain crises, acroparesthesia, hypohidrosis, gastrointestinal symptoms, angiokeratoma, and corneal abnormalities. Severe morbidity and mortality follow in adult life due to renal failure, cardiac involvement, and stroke (78,80).

Diagnosis is secured by measurement of α-GAL-A activity in males and a gene screening in females. For females genetic testing is the method of choice because of the high risk of false-negative results (X-linked monogenetic disease).

Causal treatment is the intravenous substitution of the α-GAL-A. Glycosphingolipid accumulation decreases with better renal and myocardial function but a major impact of cerebrovascular complications has not been acknowledged yet. Appropriate antiplatelet therapy with clopidogrel or ASS/dipyramidole should be administered (77).

MELAS

Mitochondrial encephalomyopathy, lactacidosis, and stroke-like episodes (MELAS) syndrome is a mitochondrial, progressive disorder with a gene transition in nucleotide 3243. MELAS is a maternally-inherited disorder (mitochondrial DNA is transmitted maternally), with an estimated prevalence of 7.59/100000 in northeast England and 236/100000 in Australia (81). Proof of mutation secures the diagnosis by obtaining skeletal muscle biopsy.

Patients with MELAS develop stroke-like episodes with focal neurological deficit before the age of 40. The pathophysiology is not yet fully understood but it differs from the diagnostic findings in cerebral ischemia such as the character of edema (vasogenic (MELAS) vs. cytotoxic) or amount of blood (hyperemia (MELAS) vs. hypoemia) in the affected brain area. Further neurological symptoms are seizures, encephalopathy, dementia, and migraine headache.

Cerebral venous thrombosis (CVT)

Thrombosis of cerebral and dural veins may cause focal neurological deficits or a life-threatening elevation of intracranial pressure by swelling edema, ischemic stroke or intracranial hemorrhage. Particularly, the largest clinical multicenter study (the ISCVT-trail) showed that about 46% of CVT are associated with ischemic stroke (93). Establishing the diagnosis and consecutive therapy is tremendously important. Compared to the past, modern neuro-imaging, in particular MRI, has simplified the diagnosis. Due to a wide spectrum of symptoms early signs may be unspecific and still, CVT is frequently overlooked (Fig. 18.4).

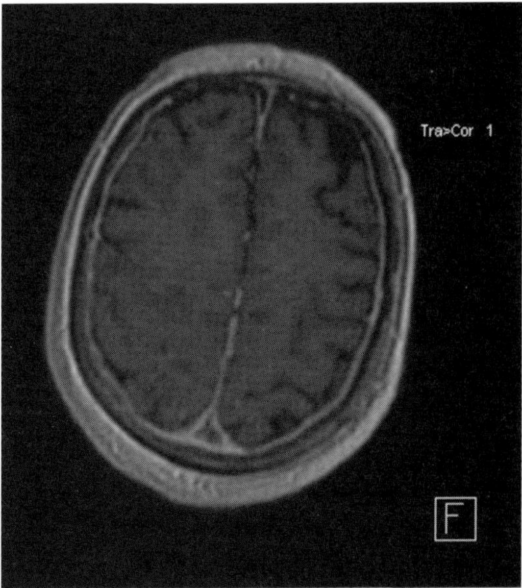

Fig. 18.4 Cerebral venous thrombosis: axial T1-post contrast agent sequence. Empty triangle sign.

CVT is an overall infrequent disease but not that uncommon among patients on specialized stroke and neurocritical-care units and may account for up to 0.5% of all strokes (82). There is an increased incidence of CVT in young female adults. The male to female ratio is 1:4 (83). Particularly young women between 20 and 35 years of age tend to develop a CVT due to their risk profile (pregnancy, puerperium, oral contraceptives, smoking). Peripartum and postpartum complications cause up to 12 CVTs in 100000 deliveries (84).

The typical complications of CVT are congestion with or without edema, venous (ischemic) infarction, bleeding, and more or less pronounced increase in intracranial pressure (ICP). An increase of cerebral blood volume with consecutively reduced perfusion pressure and also a decreased resorption of cerebral spinal fluid (CSF) due to the thrombosed sinus(es) may contribute to ICP increases (83,85–87).

Clinical symptoms are numerous; often they may mimic other neurological disorders. The most common symptoms alone or in combination are headache (90%), seizures (> 40%), focal neurological deficits (60%), reduced consciousness, and papilledema also depending on the location of the occlusion (82).

Especially in the context of known predisposing conditions awareness of CVT as a potential cause of these symptoms should be increased. If suspected, the first diagnostic step should be diagnostic imaging using a modality in keeping with the times, i.e. CT venography or MRI including T1, T2, FLAIR, T2*, and MR-venography (82,88). Before contemplating the diagnosis of CVT, careful evaluation of other sinus abnormalities or variations such as aplasia, hypoplasia, and paccioni-granulations (as opposed to floating thrombus) should be taken into account. Indirect signs to look for are the hyperdense sinus on plain CT and the empty triangle sign on contrast-enhanced CT scans. Hyperdensity is caused by thrombus (in analogy to the hyperdense middle cerebral artery sign) and the empty triangle by a dark clot in the confluens sinuum surrounded by contrast. Other imaging signs include atypical bleedings and hypodense edema. Especially, deep internal vein thrombosis with bithalamic edema or bleedings can be mistaken for basilar artery embolism with bilateral thalamic infarctions. Plain CT can hint towards, if not make the diagnosis in, up to 80% of patients, and this sensitivity is substantially increased by contrast enhancement. Multisequence MRI has a near 100% diagnostic accuracy (sensitivity and specificity).

Additional lab values may be helpful; however, measurement of d-dimers (< 500 ng/ml) despite its high negative predictive value in deep venous thrombosis (DVT), neither proves nor rules out CVT (89–92).

The largest study for CVT to date is the prospective multicenter observational (non-randomized) IVCST study (International Study on Cerebral Vein and Dural Sinus Thrombosis) with 624 patients. It showed that case fatality of CVT is not as high (less than 10%) as previously assumed, probably because of a lack of diagnosis of less severe forms in the past. The median delay of onset of symptoms to the diagnosis was 7 days (93). Death was most frequently caused by transtentorial herniation due to intractable ICP increase. The new appearance or worsening of an initially present focal deficit was associated with a poor outcome and increased mortality. On the other hand, nearly 80% of patients achieved an outcome of 0 or 1 points on the modified Rankin Score (mRS) over a median of 16 months. Recurrence rates of CVT appear to be as low as 5% (94).

In the following, treatment strategies have been established and have recently been published as guidelines for CVT by the EFNS in 2010 (95). Initially, patients with CVT should be treated with heparin after considering contraindications: either unfractioned intravenous heparin with at least twofold activated partial thromboplastin time or low molecular weight heparin (LMWH), body-weight adjusted (96,97). In uncomplicated CVT cases LMWH should be preferred due to increased mobility and less laboratory monitoring. The basic principle of anticoagulant therapy is the prevention of thrombus extension, the promotion of thrombus resolution, suppression of prothrombotic state, and the avoidance of pulmonary embolism with concomitant extracranial deep vein thrombosis. ICH due to CVT is, in general, no contraindication for heparin. However, deterioration or promotion of ICH (in 40–50% of patients with CVT (93)) may be reasons to discontinue anticoagulant therapy. Current data show that LMWH may be superior to unfractioned heparin in particular in patients with hemorrhage or ischemia due to CVT (Ferro, Bousser *et al.*, unpublished).

There is insufficient evidence from randomized controlled trials (RCTs) for treatment with intravenous or local intra-arterial thrombolysis. Severe cases with CVT at admission (i.e. comatose patients) can be treated with systemic, intra-arterial or endovascular (and subsequent thrombectomy) thrombolytics due to the high risk of death. However, the outcome is poor and is associated with a high morbidity and mortality (93,98,99). If a patient under adequate heparin therapy worsens, thrombolysis/thrombectomy may be a therapeutic option in selected cases and specialized centers, although patients with large infarcts and impending herniation may not benefit (95).

After acute antithrombotic treatment, an oral anticoagulation (OAC) with vitamin-K-antagonists should be administered. The international normalized ratio (INR) for therapy monitoring ranges between two and three. A definite duration of treatment with OAC has not been established yet. Analogous to a first incidence of extracerebral vein thrombosis patients should be treated with warfarin for 3 months if CVT was secondary to a transient risk factor. The duration of OAC extends from 6 to 12 months if the cause is idiopathic or due to 'mild' thrombophilia (heterozygous factor V Leiden, prothrombin G20210A mutation and high levels of factor VIII). Long-term administration is indicated if patients experienced two or more episodes of CVT or extracerebral vein thrombosis. 'Severe' thrombophilia (antithrombin, protein C or protein S deficiency, homozygous factor V Leiden or prothrombin G20210A mutation, antiphospholipid antibodies) also requires life-long OAC (95, 100). After discontinuation of OAC regular follow-up visits should be arranged.

Symptomatic treatment contains the medication of anti-epileptic drugs, control of ICP elevation, and control of pain (headache) and psychomotor agitation (95).

Prophylactic anti-epileptic medication appears reasonable albeit unproven in patients with focal neurological deficits and/or supratentorial lesions in CT or MRI scans. However, there is no recommendation for treatment duration (95).

Elevated intracranial pressure with threatened vision may profit from one or repeated lumbar punctures to obtain a normal closing pressure (95). In case of chronic (recurrent) increased intracranial pressure, shunting procedures may be a therapeutic option. Current data cannot support the administration of steroids (101). General principles of antiedema strategies may be useful, such as 30% head elevation, hyperventilation ($paCO_2$ of 30–35 mmHg), and hyperosmotic drugs (95).

Facing herniation due to extensive ICH and subsequent increased intracranial pressure, decompressive surgery turns out to be the last treatment option. Case series of hemicraniectomy after CVT showed a considerably good survival rate and clinical outcome with minor neurological deficits (102,103).

Due to modern neuro-imaging, advanced neurocritical care, and anticoagulant therapy, mortality of CVT improved from 30–50% to 8.3% and outcome could also be significantly improved (see above) (93). Poor outcome predictors are: older age (> 37 years old), male sex, initial presentation with coma, seizures, focal neurological deficits, ICH, posterior fossa lesions, cancer or infections (93,104).

Perioperative stroke

Ischemic stroke before, during, and after surgical procedures is a dreaded complication. Depending on the procedure the incidence is very variable. The risk of stroke is low in general surgery (0.08–0.7%) whereas in vascular and cardiac surgery, in particular combined procedures, the rate increases up to 9%. A neuroradiological study showed that after neurosurgical clipping one symptomatic ischemic event (2%) was detected whereas MRI lesions were seen in 9.8% (105). Post-interventional risk of symptomatic stroke after coiling procedures was up to 5.6%. Silent MRI-lesions afterwards were seen in 40–60% (106). The predominant perioperative ischemic stroke pattern is embolic with 62% compared to only 9% due to frank hypoperfusion (107). It is well studied that hypotension in carotid surgery with general anesthesia does not severely affect the cerebral perfusion (107). Changes in medication before surgery such as termination of antiplatelets or oral anticoagulation or statin therapy with its rebound phenomenon do moreover increase the risk of stroke prior to the first cut and during the perioperative period (108,109). Embolism is often attributed to postoperative atrial fibrillation, myocardial infarction, and hypercoagulability (surgical trauma, tissue injury, bed rest, dehydration) (110). Postoperative hypercoagulability causing an increased rate of strokes is seen more frequently in urgent surgeries compared to elective procedures (110). Hereby the risk of prolonged hospital stay, physical and mental disabilities, and the risk of death are increased.

Uncommon causes of perioperative stroke are fat embolism after orthopedic surgery or with polytrauma patients or air embolism after endoscopic procedures, intravascular interventions, and cardiopulmonary bypass. Furthermore abdominal aortic interventions may cause spinal infarcts (110).

A strong predictor for perioperative stroke is a history of previous stroke or TIA (111). Hence, the physician must take a detailed medical history of any vascular incidence, in particular within the last 6 months. Furthermore any cause of stroke should be identified and sufficiently treated before surgery. The vascular reserve is fragile in the first days after stroke, there should be a sufficient period of time after stroke and upcoming surgery in order to stabilize cardiovascular and neurological status (110). This does not hold true for some procedures such as carotid endarterectomy for symptomatic stenosis.

Perioperative discontinuation of OAK should be kept as short as possible. Bridging therapy with overlapping heparin treatment is recommended, especially in patients with high risk of thromboembolism.

During the postoperative stage any systolic dysfunction and arrhythmias are associated with an increased incidence of stroke (110,112). Blood pressure, acid-base status, electrolytes, glucose level, and heart rate should be closely monitored to directly detect signs of cardiorespiratory decompensation.

Intravenous administration of thrombolysis is not recommended after surgery due to an increased risk of bleeding. The risk of intracranial hemorrhage after t-PA occurs in 25% of patients; however, only 8% experienced a deterioration of symptoms (110). However, intra-arterial application of t-PA and endovascular treatment are a therapeutic option.

Stroke in pregnancy

The incidence of stroke in pregnancy is estimated between 34.2 per 100000 deliveries with an approximately threefold risk compared to non-pregnant women (113). It is a rare and feared complication and contributes to more than 12% of maternal death (114). However, the incidence of non-obstetric adverse events such as stroke has decreased because of better awareness of ischemic strokes. The risk of arterial occlusion is higher than stroke due to CVT. Ischemic events occur more often with 18 versus 8 hemorrhagic strokes per 100000 deliveries (115). Predominant pregnancy-related strokes are found at the end of pregnancy and post-partum (116).

The most important risk factors are age beyond 35 years old, black race, alcohol and substance abuse, electrolyte dysregulation, thrombophilia, multiple gestation, greater parity, and postpartum infection (113,114).

Pre-eclampsia consists of new onset of arterial hypertension (> 140/90 mmHg) and proteinuria (> 0.3 g/l protein in 24 h collection urine) after 20 weeks, gestation. Eclampsia presents with symptoms of pre-eclampsia and new onset of seizures (focal motoric seizures and grand mal seizures). Ischemic stroke, which is pregnancy-related, is associated with pre-eclampsia and eclampsia (25–45%) throughout the pregnancy and postpartum. Women with a history of pre-eclampsia are more likely to have a non-pregnancy-related stroke (116,117).

Diagnostic investigation should be performed as in non-pregnant patients. The underlying specific syndromes may be cerebral venous thrombosis with the occlusion of cerebral veins or sinus, SAH, postpartum cerebral angiopathy, paradoxical embolism, and peripartum cardiomyopathy. Each syndrome with its own clinical symptom complex and own field of therapeutic pathways has to be identified and appropriately treated.

As a diagnostic tool CT scans are not an option because of the ionizing radiation and the danger of fetal malformation, induction of cancer and growth and mental retardation. The imaging modality of choice is MRI. MR contrast agents easily cross the blood–placenta barrier. Therefore only in cases with great risk/benefit ratio gadolinium should be used (118).

Recent recommendations for treatment of CVT with subsequent ischemic stroke suggest a relatively safe administration of low-dose aspirin (80–100 mg) after the first trimester. However, an increased rate of still birth has been reported (119). Warfarin is contraindicated in the first trimenon due to teratogenicity, and there is a relative contraindication around delivery because of difficulty to control INR. Dose-adjusted unfractioned heparin throughout the entire pregnancy can be administered. It does not pass the blood–placenta barrier. LWMH with factor Xa-monitoring is also an option (114,120). Osteoporosis with constant application has to be mentioned. Bleeding with heparin occurs in up to 10%, the possibility of heparin-induced thrombosis and thrombocytopenia needs to be considered. Practically with an increased risk of stroke the physician can administer low-dose heparin in the first trimester and peripartum. For the second and third trimenon anticoagulation can be adjusted to aspirin because long-term use of heparin may cause osteoporosis. Benefit and risk must be well balanced.

IV thrombolysis with t-PA is well established in ischemic stroke. No data from randomized trials exist or guidelines for treatment are available for t-PA in pregnancy. There are only case reports and cases concerning thrombolysis in pregnant women. Potential risks are pre-term labor, placental abruption, fetal death, postpartum hemorrhage, and possible teratogenicity (114). About 50% of patients with pregnancy-related stroke survive with residual neurological deficit (121). An individual consideration of thrombolytics in certain patients is possible; however, a general recommendation about the administration of t-PA cannot be provided due to the lack of evidence.

Spinal cord infarction

Epidemiological data about spinal cord infarction is rare but estimates suggest an incidental rate of 1% of all strokes (122). Perioperative spinal infarction was excluded as the most common cause during major surgery, therefore the incidence may be underestimated. Typically adults are affected but patients of any age can develop spinal infarction.

Several etiologies lead to a spinal cord infarction. Diseases and manipulations at the aorta such as aortic dissection and aortic surgery are most common. Furthermore abdominal surgery (i.e. hepatectomy, cesarean section, bowel resection, spine surgery), systemic hypotension (i.e. after cardiac arrest, major bleeding) have been reported. Some cases describe a vascular malformation. In 44–74% the cause remains idiopathic (123). Vascular risk factors, such as arteriosclerosis and microangiopathic changes are discussed.

Clinical presentation contains rapid onset of para- or tetraparesis in combination with or without sensory deficits (anterior and/or posterior spinal artery). MRI is the preferred imaging modality.

Specific treatment is limited. Infarction between C1–C5 may cause dangerous dysrhythmia, blood pressure fluctuation or other vegetative dysregulation due to the disconnection of the autonomic tracts and nuclei in the spinal cord. Patients with paraparesis should be administered with LWMH for thrombosis prophylaxis.

In case series a few patients make improvements with independent gait but about half of affected patients remain wheelchair bound (124). Poor prognostic factors are: severe impairment at presentation, female sex, older age, and lack of improvement within 24 hours (124).

Hematologic disorders

Procoagulatory states or genetically determined thrombophilia, particularly in patients of young age, may cause first time and repetitive ischemic strokes. Often, younger patients already have the diagnosis of coagulopathy with adequate anticoagulation therapy when they present with re-stroke. Here, diagnostic effort should be made to rule out paradoxical emboli. The scientific data are, however, heterogeneous. Some suggest an association between thrombophilia and right to left shunt in stroke patients, others limit the combination to prothrombin gene mutation and paradoxical embolism in stroke patients (125,126). Studies did not find an association between factor V Leiden and stroke (regardless of age) (127). The prothrombin-G20210A-mutation (factor II) implies an increased risk of ischemic strokes in younger patients (128). Currently no conclusive evidence exists that inherited thrombophilias are associated with arterial thromboembolism (129). Despite conflicting data the relative effect of thrombophila is strong in the young who lack the usual risk factors leading to stroke.

Procoagulatory states can be distinguished between (1) deficiency of coagulation factors or (2) increased activation/quantity of coagulation factors, and (3) other states. Ad (1): AT-III-deficiency, APC-resistance, protein-S deficiency, plasminogen, plasminogenactivator;

Ad (2): coagulation factor overexpression (factor V and VIII), hyperfibrinogemia, paraproteinemia, cryoglobulinemia, prothrombin-G20210A-mutation;

Ad (3): malignancy associated procoagulatory states (multiple myeloma, Waldenström disease), immunologic prothrombotic states, antiphospholipid antibody syndrome (APS), Sneddon syndrome, thrombotic thrombocytopenic purpura (TTP).

The most common inherited risk factor for thrombophilia is the **factor V Leiden** point mutation. The mutated factor V cannot be inactivated by activated protein C (APC) which leads to **APC resistance** and subsequent thrombophilia. Diagnostic test of choice is a DNA sequence using PCR. Treatment is oral anticoagulation.

The **antiphospholipid syndrome** (APS) is an acquired thrombophilic autoimmune condition. Heterogeneous antiphospholipid antibodies are present which are directed against phospholipid binding proteins. Arterial and venous thrombosis are common with obstetric adverse events. Neurological manifestations are CVT, ischemic stroke, and neuropsychiatric and movement disorders. Lupus anticoagulant, anticardiolipin, and anti-b2GP-1 ELISAs are important diagnostic tests whereas the lupus anticoagulant is the strongest predictor for APS (130). Oral anticoagulation is the best treatment option for new onset or recurrent stroke.

The **prothrombin-G20210A-mutation** (factor II) is a congenital risk factor for ischemic stroke with a 3.8-fold risk for heterogeneous genotypes and estimated 208-fold increased risk for homozygous genotypes (128). The diagnostic test is the evidence of the mutant-II-allele. Treatment of choice is oral anticoagulation.

Illicit drugs

Cocaine and its alkaloid derivate 'crack', methamphetamines, LSD, and diacetylmorphine (heroine) induce an increase of blood pressure, narrowing of blood vessels, vasospasm, vasculitis, and an interaction with coagulation factors. This may result in ischemic or hemorrhagic stroke, or both.

REFERENCES

1. Kuhlencordt PJ, Roling J, Hoffmann U. Cerebrovascular diseases. *Internist* (Berl). 2009;**50**(8):945–51.
2. Leys D, Bandu L, Henon H, *et al.* Clinical outcome in 287 consecutive young adults (15 to 45 years) with ischemic stroke. *Neurology.* 2002;**59**(1):26–33.
3. Lee VH, Brown RD, Jr., Mandrekar JN, Mokri B. Incidence and outcome of cervical artery dissection: a population-based study. *Neurology.* 2006;**67**(10):1809–12.
4. Debette S, Leys D. Cervical-artery dissections: predisposing factors, diagnosis, and outcome. *Lancet Neurol.* 2009;**8**(7):668–78.
5. Touze E, Gauvrit JY, Moulin T, *et al.* Risk of stroke and recurrent dissection after a cervical artery dissection: a multicenter study. *Neurology.* 2003;**61**(10):1347–51.
6. Beletsky V, Nadareishvili Z, Lynch J, *et al.* Cervical arterial dissection: time for a therapeutic trial? *Stroke.* 2003;**34**(12):2856–60.
7. Schievink WI, Mokri B, O'Fallon WM. Recurrent spontaneous cervical-artery dissection. *N Engl J Med.* 1994;**330**(6):393–7.
8. Arnold M, Kappeler L, Georgiadis D, *et al.* Gender differences in spontaneous cervical artery dissection. *Neurology.* 2006;**67**(6):1050–2.
9. de Bray JM, Marc G, Pautot V, *et al.* Fibromuscular dysplasia may herald symptomatic recurrence of cervical artery dissection. *Cerebrovasc Dis.* 2007;**23**(5–6):448–52.
10. Tzourio C, Cohen A, Lamisse N, Biousse V, Bousser MG. Aortic root dilatation in patients with spontaneous cervical artery dissection. *Circulation.* 1997;**95**(10):2351–3.
11. Guillon B, Tzourio C, Biousse V, *et al.* Arterial wall properties in carotid artery dissection: an ultrasound study. *Neurology.* 2000;**55**(5):663–6.
12. Calvet D, Boutouyrie P, Touze E, *et al.* Increased stiffness of the carotid wall material in patients with spontaneous cervical artery dissection. *Stroke.* 2004;**35**(9):2078–82.
13. Grond-Ginsbach C, Debette S. The association of connective tissue disorders with cervical artery dissections. *Curr Mol Med.* 2009;**9**(2):210–14.
14. Dittrich R, Rohsbach D, Heidbreder A, *et al.* Mild mechanical traumas are possible risk factors for cervical artery dissection. *Cerebrovasc Dis.* 2007;**23**(4):275–81.
15. Ernst E. Adverse effects of spinal manipulation: a systematic review. *J R Soc Med.* 2007;**100**(7):330–8.
16. Maroon JC, Gardner P, Abla AA, El-Kadi H, Bost J. 'Golfer's stroke': golf-induced stroke from vertebral artery dissection. *Surg Neurol.* 2007;**67**(2):163–8; discussion 168.

17. Caso V, Paciaroni M, Bogousslavsky J. Environmental factors and cervical artery dissection. *Front Neurol Neurosci.* 2005;**20**:44–53.
18. Biffl WL, Ray CE, Jr., Moore EE, *et al.* Treatment-related outcomes from blunt cerebrovascular injuries: importance of routine follow-up arteriography. *Ann Surg.* 2002;**235**(5):699–706.
19. Sturzenegger M, Huber P. Cranial nerve palsies in spontaneous carotid artery dissection. *J Neurol Neurosurg Psychiatry.* 1993;**56**(11):1191–9.
20. Arnold M, Cumurciuc R, Stapf C, *et al.* Pain as the only symptom of cervical artery dissection. *J Neurol Neurosurg Psychiatry.* 2006;**77**(9):1021–4.
21. Guidelines for management of ischaemic stroke and transient ischaemic attack 2008. *Cerebrovasc Dis.* 2008;**25**(5):457–507.
22. Provenzale JM. MRI and MRA for evaluation of dissection of craniocerebral arteries: lessons from the medical literature. *Emerg Radiol.* 2009;**16**(3):185–93.
23. Georgiadis D, Lanczik O, Schwab S, *et al.* IV thrombolysis in patients with acute stroke due to spontaneous carotid dissection. *Neurology.* 2005;**64**(9):1612–14.
24. Arnold M, Nedeltchev K, Sturzenegger M, *et al.* Thrombolysis in patients with acute stroke caused by cervical artery dissection: analysis of 9 patients and review of the literature. *Arch Neurol.* 2002;**59**(4):549–53.
25. Metso TM, Metso AJ, Helenius J, *et al.* Prognosis and safety of anticoagulation in intracranial artery dissections in adults. *Stroke.* 2007;**38**(6):1837–42.
26. Engelter ST, Brandt T, Debette S, *et al.* Antiplatelets versus anticoagulation in cervical artery dissection. *Stroke.* 2007;**38**(9):2605–11.
27. Georgiadis D, Arnold M, von Buedingen HC, *et al.* Aspirin vs anticoagulation in carotid artery dissection: a study of 298 patients. *Neurology.* 2009;**72**(21):1810–15.
28. Nedeltchev K, Bickel S, Arnold M, *et al.* R2-recanalization of spontaneous carotid artery dissection. *Stroke.* 2009;**40**(2):499–504.
29. Ferro JM. Vasculitis of the central nervous system. *J Neurol.* 1998;**245**(12):766–76.
30. Montalban J, Rio J, Khamastha M, *et al.* Value of immunologic testing in stroke patients. A prospective multicenter study. *Stroke.* 1994;**25**(12):2412–15.
31. Jennette JC, Falk RJ, Andrassy K, *et al.* Nomenclature of systemic vasculitides. Proposal of an international consensus conference. *Arthritis Rheum.* 1994;**37**(2):187–92.
32. Cravioto H, Feigin I. Noninfectious granulomatous angiitis with a predilection for the nervous system. *Neurology.* 1959;**9**:599–609.
33. Birnbaum J, Hellmann DB. Primary angiitis of the central nervous system. *Arch Neurol.* 2009;**66**(6):704–9.
34. Salvarani C, Brown RD, Jr., Calamia KT, *et al.* Primary central nervous system vasculitis: analysis of 101 patients. *Ann Neurol.* 2007;**62**(5):442–51.
35. Ay H, Sahin G, Saatci I, Soylemezoglu F, Saribas O. Primary angiitis of the central nervous system and silent cortical hemorrhages. *AJNR Am J Neuroradiol.* 2002;**23**(9):1561–3.
36. Alhalabi M, Moore PM. Serial angiography in isolated angiitis of the central nervous system. *Neurology.* 1994;**44**(7):1221–6.
37. Katchanov J, Heuschmann PU, Endres M, Weber JR. Cerebral infarction in bacterial meningitis: predictive factors and outcome. *J Neurol.* 2010;**257**(5):716–20.
38. Kastenbauer S, Pfister HW. Pneumococcal meningitis in adults: spectrum of complications and prognostic factors in a series of 87 cases. *Brain.* 2003;126(Pt 5):1015–25.
39. van de Beek D, Patel R, Wijdicks EF. Meningococcal meningitis with brainstem infarction. *Arch Neurol.* 2007;**64**(9):1350–1.
40. Igarashi M, Gilmartin RC, Gerald B, Wilburn F, Jabbour JT. Cerebral arteritis and bacterial meningitis. *Arch Neurol.* 1984;**41**(5):531–5.
41. Bentley P, Qadri F, Wild EJ, Hirsch NP, Howard RS. Vasculitic presentation of staphylococcal meningitis. *Arch Neurol.* 2007;**64**(12):1788–9.
42. Pfister HW, Borasio GD, Dirnagl U, Bauer M, Einhaupl KM. Cerebrovascular complications of bacterial meningitis in adults. *Neurology.* 1992;**42**(8):1497–504.
43. Pfister HW, Feiden W, Einhaupl KM. Spectrum of complications during bacterial meningitis in adults. Results of a prospective clinical study. *Arch Neurol.* 1993;**50**(6):575–81.
44. van de Beek D. Corticosteroids for acute adult bacterial meningitis. *Med Mal Infect.* 2009;**39**(7–8):531–8.
45. de Gans J, van de Beek D. Dexamethasone in adults with bacterial meningitis. *N Engl J Med.* 2002;**347**(20):1549–56.
46. Oxman MN, Levin MJ. Vaccination against herpes zoster and postherpetic neuralgia. *J Infect Dis.* 2008;**197** Suppl 2: S228–36.
47. Nagel MA, Cohrs RJ, Mahalingam R, *et al.* The varicella zoster virus vasculopathies: clinical, CSF, imaging, and virologic features. *Neurology.* 2008;**70**(11):853–60.
48. Gilden D, Cohrs RJ, Mahalingam R, Nagel MA. Varicella zoster virus vasculopathies: diverse clinical manifestations, laboratory features, pathogenesis, and treatment. *Lancet Neurol.* 2009;**8**(8):731–40.
49. Steiner I, Kennedy PG, Pachner AR. The neurotropic herpes viruses: herpes simplex and varicella-zoster. *Lancet Neurol.* 2007;**6**(11):1015–28.

50. Machado EB, Michet CJ, Ballard DJ, *et al.* Trends in incidence and clinical presentation of temporal arteritis in Olmsted County, Minnesota, 1950–85. *Arthritis Rheum.* 1988;**31**(6):745–9.
51. Tanganelli P. Secondary headaches in the elderly. *Neurol Sci.* 2010;**31** Suppl 1:S73–6.
52. Hunder GG, Bloch DA, Michel BA, *et al.* The American College of Rheumatology 1990 criteria for the classification of giant cell arteritis. *Arthritis Rheum.* 1990;**33**(8):1122–8.
53. Nordborg E, Nordborg C. Giant cell arteritis: strategies in diagnosis and treatment. *Curr Opin Rheumatol.* 2004;**16** (1):25–30.
54. Kerr GS, Hallahan CW, Giordano J, *et al.* Takayasu arteritis. *Ann Intern Med.* 1994;**120**(11):919–29.
55. Hall S, Barr W, Lie JT, *et al.* Takayasu arteritis. A study of 32 North American patients. *Medicine (Baltimore).* 1985;**64** (2):89–99.
56. Guillevin L, Lhote F, Gayraud M, *et al.* Prognostic factors in polyarteritis nodosa and Churg-Strauss syndrome. A prospective study in 342 patients. *Medicine (Baltimore).* 1996;**75**(1):17–28.
57. Pagnoux C, Seror R, Henegar C, *et al.* Clinical features and outcomes in 348 patients with polyarteritis nodosa: a systematic retrospective study of patients diagnosed between 1963 and 2005 and entered into the French Vasculitis Study Group Database. *Arthritis Rheum.* 2010;**62**(2):616–26.
58. Siva A, Saip S. The spectrum of nervous system involvement in Behcet's syndrome and its differential diagnosis. *J Neurol.* 2009;**256**(4):513–29.
59. Yazici H, Fresko I, Yurdakul S. Behcet's syndrome: disease manifestations, management, and advances in treatment. *Nat Clin Pract Rheumatol.* 2007;**3**(3):148–55.
60. Al-Araji A, Kidd DP. Neuro-Behcet's disease: epidemiology, clinical characteristics, and management. *Lancet Neurol.* 2009;**8**(2):192–204.
61. Wechsler B, Dell'Isola B, Vidailhet M, *et al.* MRI in 31 patients with Behcet's disease and neurological involvement: prospective study with clinical correlation. *J Neurol Neurosurg Psychiatry.* 1993;**56**(7):793–8.
62. Belizna CC, Hamidou MA, Levesque H, Guillevin L, Shoenfeld Y. Infection and vasculitis. *Rheumatology (Oxford).* 2009;**48**(5):475–82.
63. Takeuchi KSK. Hypogenesis of bilateral internal carotid arteries. *No To Shinkei.* 1957;**9**:37–43.
64. Suzuki J, Takaku A. Cerebrovascular 'moyamoya' disease. Disease showing abnormal net-like vessels in base of brain. *Arch Neurol.* 1969;**20**(3):288–99.
65. Kraemer M, Heienbrok W, Berlit P. Moyamoya disease in Europeans. *Stroke.* 2008;**39**(12):3193–200.
66. Fukui M. Guidelines for the diagnosis and treatment of spontaneous occlusion of the circle of Willis ('moyamoya' disease). Research Committee on Spontaneous Occlusion of the Circle of Willis (Moyamoya Disease) of the Ministry of Health and Welfare, Japan. *Clin Neurol Neurosurg.* 1997;**99** Suppl 2:S238–40.
67. Slovut DP, Olin JW. Fibromuscular dysplasia. *N Engl J Med.* 2004;**350**(18):1862–71.
68. Lassiter FD. The string-of-beads sign. *Radiology.* 1998;**206** (2):437–8.
69. Olin JW, Pierce M. Contemporary management of fibromuscular dysplasia. *Curr Opin Cardiol.* 2008;**23**(6):527–36.
70. Call GK, Fleming MC, Sealfon S, *et al.* Reversible cerebral segmental vasoconstriction. *Stroke.* 1988;**19**(9):1159–70.
71. Joutel A, Corpechot C, Ducros A, *et al.* Notch3 mutations in CADASIL, a hereditary adult-onset condition causing stroke and dementia. *Nature.* 1996;**383**(6602):707–10.
72. Tournier-Lasserve E, Joutel A, Melki J, *et al.* Cerebral autosomal dominant arteriopathy with subcortical infarcts and leukoencephalopathy maps to chromosome 19q12. *Nat Genet.* 1993;**3**(3):256–9.
73. Razvi SS, Davidson R, Bone I, Muir KW. The prevalence of cerebral autosomal dominant arteriopathy with subcortical infarcts and leucoencephalopathy (CADASIL) in the west of Scotland. *J Neurol Neurosurg Psychiatry.* 2005;**76** (5):739–41.
74. Choi JC. Cerebral autosomal dominant arteriopathy with subcortical infarcts and leukoencephalopathy: a genetic cause of cerebral small vessel disease. *J Clin Neurol.* 2010;**6**(1):1–9.
75. Chabriat H, Vahedi K, Iba-Zizen MT, *et al.* Clinical spectrum of CADASIL: a study of 7 families. Cerebral autosomal dominant arteriopathy with subcortical infarcts and leukoencephalopathy. *Lancet.* 1995;**346**(8980):934–9.
76. Singhal S, Bevan S, Barrick T, Rich P, Markus HS. The influence of genetic and cardiovascular risk factors on the CADASIL phenotype. *Brain.* 2004;**127**(Pt 9):2031–8.
77. Rolfs A, Bottcher T, Zschiesche M, *et al.* Prevalence of Fabry disease in patients with cryptogenic stroke: a prospective study. *Lancet.* 2005;**366**(9499):1794–6.
78. Brouns R, Thijs V, Eyskens F, *et al.* Belgian Fabry study: prevalence of Fabry disease in a cohort of 1000 young patients with cerebrovascular disease. *Stroke.* 2010;**41** (5):863–8.
79. Bogousslavsky J, Pierre P. Ischemic stroke in patients under age 45. *Neurol Clin.* 1992;**10**(1):113–24.
80. Brady RO, Schiffmann R. Clinical features of and recent advances in therapy for Fabry disease. *JAMA.* 2000;**284** (21):2771–5.

81. Manwaring N, Jones MM, Wang JJ, *et al.* Population prevalence of the MELAS A3243G mutation. *Mitochondrion.* 2007;**7**(3):230–3.
82. Bousser MG, Ferro JM. Cerebral venous thrombosis: an update. *Lancet Neurol.* 2007;**6**(2):162–70.
83. Stam J. Thrombosis of the cerebral veins and sinuses. *N Engl J Med.* 2005;**352**(17):1791–8.
84. Agnelli G, Verso M. Epidemiology of cerebral vein and sinus thrombosis. *Front Neurol Neurosci.* 2008;**23**:16–22.
85. Villringer A, Mehraein S, Einhaupl KM. Pathophysiological aspects of cerebral sinus venous thrombosis (SVT). *J Neuroradiol.* 1994;**21**(2):72–80.
86. Stam J. Cerebral venous and sinus thrombosis: incidence and causes. *Adv Neurol.* 2003;**92**:225–32.
87. Canhao P, Ferro JM, Lindgren AG, *et al.* Causes and predictors of death in cerebral venous thrombosis. *Stroke.* 2005;**36**(8):1720–5.
88. Masuhr F, Mehraein S, Einhaupl K. Cerebral venous and sinus thrombosis. *J Neurol.* 2004;**251**(1):11–23.
89. Lalive PH, de Moerloose P, Lovblad K, *et al.* Is measurement of D-dimer useful in the diagnosis of cerebral venous thrombosis? *Neurology.* 2003;**61**(8):1057–60.
90. Tardy B, Tardy-Poncet B, Viallon A, *et al.* D-dimer levels in patients with suspected acute cerebral venous thrombosis. *Am J Med.* 2002;**113**(3):238–41.
91. Kosinski CM, Mull M, Schwarz M, *et al.* Do normal D-dimer levels reliably exclude cerebral sinus thrombosis? *Stroke.* 2004;**35**(12):2820–5.
92. Crassard I, Soria C, Tzourio C, *et al.* A negative D-dimer assay does not rule out cerebral venous thrombosis: a series of seventy-three patients. *Stroke.* 2005;**36**(8):1716–19.
93. Ferro JM, Canhao P, Stam J, Bousser MG, Barinagarrementeria F. Prognosis of cerebral vein and dural sinus thrombosis: results of the International Study on Cerebral Vein and Dural Sinus Thrombosis (ISCVT). *Stroke.* 2004;**35**(3):664–70.
94. Gosk-Bierska I, Wysokinski W, Brown RD, Jr., *et al.* Cerebral venous sinus thrombosis: Incidence of venous thrombosis recurrence and survival. *Neurology.* 2006;**67** (5):814–19.
95. Einhaupl K, Stam J, Bousser MG, et al. EFNS guideline on the treatment of cerebral venous and sinus thrombosis in adult patients. *Eur J Neurol.* 2010 Apr 7.
96. de Bruijn SF, Stam J. Randomized, placebo-controlled trial of anticoagulant treatment with low-molecular-weight heparin for cerebral sinus thrombosis. *Stroke.* 1999;**30**(3):484–8.
97. Einhaupl KM, Villringer A, Meister W, *et al.* Heparin treatment in sinus venous thrombosis. *Lancet.* 1991;**338** (8767):597–600.
98. Canhao P, Falcao F, Ferro JM. Thrombolytics for cerebral sinus thrombosis: a systematic review. *Cerebrovasc Dis.* 2003;**15**(3):159–66.
99. Stam J, Majoie CB, van Delden OM, van Lienden KP, Reekers JA. Endovascular thrombectomy and thrombolysis for severe cerebral sinus thrombosis: a prospective study. *Stroke.* 2008;**39**(5):1487–90.
100. Lijfering WM, Brouwer JL, Veeger NJ, *et al.* Selective testing for thrombophilia in patients with first venous thrombosis: results from a retrospective family cohort study on absolute thrombotic risk for currently known thrombophilic defects in 2479 relatives. *Blood.* 2009;**113** (21):5314–22.
101. Canhao P, Cortesao A, Cabral M, *et al.* Are steroids useful to treat cerebral venous thrombosis? *Stroke.* 2008;**39** (1):105–10.
102. Coutinho JM, Majoie CB, Coert BA, Stam J. Decompressive hemicraniectomy in cerebral sinus thrombosis: consecutive case series and review of the literature. *Stroke.* 2009;**40**(6):2233–5.
103. Theaudin M, Crassard I, Bresson D, *et al.* Should decompressive surgery be performed in malignant cerebral venous thrombosis? A series of 12 patients. *Stroke.* 2010;**41**(4):727–31.
104. Filippidis A, Kapsalaki E, Patramani G, Fountas KN. Cerebral venous sinus thrombosis: review of the demographics, pathophysiology, current diagnosis, and treatment. *Neurosurg Focus.* 2009;**27**(5):E3.
105. Krayenbuhl N, Erdem E, Oinas M, Krisht AF. Symptomatic and silent ischemia associated with microsurgical clipping of intracranial aneurysms: evaluation with diffusion-weighted MRI. *Stroke.* 2009;**40**(1):129–33.
106. Qureshi AI, Luft AR, Sharma M, Guterman LR, Hopkins LN. Prevention and treatment of thromboembolic and ischemic complications associated with endovascular procedures: Part II-Clinical aspects and recommendations. *Neurosurgery.* 2000;**46**(6):1360–75; discussion 1375–6.
107. Likosky DS, Marrin CA, Caplan LR, *et al.* Determination of etiologic mechanisms of strokes secondary to coronary artery bypass graft surgery. *Stroke.* 2003;**34**(12):2830–4.
108. Maulaz AB, Bezerra DC, Michel P, Bogousslavsky J. Effect of discontinuing aspirin therapy on the risk of brain ischemic stroke. *Arch Neurol.* 2005;**62**(8):1217–20.
109. Genewein U, Haeberli A, Straub PW, Beer JH. Rebound after cessation of oral anticoagulant therapy: the biochemical evidence. *Br J Haematol.* 1996;**92**(2):479–85.
110. Selim M. Perioperative stroke. *N Engl J Med.* 2007;**356** (7):706–13.

111. Hogue CW, Jr., Murphy SF, Schechtman KB, Davila-Roman VG. Risk factors for early or delayed stroke after cardiac surgery. *Circulation.* 1999;**100**(6):642–7.
112. Bucerius J, Gummert JF, Borger MA, *et al.* Stroke after cardiac surgery: a risk factor analysis of 16,184 consecutive adult patients. *Ann Thorac Surg.* 2003;**75**(2):472–8.
113. James AH, Bushnell CD, Jamison MG, Myers ER. Incidence and risk factors for stroke in pregnancy and the puerperium. *Obstet Gynecol.* 2005;**106**(3):509–16.
114. Treadwell SD, Thanvi B, Robinson TG. Stroke in pregnancy and the puerperium. *Postgrad Med J.* 2008;**84**(991):238–45.
115. Jaigobin C, Silver FL. Stroke and pregnancy. *Stroke.* 2000;**31**(12):2948–51.
116. Kittner SJ, Stern BJ, Feeser BR, *et al.* Pregnancy and the risk of stroke. *N Engl J Med.* 1996;**335**(11):768–74.
117. Brown DW, Dueker N, Jamieson DJ, *et al.* Pre-eclampsia and the risk of ischemic stroke among young women: results from the Stroke Prevention in Young Women Study. *Stroke.* 2006;**37**(4):1055–9.
118. Kanal E, Barkovich AJ, Bell C, *et al.* ACR guidance document for safe MR practices: 2007. *AJR Am J Roentgenol.* 2007;**188**(6):1447–74.
119. Sibai BM, Schneider JM, Morrison JC, *et al.* The late postpartum eclampsia controversy. *Obstet Gynecol.* 1980;**55**(1):74–8.
120. Bates SM, Greer IA, Hirsh J, Ginsberg JS. Use of antithrombotic agents during pregnancy: the Seventh ACCP Conference on Antithrombotic and Thrombolytic Therapy. *Chest.* 2004;**126**(3 Suppl):627S-44S.
121. Turan TN, Stern BJ. Stroke in pregnancy. *Neurol Clin.* 2004;**22**(4):821–40.
122. Sandson TA, Friedman JH. Spinal cord infarction. Report of 8 cases and review of the literature. *Medicine (Baltimore).* 1989;**68**(5):282–92.
123. Masson C, Pruvo JP, Meder JF, *et al.* Spinal cord infarction: clinical and magnetic resonance imaging findings and short term outcome. *J Neurol Neurosurg Psychiatry.* 2004;**75**(10):1431–5.
124. Cheshire WP, Santos CC, Massey EW, Howard JF, Jr. Spinal cord infarction: etiology and outcome. *Neurology.* 1996;**47**(2):321–30.
125. Lichy C, Reuner KH, Buggle F, *et al.* Prothrombin G20210A mutation, but not factor V Leiden, is a risk factor in patients with persistent foramen ovale and otherwise unexplained cerebral ischemia. *Cerebrovasc Dis.* 2003;**16**(1):83–7.
126. Karttunen V, Hiltunen L, Rasi V, Vahtera E, Hillbom M. Factor V Leiden and prothrombin gene mutation may predispose to paradoxical embolism in subjects with patent foramen ovale. *Blood Coagul Fibrinolysis.* 2003;**14**(3):261–8.
127. Voetsch B, Damasceno BP, Camargo EC, *et al.* Inherited thrombophilia as a risk factor for the development of ischemic stroke in young adults. *Thromb Haemost.* 2000;**83**(2):229–33.
128. De Stefano V, Chiusolo P, Paciaroni K, *et al.* Prothrombin G20210A mutant genotype is a risk factor for cerebrovascular ischemic disease in young patients. *Blood.* 1998;**91**(10):3562–5.
129. Austin S, Cohen H, Losseff N. Haematology and neurology. *J Neurol Neurosurg Psychiatry.* 2007;**78**(4):334–41.
130. Galli M, Luciani D, Bertolini G, Barbui T. Lupus anticoagulants are stronger risk factors for thrombosis than anticardiolipin antibodies in the antiphospholipid syndrome: a systematic review of the literature. *Blood.* 2003;**101**(5):1827–32.

19

Blood pressure management in acute ischemic stroke

Sandeep Ankolekar and Philip Bath

Introduction

Of the many physiological disturbances that occur in acute ischemic stroke, changes in blood pressure (BP) are the most common – 80% of patients have a high BP (systolic BP [SBP] >140 mmHg) and 5% have a low or low-normal BP (SBP <120 mmHg) [1]. Importantly, both situations are associated with a poor outcome [1]. Whether BP levels, per se, modulate outcome is unclear, and ultimately, this question will only be answered by randomized controlled trials.

Pathophysiological considerations

Cerebral autoregulation

Blood flow to the brain is tightly controlled over a narrow range of 50–70 ml/100 g/min irrespective of BP which may span a wide range (mean arterial pressure (MAP) 60–150 mmHg) [2]. This cerebral autoregulation is achieved by altering cerebrovascular resistance via arteriolar constriction; higher pressures result in vasoconstriction and hence reduction of blood flow and lower pressures lead to reflex vasodilatation. The mechanisms underlying this alteration are not fully understood; proposed hypotheses include (i) myogenic – higher pressures activate the smooth muscle stretch reflex resulting in vasoconstriction and hence reduction of blood flow, while lower pressures lead to reflex vasodilatation [3]; (ii) metabolic – reduced blood flow stimulates release of vasoactive substances that cause vasodilatation [4]; and (iii) the neurogenic theory – perivascular nerves modulate vasoconstriction and dilatation [2].

In acute stroke, autoregulation is impaired [5], a consequence of regional disequilibrium in the area of ischemia due to acidosis, hypoxia, and release of vasodilatory factors [6,7]. While such changes may benefit regional circulation, the loss of autoregulation means that brain blood flow becomes directly dependent on systemic BP [5]. Importantly, in patients with chronic hypertension, the normal ability to autoregulate works at higher levels of BP [8], presumably due to structural changes in the cerebral vessels, such that BP in the 'normal' range may still lead to hypo-perfusion.

Causes of changes in blood pressure

The mechanisms underlying high BP in acute stroke are multi-factorial. Pre-existing hypertension may be present in more than 50% of patients [9] and was found to be the strongest predictor of admission BP [10]. This could reflect previously unrecognized, or inadequately treated, chronic hypertension. However, several other factors may also be relevant. Stroke affects important regions in the cerebral cortex, e.g. insular cortex [11], and brain stem that control pressure. This may lead to hypo- or hypertension via modulation of the baroreceptor reflex, sympathetic autonomic system, and renin-angiotensin-aldosterone system. The

Critical Care of the Stroke Patient, ed. Stefan Schwab, Daniel Hanley, and A. David Mendelow. Published by Cambridge University Press.

Cushing reflex may also play a part if intracranial pressure rises secondary to cerebral edema.

Elevations in BP may also be caused, or sustained, by other contributing factors after hospital admission including pain (e.g. secondary to urinary retention), infection, patient mobilization and other nursing care, headache, and other physiological disturbances such as acidosis and hypercapnia.

Low BP in acute stroke is less common but, like high BP, is associated with poor outcome [1]. Possible explanations include dehydration and hypovolemia, low cardiac output states secondary to cardiac failure, ischemia or arrhythmias, and aortic dissection [12]. Larger ischemic strokes are associated with low BP [1], although the cause for this is less clear.

Possible mechanisms of poor outcome with altered BP

High BP is associated with increased early death, and late death or dependency. Both relationships are independent of prognostic factors such as age, sex, stroke severity, level of consciousness, and atrial fibrillation [1,13]. High BP is also associated with intermediate complications including cerebral edema and early recurrence [1,14]. While it is plausible that hemorrhagic transformation of an infarct is more likely with high BP, and experimental studies support this, the association was not present in several observations studies [1,14].

Low BP is also associated independently with a poor outcome [1]. Patients with total anterior circulation and concomitant coronary events have a lower BP [1], although whether this is a causal association remains unclear. Low BP may also reflect a low output state secondary to myocardial ischemia or severe sepsis. Either way, low BP could worsen cerebral and cardiac perfusion leading to infarction, as supported by a possible 'J'-shaped relationship between BP and stroke recurrence [1,14].

Course of BP in acute stroke

Predicting trends in individual patients is difficult since BP fluctuates significantly in the first few days to weeks after acute stroke (see Fig. 19.1). Some of these

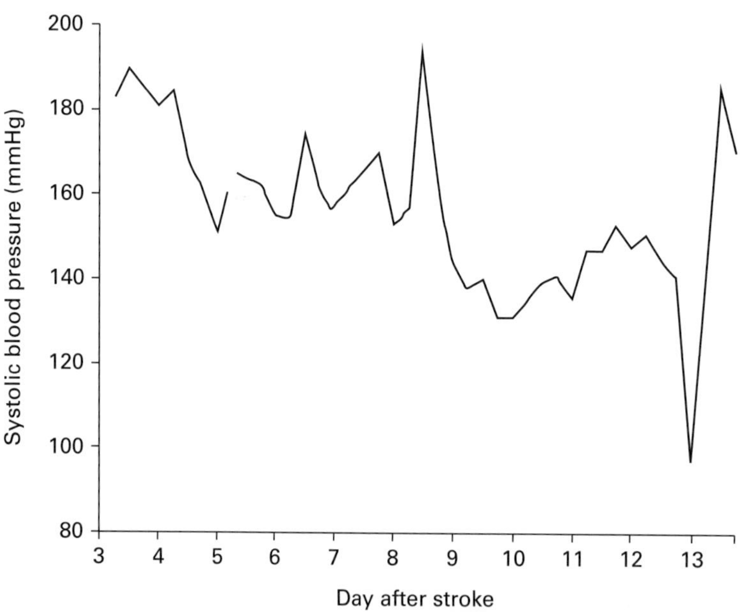

Fig. 19.1 BP fluctuation in the first 2 weeks after stroke (readings taken from a patient in an acute stroke ward).

fluctuations perhaps represent measurement issues rather than real changes. However, the natural history is for BP to decline during the first few hours and days after stroke with the greatest decline occurring in those with the highest admission values [15]. Nevertheless, BP levels remain in the hypertensive range in one-third of patients, and some of these will need detailed investigations for secondary causes of hypertension (see Section 3). Secondary prevention with BP lowering will be relevant to most patients irrespective of BP level [16].

Investigations

All patients with acute stroke and high BP should be reviewed for associated conditions that may increase BP. Investigations into the secondary causes of hypertension are generally not necessary unless the BP is especially high and remains so in the subacute stage of stroke, is very variable, or if there is evidence of target organ damage in the kidneys or heart suggesting chronicity. Such investigations should follow national and international guidelines for hypertension and may include biochemical measurement of 24-hour urinary catecholamines and cortisol, serum renin and aldosterone, and imaging of the renal vessels, kidneys and adrenal glands [17,18].

Management of hypertension

Management of high BP in acute stroke is controversial, as acknowledged by several guidelines and consensus statements [19–22]. Several important questions need answers:

- Should high BP be lowered therapeutically?
- If so, how should antihypertensive medications be administered in respect of drug class and route of administration?
- Should pre-stroke antihypertensive therapy be continued or stopped?
- What other support should be provided to patients with high BP?

Should high BP be lowered in acute stroke?

Analyses from observational studies suggest that high BP is associated independently with increased mortality, morbidity, and recurrence in patients with acute ischemic stroke [1,13,14]. However, the ischemic penumbra remains viable for several hours or even days after an acute arterial occlusion and is susceptible to further injury; such injury might be exacerbated if BP is lowered in the presence of dysfunctional cerebral autoregulation [6]. So, from an epidemiological perspective, BP should be lowered, and from a pathophysiological view, it should not. It is reassuring that a meta-analysis of 11 small trials reviewing the effect of antihypertensive agents on cerebral blood flow and velocity in acute ischemic stroke found little evidence that these agents reduce cerebral blood flow despite lowering blood pressure [23]. In non-randomized studies, before and after comparisons showed an increase in cerebral blood flow with calcium channel blockers (CCB). However, as all the studies were small, definitive conclusions could not be made [23].

The equipoise demands that data from large definitive randomized controlled clinical trials be collected, and recently completed clinical trials in both ischemic and hemorrhagic stroke have not shown definitive evidence for the benefits of BP lowering [24,25].

Stop versus continue pre-existing antihypertensive agents

More than half of patients with acute stroke have pre-existing high BP [9] and most are on BP-lowering agents. It is unclear whether such medications should be continued or stopped in the acute period, although most patients will need to take antihypertensives long term for secondary prevention [16]. The question is complex since some antihypertensive classes might be beneficial (e.g. angiotensin receptor antagonists [26] and others harmful (ß-receptor antagonists [27] during the acute and subacute phases of stroke.

The 'Continue Or Stop post-Stroke Antihypertensives Collaborative Study' (COSSACS) is the only completed trial to have addressed this question [28]. This multicentre trial enrolled 763 patients and found no difference in death or dependency at 2 weeks (primary outcome) between those who continued versus those who stopped their pre-stroke antihypertensive medications. Continuing antihypertensive medication led to a 13/8 mmHg lower BP at 2 weeks as compared to stopping it [28]. However, the study closed early due to limited recruitment and so was underpowered for assessing the effect of the interventions on functional outcome. The ongoing 'Efficacy of Nitric Oxide in Stroke' (ENOS) is also examining this question. In a preliminary analysis based on 168 participants, BP was lower by 8.6/2.3 mmHg at 1 week in those who continued their pre-stroke BP-lowering treatment [29].

Supportive treatment

All patients with high BP in acute stroke should be reviewed for easily treatable associated conditions that can increase BP such as dehydration, headache, urinary retention, pain, hypercapnia, and acidosis. Guidelines support correcting and treating such conditions when possible.

Concurrent hypertensive emergencies

Stroke may present with concomitant myocardial infarction, unstable angina, acute left ventricular failure, and aortic dissection, some of which may be the underlying cause for the stroke. No trials have specifically looked at managing BP when these conditions present with acute stroke. It is, however, generally agreed that such conditions on their own should be actively treated and current guidelines support this view [19,21,22]. Nevertheless, a recent Cochrane Collaboration review of 15 randomized controlled trials (869 patients) found no evidence of benefit with antihypertensive medications in preventing morbidity and mortality in hypertensive emergencies [30]. A second systematic review was also inconclusive [31].

Optimal BP targets in acute ischemic stroke

Several studies have confirmed a U-shaped relation between acute BP and outcome such that the best outcomes are noted between systolic BPs of 140–160 mmHg [1]. Observation from thrombolysis registers in acute stroke have also noted that the most favorable results for mortality and independence occur at baseline systolic BPs around 141–150 mmHg [32].

In the absence of good evidence for target levels for BP control in acute ischemic stroke, national and international guidelines vary in their recommendations. Different cut-off values are recommended depending on whether patients are eligible for intravenous thrombolysis, these being driven by the non-evidence-based targets used in randomized trials assessing thrombolysis in acute stroke. Observational quality care studies in North America indirectly support these guidelines as they showed improved outcomes and reduced rates of intracerebral hemorrhage (ICH) from 16% to 6% when the suggested BP recommendations were followed [33,34].

Outside the setting of thrombolysis, lowering BP may be most effective when baseline BP is very high, e.g. ACCESS was positive on a secondary prevention outcome with a baseline BP of 189/99 mmHg (although the improved outcome was not related to the difference in BP between those receiving candesartan or placebo) [26] whereas PRoFESS acute was neutral with a modest elevation of BP at baseline (mean BP 147/84) [35].

A meta-analysis of 37 clinical trials covering 13 different drug classes involving 9008 patients concluded that although poor outcome was not significantly reduced at any level of change in BP, the lowest odds of early death occurred with a reduction in BP by 8.1 mmHg, and of death or dependency at the end of follow up with a reduction of 14.6 mgHg (see Fig. 19.2) [36].

Table 19.1 summarizes the antihypertensive medications used in acute stroke and Table 19.2 summarizes the recommendations from the American Heart Association (AHA)/American Stroke Association (ASA) [21], European Stroke Organisation (ESO) [19] and the National Clinical Guidelines for Stroke UK [22].

BP management after thrombolysis

Observational studies of BP management after thrombolysis are conflicting. Data on 624 patients from the

Table 19.1 BP management guidelines for acute ischemic stroke from AHA/ASA, ESO (Europe), and UK.

	Target SBP (mmHg)	Target DBP (mmHg)	Recommended drugs
Patients suitable for thrombolysis			
AHA/ASA	>185	>110	IV labetalol or nicardipine
ESO	>185	>110	no recommendations
UK	>185	>110	no recommendations
During and after thrombolysis			
AHA/ASA[±]	180	105	IV labetalol or nicardipine; nitroprusside [§]
ESO	no recommendations	no recommendations	no recommendations
UK	no recommendations	no recommendations	no recommendations
Non-thrombolysis patients			
AHA/ASA*	>220	>220	same as above
ESO*	>120	>120	no recommendations
UK*	no recommendations	no recommendations	no recommendations

IV: intravenous; [±] AHA/ASA recommends BP monitoring every 15 minutes for 2 hours from the start of thrombolyis, then every 30 minutes for 6 hours and every hour for 16 hours.

[§] If BP is not controlled with labetalol or nicardipine or if diastolic BP >140 mmHg.

*Antihypertensives if concomitant medical hypertensive emergencies e.g. aortic dissection.

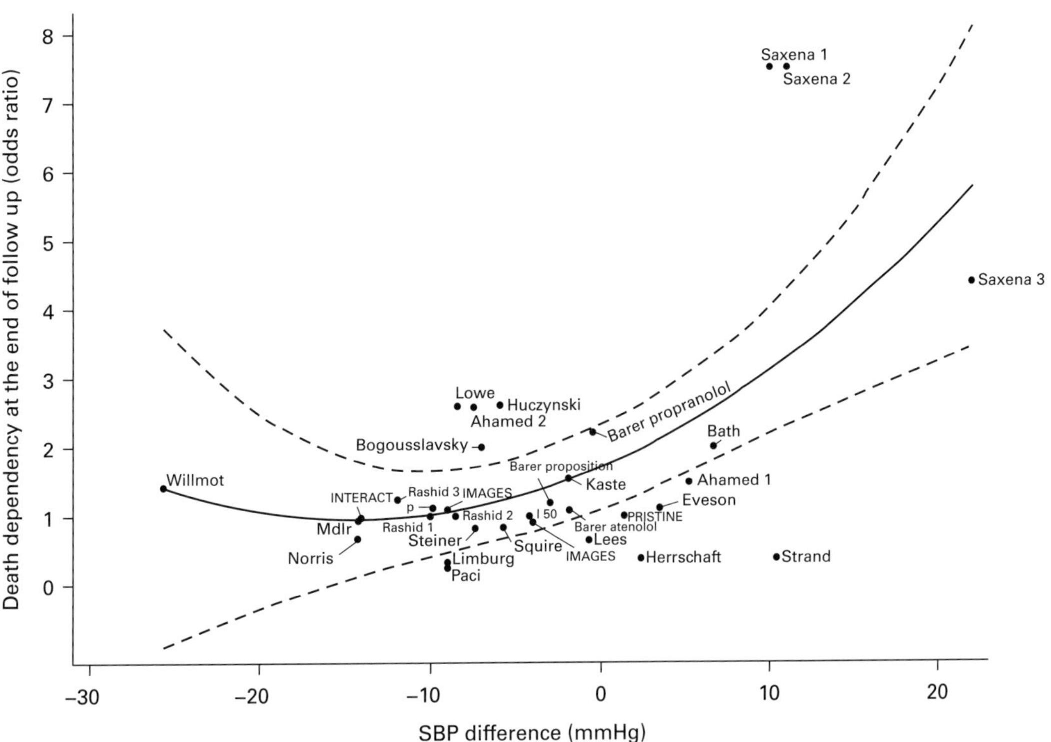

Fig. 19.2 Relationship between treatment SBP difference (active-control) and death or dependency at end of follow-up. (Reprinted from [36] with permission from Wolters Kluwer Health).

Table 19.2 Antihypertensive drugs used in acute stroke. (Information from Martindale: The complete drug reference; British National Formulary; summary of product characteristics and other sources for individual drugs).

Drug	Time to onset	Duration of action	Loading dose	Maintenance dose	Effect on CBF	Effect on ICP	Side effects	Contra-indications
Intravenous								
Enalaprilat	15 m	6–12 h	1.25 mg	1.25–5 mg every 6 h	No effect	No effect	Headache, dizziness and nausea	Hypersensitivity, angioedema
Hydralazine	10–20 m	1–4 h	5–20 mg	5–20 mg every 30 m	Increase	Increase	Headache, anorexia, GI disturbance, tachycardia, angina	Hypersensitivity, coronary artery disease
Labetalol	5–10 m	3–6 h	10–20 mg	10 mg every 20 m or 2–8 mg/m	No effect	No effect	GI disturbance, bronchospasm, flushing	Asthma, heart block
Nicardipine	5–10 m	15–30 m±	5–15 mg	5–15 mg/h	Increase	No effect	Headache, flushing, tachycardia	Hypersensitivity, aortic stenosis
Nitroglycerine	2–5 m	5–10 m	5 μg/m	20–400 μg/m	Increase	No effect	Headache, dizziness, methemoglobinemia	Hypersensitivity, aortic stenosis
Nitroprusside	seconds	1–10 m	0.2–10 μg/m	0.2–10 μg/m	Increase	Increase	Hypotension, flushing, thiocyanate toxicity	Hypertension, hypovolemia
Transdermal								
Glyceryl trinitrate [49]	30–60 m	24 h	5–15 mg/d	5–15 mg/d	Increase	No effect	Headache, dizziness and methemoglobinemia	Hypersensitivity, aortic stenosis
Sublingual								
Lisinopril [40]	-	12 h	5 mg	5–10 mg	No effect	No effect	Headache, nausea and dizziness	Hypersensitivity, angioedema
Oral								
Candesartan [26]	2 h	12–24 h	4 mg	8–16 mg	Increase	No effect	Headache, arthralgia, rash, hepatitis	Cholestasis
Lisinopril [40]	24 h	4–6 h	5 mg	5–15 mg	No effect	No effect	Headache, cough, agranulocytosis	Hypersensitivity, angioedema
Labetalol [40]	1 h	12–24 h	50 mg	100–300 mg	No effect	No effect	Headache, nausea, dizziness	Asthma, heart block

CBF: cerebral blood flow; ICP: intracranial pressure; m: minutes; h: hours; mg: milligram; μg: microgram; d: day; ± may be up to 4 hours.

NINDS thrombolysis study showed that amongst patients randomized to alteplase, hypertensive patients receiving antihypertensive therapy were less likely to have a favorable outcome at 3 months (P<0.01) than those who were hypertensive and did not receive antihypertensive therapy [37]. There was no difference among both groups in the hypertensive placebo patients.

However, data from the SITS-MOST register of over 10000 patients differ. Here, antihypertensive therapy after intravenous thrombolysis in patients with either a history of hypertension, or moderately elevated BP without a history of hypertension, did not seem to affect outcomes adversely. In contrast, withholding antihypertensive therapy in patients with a history of hypertension was associated with high mortality, a high symptomatic hemorrhage rate, and a low rate of functional independence [32].

Intracerebral hemorrhage

While not of direct relevance to acute ischemic stroke, the second Intensive Blood Pressure Reduction in Acute Cerebral Hemorrhage Trial (INTERACT-2) compared BP targets, i.e. whether SBP should be lowered rapidly to below 140 mmHg (versus <180 mmHg) in patients with primary intracerebral hemorrhage (PICH) within 6 hours of symptom onset [25]. Intensive lowering of BP did not result in a significant reduction in the primary outcome of death or severe disability, although an ordinal analysis indicated improvement in functional outcomes.

Which antihypertensive agent?

A variety of antihypertensive drug classes exist, and each may have advantages or disadvantages during the acute stroke phase. Unfortunately, there are no randomized data for several drug classes – alpha adrenergic receptor antagonists (e.g. prazosin, doxazosin) and centrally-acting agents (alpha methyldopa, moxonidine). Theoretical concerns that alpha adrenergic receptor antagonists impair functional recovery [38] may preclude future trials with these agents.

Alpha receptor antagonists

Urapidil, an alpha$_1$-adrenoceptor antagonist and 5-HT$_{1A}$ receptor agonist, was the most frequently used first-line agent in the INTERACT-2 trial in patients with hyperacute spontaneous intracerebral hemorrhage [25]. Its use in trials in ischemic stroke has yet to be described.

Angiotensin converting enzyme inhibitors

Three different ACE inhibitors have been studied across five small trials. Both lisinopril and perindopril reduced BP at 24 hours without reducing cerebral blood flow, although no change in functional outcome was noted [39,40]. Captopril has only been studied in three patients and the data are inconclusive. In a Cochrane Collaboration systematic review, participants treated with ACE-I (versus none or placebo) tended to have a lower BP of 6/5 mmHg at 24 hours [41]. The CHHIPS study randomized 179 acute stroke patients (both ischemic and hemorrhagic) to receive lisinopril (oral or sublingual), labetalol (oral or intravenous) or placebo [40]. There was no difference between the groups on the primary outcome of death and dependency at 2 weeks, and although the trial was small, the active treatment group had a just statistically significant lower death rate at 90 days.

Angiotensin receptor antagonists (ARA)

The ACCESS trial studying oral candesartan intended to include 500 participants but was stopped prematurely after 342 patients were recruited due to a significant reduction in the secondary outcome of combined death, cerebral, and cerebrovascular events at 1 year, although there was no effect of treatment on functional outcome (the primary outcome) [26]. However, the much larger Scandinavian Candesartan in Acute Stroke Trial (SCAST), which recruited over 2000 patients with acute stroke and systolic blood pressure (SBP) >140 mmHg was neutral and showed no benefit of using candesartan for the first 7 days after an acute stroke on both primary endpoints of composite vascular events and functional dependency at 6 months; a trend towards worse functional outcome was noted for the candesartan-treated patients [42]. A subgroup analysis of the PROFESS trial involving 1360 patients recruited within 72 hours of ischemic stroke also was not associated with any change in functional dependency at 30 days [35]. It is, however, unclear whether the above results are generalizable to BP lowering in acute stroke, not least because the effect on BP was very modest at 5/2 mmHg in ACCESS and SCAST and 6/2 mmHg in the PROFESS subgroup analysis.

Beta-adrenergic receptor antagonists

Beta-receptor antagonists might, theoretically, be attractive for lowering BP since they reduce metabolic demand in ischemic regions. However, the BEST randomized trial showed a trend towards increased death and disability in those 302 patients with acute stroke who were randomized to either oral atenolol or slow release propranolol, as compared to placebo [27]. Labetalol, a mixed alpha- and beta-receptor antagonist, was used as one of the active drugs (along with lisinopril – see 'Angiotensin converting enzyme inhibitors') in the CHHIPS trial and was just positive on the secondary outcome of death at day 90 [40].

Calcium channel blockers (CCB)

Trials of CCBs have variably tested nimodipine, isradipine or flunarizine in acute stroke, mostly for putative neuroprotection properties rather than to lower BP. Individuals studies found that intravenous nimodipine worsened outcome [43]. Importantly, the INWEST trial noted that functional outcome worsened in parallel with the degree of fall in BP [43,44].

Several meta-analyses sum up the existing data. First, a Cochrane Collaboration review found that, when given within the first 24 hours after stroke, CCBs reduced BP by 32/13 mmHg when given intravenously, and 13/6 mmHg when administered orally [41]. Second, another Cochrane Collaboration review assessed 28 acute stroke trials (7521 patients) and found no difference between active treatment and controls in respect of subsequent functional outcome or death [45]. However, poor outcomes were more likely with intravenous treatment, earlier administration (<12 hours of stroke onset) and higher doses [45].

Last, a systematic review of nicardipine in cerebrovascular disease noted that it improved hemodynamic and neuronal function in ischemic regions in spite of its hypotensive activity [46].

Diuretics

Only one small trial has specifically looked at diuretics in acute ischemic stroke. Oral bendroflumethiazide did not significantly alter BP, cerebral autoregulation or cardiac receptor baroreceptor sensitivity within the first 7 days of stroke [47]. However, thiazide diuretics are known to have a slow onset in respect of lowering BP, typically over several days, so these results are unsurprising.

Nitric oxide donors

Transdermal glyceryl trinitrate (GTN) has been tested in three small randomized trials involving a total of 145 patients. GTN reduced BP at 1 hour by 23/4 mmHg and over 24 hours by 13.0/5.2 mmHg [48,49]. Importantly, it did not alter cerebral blood flow, cerebral blood flow velocity or platelet function. These studies were too small to provide any definite conclusions on the effect of GTN on outcome, but a large multicentre study is currently ongoing (see 'ENOS').

Route of administration

Up to 50% of patients with acute stroke have dysphagia so that safe swallowing is compromised. Although enteral feeding is possible, nasogastric tubes are often unreliable as insertion may be difficult and confused patients often repeatedly pull the tubes out. Further, long-acting formulations of inherently short-acting drugs cannot be administered down the tubes without changing the release characteristics. As a result, oral administration of BP-lowering drugs, especially modified release versions, is unreliable.

Intravenous administration of drugs can provide rapid BP titration but requires frequent and close monitoring, ideally on an intensive care or high-dependency unit. Sublingual administration can be effective and was used in the CHHIPS trial with lisinopril [40]. Sublingual administration of short-acting drugs such as nifedipine should not be used in view of the profound and transient BP reductions.

Transdermal administration of drugs, as for glyceryl trinitrate, in acute stroke patients appears promising as it allows blood pressure response to be titrated and the drug to be withdrawn if necessary.

Ongoing randomized controlled trials

ENOS

The Efficacy of a Nitric Oxide in Stroke (ENOS, http://www.enos.ac.uk/ accessed 08 June 2013) trial is a prospective multicentre randomized controlled trial assessing the safety and efficacy of lowering BP with transdermal GTN in acute stroke with treatment started within 48 hours of the onset of ischemic stroke or primary intracerebral hemorrhage (PICH). The primary outcome is death or dependency at 3 months. In a factorial design, ENOS is also testing continuing versus stopping pre-existing antihypertensive therapy in acute stroke. ENOS has reported an interim finding that lowering BP in the presence of severe ipsilateral carotid stenosis does not appear to be hazardous [50].

ENCHANTED

The Enhanced Control of Hypertension and Thrombolysis Stroke Study (ENCHANTED, http://www.enchanted.org.au/accessed 08 June 2013) is an international collaborative, quasi-factorial randomized controlled trial with two parts. Part A will compare low-dose (0.6 mg/kg) recombinant tissue plasminogen activator (rtPA) with standard-dose (0.9 mg/kg) rtPA and Part B will compare intensive BP lowering with conservative and current guideline-based BP lowering in hyperacute ischemic stroke. The primary outcome is combined death and any disability at 90 days.

Management of hypotension

Supportive treatment

Guidelines recommend that co-existing conditions causing hypotension in the setting of acute stroke should be actively sought and corrected [21]. Measures include fluid replacement with normal saline, antiarrhythmic agents, treatment of cardiac ischemia or failure, and treatment of sepsis, as appropriate. These should be instituted promptly.

Volume expansion

Acute stroke may be associated with increased blood viscosity and hemodilution might improve outcome. A Cochrane Collaboration review of hemodilution and volume expansion in acute stroke (<72 hours of stroke onset) assessed 18 trials; these studied a variety of agents including dextran 40, hydroxyethyl starch and albumin. However, no effect on death at 4 weeks or death and dependency at 3–6 months was observed [51].

Raising BP

As cerebral autoregulation is lost following stroke, such that cerebral blood flow becomes dependent on systemic BP, some researchers have hypothesized that BP should be increased to improve cerebral perfusion [52]. A systematic review of the available literature noted that several agents have been used to elevate BP including a variety of sympathomimetics: phenylephrine, norepinephrine, epinephrine, dopamine, and dobutamine. Only one randomized controlled trial was found. However, because of the small numbers, and varying entry and outcome criteria, a meta-analysis of outcome variables was not possible. Although no conclusions could be drawn, the reviewers felt that hypotensive strokes with ipsilateral large vessel occlusion and no obvious contraindications to pressor therapy may benefit from such agents and suggested that phenylephrine was the most promising [53]. Nevertheless, sympathomimetics activate platelets which may not be appropriate in acute ischemic stroke.

Summary

High BP is common in acute ischemic stroke and is caused by a variety of conditions. Both high and low BP are associated independently with a poor outcome so lowering a high BP might be beneficial. Since cerebral autoregulation is dysfunctional in acute stroke, lowering an elevated BP might, alternatively, be hazardous. The randomized controlled trials, to date, have either been small or neutral and the management of high BP remains unclear. Ongoing trials will, hopefully, provide clarity to this uncertainty.

REFERENCES

1. Leonardi-Bee J, Bath PMW, Phillips SJ, Sandercock PAG, for the IST Collaborative Group. Blood pressure and clinical outcomes in the International Stroke Trial. *Stroke.* 2002;**33**:1315–20.
2. Paulson OB, Strandgaard S, Edvinsson L. Cerebral autoregulation. *Cerebrovasular Brain Metab Rev.* 1990;**2** (2):161–92.
3. Symon L, Held K, Dorsch NW. A study of regional autoregulation in the cerebral circulation to increased perfusion pressure in normocapnia and hypercapnia. *Stroke.* 1973;**4**(2):139–47.
4. Aaslid R, Lindegaard K, Sorteberg W, Nornes H. Cerebral autoregulation dynamics in humans. *Stroke.* 1989;**20** (1):45–52.
5. Meyer JS, Shimazu K, Fukuuchi Y, *et al.* Impaired neurogenic cerebrovascular control and dysautoregulation after stroke. *Stroke.* 1973;**4**:169–86.
6. Olsen TS, Larsen B, Herning M, Skriver EB, Lassen NA. Blood flow and vascular reactivity in collaterally perfused brain tissue. Evidence of an ischemic penumbra in patients with acute stroke. *Stroke.* 1983;**14**(3):332–41.
7. Dohmen C, Bosche B, Graf R, *et al.* Identification and clinical impact of impaired cerebrovascular autoregulation in patients with malignant middle cerebral artery infarction. *Stroke.* 2007;**38**(1):56–61.
8. Strandgaard S, Olesen J, Skinhoj E, Lassen NA. Autoregulation of brain circulation in severe arterial hypertension. *BMJ.* 1973;**3**:507–10.
9. Arboix A, Roig H, Rossich R, Martinez EM, Garcia-Eroles L. Differences between hypertensive and non-hypertensive ischemic stroke. *Eur J Neurol.* 2004;**11**(10):687–92.
10. Carlberg B, Asplund K, Hagg E. Factors influencing admission blood pressure levels in patients with acute stroke. *Stroke.* 1991;**4**:527–30.
11. Meyer S, Strittmatter M, Fischer C, Georg T, Schmitz B. Lateralization in autonomic dysfunction in ischemic stroke involving the insular cortex. *Neuroreport.* 2004;**15** (2):357–61.
12. Sprigg N, Bath PMW. Management of blood pressure in acute stroke. *Practical Neurology.* 2005;**5**:218–23.
13. Willmot M, Leonardi-Bee J, Bath PM. High blood pressure in acute stroke and subsequent outcome: a systematic review. *Hypertension.* 2004;**43**(1):18–24.
14. Sprigg N, Gray LJ, Bath PM, *et al.* Relationship between outcome and baseline blood pressure and other haemodynamic measures in acute ischaemic stroke: data from the TAIST trial. *J Hypertens.* 2006;**24**(7):1413–17.
15. Britton M, Carlsson A, de Faire U. Blood pressure in patients with acute stroke and matched controls. *Stroke.* 1986;**17**:861–4.
16. Rashid P, Leonardi-Bee J, Bath P. Blood pressure reduction and the secondary prevention of stroke and other vascular events: a systematic review. *Stroke.* 2003;**34**:2741–9.
17. Chobanian AV, Bakris GL, Black HR, *et al.* The Seventh Report of the Joint National Committee on Prevention, Detection, Evaluation, and Treatment of High Blood Pressure: the JNC 7 report. *JAMA.* 2003;**289**(19):2560–72.
18. Mancia G, De Backer G, Dominiczak A, *et al.* 2007 Guidelines for the management of arterial hypertension: The Task Force for the Management of Arterial Hypertension of the European Society of Hypertension (ESH) and of the European Society of Cardiology (ESC). *Eur Heart J.* 2007;**28**(12):1462–536.
19. The European Stroke Organisation (ESO) Executive Committee and the ESO Writing Committee. Guidelines for management of ischaemic stroke and transient ischaemic attack 2008. *Cerebrovascular Diseases.* 2008;**25**:457–507.
20. Bath P, Chalmers J, Powers W, *et al.* International Society of Hypertension (ISH): statement on the management of blood pressure in acute stroke. *J Hypertension.* 2003;**21** (4):665–72.
21. Jauch EC, Saver JL, Adams HP, *et al.* Guidelines for the early management of patients with acute ischemic stroke: A guideline for healthcare professionals from the American Heart Association/American Stroke Association. *Stroke.* 2013;**44**(3):870–947.
22. Intercollegiate Stroke Working Party. *National Clinical Guideline for Stroke.* London: Royal College of Physicians; 2012.
23. Sare GM, Gray LJ, Bath PMW. Effect of antihypertensive agents on cerebral blood flow and flow velocity in acute ischaemic stroke: systematic review of controlled studies. *J Hypertension.* 2008;**26**:1058–64.
24. Sandset EC, Bath PM, Boysen G, *et al.* The angiotensin-receptor blocker candesartan for treatment of acute stroke

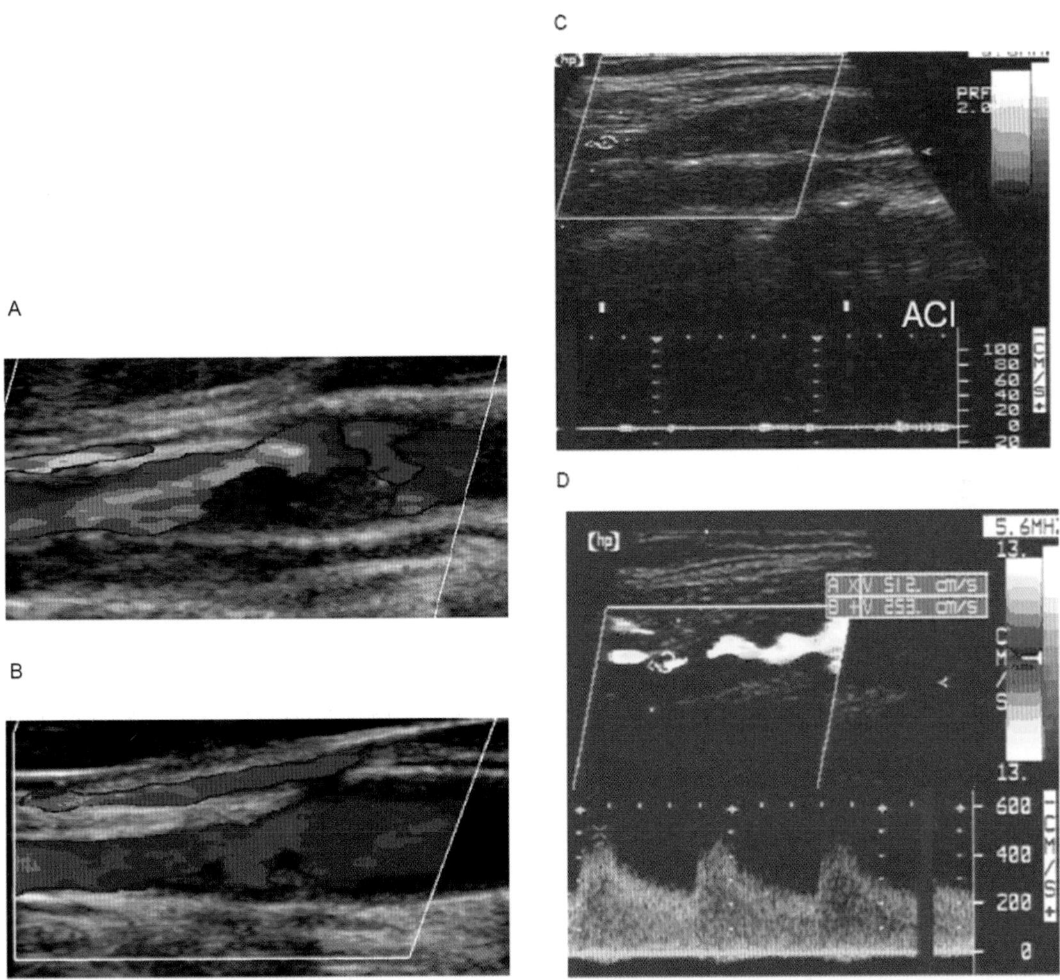

Fig. 5.1 A–D Thrombus at the carotid bulb of a 41-year-old female patient suffering from acute ischemic MCA stroke. **A.** initial investigation (day one), **B.** Follow-up investigation on day eight. A regression of thrombus volume is visible. **C and D.** Internal carotid artery of a 49-year-old male patient suffering from MCA ischemic stroke. **C.** Color-duplex scan two hours after symptom onset (severe MCA stroke). **D.** Follow-up investigation after 24 hours. Recanalization with a tight stenosis of the artery could be detected.

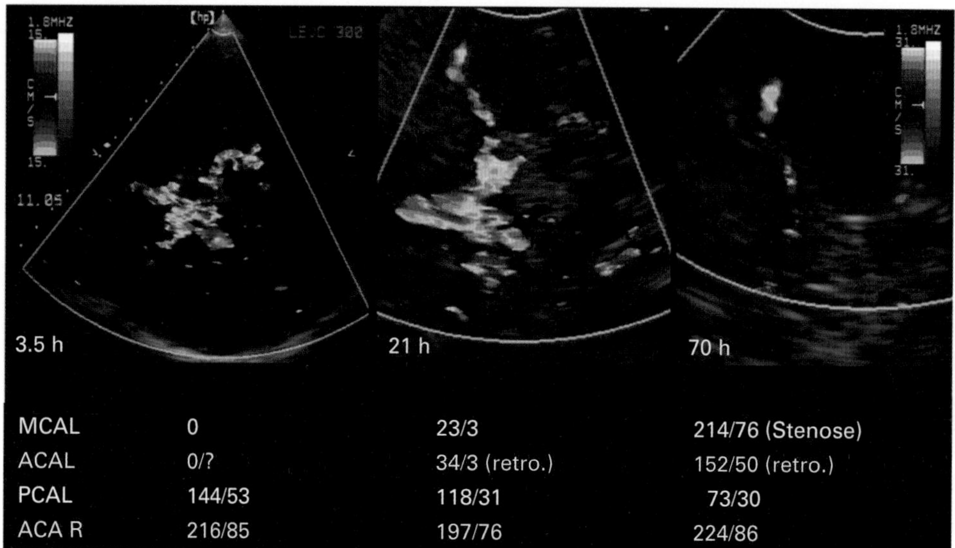

Fig. 5.2 TCCD (axial imaging plane, left side = frontal; right side = occipital) follow-up of a 76-year-old male patient suffering from acute MCA occlusion at the left side. TCCD images are given 3.5, 21, and 70 hours after symptom onset. At 3.5 hours 5 ml Levovist^{TM} 300. Below the images blood flow velocities [cm/s] in the basal cerebral arteries are displayed. MCA reopening, and a residual stenosis could be diagnosed. ACA collateral flow improved over time and PCA collateral flow decreased.

MCA, middle cerebral artery; ACA, anterior cerebral artery; PCA, posterior cerebral artery; L, left; R, right.

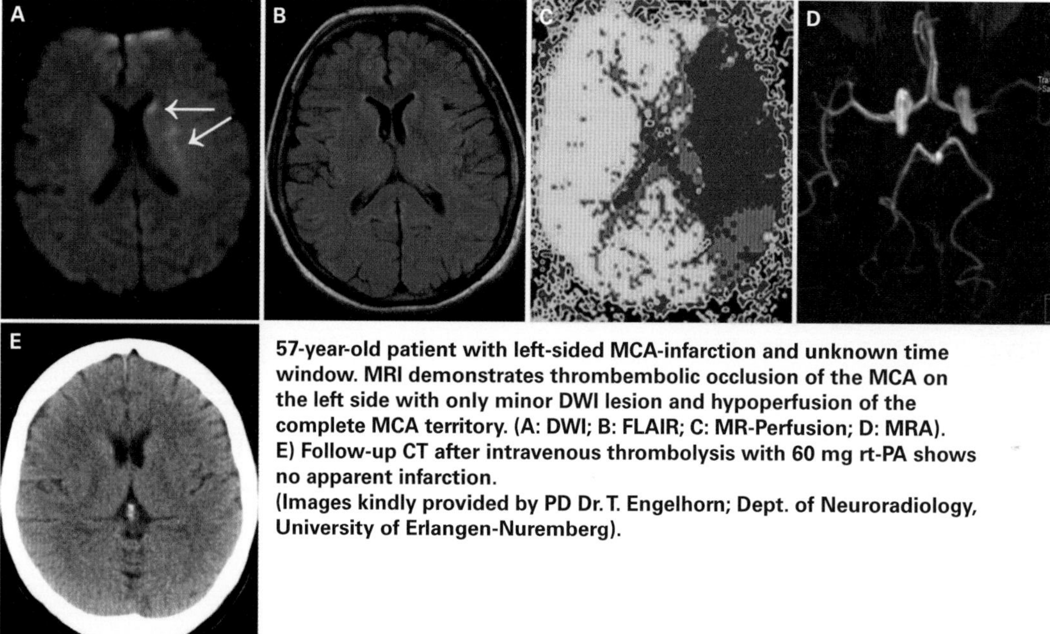

Fig. 13.1 Case presentation MRI-based thrombolysis.

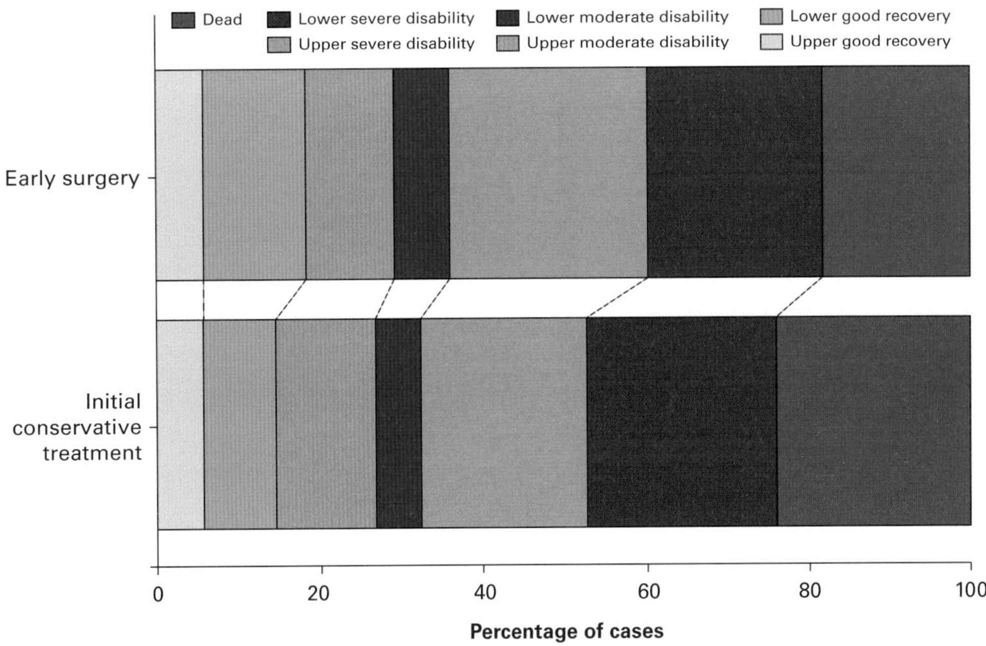

Fig. 22a.6 Glasgow Outcome Scale at 6 months for STICH II patients.

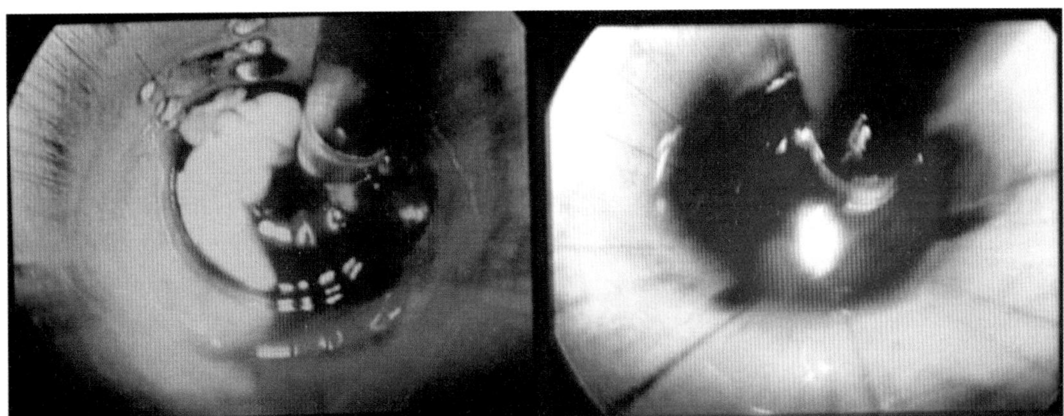

Fig. 22c.5 Intraoperative endoscopic views of a spontaneous intracerebral hemorrhage are shown.

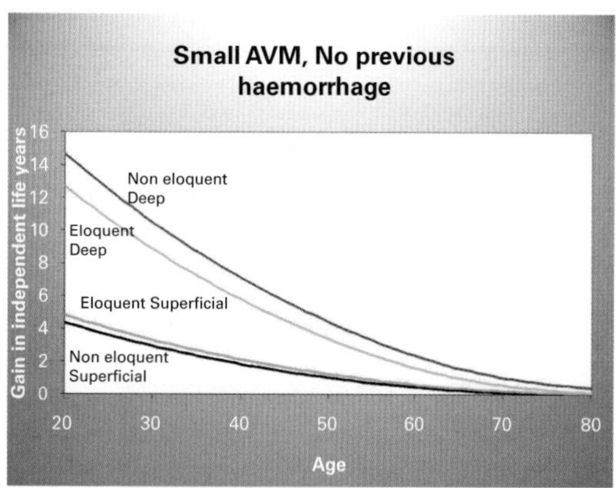

Fig. 26.2 The gain in independent life years (free of disability) in years (Y axis) plotted against age at intervention (X axis) for small (<3 cm) AVMs that are non-eloquent and deep, eloquent and deep, eloquent and superficial, and non-eloquent and superficial. (Life expectancy calculated from 2001 UK census and interventional outcomes calculated from literature review by R Vindelacheruvu 2010(6)).

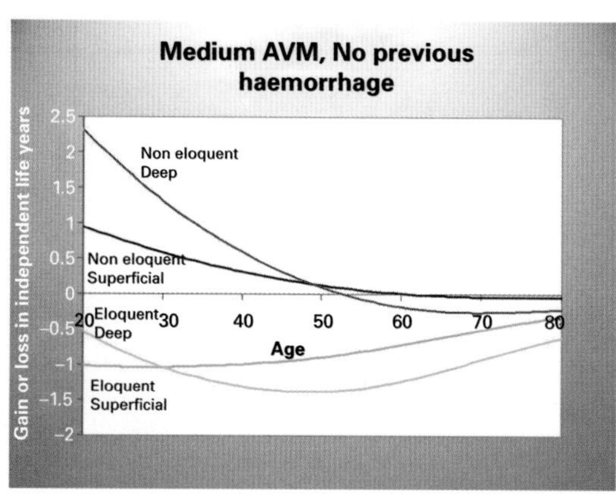

Fig. 26.3 The gain or loss in independent life years plotted against age for medium (3 to 6 cm) unruptured AVMs in the same four categories.

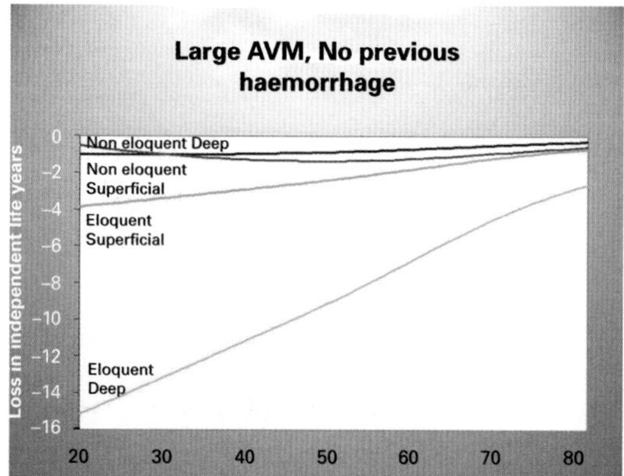

Fig. 26.4 The loss in independent life years plotted against age for large (>6 cm) unruptured AVMs in the same four categories.

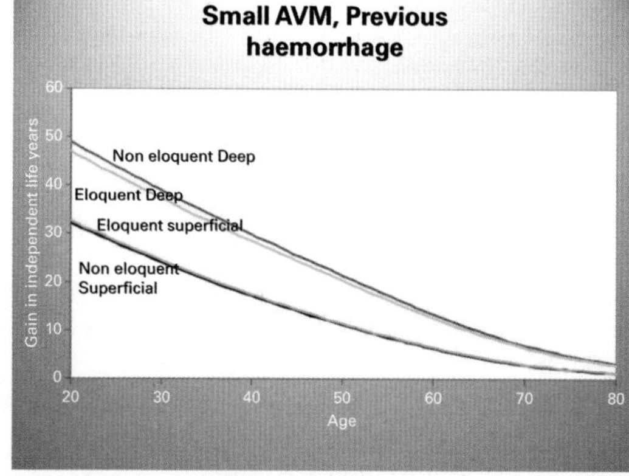

Fig. 26.5 The gain in independent life years plotted against age for small (<3 cm) ruptured AVMs in the same four categories.

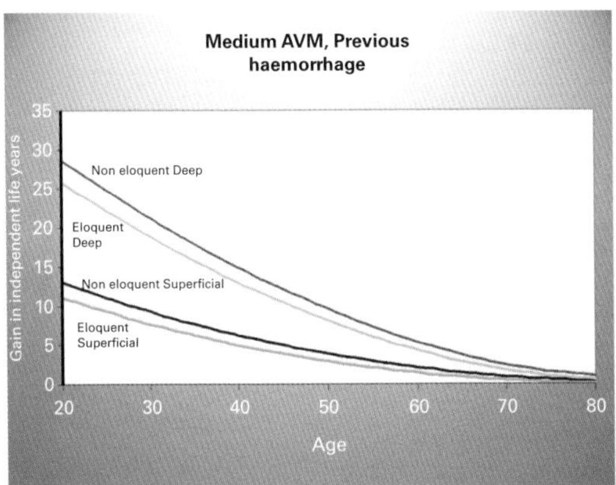

Fig. 26.6 The gain in independent life years plotted against age for medium (3 to 6 cm) ruptured AVMs in the same four categories.

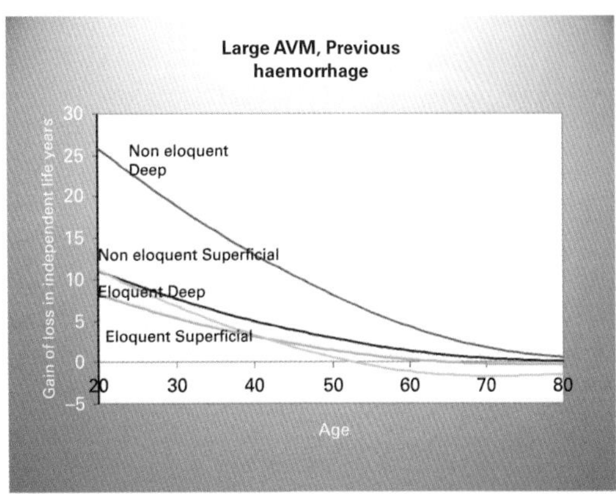

Fig. 26.7 The gain or loss in independent life years plotted against age for large (>6 cm) ruptured AVMs in the same four categories.

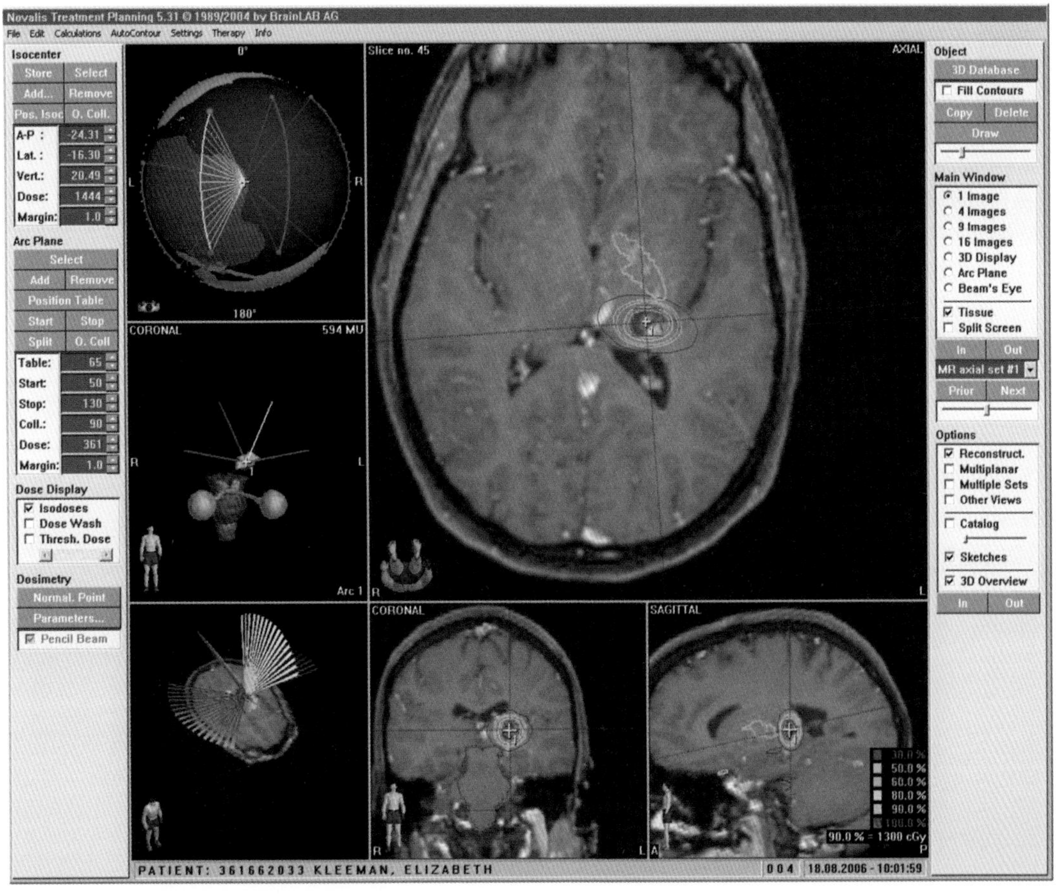

Fig. 28.9 Stereotactic radiosurgery using linear accelerator and micromultileaf collimator (13 Gy to 90% isodose line at lesion periphery) targeting posterior capsular CCM lesion. The patient had suffered from repeated symptomatic hemorrhages with partial hemisensory residual deficit during the 2 years preceding treatment. Patient had no further hemorrhagic episodes or symptom exacerbations in 4 years of follow up after radiosurgery.

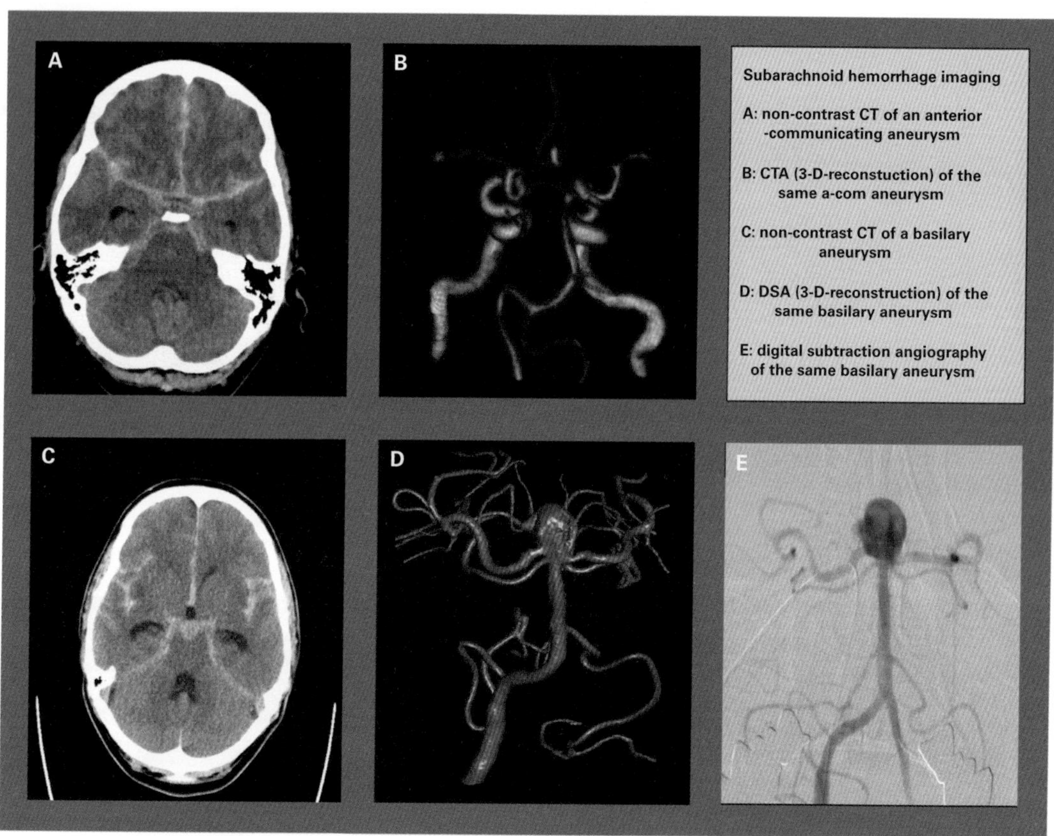

Fig. 29.1 CT/A and DSA imaging of two aneurysms.

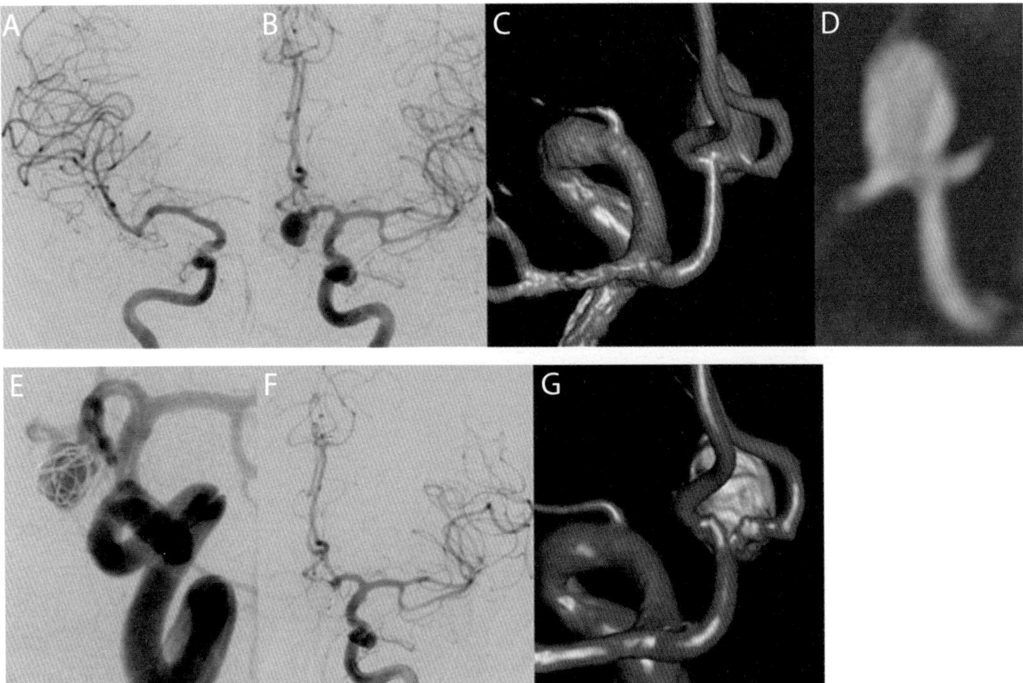

Fig. 31.1 Endovascular coil embolization of an acutely ruptured Acom aneurysm using detachable platinum coils. Note the superiority of 3D rotational angiography in displaying the angioarchitecture of the aneurysm neck.

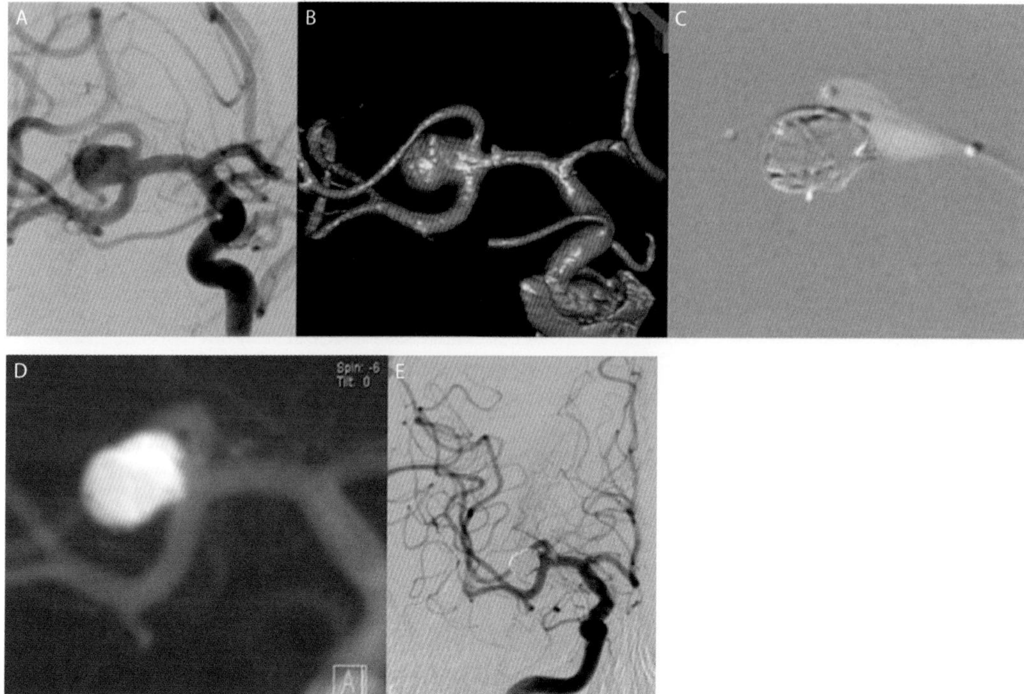

Fig. 31.2 Endovascular coil embolization of an acutely ruptured MCA aneurysm using the 'balloon-remodeling-technique' with an additional balloon placed in the superior branch of the MCA thus narrowing the broad aneurysm neck resulting in dense coil packing and complete aneurysm occlusion.

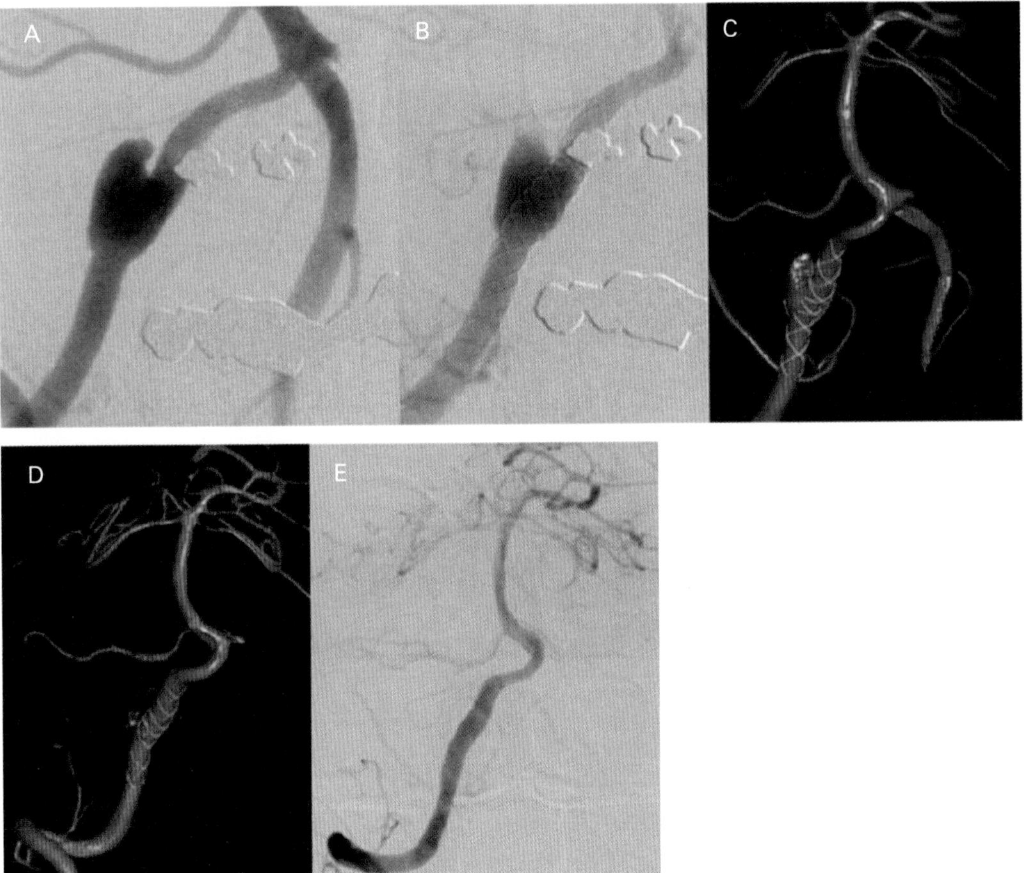

Fig. 31.5 Endovascular therapy of a dissecting fusiform aneurysm of the distal vertebral artery using a flow diverting stent (Silk) resulting in complete aneurysm obliteration at 6-month angiographic follow-up.

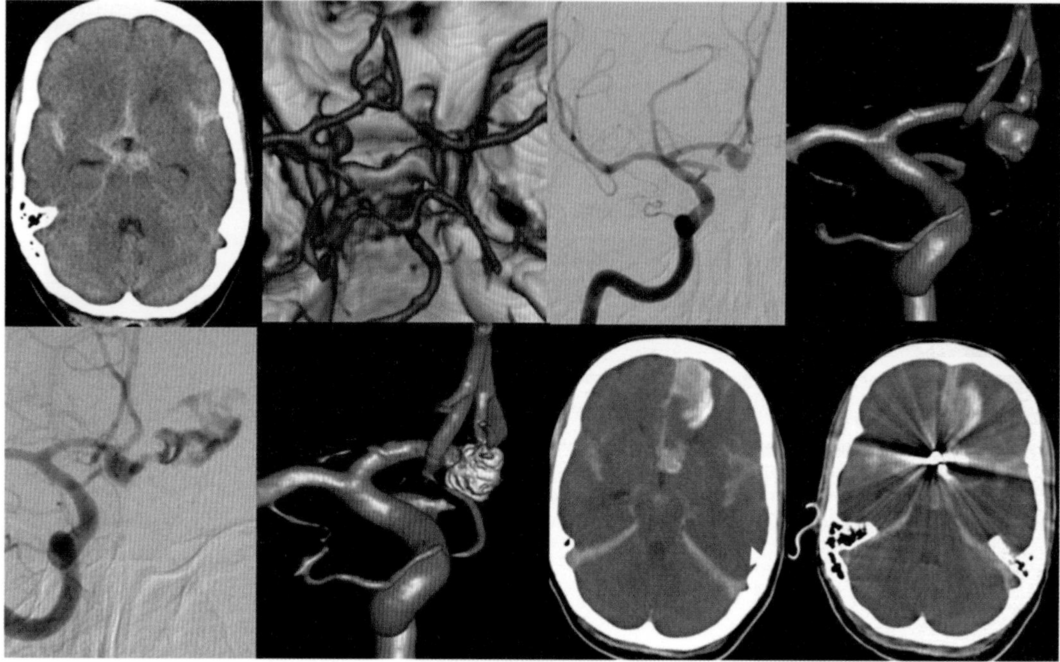

Fig. 31.6 Perforation of an acutely ruptured Acom aneurysm during diagnostic angiography prior to endovascular coil embolization. Immediate subsequent coil embolization resulted in complete aneurysm occlusion. Flat-panel-detector CT imaging (DYNA-CT) within the angio suite revealed the additional hemorrhage in the left frontal lobe.

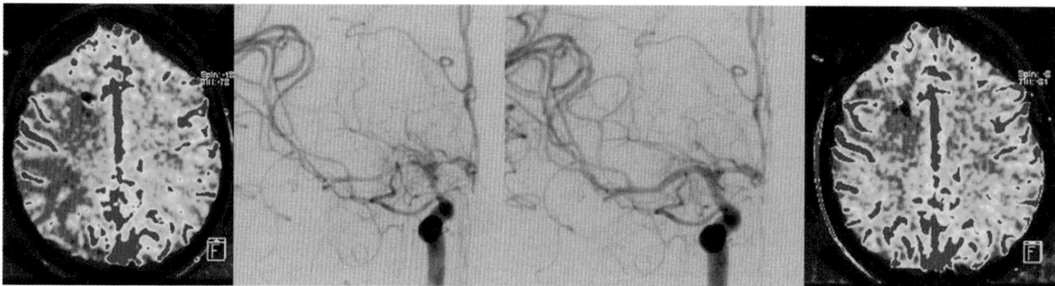

Fig. 31.7 Endovascular treatment of severe cerebral vasospasm in a patient with an acutely ruptured Acom aneurysm using intra-arterial nimodipine. Note perfusion CT imaging before and after administration of the vasoreactive drug resulting in a significantly improved brain perfusion.

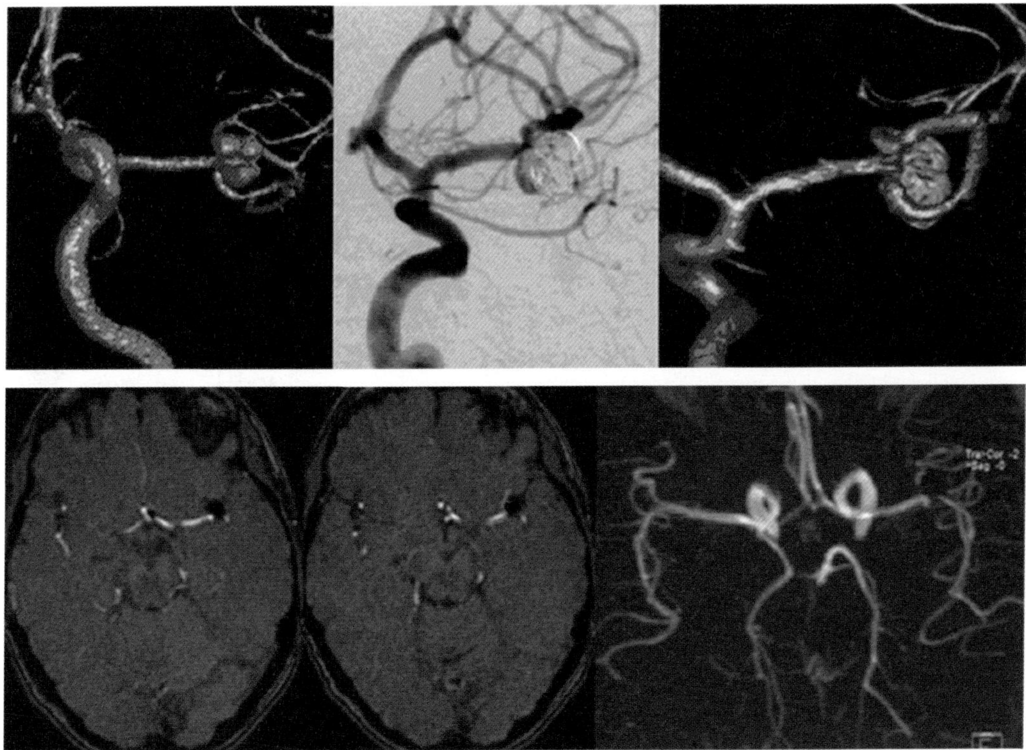

Fig. 31.8 Noninvasive follow-up of a completely embolized MCA aneurysm using TOF-MR angiography 6 months after therapy. Note the additional small aneurysm at the Acom also treated by coil embolization.

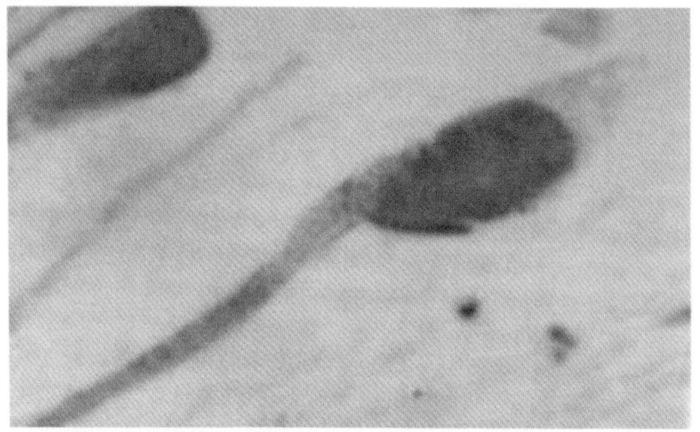

Fig. 36.5 Axonal retraction balls (reprinted with permission from Reilly and Bullock 2e).

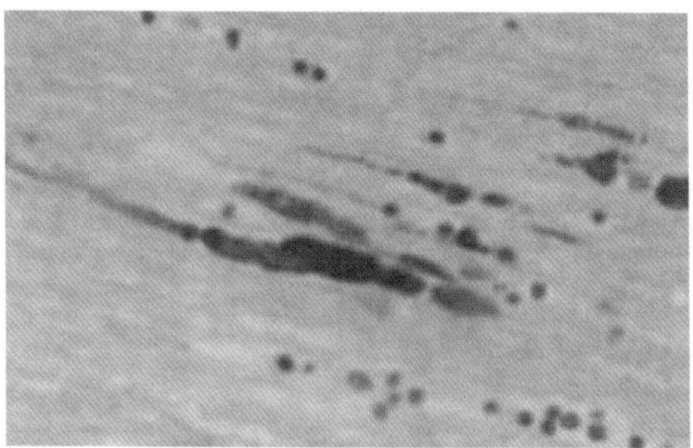

Fig. 36.6 Axonal swelling in the corpus callosum (reprinted with permission from Reilly and Bullock 2e).

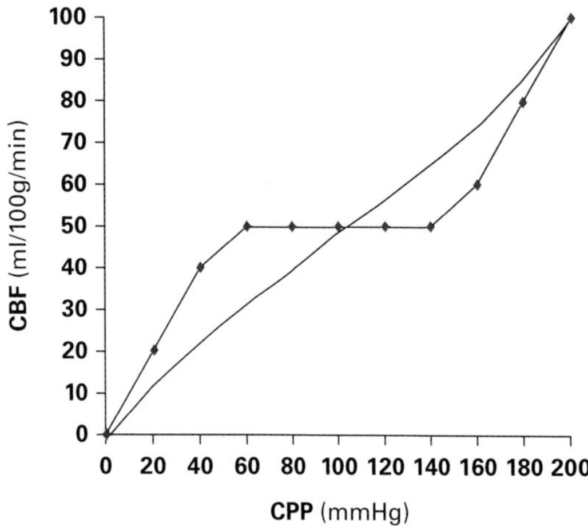

Fig. 36.15 The normal autoregulation curve (red dots) and how it alters after head injury (straight line). (CPP = BP - ICP).

(SCAST): a randomised, placebo-controlled, double-blind trial. *Lancet*. 2011;**377**(9767):741–50.
25. Anderson CS, Heeley E, Huang Y, *et al.* Rapid blood-pressure lowering in patients with acute intracerebral hemorrhage. *N Engl J Med*. 2013.
26. Schrader J, Luders S, Kulchewski A, *et al.* The ACCESS Study. Evaluation of acute candesartan therapy in stroke survivors. *Stroke*. 2003;**34**:1699–703.
27. Barer DH, Cruickshank JM, Ebrahim SB, Mitchell JR. Low dose beta blockade in acute stroke ("BEST" trial): an evaluation. *Br Med J*. 1988;**296**:737–41.
28. Robinson TG, Potter JF, Ford GA, *et al.* Effects of antihypertensive treatment after acute stroke in the Continue or Stop Post-Stroke Antihypertensives Collaborative Study (COSSACS): a prospective, randomised, open, blinded-endpoint trial. *Lancet Neurol*. 2010;**9**(8):767–75.
29. Gray L, Sprigg N, Bath P. ENOS Trial Investigators. Continuing prior antihypertensive medication in acute stroke lowers blood pressure: Data from the continue vs stop arm of the 'Efficacy of Nitric Oxide in Stroke' (ENOS) trial. *J Neurological Sci*. 2005;**238**(supplement 1):S69.
30. Perez MI, Musini VM. Pharmacological interventions for hypertensive emergencies. *Cochrane Database Syst Rev*. 2008(1):CD003653.
31. Cherney D, Straus S. Management of patients with hypertensive urgencies and emergencies: a systematic review of the literature. *J Gen Intern Med*. 2002;**17** (12):937–45.
32. Ahmed N, Wahlgren N, Brainin M, *et al.* Relationship of blood pressure, antihypertensive therapy, and outcome in ischemic stroke treated with intravenous thrombolysis retrospective analysis from Safe Implementation of Thrombolysis in Stroke-International Stroke Thrombolysis Register (SITS-ISTR). *Stroke*. 2009;**40**(7):2442–9.
33. Katzan IL, Furlan AJ, Lloyd LE, *et al.* Use of tissue-type plasminogen activator for acute ischemic stroke – The Cleveland area experience. *JAMA*. 2000;**283**(9):1151–8.
34. Katzan IL, Hammer MD, Furlan AJ, Hixson ED, Nadzam DM. Quality improvement and tissue-type plasminogen activator for acute ischemic stroke – A Cleveland update. *Stroke*. 2003;**34**(3):799–800.
35. Bath PM, Martin RH, Palesch Y, *et al.* Effect of telmisartan on functional outcome, recurrence, and blood pressure in patients with acute mild ischemic stroke: a PRoFESS subgroup analysis. *Stroke*. 2009;**40**(11):3541–6.
36. Geeganage C, Bath PMW. Relationship between therapeutic changes in blood pressure and outcomes in acute stroke. A metaregression. *Hypertension*. 2009;**54**:775–81.
37. Brott T, Lu M, Kothari R, *et al.* Hypertension and its treatment in the NINDS rt-PA stroke trial. *Stroke*. 1998;**29**:1504–9.
38. Goldstein LB, Matchar DB, Morgenlander JC, Davis JN. Influence of drugs on the recovery of sensorimotor function after stroke. *Neurorehabilitation Neural Repair*. 1990;**4**(3):137–44.
39. Sare GM, Geeganage C, Bath PM. High blood pressure in acute ischaemic stroke – broadening therapeutic horizons. *Cerebrovascular Dis*. 2009;**27 supplement (1)**: 156–61.
40. Potter JF, Robinson TG, Ford GA, *et al.* Controlling hypertension and hypotension immediately post-stroke (CHHIPS): a randomised, placebo-controlled, double-blind pilot trial. *Lancet Neurol*. 2009;**8**(1):48–56.
41. Geeganage C, Bath PM. Interventions for deliberately altering blood pressure in acute stroke. *Cochrane Database Syst Rev*. 2008(4):CD000039.
42. Else CS, Philip MWB, Gudrun B, *et al.* The angiotensin-receptor blocker candesartan for treatment of acute stroke (SCAST): a randomised, placebo-controlled, double-blind trial. *Lancet*. 2011;**377**:741–50.
43. Wahlgren NG, MacMahon DG, de Keyser J, Indredavik B, Ryman T. INWEST Study Group. Intravenous Nimodipine West European Stroke Trial (INWEST) of nimodipine in the treatment of acute ischaemic stroke. *Cerebrovascular Diseases*. 1994;**4**:204–10.
44. Ahmed N, Nasman P, Wahlgren NG. Effect of intravenous nimodipine on blood pressure and outcome after acute stroke. *Stroke*. 2000;**31**:1250–5.
45. Horn J, Limburg M. Calcium antagonists for acute ischemic stroke. *Cochrane Database Syst Rev*. 2000(2):CD001928.
46. Amenta F, Lanari A, Mignini F, *et al.* Nicardipine use in cerebrovascular disease: a review of controlled clinical studies. *J Neurol Sci*. 2009;**283**(1–2):219–23.
47. Eames PJ, Robinson TG, Panerai RB, Potter JF. Bendrofluazide fails to reduce elevated blood pressure levels in the immediate post stroke period. *Cerebrovascular Diseases*. 2005;**19**:253–9.
48. Bath PMW, Pathansali R, Iddenden R, Bath FJ. The effect of transdermal glyceryl trinitrate, a nitric oxide donor, on blood pressure and platelet function in acute stroke. *Cerebrovasc Dis*. 2001;**11**:265–72.
49. Willmot M, Ghadami A, Whysall B, *et al.* Transdermal glyceryl trinitrate lowers blood pressure and maintains cerebral blood flow in recent stroke. *Hypertension*. 2006;**47**(6):1209–15.
50. Sare GM, Gray LJ, Wardlaw J, Chen C, Bath PMW. ENOS Trial Investigators. Is lowering blood pressure hazardous in patients with significant ipsilateral carotid stenosis and

acute ischaemic stroke? Interim assessment in the 'Efficacy of Nitric Oxide in Stroke' Trial. *Blood Pressure Monitoring*. 2009;**14**(1):20–5.

51. Asplund K. Haemodilution for acute ischaemic stroke. *Cochrane Database Syst Rev*. 2002(4):CD000103.

52. Sandercock PAG, Willems H. Medical treatment of acute ischaemic stroke. *Lancet*. 1992;**339**:537–9.

53. Mistri AK, Robinson TG, Potter JF. Pressor therapy in acute ischemic stroke: Systematic review. *Stroke*. 2006;**37**(6):1565–71.

SECTION 4

Critical Care of Intracranial Hemorrhage

20

Management of intracranial hemorrhage: early expansion and second bleeds

Corina Epple and Thorsten Steiner

Introduction

Spontaneous intracerebral hemorrhage (SICH) accounts for about 15% of all strokes, and although mortality could be reduced during the last 10 years it is still about 20–30% (approaching 50%) within 3 months and severe disability in the majority of survivors [1]. Half of these deaths occur within the acute phase, especially in the first 2 days. Volume of SICH, together with conscious state, were both recognized as critical prognostic determinants [2]. For a long time it was erroneously believed that the volume of a cerebral hematoma was usually maximal at onset. Frequently observed deterioration during the first day was attributed to developing cerebral edema and mass effect surrounding the hemorrhage. However, serial CT (computed tomography) scans showed that clinical deterioration is often attributed to hematoma expansion and this is also a reason for high mortality [3,4].

Increase of hematoma volume is a frequent complication in SICH and was observed in more than 70% of cases, when defined as any increase in parenchymal volume or intraventricular invasion. In the Cincinnati study Brott and co-workers [4,5] found the majority of relevant growth, i.e. 26% (defined as an increase of more than 33% of the hematoma volume on admission CT or absolute change in hematoma volume of >12.5 ml), to occur within 4 hours after symptom onset, while an additional 12% of patients developed growth within the following 21 hours. In summary 38% of cases exhibited significant growth within the first 24 hours. This suggests that growth occurs early in the course of SICH (when most of the patients are carried between CT, MRI (magnetic resonance tomography), stroke unit, ICU or emergency room getting their diagnostic studies for acute evaluation) and early CT scan repetition is warranted to detect it [5–8]. These findings demonstrate that, like ischemic stroke, SICH is a dynamic process where the treatment goal is limitation of hematoma volume. The dynamic nature of SICH during the first several hours represents an opportunity and a challenge to physicians.

Hematoma volume at presentation, hematoma growth (as defined by Brott *et al.*) and the development of intraventricular hemorrhage (IVH) were shown to be crucial and independent predictors of early neurological deterioration and are associated with increased mortality and poor functional outcome [9]. A pooled individual patient meta-analysis showed that for each 10% increase in SICH growth, there was a 5% increased hazard of death, a 16% greater likelihood of worsening by 1 point on the mRS (modified Rankin Scale), or 18% of moving from independence to assisted independence or from assisted independence to poor outcome on the Barthel Index [8]. These findings indicate that early extension of the initial hematoma boundaries has substantial clinical implications (Fig. 20.1).

Critical Care of the Stroke Patient, ed. Stefan Schwab, Daniel Hanley, and A. David Mendelow. Published by Cambridge University Press.

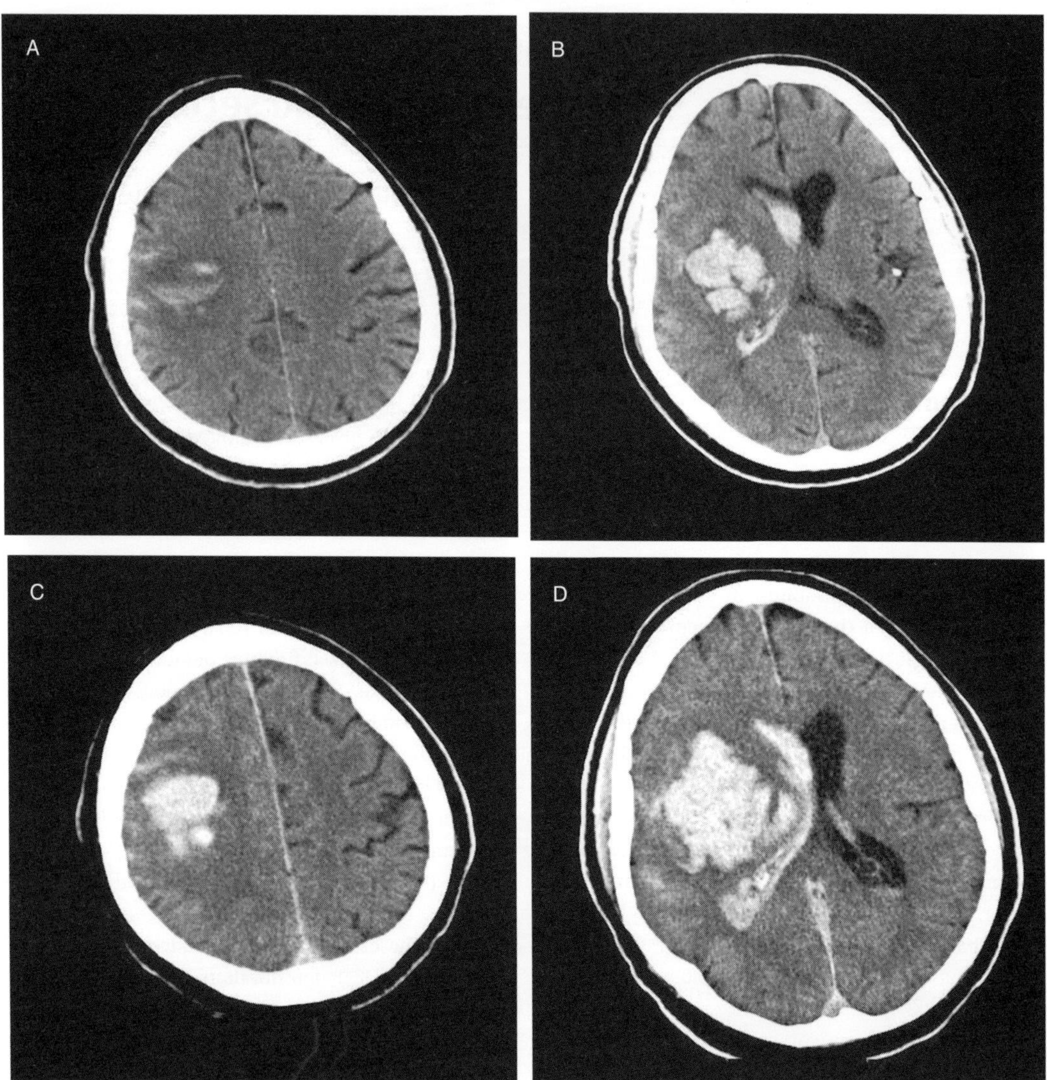

Fig. 20.1: 64-year-old man with acute left-sided hemiparesis and dysarthria; NIHSSS 9; prior ASS use, hypertension not treated. **A and B**: CCT shows a SICH with IVH with hematoma volume 44 ml 1 hour after onset. **C and D:** 2 hours later the patient developed a clinical deterioration (NIHSSS 18) with SBP>180 mmHg despite treatment with i.v. drugs. CCT shows a hematoma expansion (hematoma volume 95 ml).

Terminology

Terms for the phenomenon of hematoma enlargement in SICH have not been used consistently in the literature. They include growth, enlargement, extension, expansion, rebleeding, etc. We therefore define hematoma expansion (HE) as all forms of extended spatial distribution of the initial hemorrhage, including intraparenchymal volume enlargement, invasion of the ventricles (not necessarily associated with change in intraparenchymal volume), transition into adjacent compartments (such as the subarachnoid space), and rebleeding adjacent to the original hemorrhage. We do not, however, include the formation of a perihematomal edema in this definition although this may play a role in the pathophysiology of HE. We further define early HE as HE occurring within the first 24 hours after onset of SICH, i.e. the vast majority of all relevant HEs. Finally, we define efforts to restrict HE as all measures that are undertaken in order to prevent or reduce HE in the first place. This does not include treating the consequences of HE such as lowering intracranial pressure, hematoma evacuation merely aimed at volume reduction or clearance of the ventricles. These definitions will be used throughout this chapter. The following is focused on prevention or attenuation of early HE, not on the sequelae and complications beyond 24 hours, acknowledging, however, that these substantially influence prognosis. Here, we summarize the risk factors of HE, present current knowledge on surgical and non-surgical approaches towards HE and finally outline future strategies [10].

Expansion of parenchymal hematomas leads to intraventricular bleeding (IVH) in about 35% up to about 50% of patients [11–13]. The presence of IVH in itself is a predictor of worse outcome, but expansion of IVH does worsen the prognosis even more [12]. Expansion of IVH occurred in 21% of patients in a prospective registry [13].

Pathophysiology behind early hematoma expansion

The pathophysiology behind early hematoma expansion is not well understood. It is not clear whether it reflects leakage or rebleeding, or both. It was C. M. Fisher who concluded from the detailed study of two brains that hypertensive ICH most likely results from rupture of lipohyalinoic arteries followed by secondary arterial ruptures at the periphery of the enlarging hematoma in a cascade or avalanche fashion. This observation of mechanical disruption and tearing of smaller vessels might account for the gradual development of ICH and can probably be considered the most relevant neuropathological correlate for the 'growing' properties of hemorrhages (like a rolling snowball) [14]. Several mechanisms of brain injury after SICH have been investigated, but most of these evolve too late to account for early hematoma expansion [15]. In addition to disruption of supportive and protective functional tissue, elevated intracranial pressure, reduced oxygen supply, and mitochondrial dysfunction in the perihematomal zone, deleterious factors in the blood or perihematomal edema might act on vessels and the blood–brain barrier (BBB) [16]. It is proposed to be a heterogeneous process that includes dysregulation of hemostasis via inflammatory cascade activation and matrix metallo-proteinases (MMP) overexpression. Animal and human studies suggest an association of inflammatory activation (increased inflammatory mediator interleukin-6 [IL-6] and tumor necrosis factor alpha [TNFα]) and degradation of components of the BBB basal membrane (with increased plasma concentration of cellular fibronectins [c-Fn]) by matrix metallo-proteinases with hematoma enlargement in SICH. MMPs probably act by enhancing extracellular matrix proteolysis, damaging the basal lamina, and degrading cellular fibronectin, a glycoprotein that is essential for hemostasis [17–19]. Furthermore, repeated or continuous bleeding can be the result of coagulopathies or anticoagulants [20]. A role for disturbed autoregulation and uncontrolled perfusion pressure in hypertension as a driving force for further bleeding is conceivable but data on this are controversial.

For the extension of parenchymal bleeding into the ventricles the most accepted explanation at this time is breakthrough from adjacent anatomical structures [12]. Every increase of 10 ml of parenchymal hemorrhage was shown to increase intraventricular blood volume by about 2.5 ml and is accompanied by worsening of prognosis.

Risk factors of early hematoma expansion

Prediction of HE at baseline would be a first step toward an effective therapy. Several smaller and larger trials have investigated various potential predictors of HE, resulting in consistent as well as inconsistent evidence on several parameters. It is important to realize that many predictor studies differ in such important aspects as time to first CT, observation period and definitions of HE. In the following we have summarized predictors that were only found in prospective trials or post-hoc analyses of randomized controlled trials that used similar definitions of HE. Predictors that neither have been disapproved of, nor have been confirmed prospectively, comprise *patient and treatment characteristics* (large hematoma volume on presentation, intraventricular invasion, early neurological deterioration, treatment with rFVII, a non-intensified blood pressure treatment, prior use of warfarin), *radiological characteristics* (shorter time between onset and first CT, hematoma density heterogeneity on admission CT, occurrence of a 'spot sign' (SpS) in CTA (CT angiography), and *laboratory characteristics* (reduced platelet activity, elevated interleukin-6, elevated cellular fibronectin). Contradictive results were found for elevated d-dimers and prior use of platelets. The latter was described as a risk factor for growth in 188 SICH patients treated with tranexamic acid and antihypertensives within 24 hours, but exact timing of CT scans is not mentioned in that study [10,21,22]. Prior antiplatelet use was linked to growth of SICH. Although this relationship between prior antiplatelet use and increased hemorrhage growth is biologically quite plausible, this observation needs to be confirmed in subsequent trials [23].

Another potential factor related to HE was a higher serum creatinine level. A biological explanation could be that creatinine is a recognized marker of longstanding hypertension with accumulated vascular injury and increased fragility of small vessels and may reflect severe renal dysfunction, which is associated with impaired platelet function [24].

Contrast extravasation on admission CT angiography (the so-called 'spot-sign', see Fig. 20.2) and a contrast extravasation in a post-contrast CT scan as a predictor of hematoma expansion were also found in retrospective and prospective studies, extended to a proposed 'spot sign score', which is used to grade the number of SpS and their maximum dimension and attenuation. This was found as an independent predictor of mortality and poor outcome among survivors in SICH, but not a predictor for HE, whereas a contrast extravasation after CT angiography indicates active bleeding and was regarded as a potential sign for predicting hematoma expansion [25–27]. The PREDICT trial, a prospective multicentre observational study (including 228 patients for primary analysis) showed that the CTA spot sign is highly predictive of HE for intraparenchymal and intraventricular hemorrhage growth, and is associated with larger hemorrhage and a poor prognosis. The usefulness of the CTA SpS should be tested in proof-of-concept trials of hemostatic drugs in patients with ICH [28] (see Fig. 20.2). History of hypertension was not found to be a significant factor (see subsequently). Further systematic and comparable validation of predictors of HE is warranted as this might prevent delay of appropriate therapy but also influence estimates on prognosis or decisions to withdraw therapy.

Therapeutic options to restrict hematoma expansion

In theory, if one could stop the bleeding during the first few hours and remove the accumulated blood without significant additional brain trauma from the operation, neurological deterioration and poor outcome could be prevented in some patients. Therapeutic options to restrict HE can be divided into surgical and nonsurgical approaches, whereas both might complement each other.

Surgical approach

Insufficient evidence exists with regard to the efficacy of surgical treatment for SICH, and whether or not surgical approaches are beneficial remains controversial. Surgical procedures with varying amounts of supportive evidence include conventional craniotomy, minimally invasive surgery (MIS), and decompressive craniectomy. The diverse methods of MIS include stereotactic guidance with aspiration and thrombolysis with alteplase or urokinase and image-guided stereotactic endoscopic aspiration. With respect to the restriction of HE, neurosurgical intervention can have the following aims: removal of the source of hemorrhage, staunching of the bleeding, and elimination of the effects of blood degradation products. The mere removal of blood by

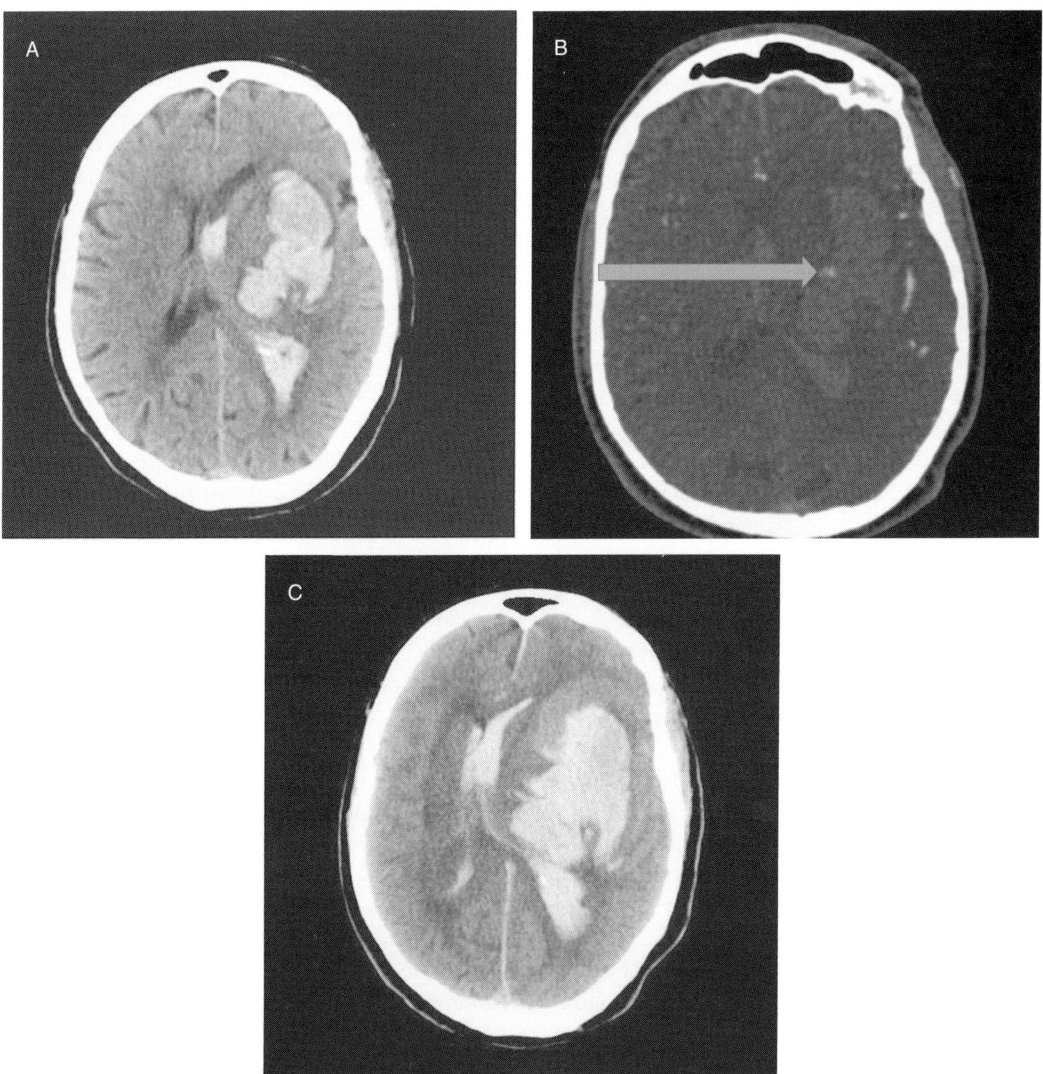

Fig. 20.2 Spot sign: **A**: baseline non-contrast CT. **B**: Baseline CT angiography with a single spot sign (see arrow). **C**: Follow up non-contrast CT 2.5 hours later showing a hematoma expansion.

open craniotomy or stereotactic aspiration, i.e. reduction of mass, cannot be regarded as a measure to restrict HE. Although it could be argued that the removal of blood leads to elimination of deleterious promoters of further bleeding or allows access to a bleeding source, these aspects were not looked at or reported specifically in most of the relevant surgical trials performed so far.

Another problem is that most surgical trials did not identify early HE or enrol enough patients early enough to allow conclusions on restriction in the sense of our definitions. Morgenstern and colleagues performed two small trials to answer the question of intervention timing. Indeed, the first study revealed better outcome for those patients operated on within 12 hours after onset. However, the follow-up study with a time window of 4 hours showed a higher mortality due to an increased rebleeding rate [29,30]. It is not clear whether early HE had an influence on these results. Release of tamponating tissue pressure at this early stage of the disease may have caused rebleeding. Some authors therefore consider combination of hemostatics with early surgery a promising alternative [31].

The Surgical Trial in Intra Cerebral Hemorrhage (STICH), currently the largest prospective trial on surgery in SICH, failed to show an outcome benefit over conservative treatment, and cannot be applied to the question of early HE restriction either, with a time window of 96 hours, mean time from ictus to surgery was 30 hours (i.e. after the majority of relevant HE should already have occurred). Furthermore, HE was not specifically identified and surgical treatment (craniotomy in 75%) was mainly directed at reduction of mass and pressure. STICH-II, the follow-up trial limited to patients with lobar SICH without IVH, was also not designed to answer the question of surgical HE restriction, and did not show a positive clinical effect of surgical hematoma evacuation within at least 50 hours after ictus at 6 months [10,32,33].

More interesting with regard to HE might be endoscopic surgery, as iatrogenic bleeding risk might be reduced in an early, less stable phase of SICH and the coagulation of oozing vessels can be combined with hematoma evacuation. Evidence, however, is very limited. Twenty years ago, a small prospective randomized trial of endoscopic vs. medical treatment of 100 SICH patients resulted in better outcome and reduced mortality for endoscopic treatment within 48 hours of onset [34]. More recently, Cho and colleagues introduced a score for basal ganglia hemorrhage and evaluated its prediction power in endoscopic versus conservative treatment of 226 patients [35]. The authors concluded that a mid-level modified intracerebral hemorrhage (MICH) score of 2–4 (based on the determinants GCS, ICH volume and IVH or hydrocephalus) favors endoscopic surgery to improve function or reduce mortality. Unfortunately, due to differences in surgical technique, radiological documentation and timing of treatment in the aforementioned surgical trials, it is difficult if not impossible to draw any conclusions on HE restriction. In fact, evidence that surgery alone can restrict expansion of SICH is presently nonexistent. Clearly, trials that are tailored more individually with regard to patient characteristics and SICH features are still necessary to elucidate the role of surgery. To date, surgery might add to medical treatment with regard to survival or independence, but this is not very robust, and thus, no general recommendation can be given with regard to surgical prevention of HE.

Nonsurgical approach

On the one hand a high blood pressure as a driving force and on the other hand the persistence of leakage, especially in a compromised coagulation, are the two major pathophysiological considerations with regard to HE that are deemed as potential treatment targets. Thus, lowering BP, antagonizing anticoagulant therapy, and applying hemostatics as conservative principles have been tested in clinical trials of reasonable quality.

Management of blood pressure

Findings on hypertension as a risk factor for rebleeding were contradictive. Many studies have shown an association between increased BP (>140/90 mmHg) in the acute phase of SICH and HE, perihematomal edema and rebleeding. The mechanism for the acute increase of blood pressure after SICH is unknown. However, it is proposed to be a multifactorial process that includes activation of the neuroendocrine systems (sympathetic nervous system, glucocorticoid system, or the renin-angiotensin axis), increased cardiac output, and stress response to conditions such as increased ICP, headache, and urinary retention [36–38]. The poor outcome associated with increased blood pressure after SICH could be minimized with blood pressure (BP) monitoring and treatment aimed at optimized cerebral perfusion while minimizing ongoing bleeding.

INTERACT (INTEnsive blood pressure Reduction in Acute Cerebral hemorrhage Trial) was the first randomized trial addressing the effect of lowering

BP in SICH and compared intensive (target SBP (systolic BP) 140 mmHg) with guideline-based (target SBP 180 mmHg) BP reduction within the first 6 hours in 404 patients with acute SICH. It yielded safety, feasibility and a trend towards reduction of HE, but no difference in outcome [39]. The choice of antihypertensive drug was at the discretion of the treating physician. INTERACT-2 was similarly designed and looked at a clinical primary endpoint of death or major disability (modified Rankin Score (mRS) of three to six) at 90 days. Though statistical significance was just missed for the primary endpoint, most other measurements do speak in favor of intensive BP lowering. The predefined ordinal analysis showed significantly lower mRS for patients with intensive BP treatment, the analyses of pre-specified subgroups (age, ethnicity, time to randomization, baseline BP, history of hypertension, baseline NIHSS, hematoma volume and location), and safety outcome did not differ in the two groups.

Based on this background, the ATACH (Antihypertensive Treatment of Acute Cerebral Hemorrhage) trial program becomes even more interesting. The first ATACH trial aimed at feasibility and safety of three levels of systolic BP reduction (BP target tiers), 1) 170–200 mmHg (n = 18); 2) 140–170 mmHg (n = 20); and 3) 110–140 mmHg (n = 22) within 6 hours after symptom onset of supratentorial ICH. This RCT included 60 patients with lobar, supratentorial SICH, a presenting SBP>170 mmHg who were treated with only intravenous nicardipin [40]. The authors reported safety and feasibility of this phase I dose-finding trial. However, ATACH-1 was not designed to address HE in the first place.

The ATACH-2 becomes particularly interesting, because it will look at the clinical effect of a stronger BP treatment (treatment trigger threshold <180 mmHg) within a shorter time frame (3 hours) compared to INTERACT-2 [41]. We should also mention another trial of intensive blood pressure reduction below a mean arterial pressure of 110 mmHg that was reported in a smaller prospective controlled trial of 42 patients with SICH and demonstrated feasibility [42].

Appreciating a slight effect of antihypertensives on HE reduction in an overall weak or equivocal context of evidence and considering that autoregulation is often preserved in the acute phase (as opposed to the post-acute phase) of SICH and furthermore aggressive lowering of BP theoretically carries the risk of cerebral ischemia in hypertensive patients, it seems reasonable to presently follow current guidelines and lower BP cautiously [43–46]. Interestingly, Gould and colleagues showed in a small RCT that BP reduction does not exacerbate perihematoma hypoperfusion. Although in this trial autoregulation was not studied <6 hours from onset (the period where BP treatment is most likely to be beneficial), this finding adds further support to the safety of early BP reduction after ICH [47] (Tables 20.1 and 20.2).

Management of temperature and blood glucose

In a pooled analysis covering 14431 patients with stroke or other brain injuries, fever is consistently associated with worse outcome across multiple outcome measures. A high body temperature after ICH may be associated with HE (biological arguments exist that fever results on a local level in blood–brain barrier breakdown and reduces cytoskeletal stability), cerebral edema, increased ICP, and early neurological deterioration [48]. Fever after ICH is associated with longer ICU and hospital stays, poor functional outcome, and increased mortality. Most infectious fevers are due to pulmonary infections and urinary tract infections. Patients with intraventricular extension of hemorrhage are thought to have more neurogenic or 'central fever' [39,48,49]. Treatment with antipyretics and cooling blankets is used for patients with a sustained fever of more than 38.3°C. No evidence is available from RCTs linking fever treatment with improved clinical outcome or reduced mortality [50]. So far there is one multicentre, randomized, prospective study available, that investigated fever in patients with acute ischemic stroke and ICH [51]. 1400 patients with acute stroke were enrolled in the PAIS trail, 11% of these (n = 273) had an ICH. Patients received prophylactic paracetamol or placebo within the first 12 hours from symptom onset. No significant effect on outcome could be attested, although the

Table 20.1 Suggested recommended guidelines for treating elevated BP in SICH (according to Morgenstern *et al.* 2010 [37]).

Systolic blood pressure (SBP)	Mean arterial pressure (MAP)	Intracranial pressure (ICP)	Recommendation
>200 mmHg	>150 mmHg		Consider aggressive reduction of BP with continuous intravenous infusion, with frequent BP monitoring every 5 minutes
>180 mmHg	>130 mmHg	Possibility of elevated ICP	Consider monitoring ICP and reducing BP using intermittent or continuous intravenous medications while maintaining a cerebral perfusion pressure ≥60 mmHg
>180 mmHg	>130 mmHg	No evidence of elevated ICP	Consider a modest reduction of BP (e.g. MAP of 110 mmHg or target BP of 160/90 mmHg) using intermittent or continuous intravenous medications to control BP and clinically re-examine the patient and BP every 15 minutes

Table 20.2 Antihypertensive drugs recommended for acute treatment of raised BP after SICH (drugs with a cerebral vasodilatation should be avoided).

Drug	Mode of action	Dosage	Comment
Labetalol	alpha-/beta-blocker	5–20 mg (intermittent boluses) every 15 min or 2 mg/min in continuous infusion (drip)	In some European countries this is not available as an i.v. drug
Uradipil	alpha-blocker	12.5–25 mg bolus or 5–40 mh/h infusion	Avoid in patients with coronary ischemia
Esmolol	beta-blocker	250 μg/kg (loading dose), then 25–300 μg/kg per min (maintenance)	Contraindicated for bradycardia, heart failure, bronchospasm
Nicardipine	vasodilatator	5–15 mg/h infusion	Contraindicated for coronary ischemia
Nitroprusside	vasodilatator	0.1–10 μg/kg per min infusion	Contraindicated for patients with high ICP
Hydralazine	vasodilatator	5–20 mg (intermittent boluses)	Avoid in patients with tachycardia or coronary ischemia
Clonidin	antisympatotonicum	25 μg bolus i.v.	Sedative; contraindicated for bradycardia

mean body temperature in the paracetamol group was significantly lower. A trend for a positive effect for patients with ICH with wide confidence intervals was shown, but the subgroup of patients with ICH was too small to derive a recommendation from these results. Meanwhile the PAIS II trail has been initiated (trial number: NTR2365) [52].

A population-based study showed an increased 7- and 30-day mortality associated with diabetes mellitus [1]. An exploratory analysis of the recombinant activated factor VII intracerebral hemorrhage trial suggested a relationship between elevated glucose and increased risk of hemorrhage growth in SICH. Certainly, serum glucose becomes elevated in response to increased stroke severity and may be a marker for larger SICH and patient stress rather than a contributing cause of HE. Whether there is a causal relationship between elevated blood glucose and hemorrhage size remains uncertain. Based on poor clinical data a normalization of blood glucose levels (>40 mg/dl and <100 mg/dl for fasting blood glucose) is recommended.

Effects of antagonization of anticoagulation and restoring of hemostasis

In particular, **recombinant coagulation factor VIIa (rFVIIa)**, licensed to treat hemophilia patients with high titer inhibitors or congenital factor VII deficiency seemed to be a promising candidate. Unfortunately, the phase III trial FAST (Factor seven for Acute hemorrhagic Stroke Trial) which included 816 patients who received either 20 or 80 μg/kg of rFVIIa or placebo, did not reveal any clinical benefit [53,54], although the trial confirmed the HE-restrictive properties of rFVIIa. However, this had no influence on functional outcome or mortality. A post-hoc analysis of the FAST data suggests a potential benefit of rFVIIa in younger patients (<70 years) with baseline hematoma volume <60 ml, IVH< 5 ml, and onset time to treatment of <2.5 hours. However, treatment with rFVIIa cannot be recommended to restrict HE in patients with SICH until these findings are confirmed in further RCTs.

Underlying hemostatic abnormalities can contribute to ICH. Patients at risk include those on anticoagulant therapy (AT), those with acquired or congenital coagulation factor deficiencies, and those with qualitative or quantitative platelet abnormalities. For patients with a **coagulation factor deficiency** and thrombocytopenia, replacement of the appropriate factor or platelets is indicated. Studies on the effect of **prior antiplatelet agent use or platelet dysfunction** on ICH hematoma growth and outcome have found conflicting results. The utility and safety of platelet transfusion or other agents in patients with a normal platelet count, but use of antiplatelet agents or platelet dysfunction, are not known. Patients undergoing treatment with AT constitute 12–14% of patients with ICH, and with increased use of AT, the proportion appears to be increasing [37,55].

The use of **vitamin-K-antagonists (VKA)**, although probably rather a contributing than a causative factor, does not only lead to a higher incidence of intracerebral hemorrhage, but also to HE in 27–54% of the cases, and well beyond the 24-hour time window that we define as early expansion. This might at least partially explain a substantial increase in mortality of up to 70%. Underlying causes of spontaneous ICH and oral anticoagulant therapy (OAC) ICH might be the same, with OAC being only a precipitating factor. It is also possible that OAC directly causes ICH by interfering with the synthesis of vitamin-K-dependent clotting factors [55–58]. Experts agree that anticoagulation has to be reversed rapidly, but the chosen ways to achieve this differ greatly [59]. There is an ongoing controversy with regard to treatment and different guidelines are inconsistent at an international level. None of the treatment regimens have been proven to be more effective than another. It is customary to discontinue oral VKA and substitute vitamin-K, but this alone is insufficient for rapid normalization of coagulation, even when given intravenously, because it requires several hours to correct the INR. Current questions arise on feasibility, safety, and efficacy of prothrombin-dependent coagulation factors in a concentrated form (PCC: prothrombin complex concentrate) versus unconcentrated 'fresh-frozen plasma (FFP)' versus single factors like recombinant coagulation factor VIIa (rFVIIa). The current data situation on these questions is inconsistent and any conclusions drawn towards preference of one of these coagulants are premature. Time to INR reversal seems to be the most important determinant, and minimizing delays in drug administration should have highest priority. A retrospective study comparing the acute treatment strategies of OAC-associated ICH using vitamin-K (VKA), FFP, and PCC with regard to hematoma growth and outcome showed that nearly all PCC-treated patients achieved an early INR reversal. The overall positive performance of PCCs compared with FFP and VKA might be because of faster INR reversal in the acute bleeding phase. This attribute of PCCs might be explained by a higher concentration of coagulation factors in PCCs compared with FFP, which contains all coagulation factors in a non-concentrated form and therefore large volumes are required to achieve effective hemostasis, while the actual content of VKA-dependent coagulation factors in each unit of FFP vary considerably. The efficacy of FFP is limited by risk of allergic and infectious transfusion reactions, processing time, and the volume required for correction with the risk of fluid overload, especially in patients with heart failure [60]. Apart from that, PCCs contain the risk of infectious diseases, even if it is small, and furthermore the risk of thrombembolism due to PCC is not clear.

The INCH (International normalized ratio (INR) Normalization in Coumadin associated intracerebral Haemorrhage) trial, a multicentre, randomized, controlled trial to compare FFP with PCC, was initiated in 2009 to answer the question of INR early reversal [61]. At present, it can only be recommended to discontinue warfarin, give vitamin-K, and rapidly reverse anticoagulation by whatever protocol is institutionally established. Current recommendations are summarized in Table 20.3.

In the case of **heparin-associated intracerebral hemorrhage**, only epidemiological data exist, insufficient to support a general recommendation concerning HE restriction [55]. Clinicians are thus left to the reasonable approach to normalize coagulation with protamine sulphate as customary. **Low-dose heparin** for prophylaxis of deep vein thrombosis does not seem to carry a relevant risk of HE [62].

Perhaps a more difficult therapeutic dilemma is how to manage patients with clinical thromboembolic complications after ICH, balancing the risk of subsequent life-threatening thromboembolism if untreated against the risk or **recurrence of ICH**. A related issue is whether or when to resume anticoagulation after ICH in patients with cardiac disease associated with high embolism risk, such as those who need mechanical valve prostheses or those with atrial fibrillation. The decision is often made on the basis of a risk–benefit analysis in the context of the individual patient. Anticoagulation has been estimated to double the

Table 20.3 Reversal of anticoagulation or in case of suspected antiplatelet use associated ICH

Drug	Indication	Dosage	Comment
Vitamin-K	OAC-reversal, hepatic dysfunction	5–10 mg i.v.	Remains an adjunct to initial therapy OAC-associated hemorrhage because normalisation of INR can take up to 24 hours
Fresh frozen plasma (FFP)	OAC-reversal, consumptive coagulopathy, hepatic dysfunction	10–20 ml/kg	Contains factors I (fibrinogen), II, V, VII, IX, X, XI, XIII, antithrombin commonly used as an adjunct to vitamin-K; acts within hours; is associated with greater volume expansion, which might precipitate heart failure, and requires much longer infusion times
Prothrombin complex concentrates (PCCs)	Factor IX defiency (hemophilia B), OAC reversal	10–50 IU/kg; max. 3000 IU	Contains various amounts of factors II, IX, X, and various amounts of VII. Be aware that not all PCCs contain all four factors. Acts within minutes; might lead to fewer complications than FFP and can be considered as an alternative to FFP
Recombinant coagulation factor VIIa (rFVIIa)	Factor VII deficiency	40–80 μg/kg	Acts within a few minutes; does not replace all clotting factors. Although the INR might be lowered, clotting might not be restored in vivo; rFVIIa is therefore not routinely recommended as a sole agent for OAC reversal in ICH
Protamine sulphate	heparin-associated ICH	max. 50 mg within 10 minutes i.v.	10 mg can inactivate 1000 IE heparin; dosage can be determined by titration
Platelet transfusions	ICH patients with history of antiplatelet use		The usefulness in ICH patients is unclear and is considered investigational

risk or recurrent ICH compared with the overall recurrence risk of ICH, and the mortality rate associated with recurrent ICH can be as high as 50% [37,63]. The risk of recurrent ICH can depend on factors such as the patient's age and the location of ICH, presence of the apolipoprotein ε2 or ε4 alleles, and greater number of microbleeds on MRI. Patients with lobar hemorrhages are at higher risk of rebleeding, probably due to suspected amyloid angiopathy [45,64]. The optimum timing of the resumption of anticoagulation is a crucial issue with conflicting evidence. Although guidelines from the American Heart Association and American Stroke Association (AHA/ASA) suggest restarting warfarin 7–10 days after ICH, the European Stroke Initiative (EUSI) after 10–14 days, there are others who suggest the optimal time point during 10–30 weeks [65].

Novel direct oral anticoagulants (DOAC) have been developed that directly inhibit the key coagulation factors II (thrombin) or factor Xa. The direct thrombin inhibitor **dabigatran-etexilate** (DE) was approved in September 2011 for stroke prevention in atrial fibrillation after the RE-LY trial had shown that DE is not inferior to warfarin in preventing stroke, with significantly reduced intracranial hemorrhage (warfarin 0.74%/year, DE 110 mg 0.23%/year and DE 150 mg 0.3%/year) [66–68]. Nevertheless intracranial hemorrhage remains the most serious and lethal complication of long-term use of oral anticoagulation, but the risk of hematoma expansion with DOACs is not known. The optimal management of dabigatran-associated ICH is unknown and no specific antidote is available. No preclinical model has been established to test potential hemostatic strategies so far. Zhou *et al.* therefore established a murine model of OAC-ICH that was sensitive to pretreatment with dabigatran and assessed the kinetics of hematoma expansion after collagenase-induced ICH in mice, and tested the efficacy of different hemostatic factors. The major findings of this study were that high doses of DE caused an early excess hematoma expansion in this model, that administration of coagulation factors (particularly PCC) prevented excess hematoma expansion caused by dabigatran, and that PCC reversed the prolongation of bleeding time and prevented excess hematoma expansion in a dose-dependent manner and was associated with improved survival. Perhaps administration of PCC or FFP increases the availability of factor II, which reconstitutes the coagulation cascade. In contrast, the inefficiency of FVIIa to reduce hematoma expansion in this study may result from its inability to counteract the inhibitive effect of dabigatran on factor II. Because the pathophysiology of ICH in patients is only partially reflected in current experimental ICH models, the efficacy and safety of this strategy must be further evaluated in appropriate clinical studies [69].

There are currently two other DOACs which have been approved for prophylaxis of embolic stroke in patients with atrial fibrillation, which are **rivaroxaban** (12/2011) and **apixaban** (11/2012), direct inhibitors of factor Xa. Rivaroxaban has been compared with warfarin in the ROCKET AF trial, which showed lower or similar rates of thromboembolic events, but less intracranial hemorrhage (warfarin 1.2%/year, rivaroxaban 0.8%/year) [70]. Similarly, therapy with apixaban (5 mg twice daily) led to significantly fewer intracranial hemorrhages (0.33%/year) than did warfarin (0.8%/year) in ARISTOTLE [6]. In addition, there is no known antidote for acute reversal of rivaroxaban or apixaban either. Eerenberg *et al.* presented a reversal of coagulation tests by PCC for rivaroxaban in volunteers, while the results for dabigatran are inconclusive because bleeding times were not assessed [71]. However, the efficacy of this treatment has not been demonstrated in clinical trials.

The discrepancy between the PCC effect on plasma coagulation assays and bleeding time raises the question of whether the coagulation tests adequately monitor the potential of PCC for reversal in cases of bleeding associated with dabigatran. In an emergency setting of ICH under DOAC, physicians face the problem that routine coagulation tests such as partial thrombin time (PTT), prothrombin time (PT, expressed as international normalized ratio (INR)) may be within normal limits. Thus, DOAC in comatose or aphasic patients might go undetected unless laboratory methods such as ecarin clotting time (ECT), thrombin time (TT), or hemoclot assays are applied.

Although data are limited, PCCs have been suggested as a plausible – but unproven – therapy for the rapid reversal of dabigatran, rivaroxaban, and apixaban's anticoagulant effects. Some of the prothrombin complex concentrate preparations contain inactivated clotting factors, whereas others (activated prothrombin complex concentrate) contain activated clotting factors. The latter preparations may be more potent but also have higher thrombogenic potential [72]. Diuresis with intravenous fluids may enhance the renal excretion of dabigatran. Dabigatran is a lipophilic molecule. In an in vitro experiment simulating the digestion of high amounts of dabigatran over 2–3 hours, 99% of the drug was adsorbed by activated charcoal [73]. Given the kinetics of dabigatran, it seems plausible to use activated carbon within 2 hours after intake of dabigatran. Also for rivaroxaban and apixaban the use of active carbon is recommended. Acute hemodialysis might also be useful if these measures do not stop the bleeding, because only about one third of dabigatran is bound to plasma proteins and can therefore not be dialyzed, although this can take hours to begin and complete. Dialysis is not suitable for apixaban and rivaroxaban, which are 85–95% bound to plasma [74].

Future strategies

Unfortunately, almost all 'classical' approaches have failed to control HE in randomized trials with regard to outcome, probably for disease-immanent but also for trial-immanent reasons. It is also possible that the critical amount of HE restriction for relevance in outcome has not been achieved so far or that long-term complications of SICH have masked the initial effect. Various hemostatic agents have been considered for use in spontaneous intracranial hemorrhage. However, most of these have not been tested in larger clinical trials, so far [75,76]. Current treatment strategies might also be double-edged swords. Surgical intervention can reduce bleeding size but also lead to decompression of tissue and thereby enhance bleeding. Nonsurgical intervention such as hemostasis might stop bleeding but also compromise normal circulation. Therefore, the right balance and possibly the combination of current treatment regimes, as well as the evaluation of alternative future strategies, seem urgent.

The following sums up several emerging treatment targets. Surgically, the combination of stereotactic minimal invasive aspiration and clot lysis with rtPA has been proposed, especially with regard to deep hematomas. A study in 15 (highly selected) patients demonstrated ICH volume reduction without the enlargement of perihematomal edema often feared [77]. Whether this approach can indeed lead to a better outcome is currently being investigated in the MISTIE (Minimally Invasive Surgery Plus rtPA for Intracerebral Hemorrhage Evacuation) trial combining stereotactic clot aspiration (starting 6 hours after clot stabilization) with different doses of rtPA (alteplase) within the first 72 hours from onset [78]. The preliminary analysis suggests that MIS plus alteplase shows greater clot resolution than does conventional medical treatment. While the early administration of rtPA in the setting of SICH will be interesting with regard to HE as an unwanted effect, this approach can hardly be seen as a measure to restrict HE, as it is primarily aimed at hematoma evacuation. More promising in that respect might be the combination of surgery with hemostatic drugs such as rFVIIa, especially in the light of frequent rebleeding in ultra-early operations [50]. The SPOTLIGHT (Spot Sign Selection of Intracerebral Hemorrhage to Guide Hemostatic Therapy; ClinicalTrial.gov identifier NCT01359202) and STOP-IT (Spot Sign for Predicting and Treating ICH Growth Study; NCT00810888) are trials that are underway to study the use of CT angiography spot sign to stratify patients most at risk of hematoma expansion and who might benefit from therapy with rFVIIa.

On the nonsurgical side, further elucidation of the way to control blood pressure is encouraged by the phase III ATACH-2 (NCT 01176565). Whether the rapid- and short-acting intravenous antihypertensive clevidipine is beneficial in the acute phase of SICH is currently being investigated in the ACCELERATE (the evaluation of patients with acute hypertension and intracerebral hemorrhage with intravenous clevidipine treatment) trial [79]. As to neuroprotectants, although so many have failed in ischemic stroke, the situation might be different in hemorrhage, and lessons from trial-immanent reasons for failure might help to more successfully apply neuroprotectants in SICH. The free radical scavenger NXY-509, having failed in ischemic stroke trials, proved safe and tolerable applied within 6 hours of SICH, but showed no improvement in outcome, however, in a safety trial design [80]. Out of other candidates, matrix metallo-proteinases (MMP) might play a relevant role in SICH development and expansion [19]. Data from a mouse model showed that inhibition of the gelatinase MMP-9 by the broad-spectrum inhibitor GM6001 had several beneficial effects, including decreased injury volume and improved functional outcome [81]. Thus, MMP inhibitors might be promising if safe and feasible in humans. This being completely unclear and most probably a question of the distant future, other ways to achieve endogenous inhibition of MMPs should be pursued. Substances which are already in clinical use for other indications and therefore potentially available for use in SICH patients have been demonstrated as neuroprotectants restricting HE in experimental animal models of ICH by an active South Korean group. These agents comprise the cytokine erythropoietin, the anticonvulsant valproic acid, and the moderate NMDA receptor antagonist memantine [82–84].

A rather nonselective way of neuroprotection, hypothermia, might have beneficial effects on blood–brain barrier damage, mitochondrial dysfunction, cerebral O_2 consumption, penumbral depolarizations, excitotoxicity, and development of perihematomal edema. Several of these factors are probably involved in the pathophysiology of HE. Hypothermia in SICH, on its own or in combination with decompressive hemicraniectomy, is currently being investigated by Kollmar and colleagues (Germany).

Conclusion

Secondary hematoma expansion of spontaneous intracerebral hemorrhage is a frequent, early and very relevant complication of this devastating disease and demands rapid restricting efforts. Some predictors of HE have been identified, but these are not always accessible treatment targets. Unfortunately, all measures to restrict HE have as yet failed to improve outcome in controlled trials. It is still reasonable though, considering data from available studies and pathophysiological concepts, to follow current guidelines and to reverse the action of prior anticoagulants quickly, to lower extreme systolic blood pressure cautiously, to aim for homeostasis in vital functions and metabolism, and to find an interdisciplinary treatment strategy with the neurosurgeon. Above all, it is paramount to create, to conduct or to randomize patients into controlled trials on this subject, because most guidelines and recommendations are based on empirical data.

REFERENCES

[1] Sacco S, Marini C, Toni D, Olivieri L, Carolei A. Incidence and 10 year survival of intracerebral hemorrhage in a population-based registry. *Stroke.* 2009;**40**:394–9.

[2] Broderick J, Brott T, Duldner JE, Tomsick T, Huster G. Volume of intracrerbral hemorrhage: A powerful and easy-to-use predictor of 30-day mortality. *Stroke.* 1993;**24**:987–93.

[3] Herbstein DJ, Schaumberg HH. Hypertensive intracerebral hematoma. An investigation of the initial hemorrhage and rebleeding using chronium cr 51-labeled erythrocytes. *Arch Neurol.* 1974;**30**:412–14.

[4] Brott T, Broderick J, Kothari R, *et al.* Early hemorrhage growth in patients with intracerebral hemorrhage. *Stroke.* 1997;**28**(1):1–5.

[5] Brott T, Broderick J, Kothari R, *et al.* Early hemorrhage growth in patients with intracerebral hemorrhage. *Stroke.* 1997;**28**:1–5.

[6] Connolly SJ, Eikelboom J, Joyner C, *et al.* Apixaban in patients with atrial fibrillation. *N Engl J Med.* 2011;**364**(9):806–17.

[7] Rosand J, Eckman MH, Knudsen KA, Singer DE, Greenberg SM. The effect of warfarin and intensity of anticoagulation on outcome of intracerebral hemorrhage. *Arch Intern Med.* 2004;**164**:880–4.

[8] Davis SM, Broderick J, Hennerici M, *et al.* Hematoma growth is a determinant of mortality and poor outcome after intracerebral hemorrhage. *Neurology.* 2006;**66**:1175–81.

[9] Leira R, Davalos A, Silva Y, *et al.* Early neurologic deterioration in intracerebral hemorrhage: Predictors and associated factors. *Neurology.* 2004;**63**:461–7.

[10] Steiner T, Bösel J. Options to restrict hematoma expansion after spontaneous intracerebral hemorrhage. *Stroke.* 2010;**40**:3275–80.

[11] Tuhrim S, Horowitz DR, Sacher M, Godbold JH. Volume of ventricular blood is an important determinant of outcome in supratentorial intracerebral hemorrhage. *Crit Care Med.* 1999;**27**(3):617–21.

[12] Steiner T, Schneider D, Mayer S, *et al.* Dynamics of intraventricular hemorrhage in patients with spontaneous intracerebral hemorrhage: risk factors, clinical impact, and effect of hemostatic therapy with recombinant activated factor VII. *Neurosurgery.* 2006;**59**:767–74.

[13] Maas MB, Nemeth AJ, Rosenberg NF, *et al.* Delayed intraventricular hemorrhage is common and worsens outcomes in intracerebral hemorrhage. *Neurology.* 2013;**80**(14):1295–9.

[14] Kase CS, Mohr JP, Caplan LR, eds. Intracerebral hemorrhage. *Stroke: Pathophysiology, Diagnosis, and Management.* 4 ed: Philadelphia: Churchill Livingstone, 2004.

[15] Xi G. Intracerebral hemorrhage: Pathophysiology and therapy. *Neurocritical Care.* 2004;**1**:5–18.

[16] Kim-Han JS, Kopp SJ, Dugan LL, Diringer MN. Perihematomal mitochondrial dysfunction after intracerebral hemorrhage. *Stroke.* 2006;**37**:2457–62.

[17] Silva Y, Leira R, Tejada J, *et al.* Molecular signatures of vascular injury are associated with early growth of intracerebral hemorrhage. *Stroke.* 2005;**36**:86–91.

[18] Florczak-Rzepka M, Grond-Ginsbach C, Montaner J, Steiner T. Matrix metalloproteinases in human spontaneous intracerebral hemorrhage - an update. *Cerebrovasc Dis.* 2012;**34**:249–62.

[19] Alvarez-Sabin J, Delgado P, Abilleira S, *et al.* Temporal profile of matrix metalloproteinases and their inhibitors after spontaneous intracerebral hemorrhage: Relationship to clinical and radiological outcome. *Stroke.* 2004;**35**:1316–22.

[20] Naidech AM, Jovanovic B, Liebling S, *et al.* Reduced platelet activity is associated with early clot growth and worse 3-month outcome after intracerebral hemorrhage. *Stroke.* 2009;**40**:2398–401.

[21] Delgado P, Alvarez-Sabin J, Abilleira S, *et al.* Plasma d-dimer predicts poor outcome after acute intracerebral hemorrhage. *Neurology.* 2006;**67**:94–8.

[22] Sorimachi T, Fujii Y, Morita K, Tanaka R. Predictors of hematoma enlargement in patients with intracerebral hemorrhage treated with rapid administration of antifibrinolytic agents and strict blood pressure control. *J Neurosurg.* 2007;**106**:250–4.

[23] Saloheimo P, Ahonen M, Juvela S, *et al.* Regular aspirin-use preceding the onset of primary intracerebral hemorrhage is an independent predictor for death. *Stroke.* 2006;**37**:129–33.

[24] Broderick JP, Diringer MN, Hill MD, *et al.* Determinants of intracerebral hemorrhage growth: An exploratory analysis. *Stroke.* 2007;**38**:1072–5.

[25] Goldstein JN, Fazen LE, Snider R, *et al.* Contrast extravasation on CT angiography predicts hematoma expansion in intracerebral hemorrhage. *Neurology.* 2007;**68**:889–94.

[26] Delgado Almandoz JE, Yoo AJ, Stone MJ, *et al.* Systematic characterization of the computed tomography angiography spot sign in primary intracerebral hemorrhage identifies patients at highest risk for hematoma expansion: The spot sign score. *Stroke.* 2009;**40**:2994–3000.

[27] Li N, Wang Y, Wang W, *et al.* Contrast extravasation on computed tomography angiography predicts clinical outcome in primary intracerebral hemorrhage, a prospective study of 139 cases. *Stroke.* 2011;**42**:3441–6.

[28] Demchuk AM, Dowlatshahi D, Rodriguez-Luna D, *et al.* Prediction of haematoma growth and outcome in patients with intracerebral haemorrhage using the CT-angiography spot sign (PREDICT): a prospective observational study. *Lancet Neurol.* 2012;**11**:307–14.

[29] Morgenstern LB, Frankowski RF, Shedden P, Pasteur W, Grotta JC. Surgical treatment for intracerebral hemorrhage (STICH): A single-center, randomized clinical trial. *Neurology.* 1998;**51**:1359–63.

[30] Morgenstern LB, Demchuk AM, Kim DH, Frankowski RF, Grotta JC. Rebleeding leads to poor outcome in ultra-early craniotomy for intracerebral hemorrhage. *Neurology.* 2001;**56**:1294–9.

[31] NINDS ICH Workshop Participants. Priorities for clinical research in intracerebral hemorrhage. Report from a National Institute of Neurologic Disorders and Stroke Workshop. *Stroke.* 2005;**36**:e23–e41.

[32] Mendelow AD, Gregson BA, Rowan EN, *et al.* Early surgery versus initial conservative treatment in patients with spontaneous supratentorial lobar intracerebral haematomas (STICH II): a randomised trial. *Lancet.* 2013; May 29.

[33] Mendelow AD, Unterberg A. Surgical treatment of intracerebral haemorrhage. *Curr Opin Crit Care.* 2007;**13**:169–74.

[34] Auer LM, Deinsberger W, Niederkorn K, *et al.* Endoscopic surgery versus medical treatment for spontaneous intracerebral hematoma: A randomized study. *J Neurosurg.* 1989;**70**:530–5.

[35] Cho DY, Chen CC, Lee WY, Lee HC, Ho LH. A new modified intracerebral hemorrhage score for treatment

decisions in basal ganglia hemorrhage – a randomized trial. *Crit Care Med.* 2008;**36**:2151–6.

[36] Qureshi AI. Acute hypertensive response in patients with stroke: pathophysiology and management. *Circulation.* 2008;**118**:176–87.

[37] Morgenstern LB, Hemphill JC 3rd, Anderson C *et al.* Nursing at AHASCaCoC. Guidelines for the management of spontaneus intracerebral hemorrhage: a guideline for healthcare professionals from the American Heart Association/American Stroke Assiciation. *Stroke.* 2010;**41**:2108–29.

[38] Ohwaki K, Yano E, Nagashima H, *et al.* Blood pressure management in acute intracerebral hemorrhage: Relationship between elevated blood pressure and hematoma enlargement. *Stroke.* 2004;**35**:1364–7.

[39] Anderson CS, Huang Y, Wang JG, *et al.* Intensive blood pressure reduction in acute cerebral haemorrhage trial (interact): A randomised pilot trial. *Lancet Neurol.* 2008;**7**:391–9.

[40] Qureshi AI, Tariq N, Divani AA *et al.*, and the ATACH investigators. Antihypertensive treatment of acute cerebral hemorrhage (ATACH). *Critical Care Medicine.* 2010;**38**:637–48.

[41] Qureshi AI, Palesch YY. Antihypertensive Treatment of Acute Cerebral Hemorrhage (ATACH) II: design, methods, and rationale. *Neurocrit Care.* 2011;**15** (3):559–76.

[42] Koch S, Romano JG, Forteza AM, Otero CM, Rabinstein AA. Rapid blood pressure reduction in acute intracerebral hemorrhage: Feasibility and safety. *Neurocrit Care.* 2008;**8**:316–21.

[43] Diedler J, Sykora M, Rupp A, *et al.* Impaired cerebral vasomotor activity in spontaneous intracerebral hemorrhage. *Stroke.* 2009;**40**:815–19.

[44] Morgenstern LB, Hemphill JC, 3rd, Anderson C, *et al.* Guidelines for the management of spontaneous intracerebral hemorrhage. A guideline for healthcare professionals from the American Heart Association/ American Stroke Association. *Stroke.* 2010;**41**:2108–29.

[45] Broderick JP, Connolly ES, Feldman E, *et al.* Guidelines for the management of spontaneous intracerebral hemorrhage in adults. 2007 update. A guideline from the American Heart Association, American Stroke Association Stroke Council, High Blood Pressure Research Council, and the Quality of Care and Outcomes in Research Interdisciplinary Working Group. *Stroke.* 2007;**38**:e391–413.

[46] Steiner T, Kaste M, Forsting M, *et al.* Recommendations for the management of intracranial haemorrhage – part 1: Spontaneous intracerebral haemorrhage. The European Stroke Initiative writing committee and the writing committee for the Eusi Executive Committee. *Cerebrovasc Dis.* 2006;**22**:294–316.

[47] Gould B, McCourt R, Asdaghi N, *et al.* Autoregulation of cerebral blood flow is preserved in primary intracerebral hemorrhage. *Stroke.* 2013;**44**:1726–8.

[48] Greer DM, Funk SE, Reaven NL, Ouzounelli M, Uman GC. Impact of fever on outcome in patients with stroke and neurologic injury: a comprehensive meta-analysis. *Stroke.* 2008;**39**:3029–35.

[49] Reith J, Jorgensen HS, Pedersen PM, *et al.* Body temperature in acute stroke: relation to stroke severity, infarct size, mortality, and outcome. *Lancet.* 1996;**347**:422–5.

[50] Balami JS, Buchan AM. Complications of intracerebral haemorrhage. *Lancet Neurol.* 2012;**11**:101–18.

[51] den Hertog HM, van der Worp HB, van Gemert HM, *et al.* The Paracetamol (Acetaminophen) In Stroke (PAIS) trial: a multicentre, randomised, placebo-controlled, phase III trial. *Lancet Neurol.* 2009;**8**:434–40.

[52] Paracetamol (Acetaminophen) in Stroke 2 (PAIS 2): A randomized clinical trial to investigate the effect of high-dose paracetamol in patients with acute stroke and a body temperature of 37.0°C or above. http://wwwtrial-registernl/trialreg/admin/rctviewasp?TC=2365, 2612012, 2010.

[53] Mayer S, Brun N, Broderick J, *et al.* Recombinant activated factor VII for acute intracerebral hemorrhage. *N Engl J Med.* 2005;**352**:777–85.

[54] Mayer S, Brun N, Broderick J, *et al.* Efficacy and safety of recombinant activated factor vii for acute intracerebral hemorrhage. *N Engl J Med.* 2008;**358**:2127–37.

[55] Flaherty ML, Kissela B, Woo D, *et al.* The increasing incidence of anticoagulant-associated intracerebral hemorrhage. *Neurology.* 2007;**68**:116–21.

[56] Flibotte JJ, Hagan N, O'Donnell J, Greenberg SM, Rosand J. Warfarin, hematoma expansion and outcome of intracerebral hemorrhage. *Neurology.* 2004;**63**:1059–64.

[57] Hart RG, Boop BS, Anderson DC. Oral anticoagulants and intracranial hemorrhage. Facts and hypotheses. *Stroke.* 1995;**26**:1471–7.

[58] Rosand J, Hylek EM, O'Donnell HC, Greenberg SM. Warfarin-associated hemorrhage and cerebral amyloid angiopathy: A genetic and pathologic study. *Neurology.* 2000;**55**:947–51.

[59] Aguilar MI, Hart RG, Kase CS, *et al.* Treatment of warfarin-associated intracerebral hemorrhage: Literature review and expert opinion. *Mayo Clin Proc.* 2007;**82**:82–92.

[60] Huttner HB, Schellinger PD, Hartmann M, *et al.* Hematoma growth and outcome in treated neurocritical care patients with intracerebral hemorrhage related to oral anticoagulant therapy. Comparison of acute treatment strategies using vitamin K, fresh frozen plasma, and prothrombin complex concentrates. *Stroke.* 2006;**37**:1465–70.

[61] Steiner T, Freiberger A, Griebe M, *et al.* International normalised ratio normalisation in patients with coumarin-related intracranial haemorrhages – the INCH trial: a randomised controlled multicentre trial to compare safety and preliminary efficacy of fresh frozen plasma and prothrombin complex – study design and protocol. *Int J Stroke.* 2011;**6**(3):271–7.

[62] Boeer A, Voth E, Henze T, Prange HW. Early heparin therapy in patients with spontaneous intracerebral haemorrhage. *J Neurol Neurosurg Psychiatry.* 1991;**54**:466–7.

[63] Eckman MH, Rosand J, Knudsen KA, Singer DE, Greenberg SM. Can patients be anticoagulated after intracerebral hemorrhage? A decision analysis. *Stroke.* 2003;**34**:1710–11.

[64] Greenberg SM, Eng JA, Ning M, Smith EE, Rosand J. Hemorrhage burden predicts recurrent intracerebral hemorrhage after lobar hemorrhage. *Stroke.* 2004;**35**:1415–20.

[65] Majeed A, Kim Y, Roberts R, Holmström M, Schulman S. Optimal timing of resumption of wafarin after intracranial hemorrhage. *Stroke.* 2010;**41**:2860–6.

[66] Connolly SJ, Ezekowitz MD, Yusuf S, *et al.* Dabigatran versus warfarin in patients with atrial fibrillation. *N Engl J Med.* 2009;**361**:1139–51.

[67] Wallentin L, Yusuf S, Ezekowitz MD, *et al.* Efficacy and safety of dabigatran compared with warfarin at different levels of international normalised ratio control for stroke prevention in atrial fibrillation: an analysis of the RE-LY trial. *Lancet.* 2010;**376**:975–83.

[68] Steiner T, Bohm M, Dichgans M, *et al.* Recommendations for the emergency management of complications associated with new direct oral anticoagulants (doac) apixaban, dabigatran, and rivaroxaban. *Clinical Res Cardiol.* 2013;**102**:399–412.

[69] Zhou W, Schwarting S, Illanes S, *et al.* Hemostatic therapy in experimental intracerebral hemorrhage associated with the direct thrombin inhibitor dabigatran. *Stroke.* 2011;**42**:3594–9.

[70] Patel MR, Mahaffey KW, Garg J, *et al.* Rivaroxaban versus warfarin in nonvalvular atrial fibrillation. *N Engl J Med.* 2011;**365**:883–91.

[71] Eerenberg ES, Kamphuisen PW, Sijpkens MK, Meijers JC, Buller HR. Reversal of rivaroxaban and dabigatran by prothrombin complex concentrate a randomized, placebo-controlled, crossover study in healthy subjects. *Circulation.* 2011: 124.

[72] Leissinger CA, Blatt PM, Hoots WK, Ewenstein B. Role of prothrombin complex concentrates in reversing warfarin anticoagulation: a review of the literature. *Am J Hematol.* 2008;**83**:137–43.

[73] van Ryn J, Stangier J, Haertter S, *et al.* Dabigatran etexilate – a novel, reversible, oral direct thrombin inhibitor: interpretation of coagulation assays and reversal of anticoagulant activity. *Thromb Haemost.* 2010;**103**(6):1116–27.

[74] van Ryn J, Stangier J, Haertter S, *et al.* Dabigatran etexilate – a novel, reversible, oral direct thrombin inhibitor: interpretation of coagulation assays and reversal of anticoagulant activity. *Thromb Haemost.* 2010;**103**:1116–27.

[75] Piriyawat P, Morgenstern LB, Yawn D, Hall CE, Grotta JC. Treatment of acute intracerebral hemorrhage with e-aminocaproic acid – a pilot study. *Neurocritical Care.* 2004;**1**:47–51.

[76] Vujkovac B, Sabovic M. Treatment of subdural and intracerebral haematomas in a haemodialysis patient with tranexamic acid. *Nephrol Dial Transplant.* 2000;**15**:107–9.

[77] Carhuapoma JR, Barrett RJ, Keyl PM, Hanley DF, Johnson RR. Stereotactic aspiration-thrombolysis of intracerebral hemorrhage and its impact on perihematoma brain edema. *Neurocrit Care.* 2008;**8**:322–9.

[78] Morgan T, Zuccarello M, Narayan R, *et al.* Preliminary findings of the minimally-invasive surgery plus rtPA for intracerebral hemorrhage evacuation (MISTIE) clinical trial. *Acta Neurochir Suppl.* 2008;**105**:147–51.

[79] The Medicines Company. Clevidipine in the treatment of patients with acute hypertension and intracerebral hemorrhage (accelerate). http://clinicaltrialsgov/show/NCT00666328; Acess date: 16.3.2009.

[80] Lyden PD, Shuaib A, Lees KR, *et al.* Safety and tolerability of nxy-059 for acute intracerebral hemorrhage: The chant trial. *Stroke.* 2007;**38**:2262–9.

[81] Wang J, Tsirka SE. Tuftsin fragment 1-3 is beneficial when delivered after the induction of intracerebral hemorrhage. *Stroke.* 2005;**36**:613–18.

[82] Lee ST, Chu K, Jung KH, *et al.* Memantine reduces hematoma expansion in experimental intracerebral hemorrhage, resulting in functional improvement. *J Cereb Blood Flow Metab.* 2006;**26**:536–44.

[83] Lee ST, Chu K, Sinn DI, *et al.* Erythropoietin reduces perihematomal inflammation and cell death with enos and stat3 activations in experimental intracerebral hemorrhage. *J Neurochem.* 2006;**96**:1728–39.

[84] Sinn DI, Kim SJ, Chu K, *et al.* Valproic acid-mediated neuroprotection in intracerebral hemorrhage via histone deacetylase inhibition and transcriptional activation. *Neurobiol Dis.* 2007;**26**:464–72.

21a

Management of acute hypertensive response in the ICH patient

Wondwossen G. Tekle and Adnan I. Qureshi

Introduction

About 37000 to 52400 people in the United States suffer from intracerebral hemorrhage (ICH) every year (1). Hypertension is the most important risk factor for spontaneous ICH accounting for about 60–70% of cases (2). Broderick *et al.* showed hypertension was the primary cause of ICH in 72% of the 188 patients evaluated in the study (3). Risk of ICH is increased in certain populations of hypertensive patients who are non-compliant with antihypertensive medication, are aged 55 years or younger, or are cigarette smokers. Hispanics, African Americans, Native Americans, and those of Asian ancestry have higher incidence of ICH related to hypertension (4–6). Nearly two-thirds of hypertensive patients have uncontrolled blood pressure (BP) (greater than 140/90 mmHg) at admission (7). Control of BP among patients with chronic hypertension reduces the incidence of intracerebral hemorrhage (8–10).

Elevated BP, termed as acute hypertensive response (AHR), is observed in over 60% of patients coming to the ER (11). A large and nationally representative survey (12) showed that over 75% of ICH patients had systolic blood pressure (SBP) > 140 and 20% greater than 180 mmHg at presentation. Patients with stroke and high initial BP are at a 1.5–5.0-fold increased risk of death or dependency and clinical deterioration (13, 14).

Pathophysiology

Cerebral autoregulation is a mechanism by which the brain maintains its normal blood flow despite fluctuations in cerebral perfusion pressure (CPP) over a range of mean arterial blood pressure (MAP) changes ranging from 60 to 150 mmHg (15). Pre-capillary arterioles in the brain are responsible for autoregulation, constricting during elevated BP and dilating during hypotension to maintain constant cerebral blood flow. CPP is the difference between MAP and intracranial pressure, and the normal range of CPP is around 60–100 mmHg.

During chronic hypertension, the autoregulation curve (Fig. 21a.1) shifts to the right in order to maintain normal flow under higher systemic BP (16). The arterioles of small and medium size adapt to the persistently elevated systemic BP, which presumably results in structural changes in the walls of these small vessels and reduction in their baseline caliber. Such changes likely stiffen the vessels and decrease their compliance, resulting in degenerative changes in arterioles and making them prone to rupture.

Breakage of elastic lamina, lipohyalinosis, granular or vesicular cellular degeneration, fibrinoid necrosis of the subendothelium with focal dilatations (microaneurysms) in the walls of cerebral vessels are among the main pathologic processes leading to vascular rupture in most cases of hypertension-related ICH (17,18).

Critical Care of the Stroke Patient, ed. Stefan Schwab, Daniel Hanley, and A. David Mendelow. Published by Cambridge University Press.

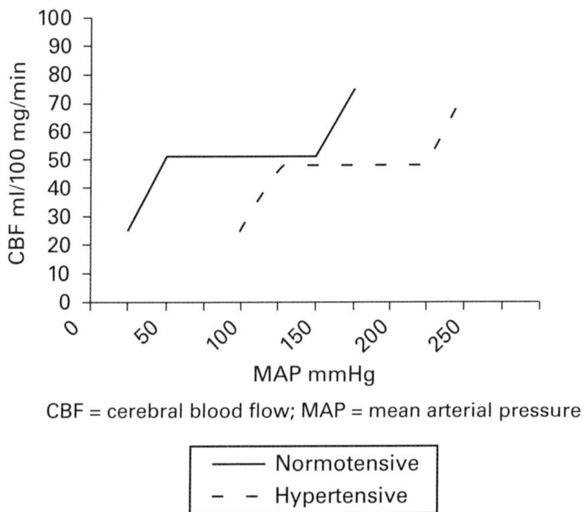

Fig. 21a.1 Cerebral autoregulation in normotensive and chronically hypertensive patients.

Degeneration of smooth muscle cells may be the result of prolonged tension or spasm of the arterial wall as a result of longstanding hypertension (15). Most bleeding in hypertension-related ICH occurs at or near the bifurcation of small arterioles, ranging between 50 and 700 μm in diameter.

Rationale for treatment of AHR in acute ICH

Elevated SBP after ICH is associated with hemorrhage growth and poor outcome (19,20), although the cause and effect relationship is unclear. SBP reduction may reduce the rate of hematoma expansion; however, conclusive evidence is still lacking. As a result, controversy remains on what should be the ideal goal of treatment for the AHR. Two recently concluded multicentre clinical trials documented the safety and tolerability of early and aggressive reduction of BP in acute phase of ICH (21,22). Large phase III trials are being planned to answer the bigger question of whether or not such treatments improve outcome.

Some of the crucial pathophysiologic and prognostic considerations pertaining to management of AHR in ICH are based on the effect of SBP reduction on regional cerebral blood flow (rCBF) and metabolism, hematoma expansion, peri-hematoma edema, and ultimately, clinical outcome.

Regional cerebral blood flow and metabolism in ICH

Evidence suggests that SBP reduction in acute ICH may be tolerated because of reduced metabolism (hibernation) (23) and preserved autoregulation (24,25) in the perihematoma region. Qureshi *et al.* described three phases for CBF and metabolic changes in the perihematoma region (23). Hibernation is seen during the first 48 hours whereby a reduction in rCBF and metabolism occurs in both ipsilateral and contralateral hemispheres. Reperfusion phase occurs between 48 hours and 14 days, and consists of a heterogeneous pattern of blood flow, including areas of normal, hypo- and hyper-cerebral perfusion. Finally, normalization phase comes after 14 days and a normal blood flow pattern is restored except in the non-viable tissue.

Powers *et al.* found that there was no change in both global and peri-hematoma rCBF and autoregulation was preserved in small- and medium-sized hematomas when MAP was reduced by a magnitude of 15% from baseline value (24). Zazulia *et al.* demonstrated decreased rCBF and oxygen extraction fraction (OEF) (26) using positron emission tomography (PET) scan in acute phase of ICH. Multiple other magnetic resonance imaging (MRI) and PET-based studies (27–30) have confirmed the absence of ischemia in the perihematomal tissue. The mechanism underlying reduction in rCBF and metabolism in the peri-hematoma is unclear; although direct inhibition of mitochondrial function has been proposed (31–33).

Some studies (34–37) suggested that an 'ischemic penumbra' may be seen when the hematoma is large and associated with elevated ICP (38). While local microvascular compression and impaired autoregulation are thought to be some of the mechanisms involved to create such an ischemic zone (34–36), it is arguable that decreasing BP could potentially impair rCBF and lead to further tissue ischemia.

In the setting of increased ICP after ICH, elevated BP may be helpful to maintain adequate cerebral perfusion pressure (CPP).

Hematoma expansion and peri-hematoma edema

Early elevation of SBP in ICH patients is associated with hematoma expansion (37,39,40) and peri-hematoma brain edema formation (41). Chen *et al.* (42) observed a persistent elevation of BP in six of their eight patients before hematoma expansion. Broderick *et al.* (43) also recorded a SBP of at least 195 mmHg during the first 6 hours after symptom onset in five out of six patients with hematoma expansion. In one observational study, hematomas enlarged in 9% of patients with systolic blood pressure maintained below 150 mmHg and in 30% of those with systolic blood pressure maintained at less than 160 mmHg or a higher threshold (44). Yet, it remains unclear whether elevated systolic BP contributes to hemorrhage expansion or elevation in SBP occurs in response to increased ICP from hemorrhage growth (44). Some prospective studies of ICH growth did not find an independent association between clinical variables such as hypertension and ICH expansion (45,46). The Recombinant Activated Factor VII Intracerebral Hemorrhage Trial (FAST) found that baseline BP was associated with ICH growth in univariate but not multivariate analyses (47). In a study of patients with ischemic stroke (48), persistently elevated SBP was associated with formation of cerebral edema, although the prognostic value of relative peri-hematomal edema remains controversial (49). The Intensive Blood Pressure Reduction in Acute Cerebral Hemorrhage Trial (INTERACT) (21) showed early intensive BP-lowering treatment attenuated hematoma growth over 72 hours in patients with ICH, but there were no appreciable effects on peri-hematomal edema.

Highlights of ATACH and INTERACT trials on safety and tolerability of early and aggressive reduction of BP in acute ICH

The ATACH (50) was a traditional phase I, dose escalation, multicentre prospective study that recruited patients with ICH and SBP >170 mmHg who present to the emergency department within 6 hours of symptom onset. Intravenous nicardipine was administered to reduce SBP to three different target SBP tiers of 170–200 mmHg, 140–170 mmHg, and 110–140 mmHg in the first, second, and third cohorts of patients respectively. Primary outcomes of interest were: (1) treatment feasibility (achieving and maintaining the systolic blood pressure goals for 18–24 hours); (2) neurologic deterioration within 24 hours; and (3) serious adverse events within 72 hours. ATACH found that the proportions of neurologic deterioration and serious adverse events were below the prespecified safety thresholds, and the 3-month mortality rate was lower than expected in all SBP tiers.

The INTERACT trial recruited 404 patients with CT-confirmed ICH and elevated SBP (150–220 mmHg) and randomly assigned to an intensive (target SBP <140 mmHg) or standard ASA guideline management of BP (target SBP <180 mmHg) using available intravenous agents. Patients had baseline and repeat CTs (24 and 72 hours) using standardized techniques with digital image analysis. Outcomes were increased in hematoma and peri-hematomal edema volumes over 72 hours. INTERACT concluded that early intensive BP-lowering treatment attenuated hematoma growth over

72 hours in intracerebral hemorrhage, but there were no appreciable effects on perihematomal edema.

Both ATACH and INTERACT trials reported that aggressive reduction of BP to less than 140 mmHg probably decreases the rate of substantial hematoma enlargement without increasing adverse events. In subgroup analyses from INTERACT, patients recruited within 3 hours and those with an initial SBP of 181 mmHg or more seemed to have the greatest benefit with aggressive lowering of SBP. No difference in rates of death and disability at 3 months were seen between patients treated with aggressive SBP reduction in ATACH or INTERACT studies, although the analyses were limited by small sample sizes.

SBP reduction and clinical outcome

In one multicentered prospective observational study, reduction in BP to <160/90 mmHg showed a trend toward improved outcome in patients treated within 6 hours of symptoms onset (51). Another single-centre study showed that reduction of BP in patients with acute ICH is safe, and suggested that aggressive reduction might reduce the risk of neurological deterioration in the first 24 hours of admission (52).

Most recently, post-hoc analysis in the Antihypertensive Treatment of Acute Cerebral Hemorrhage Study (ATACH) (53) found a non-significant relationship between SBP reduction and the outcome measures, namely hematoma expansion (defined as an increased intraparenchymal hemorrhage volume >33% on 24 hours vs. baseline computed tomographic [CT] images), higher peri-hematomal edema ratio (defined as a >40% increased ratio of edema volume to hematoma volume on 24 hours vs. baseline CT images), and poor 3-month outcome (defined as a modified Rankin Scale score of 4–6). Although ATACH was primarily a safety study and was not powered for such end points, the investigators found that greater SBP reduction at all time points within 24 hours of symptom onset was actually associated with reduction in hematoma expansion and lower rates of death and disability. This consistently favorable direction of these associations supports further studies with an adequately powered randomized controlled design to evaluate the efficacy of aggressive pharmacologic SBP reduction.

American Stroke Association Stroke Council and the European Stroke Initiative guidelines (Table 21a.1)

The current American Stroke Association Stroke Council (54) and the European Stroke Initiative guidelines (55) recommend maintaining SBP <180 mmHg in the acute period using short half-life IV antihypertensive medication. Both guidelines consider the possibility of more aggressive SBP lowering in the absence of clinical signs of elevated intracranial pressure (56) or chronic hypertension (50). Recent data suggest a greater therapeutic benefit with more aggressive lowering of blood pressure (56). Because the effect on clinical outcome has not been fully assessed, the more conservative targets set in the ASA Stroke Council (54).

Table 21a.1 AHA/ASA recommendations for management of BP during acute ICH.

1. If SBP is >200 mmHg or MAP is >150 mmHg, then consider aggressive reduction of BP with continuous intravenous infusion, with frequent BP monitoring every 5 minutes.
2. If SBP is >180 mmHg or MAP is >130 mmHg and there is evidence of or suspicion of elevated ICP, then consider monitoring ICP and reducing BP using intermittent or continuous intravenous medications to keep cerebral perfusion pressure >60 to 80 mmHg
3. If SBP is >180 mmHg or MAP is >130 mmHg and there is no evidence of or suspicion of elevated ICP, then consider a modest reduction of BP (e.g. MAP of 110 mmHg or target BP of 160/90 mmHg) using intermittent or continuous intravenous medications to control BP, and clinically re-examine the patient every 15 minutes.

SBP indicates systolic blood pressure; MAP, mean arterial pressure. Reproduced with permission [54].

and the EUSI guidelines (55) should be followed. Great caution is advised about lowering BP too aggressively without concomitant management of cerebral perfusion pressure.

Frequent or continuous BP monitoring is necessary in all patients with ICH. Even though BP can be monitored adequately with an inflatable cuff in most patients with acute hypertensive response, intra-arterial monitoring should be considered in patients who require frequent titration with intravenous antihypertensive agents and in patients whose neurological status is deteriorating. ICP monitoring may be necessary in patients with a suspected increased ICP, to measure and preserve cerebral perfusion pressure during systemic BP lowering. Patients with a poor level of consciousness, midline shift, or compression of basal cisterns on computed tomographic scan may be considered for ICP monitoring when being treated with antihypertensive agents.

The AHA guideline also recommends BP management tailored to the individual patient factors such as pre-morbid BP, presumed cause of hemorrhage, age, and elevated ICP. MAP should be maintained between 90 and 130 mmHg. As there is no evidence-based guideline on how low the BP can be in ICH, particularly those with no history of chronic hypertension, it is recommended that SBP be maintained above 90 mmHg in all cases of ICH (57).

The European Union Stroke Initiative (EUSI) BP management recommendation (55) takes into account the patient's premorbid BP status, and it is summarized as follows:

- Patients with known hypertension or signs of chronic hypertension (e.g. electrocardiogram or retinal changes), an upper limit of SBP of 180 mmHg and a diastolic BP of 105 mmHg, and target BP is 160/100 mmHg (or MAP 120 mmHg).
- Patients without known history of hypertension, the upper limits are 160/95 mmHg, and the target BP is 150/90 mmHg (or MAP 110 mmHg).
- The mean BP reduction should always be limited to <= 20% of baseline.

If the patient has an ICP monitor, CPP should be monitored and maintained >70 mmHg by titrating the MAP. The consensus to keep CPP >70 mmHg is derived from experience in traumatic brain injury and ICH which suggests that maintaining CPP >60 mmHg is associated with better outcome (58,59). The Brain Trauma Foundation (60) recommends maintaining cerebral perfusion pressure >70 mmHg to enhance perfusion to ischemic regions of the brain after severe traumatic injury. However, it is worth noting that this global measure of CPP can underestimate the localized pressure, perfusion, and autoregulatory changes in focal ICH. Until more sensitive measures based on direct local blood flow and metabolism parameters are discovered for routine clinical use, the standard CPP measurement should be utilized.

Antihypertensive agents and regimens

The goal of pharmacologic reduction of AHR should be to achieve good BP control without promoting cerebral vasodilatation and increased cerebral blood volume (CBV). The agents that are recommended by the ASA for acute hypertensive response are either intravenous or transdermal agents with rapid onset and short duration of action to allow precise titration. Table 21a.2 summarizes some of the characteristics of these agents. Indirect comparisons suggest that intermittent intravenous bolus regimens of anti-hypertensives produce more variable BP control than do continuous infusion regimens (63).

A multicentre prospective observational study (63) reported the use of intravenous labetalol, hydralazine, and/or nitroprusside for maintaining BP >160/90 mmHg within 24 hours of symptom onset among patients with ICH. Low rates of neurological deterioration and hematoma expansion were observed in treated patients. Patients treated within 6 hours of symptom onset were more likely to be functionally independent at 1 month than patients who were treated between 6 and 24 hours.

Another study (78) evaluated the tolerability and safety of intravenous nicardipine infusion within 24 hours of symptom onset to reduce and maintain MAP <130 mmHg, consistent with previous ASA guidelines. The primary outcome of tolerability was achieved in 86% of the patients. Low rates of neurological

Table 21a.2 Pharmacological characteristics of antihypertensive agents recommended in the Stroke Council, American Heart Association's statement for healthcare professionals.

Agent	Mechanism of action	CBF	ICP	Autoregulation	Platelet activity‡	Cardiac contractility‡	Dose	Onset of action	Half-life	Ischemic stroke	ICH
Labetalol	α- and β-adrenergic blocker	. . .	. . .	. . .	–	. . .	5–20 mg bolus every 15 min up to 300 mg	5–10 min	3–6 h	SS, CS (62), ES (65)	SS, CS (63,64), ES (66)
Hydralazine	Direct relaxation of arteriolar smooth muscle	++	++	–	–	. . .	5–20 mg bolus every 15 min	10–20 min	1–4 h	SS, ES (67)	SS, CS (63)
Nitroprusside	Releases nitric oxide	++	++	–	–	. . .	Infusion of 0.2 to 10 $\mu g \cdot kg^{-1} \cdot min^{-1}$	Within seconds	2–5 min	SS, CS (62), ES (68)	SS, CS (63)
Nitroglycerine	Releases nitric oxide	+	. . .	. . .	–	. . .	20–400 μg/min	1–2 min	3–5 min		SS, CS (69)
Nitropaste	Releases nitric oxide	+	. . .	. . .	–	. . .	0.2–0.4 mg/h up to 0.8 mg/h	1–2 min	3–5 min	SS, CS (70)	SS, CS (70)
Nicardipine	Calcium channel blocker	+	. . .	–	–	. . .	5–15 mg/h	5–10 min	0.5–4 h	SS, CS (71)	SS, CS (72,73)
Esmolol†	β-adrenergic blocker	. . .	. . .	. . .	+	–	250 μg/kg bolus followed by 25 to 300 $\mu g \cdot kg^{-1} \cdot min^{-1}$	5 min	9 min		SS
Enalapril*	ACE inhibitor	. . .	. . .	++	–	. . .	1.25–5 mg every 6 h	15 min	1–4 h	CS (74), ES (67)	SS, ES (75)

Reprinted with permission (61).

CBF indicates cerebral blood flow; SS, scientific statement; CS, clinical study; ES, experimental study; ACE, angiotensin-converting enzyme; + increase or favorable effects; ++ substantial increase or favorable effects; – decrease or negative effects; . . . no documented direct effect.

No conclusive evidence is present at this point to avoid any particular class of antihypertensive medication (including β-blockers (76)). In general, medications with slow onset of action, long half-lives, or those known to cause precipitous BP reduction (sublingual nifedipine (77)) should be avoided in the first 24 hours because they cannot be titrated to ensure controlled BP reduction.

*Data predominantly derived from other ACE inhibitors.

†Limited data available.

‡Not derived from studies performed in acute stroke settings and unclear direct relevance.

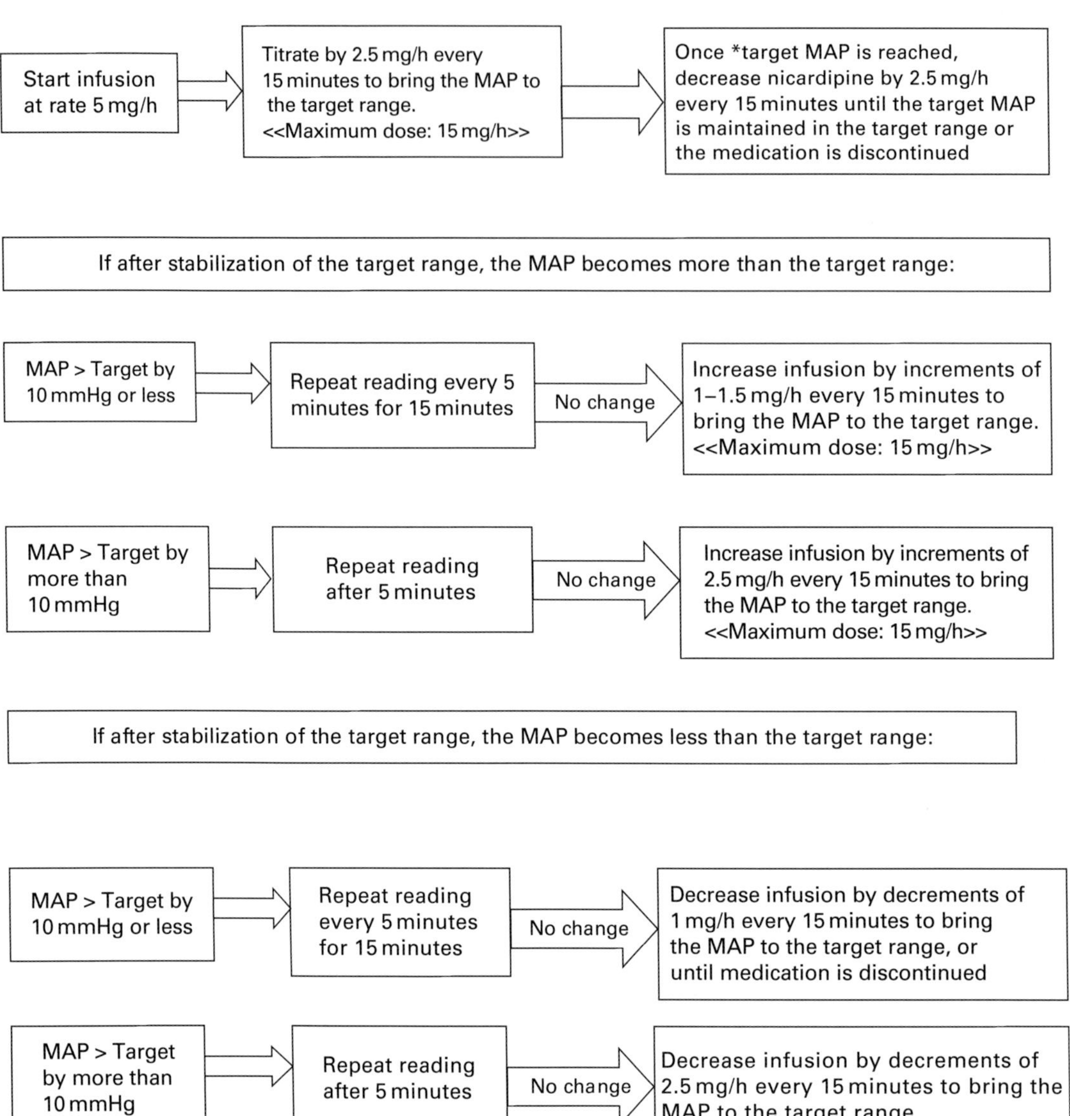

Fig. 21a.2 Nicardapine infusion protocol.

deterioration and hematoma expansion were observed among treated patients. Recently, INTERACT and ATACH trials also showed the feasibility and tolerability of IV nicardipine and other anti-hypertensive infusion protocols. Figure 21a.2 shows nicardipine infusion protocol used by our centre.

Management of hypertension with oral medications in the immediate post-ICH period

A number of clinical trials have shown the benefit of treating hypertension in the immediate post-stroke

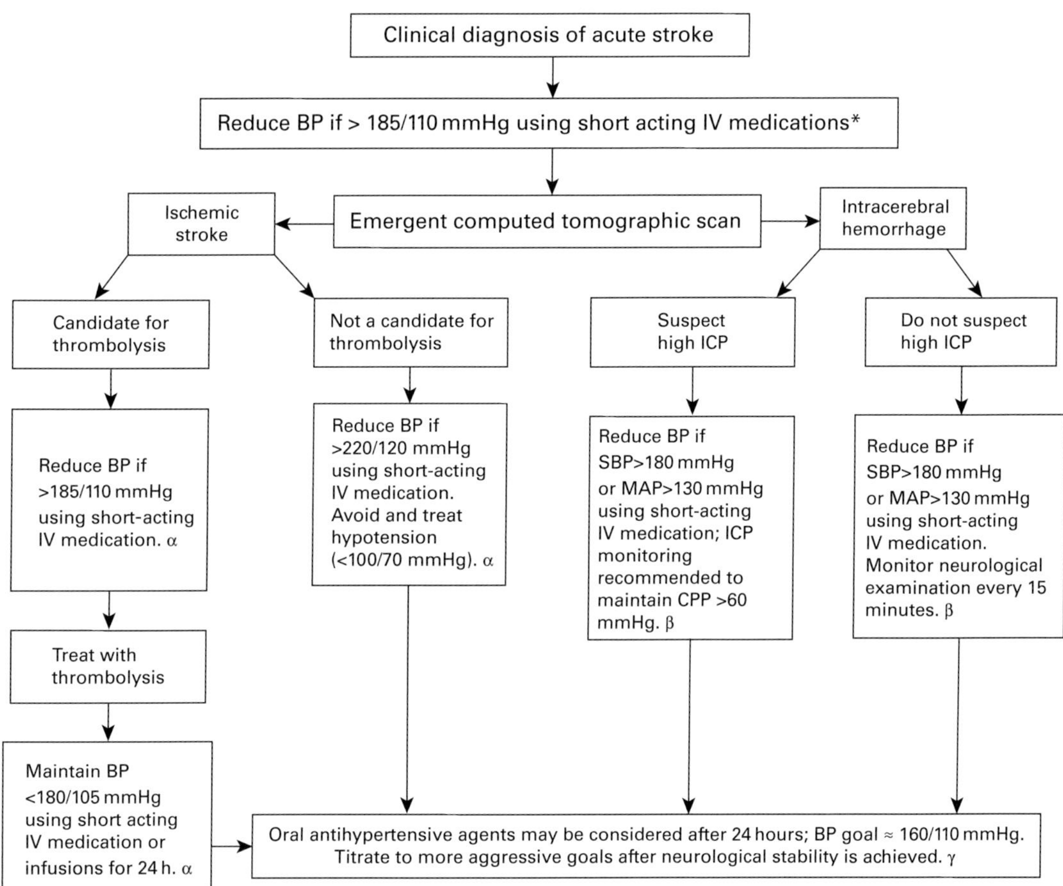

Fig. 21a.3 Algorithm for treatment of acute hypertensive response among patients with stroke and stroke subtypes. IV indicates intravenous; SBP, systolic BP; DBP, diastolic BP; and CPP, cerebral perfusion pressure. *Based on the NINDS rtPA prethrombolytic protocol (62) for patients with acute ischemic stroke, for short-term BP management by Emergency Medical Services without delaying early diagnosis and differentiation. The Emergency Medical Services BP management practices vary considerably in the absence of distinction between ischemic stroke and ICH (83). α Based on recommendations of the ASA, Stroke Council (54,84), and/or European Stroke Initiative (85). β The recommended BP treatment threshold is similar to the existing ASA and European Stroke Initiative recommendations for patients with ICH (54,85). γ Based on recommendations of JNC 7 (7) and the ACCESS protocol (82). Reprinted with permission from (61).

period (79–81). Oral anti-hypertensive medications can be started within 24–72 hours if the patient's condition is stable, because most of the acute processes, such as hematoma expansion and ischemic penumbra are uncommon after the first 24 hours (61). ACCESS trial (82) results supported this early initiation and gradual titration to more aggressive BP treatment targets. Figure 21a.3 illustrates an algorithm for treatment of AHR in stroke subtypes and transitioning to oral anti-hypertensive medications.

The seventh report of the Joint National Committee on Prevention, Detection, Evaluation, and Treatment of High Blood Pressure (JNC 7) recommends that BP be maintained at intermediate levels (around 160/100 mmHg) until neurological stability is achieved. Special circumstances such as elevated ICP, progressive cerebral edema, ongoing cerebral ischemia due to occlusive vessel disease or symptomatic cerebral vasospasm, and postoperative cerebral changes require individualized management. After the first week, or when neurological stability is achieved, a more aggressive treatment can be initiated for secondary prevention of recurrent stroke.

A systematic review (86) of seven randomized, controlled trials involving patients with prior stroke or transient ischemic attack showed angiotensin-converting enzyme inhibitors and diuretics, separately and in combination, but not β-blockers, reduced vascular events. Another estimate of stroke reduction with different anti-hypertensive medications (angiotensin-converting enzyme inhibitors, calcium antagonists, angiotensin receptor blockers, and diuretics or β-blockers) using data from 29 randomized trials (87) directed toward primary prevention suggested that the greatest reduction was observed with angiotensin receptor blockers, with small (borderline significance) differences between the other different classes of anti-hypertensive medication.

The JNC-7 provides a guideline for long-term hypertension management (7). Below is the summary of some of the most important points.

- Thiazide-type diuretics should be used as initial therapy for most patients, either alone or in combination with one of the other classes (ACEIs, ARBs, BBs, and CCBs) that have also been shown to reduce one or more hypertensive complications in randomized controlled outcome trials.
- Selection of one of these other agents as initial therapy is recommended when a diuretic cannot be used or when a compelling indication is present that requires the use of a specific drug. Compelling indications for specific therapy involve high-risk conditions that can be direct sequelae of hypertension (HF, ischemic heart disease, chronic kidney disease, recurrent stroke) or commonly associated with hypertension (diabetes, high coronary disease risk). Therapeutic decisions in such individuals should be directed at both the compelling indication and BP lowering.
- More than two-thirds of hypertensive individuals cannot be controlled on one drug and will require two or more anti-hypertensive agents selected from different drug classes. If BP is more than 20/10 mmHg above the goal BP, consideration should be given to initiating therapy with two agents, one of which usually should be a thiazide-type diuretic. The initiation of therapy with more than one drug increases the likelihood of achieving BP goal in a more timely fashion. The use of multidrug combinations often produces greater BP reduction at lower doses of the component agents, resulting in fewer side effects.

REFERENCES

1. Qureshi AI, Tuhrim S, Broderick JP, *et al.* Spontaneous intracerebral hemorrhage. *N Engl J Med* 2001;**344**:1450–60.
2. Brott T, Thalinger K, Hertzberg V. Hypertension as a risk factor for spontaneous intracerebral hemorrhage. *Stroke* 1986;**17**:1078–83.
3. Broderick JP, Brott T, Tomsick T, Miller R, Huster G. Intracerebral hemorrhage more than twice as common as subarachnoid hemorrhage. *J Neurosurg* 1993;**78**(2):188–91.
4. Thrift AG, McNeil JJ, Forbes A, Donnan GA. Three important subgroups of hypertensive persons at greater risk of intracerebral hemorrhage. *Hypertension* 1998;**31**:1223–9.
5. Qureshi AI, Suri MAK, Safdar K, *et al.* Intracerebral hemorrhage in blacks: risk factors, subtypes, and outcome. *Stroke* 1997;**28**:961–4.
6. Ariesen MJ, Claus SP, Rinkel GJ, Algra A. Risk factors for intracerebral hemorrhage in the general population: a systematic review. *Stroke* 2003;**34**(8):2060–5.
7. Chobanian AV, Bakris GL, Black HR, *et al.* The Seventh Report of the Joint National Committee on Prevention, Detection, Evaluation, and Treatment of High Blood Pressure: the JNC 7 Report. *JAMA* 2003;**289**(19):2560–72.
8. Furlan AJ, Whisnant JP, Elveback LR. The decreasing incidence of primary intracerebral hemorrhage: a population study. *Ann Neurol* 2003;**5**:367–73.
9. Hypertension Detection and Follow-up Program Cooperative Group. Five-year findings of the Hypertension Detection and Follow-up Program. III. Reduction in stroke incidence among persons with high blood pressure. *JAMA* 2003;**247**:2560–638.
10. SHEP Cooperative Research Group. Prevention of stroke by antihypertensive drug treatment in older persons with isolated systolic hypertension: final results of the Systolic Hypertension in the Elderly Program (SHEP). *JAMA* 2003;**265**:3255–64.

11. Qureshi AI. Acute hypertensive response in patients with stroke: pathophysiology and management. *Circulation* 2008;**118**:176–87.
12. Qureshi AI, Ezzeddine MA, Nasar A, *et al.* Prevalence of elevated blood pressure in 563,704 adult patients with stroke presenting to the ED in the United States. *Am J Emerg Med* 2003;**25**:2560–38.
13. Willmot M, Leonardi-Bee J, Bath PM. High blood pressure in acute stroke and subsequent outcome: a systematic review. *Hypertension* 2004;**43**:18–24.
14. Kazui SMK, Sawada T, Yamaguchi T. Predisposing factors to enlargement of spontaneous intracerebral hematoma. *Stroke* 2003;**28**:2370–5.
15. Paulson OB, Strandgaard S, Edvinsson L. Cerebral autoregulation. *Cerebrovasc Brain Metab Rev* 1990;**2**:161–92.
16. Strandgaard S. Autoregulation of cerebral blood flow in hypertensive patients: the modifying influence of prolonged antihypertensive treatment on the tolerance to acute, drug-induced hypotension. *Circulation* 1976;**53**:720–7.
17. Takebayashi S, Kaneko M. Electron microscopic studies of ruptured arteries in hypertensive intracerebral hemorrhage. *Stroke* 2003;**14**:28–36.
18. Mizutani T, Kojima H, Miki Y. Arterial dissections of penetrating cerebral arteries causing hypertension-induced cerebral hemorrhage. *J Neurosurg* 2003;**93**:859–62.
19. Leira R, Dávalos A, Silva Y, *et al.* Stroke Project, Cerebrovascular Diseases Group of the Spanish Neurological Society. Early neurologic deterioration in intracerebral hemorrhage: predictors and associated factors. *Neurology* 2004;**63**:461–7.
20. Fogelholm, R, Avikainen S, Murros, K. Prognostic value and determinants of first-day mean arterial pressure in spontaneous supratentorial intracerebral hemorrhage. *Stroke* 1997;**28**:1396–1400.
21. Anderson CS, Huang Y, Arima H, *et al.* Effects of early intensive blood pressure-lowering treatment on the growth of hematoma and perihematomal edema in acute intracerebral hemorrhage: the Intensive Blood Pressure Reduction in Acute Cerebral Haemorrhage Trial (INTERACT). *Stroke* 2003;**41**(2):307–12.
22. Qureshi AI, Tariq N, Divani AA, *et al.* Antihypertensive Treatment of Acute Cerebral Hemorrhage (ATACH). *Crit Care Med* 2003;**38**(2):637–48.
23. Qureshi AI, Hanel RA, Kirmani JF, Yahia AM, Hopkins LN. Cerebral blood flow changes associated with intracerebral hemorrhage. *Neurosurg Clin N Am* 2002;**13**(3):355–70.
24. Powers WJ, Zazulia AR, Videen TO, *et al.* Autoregulation of cerebral blood flow surrounding acute (6 to 22 hours) intracerebral hemorrhage. *Neurology* 2003;**57**(1):18–24.
25. Qureshi AI, Wilson DA, Hanley DF, Traystman RJ. No evidence for an ischemic penumbra in massive experimental intracerebral hemorrhage. *Neurology* 1999;**52** (2):266–72.
26. Zazulia AR, Diringer MN, Videen TO, *et al.* Hypoperfusion without ischemia surrounding acute intracerebral hemorrhage. *J Cereb Blood Flow Metab* 2001;**21**(7):804–10.
27. Schellinger PD, Fiebach JB, Hoffmann K, *et al.* Stroke MRI in intracerebral hemorrhage: is there a perihemorrhagic penumbra? *Stroke* 2003;**34**:1674–9.
28. Hirano T, Read SJ, Abbott DF, *et al.* No evidence of hypoxic tissue on 18F-fluoromisonidazole PET after intracerebral hemorrhage. *Neurology* 2003;**53**(9):2179–82.
29. Carhuapoma JR, Wang PY, Beauchamp NJ, *et al.* Diffusion-weighted MRI and proton MR spectroscopic imaging in the study of secondary neuronal injury after intracerebral hemorrhage. *Stroke* 2003;**31**(3):726–32.
30. Zazulia AR, Diringer MN, Videen TO, *et al.* Hypoperfusion without ischemia surrounding acute intracerebral hemorrhage. *J Cereb Blood Flow Metab* 2001;**21**(7):804–10.
31. Nath FP, Kelly PT, Jenkins A, *et al.* Effects of experimental intracerebral hemorrhage on blood flow, capillary permeability, and histochemistry. *J Neurosurg* 2003;**66** (4):555–62.
32. Yang GY, Betz AL, Chenevert TL, Brunberg JA, Hoff JT. Experimental intracerebral hemorrhage: relationship between brain edema, blood flow, and blood-brain barrier permeability in rats. *J Neurosurg* 1994;**81**(1):93–102.
33. Nath FP, Jenkins A, Mendelow AD, Graham DI, Teasdale GM. Early hemodynamic changes in experimental intracerebral hemorrhage. *J Neurosurg* 1986;**65**(5):697–703.
34. Nath FP, Kelly PT, Jenkins A, *et al.* Effects of experimental intracerebral hemorrhage on blood flow, capillary permeability, and histochemistry. *J Neurosurg* 2003;**66**(4):555–62.
35. Bullock R, Brock-Utne J, van Dellen J, Blake G. Intracerebral hemorrhage in a primate model: effect on regional cerebral blood flow. *Surg Neurol* 2003;**29** (2):101–7.
36. Mendelow AD, Bullock R, Teasdale GM, Graham DI, McCulloch J. Intracranial haemorrhage induced at arterial pressure in the rat: Part 2. Short term changes in local cerebral blood flow measured by autoradiography. *Neurol Res* 2003;**6**(4):189–93.
37. Broderick JP, Brott TG, Tomsick T, *et al.* Ultra-early evaluation of intracerebral hemorrhage. *J Neurosurg* 1990;**72**:195–9.
38. Kidwell CS, Saver JL, Mattiello J, *et al.* Diffusion-perfusion MR evaluation of perihematomal injury in hyperacute intracerebral hemorrhage. *Neurology* 2003;**57**:1611–17.

39. Kazui S, Minematsu K, Yamamoto H, Sawada T, Yamaguchi T. Predisposing factors to enlargement of spontaneous intracerebral hematoma. *Stroke* 1997;**28** (12):2370–5.
40. Dandapani BK, Suzuki S, Kelley RE, Reyes-Iglesias Y, Duncan RC. Relation between blood pressure and outcome in intracerebral hemorrhage. *Stroke* 1995;**26**(1):21–4.
41. Qureshi AI, Tuhrim S, Broderick JP, *et al.* Spontaneous intracerebral hemorrhage. *New Engl J Med* 2001;**344** (19):1450–60.
42. Chen ST, Chen SD, Hsu CY, Hogan EL. Progression of hypertensive intracerebral hemorrhage. *Neurology* 1989;**39**(11):1509–14.
43. Broderick JP, Brott TG, Tomsick T, Barsan W, Spilker J. Ultra-early evaluation of intracerebral hemorrhage. *J Neurosurg* 1990;**72**(2):195–9.
44. Ohwaki K, Yano E, Nagashima H, *et al.* Blood pressure management in acute intracerebral hemorrhage: relationship between elevated blood pressure and hematoma enlargement. *Stroke* 2004;**35**:1364–7.
45. Brott T, Broderick J, Kothari R, *et al.* Early hemorrhage growth in patients with intracerebral hemorrhage. *Stroke* 1997;**28**:1–5.
46. Jauch EC, Lindsell CJ, Adeoye O, *et al.* Lack of evidence for an association between hemodynamic variables and hematoma growth in spontaneous intracerebral hemorrhage. *Stroke* 2006;**37**:2061–5.
47. Broderick JP, Diringer MN, Hill MD, *et al.* Determinants of intracerebral hemorrhage growth: an exploratory analysis. *Stroke* 2007;**38**:1072–5.
48. Vemmos KN, Tsivgoulis G, Spengos K, *et al.* Association between 24-h blood pressure monitoring variables and brain oedema in patients with hyperacute stroke. *J Hypertens* 2003;**21**(11):2167–73.
49. Gebel JM Jr, Jauch EC, Brott TG, *et al.* Relative edema volume is a predictor of outcome in patients with hyperacute spontaneous intracerebral hemorrhage. *Stroke* 2002;**33**(11):2636–41.
50. Qureshi AI. Antihypertensive treatment of acute cerebral hemorrhage (ATACH): rationale and design. *Neurocrit Care* 2007;**6**:56–66.
51. Qureshi AI, Mohammad YM, Yahia AM, *et al.* A prospective multicenter study to evaluate the feasibility and safety of aggressive antihypertensive treatment in patients with acute intracerebral hemorrhage. *J Intensive Care Med* 2005;**20**:34–42.
52. Suri MF, Suarez JI, Rodrigue TC, *et al.* Effect of treatment of elevated blood pressure on neurological deterioration in patients with acute intracerebral hemorrhage. *Neurocrit Care* 2003;**9**:177–82.
53. Qureshi AI, Palesch YY, Martin R, *et al.* Effect of systolic blood pressure reduction on hematoma expansion, perihematomal edema, and 3-month outcome among patients with intracerebral hemorrhage: results from the antihypertensive treatment of acute cerebral hemorrhage study. *Arch Neurol* 2003;**67**(5):570–6.
54. Broderick J, Connolly S, Feldmann E, *et al.* Guidelines for the management of spontaneous intracerebral hemorrhage in adults: 2007 update: A guideline from the American Heart Association/American Stroke Association Stroke Council, High Blood Pressure Research Council, and the Quality of Care and Outcomes in Research Interdisciplinary Working Group Stroke. *Stroke* 2007;**38**:2001–23.
55. Steiner T, Kaste M, Forsting M, *et al.* Recommendations for the management of intracranial haemorrhage – part I: Spontaneous intracerebral haemorrhage. The European Stroke Initiative Writing Committee and the Writing Committee for the EUSI Executive Committee. *Cerebrovasc Dis* 2006;**22**:294–316.
56. Ohwaki K, Yano E, Nagashima H, *et al.* Blood pressure management in acute intracerebral hemorrhage: relationship between elevated blood pressure and hematoma enlargement. *Stroke* 2004;**35**:1364–7.
57. Mayer SA, Rincon F. Treatment of intracerebral haemorrhage. *Lancet Neurol* 2003;**4**:662–72.
58. Robertson CS, Valadka AB, Hannay HJ, *et al.* Prevention of secondary ischemic insults after severe head injury. *Crit Care Med* 1999;**27**:2086–95.
59. Fernandes HM, Siddique S, Banister K, *et al.* Continuous monitoring of ICP and CPP following ICH and its relationship to clinical, radiological and surgical parameters. *Acta Neurochir* Suppl. 2000;**76**:463–6.
60. The Brain Trauma Foundation, The American Association of Neurological Surgeons, The Joint Section on Neurotrauma and Critical Care. Guidelines for cerebral perfusion pressure. *J Neurotrauma* 2003;**17**:507–11.
61. Qureshi AI. Acute hypertensive response in patients with stroke: Pathophysiology and management. *Circulation* 2008;**118**;176–87.
62. Brott T, Lu M, Kothari R, *et al.* Hypertension and its treatment in the NINDS rt-PA stroke trial. *Stroke.* 1998;**29**:1504–9.
63. Qureshi AI, Mohammad YM, Yahia AM, *et al.* A prospective multicenter study to evaluate the feasibility and safety of aggressive antihypertensive treatment in patients with acute intracerebral hemorrhage. *J Intensive Care Med* 2005;**20**:34–42.

64. Patel RV, Kertland HR, Jahns BE, *et al.* Labetalol: response and safety in critically ill hemorrhagic stroke patients. *Ann Pharmacother* 1993;**27**:180–1.
65. Fagan SC, Bowes MP, Lyden PD, Zivin JA. Acute hypertension promotes hemorrhagic transformation in a rabbit embolic stroke model: effect of labetalol. *Exp Neurol* 1998;**150**:153–8.
66. Qureshi AI, Wilson DA, Hanley DF, Traystman RJ. Pharmacologic reduction of mean arterial pressure does not adversely affect regional cerebral blood flow and intracranial pressure in experimental intracerebral hemorrhage. *Crit Care Med* 1999;**27**:965–71.
67. Elewa HF, Kozak A, Johnson MH, Ergul A, Fagan SC. Blood pressure lowering after experimental cerebral ischemia provides neurovascular protection. *J Hypertens* 2007;**25**:855–9.
68. Zhang F, Iadecola C. Nitroprusside improves blood flow and reduces brain damage after focal ischemia. *Neuroreport* 1993;**4**:559–62.
69. Kuroda K, Kuwata N, Sato N, *et al.* Changes in cerebral blood flow accompanied with reduction of blood pressure treatment in patients with hypertensive intracerebral hemorrhages. *Neurol Res* 997;**19**:169–73.
70. Willmot M, Ghadami A, Whysall B, *et al.* Transdermal glyceryl trinitrate lowers blood pressure and maintains cerebral blood flow in recent stroke. *Hypertension* 2006;**47**:1209–15.
71. Horn J, Limburg M. Calcium antagonists for acute ischemic stroke. *Cochrane Database Syst Rev* 2000;(**2**):CD001928.
72. Powers WJ, Zazulia AR, Videen TO, *et al.* Autoregulation of cerebral blood flow surrounding acute (6 to 22 hours) intracerebral hemorrhage. *Neurology* 2001;**57**:18–24.
73. Qureshi AI, Harris-Lane P, Kirmani JF, *et al.* Treatment of acute hypertension in patients with intracerebral hemorrhage using American Heart Association guidelines. *Crit Care Med* 2006;**34**:1975–80.
74. Waldemar G, Vorstrup S, Andersen AR, Pedersen H, Paulson OB. Angiotensin-converting enzyme inhibition and regional cerebral blood flow in acute stroke. *J Cardiovasc Pharmacol* 1989;**14**:722–9.
75. Smeda J, Vasdev S, King SR. Effect of poststroke captopril treatment on mortality associated with hemorrhagic stroke in stroke-prone rats. *J Pharmacol Exp Ther* 1999;**291**:569–75.
76. Dziedzic T, Slowik A, Pera J, Szczudlik A. Beta-blockers reduce the risk of early death in ischemic stroke. *J Neurol Sci* 2007;**252**:53–6.
77. Rehman F, Mansoor GA, White WB. 'Inappropriate' physician habits in prescribing oral nifedipine capsules in hospitalized patients. *Am J Hypertens* 1996;**9**:1035–9.
78. Qureshi AI, Harris-Lane P, Kirmani JF, *et al.* Treatment of acute hypertension in patients with intracerebral hemorrhage using American Heart Association guidelines. *Crit Care Med* 2006;**34**:1975–80.
79. Gueyffier F, Boissel JP, Boutitie F, *et al.* Effect of antihypertensive treatment in patients having already suffered from stroke: gathering the evidence: the INDANA (Individual Data Analysis of Antihypertensive Intervention Trials) Project Collaborators. *Stroke* 2003;**28**:2557–62.
80. Rezaiefar P, Pottie K. Blood pressure and secondary prevention of strokes: how low should we go? Randomised trial of a perindopril-based blood-pressure-lowering regimen among 6,105 individuals with previous stroke or transient ischaemic attack. *Can Fam Physician* 2003;**48**:1625–9.
81. Arima H, Chalmers J, Woodward M, *et al.* Lower target blood pressures are safe and effective for the prevention of recurrent stroke: the PROGRESS trial. *J Hypertens* 2003;**24**:1201–8.
82. Schrader J, Luders S, Kulschewski A, *et al.* The ACCESS Study: evaluation of acute candesartan cilexetil therapy in stroke survivors. *Stroke* 2003;**34**:1699–1703.
83. Moon JS, Janjua N, Ahmed S, *et al.* Prehospital neurologic deterioration in patients with intraparenchymal hemorrhage. *Crit Care Med* 2008;**36**: 172–5.
84. Adams HP Jr, Del Zoppo G, Alberts MJ, *et al.* Guidelines for the early management of patients with ischemic stroke. *Circulation* 2007;**115**:e478–534.
85. Steiner T, Kaste M, Forsting M, *et al.* Recommendations for the management of intracranial haemorrhage, part I: spontaneous intracerebral haemorrhage: the European Stroke Initiative Writing Committee and the Writing Committee for the EUSI Executive Committee [correction *Cerebrovasc Dis* 2006;22:461]. *Cerebrovasc Dis* 2003;**22**:294–316.
86. Rashid P, Leonardi-Bee J, Bath P. Blood pressure reduction and secondary prevention of stroke and other vascular events: a systematic review. *Stroke* 2003;**34**:2741–8.
87. Turnbull F. Blood Pressure Lowering Treatment Trialists' Collaboration. Effects of different blood-pressure-lowering regimens on major cardiovascular events: results of prospectively-designed overviews of randomized trials. *Lancet* 2003;**362**:1527–35.

21b

Respiratory care of the ICH patient

Omar Ayoub and Jeanne Teitelbaum

Introduction

The overall incidence of intracerebral hemorrhage (ICH) is estimated to be 12–15 cases per 100000 population [1]. ICH represents around 15–30% of the overall stroke admissions to the hospital and results in significant disability, morbidity, and 30–50% mortality [2].

The most common cause of death in patients admitted with ICH was found to be withdrawal of life-sustaining interventions, and this accounted for 68% of the overall mortality. Indeed, the frequency of use of 'do not resuscitate' orders is highly associated with the odds of dying in hospital from ICH [3]. When aggressive management is instituted, patients who are treated in the neurologic intensive care unit have a lower mortality rate than those hospitalized in a general ICU [4]. The effect on morbidity, however, is related to the cause of respiratory failure. When the problem is that of incomplete airway protection due to structural weakness or dysfunction, the intubation and ventilation will improve both morbidity and mortality; when intubation and ventilation are instituted because of a low GCS, the aggressive approach to ventilation will not change overall outcome [5].

This chapter will address airway assessment and management in the critically ill patient with ICH, focusing on methods of assessment, indications for intubation, ventilation and tracheostomy, methods of ventilation, and the indications and implementation of successful weaning from the ventilator.

Indications for intubation and ventilation

Among patients admitted to ICUs, 20% will have an acute neurological disorder as the principal indication for instituting mechanical ventilation (MV), with half of these patients receiving MV for neuromuscular disease and the other half for coma or central nervous system dysfunction [6].

Ventilatory support is needed to maintain proper oxygenation to tissues, particularly the injured brain cells, in order to prevent further neurologic and systemic injury resulting from hypoxia or hypercapnea.

The decision to intubate and mechanically ventilate the patient depends on the clinical picture, even before imaging. The general indications for intubation in this particular subset of patients includes decreased level of consciousness with a GCS of 8 or less, raised ICP, inability to protect the airway, anticipation of decline, co-existing pulmonary indications and as a temporizing measure prior to surgical intervention.

In the next sections, we will go over the different indications and physiological rationale for intubation and MV in patients with ICH.

Decreased respiratory drive

The major causes for decreased respiratory drive after ICH are a decreased level of consciousness (LOC) and damage to the brainstem with or without abnormal

Critical Care of the Stroke Patient, ed. Stefan Schwab, Daniel Hanley, and A. David Mendelow. Published by Cambridge University Press.

LOC. Regardless of the cause of encephalopathy, there is an association between reduced level of consciousness and depression of the respiratory drive, hypoventilation and lack of airway protection [7]. Although the main reason for coma would be through intracranial hypertension (ICHT) and subsequent herniation, this could occur with normal or only slightly increased ICP as well. The causes of coma without ICHT include brainstem hemorrhage, cerebellar hemorrhage, relatively small mesial temporal hemorrhage with uncal herniation but without massive change in global ICP, and concomitant toxic or metabolic encephalopathy.

For the obtunded or comatose patient with decreased respiratory drive, intubation is not only to maintain airway but also to provide ventilation. If there is increased ICP, ventilation assures not only normocapnea but is used as a method to lower ICP through hyperventilation.

High ICP

Mechanical ventilation is used routinely in the management of high ICP to correct hypoxemia, hypercarbia, and acidosis that usually occur in conjunction with intracranial hypertension. Almost invariably, these patients require MV because of the accompanying decrease in their level of consciousness. The high ICP seen in hemorrhagic stroke is due to the mass effect of the hematoma as well as the surrounding edema. MV in this scenario is used not only to protect the airway and assure oxygenation but also to stabilize and reduce ICP.

Hyperventilation

If there is clinical or objective evidence of herniation, therapeutic hyperventilation is indicated and proven effective in ICH while completing the investigation and beginning other methods of ICP reduction. CO_2 is a potent modulator of CBF and hence of ICP. Hypocapnea results in vasoconstriction of the cerebral vessels, and as a result CBF and CBV will decrease leading to a decrease in ICP. The range in which $PaCO_2$ has the greatest impact on cerebral vessel caliber is 20–60 mmHg. Within this range, CBF changes 3% for every 1 mmHg change in $PaCO_2$ [8]. A decrease in CO_2 tension by 10 mmHg can produce sufficient reduction in CBV to effect a profound decrease in ICP.

Experimental studies have shown that the change in caliber of blood vessels is a direct effect of extracellular pH rather than an effect of CO_2 or bicarbonate [9]. This explains the lack of efficacy of prolonged hyperventilation in the treatment of high ICP, as the extracellular pH of the brain tends to normalize within hours (10–20 hours) of therapy, with rebound vasodilatation when hyperventilation is discontinued [10].

Current guidelines recommend against prophylactic hyperventilation, and therapeutic hyperventilation should be used only for short periods of time, targeting a modest reduction in PCO_2 to approximately 30 to 35 mmHg [11]. Lower levels of CO_2 may result in brain hypoxia, but results are very contradictory, and during the hyper-acute phase of herniation, there is likely no danger in temporarily decreasing PCO_2 as low as 25 mmHg [12,13].

The present guidelines do not address exact length of use, exact mechanical parameters, or the duration of hyperventilation. Eminence-based recommendations are as follows:

- Use in the presence of severe ICHT, as a first measure while instituting osmotic agents and assessing the use of other measures (decompression, EVD)
- The PCO_2 should be lowered by at least 10 mmHg to reach a level of 30 mmHg. Go to 25 mmHg of PCO_2 if there is still uncontrolled ICHT.
- Set the ventilator to give tidal volumes of 12–15 cc/kg at a rate of 12–14 breaths per minute while monitoring blood gases and end-tidal CO_2. If the goal is not attained, increase the rate as necessary to 16 and up to 20 per minute. Work quickly, as the effect is almost immediate and the dangers of herniation may be imminent.
- Hyperventilation is a temporizing measure, to be used for impending herniation and removed as soon as other measures of ICP control have been instituted. If used for less than 1 hour, it can be stopped without worry of rebound. If in place for more than 6 hours, weaning must be progressive to avoid rebound. Prolonged hyperventilation, and levels below 25 mmHg for 5 days, are deleterious, especially in trauma.

Poor airway protection

This is often seen in conjunction with abnormal drive in the comatose patient, but can be seen in isolation as well.

In the comatose patient, the oropharyngeal muscle tone is significantly decreased, leading to posterior displacement of the tongue and airway obstruction [14]. As well, airway patency may be compromised by foreign objects, secretions, orofacial fractures, or soft tissue edema that are associated with cervical injuries, on top of traumatic ICH.

In addition to damage due to ICH, patients may have associated systemic disorders that can compromise ventilation and oxygenation, such as drug or alcohol overdose, aspiration pneumonia, pulmonary contusions, fat emboli, pneumothorax, flail chest, and pulmonary edema.

Even without intracranial hypertension or lowered level of consciousness there can be an impaired ability to protect the airway and to assure ventilation. This can occur with brainstem or hemispheric damage.

Extensive hemispheric damage can lead to dysphagia with aspiration and eventual respiratory insufficiency. If continuous aspiration is occurring despite nasogastric feeding and suction, the airway will need to be protected by intubation and possibly tracheostomy if the situation does not improve. Ventilation is only necessary if pneumonia is severe and impedes spontaneous efficient breathing.

Brainstem hemorrhage affecting the dorsomedial and ventrolateral medulla will affect the centers for automatic respiratory drive and rhythmic breathing, leading to hypoventilation. A lesion in the pontine pneumotaxic centers on the other hand can impair the ability to modulate respiratory frequency, and fine control of the respiratory function [14].

Aerodynamic studies of patients with brainstem stroke show abnormal inspiration phase volume, peak inspiratory flow, duration of glottic closure, and delayed onset to peak of the expulsive phase, all of which can contribute to ineffective cough and an increased risk for aspiration pneumonia [15].

Also, through damage to the cranial nerves and their nuclei, patients with brainstem dysfunction have marked abnormalities of their cough reflex, swallowing, and phonation, all of which can affect respiration indirectly or lead to complications that mandate prolonged respiratory support.

Anticipation of decline

On occasion, it may be necessary to intubate and ventilate a patient prior to the onset of respiratory distress, to avoid aspiration, hypoxia, and worsening intracranial hypertension in a patient that is actively deteriorating or very likely to do so. Although intubation does have associated risks (hypotension, esophageal intubation, aspiration) and it is known to be associated with longer ICU stay, these complications are even more frequent if the intubation is done in a hurried fashion in a decompensated patient. A patient who presents early after an ICH and is already showing a change in level of consciousness, or in whom there is already some degree of shift and hydrocephalus on CT is likely to require this type of early intubation.

Pulmonary indications

Patients who have acute neurologic disorders are at increased risk for major pulmonary complications [16]. These include: risk of pneumonia, pulmonary embolism, hypoxemic respiratory failure, neurogenic pulmonary edema, and acute respiratory distress syndrome (ARDS).

Also, early intubation may be required in the subset of patients who have pre-existing pulmonary disease, who may get cardiopulmonary decompensation as a result of overlying acute brain process [17].

Types of intubation and ventilation available

The standard method of establishing a patent airway is by orotracheal intubation, but other techniques can be used. These include:

- Bag-valve mask ventilation
- BIPAP
- Nasotracheal intubation
- Laryngeal mask
- Surgical cricothyrotomy
- Oro-tracheal intubation

It is crucial to have a good assessment of the airway looking for signs of difficulties. 'Difficult airway' is defined by the American Society of Anesthesiology as the existence of clinical factors that complicate either ventilation using face-mask or intubation performed by an experienced clinician. In most cases, oro-tracheal intubation will be accomplished using rapid sequence intubation technique (RSI). The purpose of RSI is to quickly and effectively induce unconsciousness and paralysis using a specific sequence of drug therapy. When compared to intubation without paralysis, it reduces the incidence of complications such as aspiration and traumatic injury to the airways [18]. The sequence or RSI can be summarized in the 'seven Ps': Preparation for the procedure, Preoxygenation, Premedication, Paralysis, Protection by Sellick maneuver, Placement of the tube, and Post-intubation management.

1. Preparation: includes rapid assessment of the patient, collecting the necessary drugs and equipment needed for the procedure.
2. Pre-oxygenation or alveolar de-nitrogenation is implemented to create a reservoir of oxygen in the lungs that prevents desaturation during attempts of intubation. Give 100% oxygen by non-rebreathing mask if awake, or by bag-valve mask ventilation if not.
3. Premedications: these are used to reduce the adverse physiological response of laryngoscopy. LOAD (lidocaine, opioids, atropine, and a defasciculating dose of paralytic agent) is the mnemonic to summarize the agents used for this purpose.
   i. Lidocaine of 1.5 mg/kg is used to attenuate the cardiovascular response to intubation, suppress the cough reflex, and mitigate the ICP response to intubation [19,20].
   ii. Opioids, specifically fentanyl, reduce the sympathetic response to intubation on top of its analgesic and sedative effect [21].
   iii. Atropine is usually used in children to blunt the vagal response and bradycardia that occur as a result of laryngoscopy.
   iv. For paralysis, a small defasciculating dose of non-depolarizing paralytic agent (e.g. rocuronium) can be used prior to the administration of succinylcholine to reduce fasciculations and the associated increase in ICP that results from it. It is not clear that this increase in ICP actually affects outcome [22].
4. Induction: After giving the LOAD, sedation is accomplished by the administration of an induction agent, followed by either depolarizing or non-depolarizing paralytic agent. There are many induction agents that can be used with different side effect profiles and pharmacological properties. Clinicians should have detailed knowledge of their properties as the choice of the right agent will depend on the clinical scenario.
   i. Propofol: rapid acting, lipid soluble induction agent that induces hypnosis on top of its anticonvulsive and antiemetic properties. It is known to depress the pharyngeal and laryngeal muscle tone and reflexes more than any other agent and may be used with opioids alone when neuromuscular paralysis is contraindicated. [23]. It has the ability to reduce the ICP by decreasing intracranial blood volume and cerebral metabolism. [24]. These mechanisms may underlie the improved outcome with its use in patients with high ICP in the setting of traumatic brain injury [25].

      Propofol has no analgesic properties, and the major side effect is drug-induced hypotension by its action on systemic vascular resistance. Hypersensitivity reaction can occur in patients with egg/soy allergy.
   ii. Etomidate: this is a non-barbiturate hypnotic agent that has a rapid onset of action, short duration, minimal histamine release after administration, and little or no effect on the systemic BP [26].

      Disadvantages include the inability to blunt the sympathetic response, lowering seizure threshold, high incidence of myoclonus, occurrence of nausea and vomiting, and suppression of the adrenal glands. It is widely used as an induction agent in patients with polytrauma given the lack of effect on systemic BP. (It is used less often in patients with high ICP because of the availability of other agents that blunt the sympathetic response in intubation, but in general it is safe to use).

   iii. Ketamine is a phencyclidine derivative that has a rapid onset of action with amnestic, analgesic, and sympathomimetic properties. It does not abate airway-protective reflexes or spontaneous ventilation and it causes bronchodilation [27].

      A recent review of the literature shows that ketamine can be used safely in patients with high ICP as long as patients are sedated and properly ventilated [28].
   iv. Sodium thiopental is a good choice for patients with status epilepticus or increased ICP because of its cerebroprotective effects. It causes cerebral vasoconstriction, reduces cerebral blood volume, and decreases ICP [29]. The major drawback of its use is the systemic hypotension that occurs with it.
   v. Midazolam can be used as an induction agent and has anticonvulsant properties. It could cause hypotension with high doses.
5. Paralysis: after the injection of the induction agent of choice, a paralytic drug should be given and should be tailored to the clinical situation. We present some of the data about paralytic agents and the advantages versus disadvantages of each of them.
   i. Depolarizing drugs: these agents act on the acetylcholine receptors as agonists, causing prolonged depolarization and resulting in muscle relaxation after a brief period of fasciculation. Succinylcholine is the prototypical drug of this class that has a rapid onset of action (30–60 seconds) and short duration of action (5–15 minutes). Spontaneous respiration may return 9–10 minutes after its use. It is usually degraded by plasma and hepatic pseudocholinesterases. Succinylcholine is given in a dose of 1.5 mg/kg because lower doses could cause relaxation of the laryngeal muscles before skeletal muscles, which could complicate intubation and put the patient at risk of aspiration. The side effect profile includes hyperkalemia, malignant hyperthermia and increased ICP [30,31]. It should be avoided in diseases that have up-regulation of the acetylcholine receptors as it may cause an exaggerated release of potassium. These disorders include stroke, multiple sclerosis, muscular dystrophies, GBS, and others. Based on the side-effect profile and the extensive risks imposed, some intensivists discourage its use with critically ill patients in the ICU [32].
   ii. Non-depolarizing agents such as rocuronium: these agents act by blocking acetylcholine receptors at the neuromuscular junction. It has a short onset of action (1–2 minutes), longer duration of activity (45–70 minutes), and the usual dose is 1 mg/kg. They do not have the side-effect profile of depolarizing agents and have been used as a substitute when the other class is contraindicated.

      In a systematic review, the use of succinylcholine was compared to rocuronium in intubation procedures. The reviewers found that the use of succinylcholine resulted in a superior intubation condition compared to rocuronium when rigorous standards were used to define excellent conditions. When these standards were less rigorously used to define adequate conditions, and when propofol was added as an induction agent, the two drugs had similar efficacy. The success rate of intubation was the same for both groups under all circumstances [33].
6. Sellick maneuver: is performed by applying pressure on the cricoid to prevent passive aspiration and gastric insufflation.
7. Placement of the endotracheal tube (ETT): this should be done under direct visualization of the vocal cords. By applying pressure at the thyroid cartilage the field of visualization can be improved. As mentioned before, preparation is the best way to intubate patients who are critically ill, especially when it comes to passing the ETT. Different devices are of help in passing the ETT into proper position that should be kept around the intubating field especially in the neuroICU setting. A lighted stylet, gum elastic bougie, laryngeal mask airway, or fiberoptic machine should be ready whenever needed, especially if there is an anticipation of difficult airway. These devices decrease the incidence of failed intubations and could be used when direct laryngoscopy is contraindicated or difficult [34].

Modes of mechanical ventilation

Basically, there are modes of ventilation that breathe for the patient and others that assist the patient and allow the initiated breath to be large enough to assure adequate ventilation.

1. Controlled modes of ventilation: these will dictate the frequency of the ventilation as well as either the volume of the breath (volume control), or the pressure at which the air is sent (pressure control). The patient's own respiratory rate does not affect the frequency of the delivered breaths, and the volume or pressure remain constant, not taking into account lung compliance. In a conscious or semi-conscious patient with some residual muscle strength, this can result in the patient fighting the ventilator. If the lungs are very stiff, fixed volume might lead to unacceptably high lung pressures and pneumothorax.

   Fixed ventilation is used in patients who have no respiratory drive or who are paralyzed. Fixed pressures are used in patients with such stiff lungs that must not receive air pushed in above a specific threshold of pressure, even if this leads to hypercarbia.
2. Assisted modes of ventilation: in this case the patient initiates the breath and the machine assists and maximizes tidal volume by supplying a set volume or a set inspiratory pressure.
   i. SIMV stands for synchronized intermittent mandatory ventilation. The machine will deliver a set number of breaths but will synchronize them with the patient's efforts and supply breaths when the spontaneous rate is below the set rate. For spontaneous breaths, the work of breathing is decreased by providing a pressure support. So, when on SIMV mode, the patient receives three different types of breath: 1 – the controlled mandatory breath; 2 – the assisted breath; and 3 – the spontaneous breath that can be pressure supported.
   ii. PS or pressure support can be used as a partial or full support mode. The patient controls all parts of the breath except the pressure limit. The patient triggers the ventilator – the ventilator delivers a flow up to a preset pressure limit (for example 10 cmH_2O) depending on the desired minute volume, the patient continues the breath for as long as they wish, and flow cycles off when a certain percentage of peak inspiratory flow (usually 25%) has been reached. Tidal volumes may vary, just as they do in normal breathing. The level of pressure support is set at the pressure that assures an adequate tidal volume.

In patients with neurological rather than pulmonary disease and preservation of respiratory drive, PS is the best choice for ventilation. If respiratory drive is compromised, SIMV works well. Many other considerations are involved when the main issue is pulmonary.

Parameters of ventilation

The literature on respiratory care and mechanical ventilation in patients with ICH is scarce. Few trials have addressed this issue, and until now we do not have guidelines for the exact parameters that should be implemented for the management of this population. Most of the current practice recommendations are based on evidence from brain trauma trials and on expert opinion.

The recommendation by The Brain Trauma Foundation for oxygenation and ventilation in brain injury patients is to prevent hypoxia by maintaining PaO_2 >60 mmHg and arterial oxygen saturation of >90%. All effort should be made to prevent hypoxia, hypercapnea, and respiratory acidosis as they have deleterious effects in patients with brain disease.

The use of positive end expiratory pressure (PEEP)

Positive pressure ventilation in general increases functional residual capacity, prevents alveolar de-recruitment, and improves oxygenation. It is very useful in cases where pulmonary abnormalities contribute to the respiratory insufficiency. However, PEEP may increase ICP in selected clinical circumstances. First, the positive pressure could be transmitted directly through the neck to the cranial cavity. Second the rise in the intrathoracic pressure causes decreased venous return to the heart and, as a result, the jugular venous pressure rises, leading to higher cerebral blood volume (CBV) and an increase in ICP. Third, the reduction in venous return causes decreased cardiac output and blood pressure with net effect of reduction of cerebral perfusion pressure. The brain reacts to this low CPP by vasodilation which will increase the overall CBV and potentially exacerbate the increase in ICP.

When these theoretical risks were translated to clinical trials, the danger of PEEP to ICP was much less obvious. The effect is not seen in lungs with poor compliance [35], it is clinically insignificant in patients with intact or partially intact autoregulation [36,37] and, in general, the preponderance of available studies suggest that a deleterious effect on ICP or CPP is quantitatively modest or non-existent, with levels of PEEP up to 15 cmH_2O) [38–41].

The use of protective mechanical ventilation

Brain directed ventilation strategies implemented the use of large tidal volumes, high-inspired oxygen, low PEEP, intravascular fluid loading, and use of vasopressors to maintain adequate CPP. All of these measures were used to ensure protection of the airways with proper oxygenation, maintenance of adequate levels of CO_2, and prevention of deleterious effects of positive pressure ventilation on ICP.

On the other hand, in the presence of severe lung disease, lung protective MV would mean the use of low tidal volume and plateau pressure to prevent alveolar overdistension, the use of PEEP to prevent atelectasis, and restricted fluid use to aid in oxygenation and to prevent ventilation-induced lung injury (VILI), which is histologically similar to the alveolar damage associated with ARDS/ALI syndromes (adult respiratory distress syndrome and acute lung injury). Not only can VILI contribute to the development of ARDS/ALI in high-risk patients, it also affects the overall morbidity and mortality in those individuals [42].

We do not know yet what are the implications and importance of VILI in patients with neurological diseases. Theoretically, the use of low tidal volume may lead to reduction in minute ventilation and hypercapnea, and this may lead to an increase in ICP. We have some preliminary data indicating that low tidal volume use is safe in patients with neurological injury and should be used if the patient's medical condition warrants it [43].

Use of other specialized methods of ventilation

Most patients with a hemorrhagic stroke will have normal or only moderately abnormal lungs, and therefore conventional modes of ventilation will be more than adequate. In the patient with severely damaged lungs, with ARDS or pulmonary fibrosis, conventional methods of ventilation may be ineffective. The use of high-frequency oscillating ventilation (HFOV), prone position, and nitric oxide may help oxygenation, but their effect on ICP and CBF are not well studied. They would not be used unless the respiratory condition demands it.

When to wean from mechanical ventilation

It is very clear that prolonged mechanical ventilation leads to an increase in mortality, morbidity, and ICU length of stay [44]. In order to expedite the weaning process, a number of variables were studied in order to determine which could predict successful weaning from the ventilator.

Ideally, there should be several parameters that could predict, accurately and with a high success rate, which patient could be weaned successfully. The American College of Chest Physicians and the American Association for Respiratory Care advocate the use of eight different parameters to enhance accuracy of successful weaning [45]. Even with rigorous application of those parameters, 13% of patients with parameters indicating success will still fail extubation. The parameters recommended by the American College of Chest Physicians were elaborated using patients intubated for respiratory distress due to pulmonary abnormalities.

Patients intubated for reasons related to abnormalities of the central nervous system are not represented, and so these parameters will be even less accurate in the patient with ICH.

In neurologically impaired patients such as stroke, fewer parameters need to be considered. The GCS is likely the best predictor of successful extubation. In a randomized study, Namen and colleagues found that successful extubation rose by 39% for each 1-point increment in the GCS and that a GCS of 8 or more is associated with the best success [46]. Coplin and collaborators [47], however, found that GCS is not a major factor in predicting extubation. Their study showed that 80% of patients with GCS of 8 could be extubated, and patients with GCS of 4 had an even higher rate of extubation success (90%). It makes sense that level of consciousness (LOC) should be an important factor in successful extubation, but clearly more studies are needed.

Besides LOC, it is also important to be sure that pharyngeal muscles are strong enough to protect the airway. Clinical evaluation of facial, pharyngeal muscles and neck flexion are an excellent gauge of airway protection.

If respiratory muscle weakness is the reason for intubation, the predictors used by pneumologists can be of some value although the studies did not include patients with neuromuscular disease (44).

Parameters predicting successful extubation in the studies mentioned include: SaO_2 of >90% on FiO_2 <0.4, PEEP <8 cmH_2O required while on the ventilator, respiratory rate (f) <35/minute, maximal inspiratory pressure less than −20 to −25 cmH_2O, tidal volume Vt >5 ml/kg, vital capacity >10 ml/kg, and f/Vt <105 breaths/min/L with no evidence of respiratory acidosis.

Three parameters that predicted failure were tidal volume of <325 ml [negative predictive value NPV =94%], negative inspiratory pressure −15 cmH_2O [NPV=100%], and f/Vt >105 breaths/min/L [NPV=95%].

For neuromuscular disease, these have been modified: maximal inspiratory pressure more negative than −30 to −35 cmH_2O, the ability to generate a Vt >5 ml/kg with a pressure support of 6 for more than 24 hours.

How to wean from mechanical ventilation

The method for weaning depends on the underlying pathology that led to the respiratory distress. We will focus on weaning the patient intubated after ICH.

The general outline to wean and liberate from a ventilator has three main steps:

1. **Assessment of patient readiness:** the patient needs to be clinically stable, no evidence of bradycardia (40) or tachycardia (>140), stable blood pressure (systolic BP of 90–160 mmHg), no overt tachypnea, and no hypoxia. Parameters of extubation mentioned above have been met.
2. **Application of spontaneous breathing trial (SBT):** three options exist to perform the SBT: 1) T-tube trial. 2) low-level pressure support ventilation (PSV), and 3) use of Automatic Tube Compensation (ATC). In pulmonary patients, there is no difference in the percentage of patients who pass the SBT or in those who will be extubated if either method was used [48]. In our patient population, the traditional spontaneous breathing trial is not reliable. If the problem was one of LOC, an awake patient who triggers the ventilator on a regular basis, coughs well, and defends his airway can be extubated without further ado. If the problem is weakness of the cranial nerves innervating the pharynx, the patient will breathe easily without the ventilator, but extubation cannot occur as long as the weakness persists. For the patient with neuromuscular weakness, fatigue can occur several hours after the ventilator's assistance has been removed. The patient will do well on a SBT of 3 hours, seem fine and then go into respiratory failure during the night. For these patients, pressure support must be gradually brought to 6 hours, and then they need to successfully remain at this level for 24 hours. Only then are they ready for extubation, again presuming that the bulbar muscles are strong.
3. **Trial of extubation**. Many studies demonstrated that 13% of those who pass the SBT and got extubated will fail and be intubated again. This number increases up to 40% if SBT is not done prior to extubation attempt. Physicians should always look for possible reversible causes of failure and correct them in order to succeed with the next trial. After

Table 21b.1

Preparation –10 min	Pre-oxygenation –5 min	Premedication –2 min	Induction/ paralysis time zero	Intubation +30–45 s
1. Rapid assessment of the patient 2. Collect drugs and equipment needed 3. Be ready for possible complications of the procedure (e.g. hypotension)	Oxygenate 100% with nonbreather/bag valve mask	Think of the LOAD: Lidocaine Opiate Atropine Defasciculating dose of non-depolarizing paralytic agent	Induction: a) Propofol b) Etomidate c) Midazolam d) Sodium Thiopental Paralysis: a) Rocuronium b) Succinylcholine	With application of Sellick maneuver pass the endotracheal tube under direct visualization of the cord

stabilization of the patient, another trial of SBT can be attempted by applying the same principles and parameters each time.

Tracheostomy: indications and timing

Long-term outcome in intensive care unit survivors after mechanical ventilation for intracerebral hemorrhage is better than that for ischemic stroke. In a retrospective study of 120 ventilated patients, survival was 57% at 3 years, and 42% of these had slight or no disability. Factors correlating with unfavorable outcome were age >65 years and a GCS below 15 at discharge [49]. In a similar retrospective study, early tracheostomy correlated with shorter ICU and hospital stays (p <0.01). [50]

Endotracheal tubes with soft cuffs can generally be maintained for two weeks. In the presence of prolonged coma or pulmonary complications, elective tracheostomy should be performed after 2 weeks.

REFERENCES

1. Gebel JM, Broderick JP. Intracerebral hemorrhage. *Neurol Clin* 2000;**18**:419–38.
2. Sacco, RL, Mayer, SA. Epidemiology of intracerebral hemorrhage. In *Intracerebral Hemorrhage.* Edited by Feldmann E. Armonk, NY: Futura Publishing Co.; 1994: 3–23.
3. Zurasky JA, Aiyagari V, Zazulia AR, Shackelford A, Diringer MN. Early mortality following spontaneous intracerebral hemorrhage. *Neurology* 2005;**64**:725–7.
4. Diringer MN, Edwards DF. Admission to a neurologic/ neurosurgical intensive care unit is associated with reduced mortality rate after intracerebral hemorrhage. *Crit Care Med* 2001;**29**:635–40.
5. Bushnell CD, Phillips-Bute BG, Laskowitz DT, *et al.* Survival and outcome after endotracheal intubation for acute stroke. *Neurology* 1999;**52**(7):1374–81.
6. Esteban A, Anzueto A, Alia I, *et al.* How is mechanical ventilation employed in the intensive care unit? An international utilization review. *Am J Respir Crit Care Med* 2000;**161(5)**:1450–8.
7. Bolton CF. Anatomy and physiology of the nervous system control of respiration. In: Bolton CF, Chen R, Wijdicks EFM, *et al.* (editors). *Neurology of breathing.* Philadelphia: Butterworth Heineman; 2004;19–35.
8. Fortune JB, Feustel PJ, Graca L, *et al.* Effect of hyperventilation, mannitol, and ventriculostomy drainage on cerebral blood flow after head injury. *J Trauma* 1995;**39 (6)**:1091–9.
9. Kontos HA, Raper AJ, Patterson JL. Analysis of vasoactivity of local pH, PCO2 and bicarbonate on pial vessels. *Stroke* 1977;**8(3)**:358–60.
10. Muizelaar JP, van der Poel HG, Li ZC, *et al.* Pial arteriolar vessel diameter and sCO2 reactivity during prolonged hyperventilation in the rabbit. *J Neurosurg* 1988;**69**(6):923–7.
11. Guidelines for the management of severe traumatic brain injury. XIV. Hyperventilation. *J Neurotrauma* 2007;**24** (Suppl 1):S87–90.
12. Muizelaar JP, Marmarou A, Ward JD, *et al.* Adverse effects of prolonged hyperventilation in patients with severe head

injury: a randomized clinical trial. *J Neurosurg* 1991;**75 (5)**:731–9.

13. Marion DW, Puccio A, Wisniewski SR, *et al.* Effect of hyperventilation on extracellular concentrations of glutamate, lactate, pyruvate, and local cerebral blood flow in patients with severe traumatic brain injury. *Crit Care Med* 2002;**30 (12)**:2619–25.
14. Bolton C. Respiration in central nervous system disorders. In: Bolton C, Chen R, Wijdicks E, *et al.*, (editors). *Neurology of Breathing.* Philadelphia: Butterworth Heinemann; 2004;151–64.
15. Smith Hammond CA, Goldstein LB, Zajac DJ, *et al.* Assessment of aspiration risk in stroke patients with quantification of voluntary cough. *Neurology* 2001;**56 (4)**:502–6.
16. Berthiaume L, Zygun D. Non-neurologic organ dysfunction in acute brain injury. *Crit Care Clin* 2006;**22** (4):753–66.
17. Deem S. Management of acute brain injury and associated respiratory issues. *Respir Care* 2006;**51**(4):357–67.
18. Li J, Murphy-Lavoie H, Bugas C, Martinez J, Preston C. Complications of emergency intubation with and without paralysis. *Am J Emerg Med* 1999;**17**:141–3.
19. Lev R. Rosen P. Prophylactic lidocaine use preintubation: a review. *J Emerg Med* 1994;**12**:499–506.
20. Yukioka H, Hayashi M, Terai T, Fujimori M. Intravenous lidocaine as a suppressant of coughing during tracheal intubation in elderly patients. *Anesth Analg* 1993;**77**:309–12.
21. Ko SH, Kim DC, Han YJ, Song HS. Small-dose fentanyl: optimal time of injection for blunting the circulatory responses to tracheal intubation. *Anesth Analg* 1998;**86**:658–61.
22. Clancy M, Halford S, Walls R, Murphy M. In patients with head injuries who undergo rapid sequence intubation using succinylcholine, does pretreatment with a competitive neuromuscular blocking agent improve outcome? A literature review. *Emerg Med J* 2001;**18**(5):373–5.
23. Wong AK, Teoh GS. Intubation without muscle relaxant: an alternative technique for rapid tracheal intubation. *Anaesth Intensive Care* 1996;**24**:224–30.
24. Merlo F, Demo P, Lacquaniti L, *et al.* Propofol in single bolus for treatment of elevated intracranial hypertension. *Minerva Anestesiol* 1991;**57**:359–63.
25. Kelly DF, Goodale DB, Williams J, *et al.* Propofol in the treatment of moderate and severe head injury: a randomized, prospective double-blinded pilot trial. *J Neurosurg* 1999;**90**:1042–52.
26. Smith DC, Bergen JM, Smithline H, Kirschner R. A trial of etomidate for rapid sequence intubation in the emergency department. *J Emerg Med* 2000;**18**:13–16.
27. Miller RD. *Anesthesia.* 5th ed. New York, NY: Churchill Livingstone, 2000.
28. Zeiler FA, Teitelbaum J, West M, Gillman LM. The ketamine effect on ICP in traumatic brain injury. *Neurocrit Care* 2014; February epub.
29. Wadbrook PS. Advances in airway pharmacology. Emerging trends and evolving controversy. *Emerg Med Clin North Am* 2000;**18**:767–88.
30. Orebaugh SL. Succinylcholine: adverse effects and alternatives in emergency medicine. *Am J Emerg Med* 1999;**17**:715–21.
31. Cottrell JE, Hartung J, Giffin JP, Shwiry B. Intracranial and hemodynamic changes after succinylcholine administration in cats. *Anesth Analg* 1983;**62**:1006–9.
32. Booij LH. Is succinylcholine appropriate or obsolete in the intensive care unit? *Crit Care* 2001;**5**:245–6.
33. Lee J, Wells G. Are intubation conditions using rocuronium equivalent to those using succinylcholine? *Acad Emerg Med* 2002;**9**:813–23.
34. Butler KH, Clyne, B. Management of the difficult airway: alternative airway techniques and adjuncts. *Emerg Med Clin North Am* 2003;**21**:259–89.
35. Caricato A, Conti G, Della Corte F, *et al.* Effects of PEEP on the intracranial system of patients with head injury and subarachnoid hemorrhage: the role of respiratory system compliance. *J Trauma* 2005;**58(3)**:571–6.
36. Mascia L, Grasso S, Fiore T, *et al.* Cerebro-pulmonary interactions during the application of low levels of positive end-expiratory pressure. *Intensive Care Med* 2005;**31(3)**:373–9.
37. Georgiadis D, Schwarz S, Baumgartner RW, *et al.* Influence of positive end-expiratory pressure on intracranial pressure and cerebral perfusion pressure in patients with acute stroke. *Stroke* 2001;**32**(9):2088–92.
38. Muench E, Bauhuf C, Roth H, *et al.* Effects of positive end-expiratory pressure on regional cerebral blood flow, intracranial pressure, and brain tissue oxygenation. *Crit Care Med* 2005;**33**(10):2367–72.
39. Georgiadis D, Schwarz S, Baumgartner RW, *et al.* Influence of positive end-expiratory pressure on intracranial pressure and cerebral perfusion pressure in patients with acute stroke. *Stroke* 2001;**32(9)**:2088–92.
40. McGuire G, Crossley D, Richards J, *et al.* Effects of varying levels of positive end-expiratory pressure on intracranial pressure and cerebral perfusion pressure. *Crit Care Med* 1997;**25(6)**:1059–62.

41. Huynh T, Messer M, Sing RF, *et al.* Positive end-expiratory pressure alters intracranial and cerebral perfusion pressure in severe traumatic brain injury. *J Trauma* 2002;**53 (3)**:488–92.
42. Gajic O, Frutos-Vivar F, Esteban A, *et al.* Ventilator settings as a risk factor for acute respiratory distress syndrome in mechanically ventilated patients. *Intensive Care Med* 2005;**31(7)**:922–6.
43. Kahn JM, Caldwell EC, Deem S, *et al.* Acute lung injury in patients with subarachnoid hemorrhage: incidence, risk factors, and outcome. *Crit Care Med* 2006;**34**(1):196–202.
44. Mutlu GM, Factor P. Complications of mechanical ventilation. *Respir Care Clin N Am* 2000;**6(2)**:213–52.
45. Khamiees M, Raju P, DeGirolamo A, *et al.* Predictors of extubation outcome in patients who have successfully completed a spontaneous breathing trial. *Chest* 2001;**120 (4)**:1262–70.
46. Namen AM, Ely EW, Tatter SB, *et al.* Predictors of successful extubation in neurosurgical patients. *Am J Respir Crit Care Med* 2001;**163**(3Pt 1):658–64.
47. Coplin WM, Pierson DJ, Cooley KD, *et al.* Implications of extubation delay in brain-injured patients meeting standard weaning criteria. *Am J Respir Crit Care Med* 2000;**161 (5)**:1530–6.
48. Matic I, Majeric-Kogler V. Comparison of pressure support and T-tube weaning from mechanical ventilation: A randomized prospective study. *Croat Med J* 2004;**45**:162–6.
49. Roch A, Michelet P, Jullien, AC. Long-term outcome in intensive care unit survivors after mechanical ventilation for intracerebral hemorrhage. *Crit Care Med* 2003;**31**:2651–6.
50. Rabinstein A, Wijdicks E. Outcome of survivors of acute stroke who require prolonged ventilatory assistance and tracheostomy. *Cerebrovasc Dis* 2004;**18**:325–31.

Nutrition in the ICH patient

Dimitre Staykov and Jürgen Bardutzky

Introduction

Malnutrition and outcome in patients with stroke

Several studies have investigated the influence of nutritional status on prognosis in patients with stroke [1–8]. The utilization of different tools for assessment of nutritional status, however, makes comparisons between those studies very difficult.

Stratton *et al.* [9] used the Malnutrition Universal Screening Tool (MUST) and showed that malnutrition correlated with worse outcome, increased hospital stay, and mortality in elderly patients. Martineau *et al.* [2] assessed the nutritional status of stroke patients using the patient-generated subjective global assessment (PG-SGA). In this retrospective study, 19% of patients were found to be malnourished on admission. Malnutrition was associated with longer hospital stay and higher complication rates. Using the same screening tool (SGA) in 185 consecutive stroke patients, Davis *et al.* [3] showed a correlation between malnutrition assessed on admission and higher mortality and unfavorable functional outcome (modified Rankin scale (mRS) 3–6) 30 days after the stroke. This trend was present, however, no longer significant, after adjustments for age, premorbid mRS and National Institute of Health Stroke Scale (NIHSS) on admission were made. A highly significant correlation between poor nutritional status and worse functional outcome (mRS 3–5), as well as mortality after 6 months was shown in the FOOD trial [4], even when adjustments were made for all important predictors of outcome after stroke. Malnourished patients also suffered more often infections, gastrointestinal bleedings and decubitus ulcers. In this trial, however, nutritional status assessment was not standardized, but rather based on estimation by the treating physician.

Some authors use laboratory parameters such as e.g. serum albumin as an addition to clinical tools for assessment of the nutritional status. Within a prospective study on patients with acute stroke, Davalos *et al.* measured the triceps skin flap, arm circumference, serum albumin, and performed indirect calorimetry on admission and 1 week later [5]. Malnourished patients had a higher incidence of infections and decubitus ulcers, furthermore, there was a trend towards association of poor nutritional status 1 week after admission with worse prognosis (death or a Barthel index <50) at 30 days. Axelsson *et al.* [6] assessed nutritional status by body weight, triceps skin flap, and arm circumference measurements. Additionally, serum albumin, pre-albumin, and trasferrin values were considered as indicators of malnutrition if they were below the normal range. Patients in whom two of those parameters were lowered suffered infections more often than non-malnourished stroke patients. Using similar assessment parameters, Finestone *et al.* [7] could show that malnourished stroke patients needed longer rehabilitation for functional recovery than non-malnourished patients. Finally, Perry and McLaren [8] could also demonstrate that poor nutritional status and

Critical Care of the Stroke Patient, ed. Stefan Schwab, Daniel Hanley, and A. David Mendelow. Published by Cambridge University Press.

malnutrition correlates with a worse quality of life after stroke.

Although the quality of the available data almost uniformly corresponds to a class III evidence, there are indications that malnutrition may cause increased hospital stay, higher morbidity, and mortality in stroke patients. Malnourished stroke patients may suffer more frequently infections and decubitus ulcers, and patients admitted to a rehabilitation facility may need longer in order to achieve a certain level of independence, as compared to non-malnourished patients. The fact that approximately every fifth stroke patient shows signs of malnutrition on admission makes treatment and avoidance of malnutrition a potential therapeutic target in such patients.

Energy demand in patients with stroke

The knowledge of the patient's energy demand is an important prerequisite for the development of an adequate nutritional regimen. To date, very few studies have investigated the baseline (BEE) and total energy expenditure (TEE) in stroke patients, particularly in patients with intracerebral hemorrhage (ICH). Stroke patients who do not require critical care have been reported to have a daily resting energy expenditure comprising approximately 1100 to 1700 kcal, or about 110% of the BEE calculated according to the formula of Harris and Benedict [5,10,11]. However, in a study on 27 stroke patients (10 with intracerebral hemorrhage and 17 with ischemic stroke), Chalela *et al.* analyzed the nitrogen balance over a period of 18 months and found that a large proportion of patients (44%) was catabolic. The authors concluded that usage of Harris-Benedict equation to estimate caloric needs led to underfeeding in those patients [12].

Within a single-center study, we investigated the energy expenditure in 34 nonseptic sedated and mechanically ventilated stroke patients during the first 5 days of treatment on a neurocritical care unit by means of continuous indirect calorimetry [13]. TEE in those patients was approximately 1600 kcal/d (20 kcal/kg body weight/d) and correlated well with the BEE, as predicted using the Harris-Benedict equation. In accordance with the study of Finestone *et al.* [10], we found no difference between patients with ischemic stroke and ICH, and neurosurgical procedures, such as craniectomy or external ventricular drainage, also did not influence energy expenditure. When comparing our results to other studies on critically ill sedated patients [14,15], the TEE values we found in stroke patients were remarkably lower. In septic stroke patients treated in the same setting, we observed an increase of TEE to a value approximating 140% of BEE. In contrast to that, stroke patients treated with moderate hypothermia (33°C) showed a decrease in TEE to a value reaching roughly 75% of BEE calculated with the Harris-Benedict equation [16].

Although the currently available data do not allow a firm conclusion on the value of energy-expenditure-oriented nutritional support, there are indications that underfeeding, as well as overfeeding may have detrimental effects on the prognosis of stroke patients. Therefore, measurement of TEE in critically ill stroke patients by means of indirect calorimetry may be of advantage for the design of an adequate individual nutrition regimen. As this method is not widely available, calculations based on the Harris-Benedict equation could be used to estimate the energy demand in nonseptic sedated stroke patients during the acute phase of treatment. In such patients, calculated BEE seems to well represent TEE of approximately 20 kcal/kg body weight/d.

Oral nutritional supplementation in nondysphagic patients

Very few studies have investigated the influence of oral nutritional supplementation on the clinical course and outcome of nondysphagic stroke patients. The FOOD study [17] included in total 4023 patients and could not demonstrate a beneficial effect of oral nutritional supplementation (360 ml/d, 1.5 kcal/ml, 62.5 g/l protein) on mortality and functional outcome. In a subgroup analysis, a nonsignificant trend towards reduction of mortality and poor outcome was found for patients who were estimated to have poor nutritional status (n = 314) and received enteral sip feeding. However, several methodological issues in the FOOD study have raised criticism and make the interpretation of those data difficult. First, the nutritional status was estimated by the treating physician and no standardized tool was used. Second, compliance for the oral nutritional supplementation comprised approximately 55%. Third, food intake was not documented, so it remains unclear if energy and protein intake was actually increased in those patients. Total food intake was calculated in an earlier study on 42 stroke patients who were able to eat within 1 week after symptom onset. Gariballa *et al.* [18] could demonstrate that energy and protein intake can be increased with enteral sip feeding (400 ml/d, 1.5 kcal/ml, 50 g/l protein). Weight loss, as well as serum albumin and iron decrease could be avoided in patients who received nutritional supplementation. The authors also reported trends towards better functional outcome and mortality in supplemented patients, however, those results did not reach significance. Those data do not allow a general recommendation for oral nutritional supplementation in non-dysphagic stroke patients. Moreover, the FOOD study has also provided some insights into the practicability of oral nutritional supplementation. Roughly one-third of the patients who received oral supplements within the FOOD study discontinued the supplement intake because of bad taste, nausea, diarrhea, or unwanted weight gain [17]. In 33 patients with diabetes, poor glycemic control led to premature stopping of oral supplementation. As hyperglycemia has been identified as a negative prognostic predictor in patients with acute stroke [19], this issue certainly deserves further critical evaluation.

However, selected patients may benefit from oral nutritional supplementation. In a meta-analysis of 35 randomized controlled trials on 3242 patients treated in hospitals or nursing homes, Milne *et al.* [20] could show that supplements may reduce complications and mortality in old and undernourished patients. In the FOOD study, the risk for decubitus ulcers was lower in patients who received enteral sip feeding, and this result was borderline statistically significant ($p = 0.057$) [17]. The effectiveness of oral nutritional supplementation for prevention of decubitus in at-risk patients has been shown in a meta-analysis by Stratton *et al.* [21]. The risk of decubitus ulcers was significantly reduced (by 25%) in elderly, postsurgical, and chronically hospitalized patients who received supplements. Although not investigated yet, stroke patients at risk of developing decubitus ulcers (elderly, undernourished, immobilized patients) may also benefit from oral nutritional supplementation.

Enteral nutrition

Enteral nutrition and prognosis in patients with stroke

Early enteral nutrition (within 24 hours after admission) has been shown to significantly reduce infection risk and hospital stay in critically ill patients [22,23]. Up to roughly one-third of patients with stroke have been reported to require nutritional support via tube feeding in the acute phase [24]. Unfortunately, very few studies have investigated the influence of tube feeding on outcome in the setting of stroke. The second part of the FOOD study [25] included 859 dysphagic stroke patients who were assigned to early enteral tube feeding (within 7 days from admission) versus no feeding for more than 7 days. Early tube feeding resulted in a trend towards reduced mortality (by 5.8%), however, this finding was not statistically significant ($p = 0.09$). On the other hand, a major methodological limitation of this study was the utilization of the so-called 'uncertainty principle' of patient enrolment, i.e. patients were randomized if the treating physician was uncertain of the necessity of early tube feeding. This selection bias with a priori exclusion of patients with a clear indication for enteral tube nutrition may have weakened the measured positive effect of enteral feeding on outcome. Another unanswered question is, if a subgroup of stroke patients particularly benefits from enteral tube feeding. Such patients could be e.g. those who are malnourished at admission, or those who are at risk of malnutrition in the course of treatment, like patients with dysphagia, disturbed consciousness, or severe neurological deficits.

Spontaneously breathing patients with dysphagia

Inadequate food intake may have different causes in patients with stroke. Apart from dysphagia, other factors such as immobility, disturbances of consciousness, neuropsychological deficits, aphasia, apraxia etc. may play a substantial role. Estimating the duration of such disturbances of food intake is difficult, because of wide individual variations.

Dysphagia is a common symptom which affects up to approximately 50% of stroke patients and carries a three- to seven-fold increased risk of aspiration pneumonia [26]. Patients with dysphagia are also at risk of developing malnutrition in the course of treatment [27]. However, a large proportion of those patients experience significant improvement within a relatively short time span. Smithard *et al.* [28] report aspiration in 51% of patients with stroke immediately after symptom onset (n = 121). The proportion of those patients observed after 7 days was 27%, within 6 weeks it decreased to 6.8% and after 6 months, it was only 2.3% [28]. This study illustrates the importance of regular assessment of dysphagia after stroke. Diagnosis and estimation of severity of dysphagia can be performed clinically (gag reflex, coughing after swallowing, dysphonia, prolonged swallowing act) or using apparative support (videofluoroscopy, x-ray, transnasal endoscopy). The available data on different screening and assessment methods for dysphagia reveal highly variable findings considering sensitivity and specificity [29]. Therefore, recommendation of a particular screening or assessment tool is usually based on expert opinion.

The question of whether enteral tube feeding can lower the incidence of complications associated with dysphagia has not been sufficiently studied yet. In the acute phase of stroke, aspiration pneumonia does not seem to be reduced with enteral tube feeding [30,31]. However, in the long-term management of stroke patients with dysphagia, nasogastric tube feeding has been shown to be associated with a significantly lower incidence of aspiration pneumonia. Nakajoh *et al.* [32] observed 100 stroke patients with dysphagia over a period of 1 year and found that patients who received oral nutrition (n = 48) developed aspiration pneumonia in 54.3% of cases, as compared to only 13.2% when enteral tube feeding was used (n = 52). A subgroup analysis of bedridden patients revealed a comparably high pneumonia rate of 64% with enteral tube feeding. Therefore, enteral tube feeding may be beneficial in patients with long-lasting dysphagia and otherwise good functional status. Tube feeding is usually recommended in patients who are expected to have dysphagia for more than 1 week [33].

From the pathophysiological point of view, an early start of enteral feeding should be beneficial in order to keep the intestinal barrier intact and prevent enteral bacteria from dislocation into the bloodstream. In support of this hypothesis, a lower incidence of sepsis episodes has been reported in surgical patients who received enteral versus parenteral feeding [34]. A retrospective study of 52 stroke patients showed that early enteral feeding (<72 hours after admission) led to a significantly lower length of hospital stay [35]. The FOOD study did not show a significant benefit for stroke patients with dysphagia who received early tube feeding; however, a trend towards reduction of mortality in those patients was reported (see above) [25].

Critically ill patients and stroke patients requiring intensive care

In critically ill patients, malnutrition has been associated with impaired immune function, impaired ventilatory drive, and weakened respiratory muscles, leading to increased infectious morbidity and mortality [36]. Owing to increased substrate metabolism, undernutrition is more likely to develop in critical illness than in uncomplicated starvation [37]. Early enteral nutrition is therefore recommended in critically ill patients who are not expected to be on full oral diet within 3 days [37]. In patients with hemodynamic instability, or high gastric residuals, minimal enteral nutrition with additional parenteral feeding should be considered [37].

The most common causes leading to mechanical ventilation in stroke patients are disturbances of consciousness, increased intracranial pressure, central respiratory failure, or respiratory complications caused by aspiration. In such patients, fast weaning off from the respirator is usually not possible and, consecutively, return to full oral diet within 1 week cannot be expected. However, early enteral nutrition in stroke patients may be difficult because of the frequent need of sedation, leading to disturbances in gastrointestinal motility. Such complications may require a combination of enteral and parenteral nutrition in order to cover the energy demand of a mechanically ventilated stroke patient.

Route of administration

Nasogastric feeding versus percutaneous endoscopic gastrostomy (PEG)

Nasogastric enteral feeding may be difficult in stroke patients, who are often confused, uncooperative, and do not tolerate the feeding tube. Percutaneous endoscopic gastrostomy (PEG) represents an interesting alternative for enteral nutrition in such cases. Enthusiasm for this method was encouraged after a small single center randomized study (n = 30) showed a significantly lower mortality rate in stroke patients treated with PEG (12.5%), as compared to nasogastric tube feeding (57%) [38]. However, those results could not be confirmed in the second part of the FOOD study [25]. Dennis *et al.* investigated the effects of nasogastric versus PEG tube feeding in 321 stroke patients and even found a significantly increased risk of death or poor outcome (defined as a modified Rankin scale of 4 or 5) in patients treated with PEG. Despite the larger sample size in the FOOD study, those results should also be interpreted with caution, because of several major methodological issues. First, as mentioned above, this part of the FOOD study also utilized the 'uncertainty principle' for enrolment, i.e. patients were included only if the treating physician was unsure of the indication of either treatment method. Second, initiation of enteral feeding was performed at different time points in both groups, because of difficulties considering early placement of a PEG. Three days after admission, only 48% of the patients in the PEG arm had a gastric tube, as compared to 86% in the nasogastric tube arm. PEG may be beneficial for mechanically ventilated patients, who require nutritional support for more than 14 days, because it may be associated with a lower risk of pneumonia [39,40].

In the clinical routine, the nasogastric tube seems to have the best practicability for early initial enteral feeding in the first 2–3 weeks after stroke. A PEG should only be recommended if the patients do not tolerate nasogastric feeding, or if a prolonged enteral feeding for more than 2–3 weeks is necessary.

Duodenal/jejunal tube

Currently there is no study on the value of jejunal feeding in patients with stroke. Available studies in other patient collectives have not demonstrated any benefit of post-pyloric, as compared to pre-pyloric feeding [37,41].

Enteral versus parenteral nutrition

Currently there is wide agreement on the recommendation of enteral over parenteral feeding whenever it is feasible [36,37,42]. This recommendation is based on the hypothesis of functional and morphological improvement of the gastrointestinal tract with enteral nutrition, and also on the reduction of bacterial dislocation and risk of infections with tube feeding. To date, those potential benefits of enteral over parenteral feeding have not been sufficiently proven in clinical studies. In meta-analysis of 27 trials including 1829 patients, Braunschweig *et al.* [39] did not find significant differences in mortality with either enteral or parenteral nutrition. A relevant clinical finding was, however, a significantly increased cumulative risk of infections with parenteral nutrition, as compared to either oral or enteral feeding. Another systematic review [43] found decreased costs to be the only advantage of enteral over parenteral nutrition. A more recent review [37] basically came to the same conclusion, showing no difference in mortality or length of hospital stay between the two regimens. Those findings were confirmed in a very large, recently published, randomized controlled trial which compared early (within 48 hours from admission) and late initiation (not before day eight) of parenteral nutrition to supplement insufficient enteral nutrition in 4640 critically ill patients [44]. Both groups received early enteral nutrition and insulin was infused to achieve normoglycemia. Patients in the late initiation group were more likely to be discharged alive earlier from the ICU and from the hospital (OR 1.06, 95%

CI 1.00–1.13, p = 0.04). Those patients also had fewer ICU infections and lower duration of ventilation and renal replacement therapy. Moreover, late initiation of parenteral nutrition was associated with a significant reduction of health care costs. Functional outcome and death rates did not differ significantly between the two groups.

Patients who tolerate enteral nutrition and can be fed approximately to the target values should not receive additional parenteral nutrition; however, in the clinical routine, there are cases in which parenteral supplementation may become necessary. Such cases are, e.g. patients who cannot be fed sufficiently enterally, or patients completely intolerant to enteral nutrition [37]. This problem occurs more frequently in critically ill patients, who usually tolerate only small amounts of enteral nutrition in the initial phase of treatment. Another recent, large, randomized controlled trial addressed the use of early parenteral nutrition versus standard care in 1372 critically ill patients with short-term relative contraindications to early enteral nutrition [45]. Early parenteral nutrition (initiated after a mean time of 44 min after randomization) resulted in higher energy and protein intake during the first days of ICU stay, as compared to the standard care group. There was no difference in day-60 all-cause mortality, ICU infection rates, ICU or hospital length of stay, although patients who received early parenteral nutrition required significantly fewer days of mechanical ventilation. This study could not detect a harmful effect of parenteral nutrition.

Immune modulating nutrition

While the biological properties of immuno-nutrients have been well studied in experimental models, the role of immune-modulating nutrition, i.e. supplementation with nutrients that have physiologic effects on immune function in the clinical setting, is still controversial. The idea of immune-modulated nutrition is based on the realization that optimal function of the immune system is impaired in the presence of malnutrition [46].

The most important substrates used include arginine, glutamine, omega-3 fatty acids, nucleotides, and antioxidants. Current evidence suggests that a fish oil immune-modulating diet without added arginine reduces mortality, secondary infections, and length of stay in patients with sepsis and acute respiratory distress syndrome [47]. Furthermore, glutamine supplementation may be beneficial in burns patients [47]. Combined formulas enriched with arginine, nucleotides, and omega-3 fatty acids seem to be superior to a standard enteral formula in upper gastrointestinal surgical patients and patients with trauma [37]. However, in severely ill intensive care unit patients who do not tolerate more than 700 ml enteral nutrition daily, immune-modulating nutrition may have negative effects [37].

The use of immune-modulating nutrition in stroke patients, or patients with ICH in particular, has not been investigated systematically.

Management of blood glucose

High blood glucose on admission has been associated with increased mortality in both diabetic and non-diabetic patients with ICH [48]. In stroke patients, targets for optimal glycemic control are still unclear, and treatment recommendations are generally based on expert opinions [33,49]. Despite the role of hyperglycemia as a negative prognostic predictor in different settings, including ischemic stroke and ICH, trials investigating tight glycemic control have brought up conflicting results, and meanwhile there is increasing evidence that intensive insulin treatment is rather detrimental in critically ill patients [50]. The NICE-SUGAR trial (Normogycemia in Intensive Care Evaluation – Survival Using Glucose Algorithm Regulation) [50] enrolled over 6000 patients, who were randomized to undergo intensive glucose control (target blood glucose 80–110 mg/dl) versus conventional glucose control (target blood glucose <180 mg/dl). The patients who were treated with intensive glucose control showed a significantly higher mortality rate (27.6% versus 24.9%), as compared to controls. A recently published post-hoc analysis from NICE-SUGAR [51] focuses on the role of hypoglycemia, which was observed more frequently in the intensive glucose control group. A moderate hypoglycemia (blood glucose 41–70 mg/dl) occurred in 74.2% of the patients in the intensive glucose control group versus

15.8% in the conventional management group. Severe hypoglycemia (blood glucose <40 mg/dl) was also more frequent in intensive glucose control patients (6.9% versus 0.5% in controls). Both moderate and severe hypoglycemia were significantly associated with higher mortality (OR 1.41 for moderate and 2.1 for severe hypoglycemia) in both groups. Although a direct causal relationship cannot be derived from this finding, more frequent hypoglycemia may be one plausible explanation of the higher mortality observed in the intensive glucose control group in this study. Based on NICE-SUGAR, tight glycemic control cannot be recommended for critically ill patients. This recommendation may possibly be transferred to patients requiring neurocritical care, as microdialysis studies have shown that tight glycemic control may impair cerebral glucose metabolism after severe brain injury [52].

A recently published French randomized controlled trial investigated the effect of tight glycemic control on infarct size in patients with ischemic stroke [53]. One-hundred-and-eighty patients with ischemic stroke (NIHSS 5–25) were randomized either to receive intensive insulin treatment (continuous insulin infusion, target blood glucose <5.5 mmol/l) or conventional subcutaneous insulin administration (every 4 hours, target blood glucose <8 mmol/l). MR imaging was performed before randomization and 1–3 days later. Functional outcome was assessed after 3 months. The primary endpoint of the trial was the difference in the proportion of patients with mean capillary glucose <7 mmol/l during the first 24 hours. The secondary endpoint was the influence of treatment allocation on infarct growth as determined on baseline and follow-up MRI. Intensive insulin treatment (IIT) led to a significantly higher proportion of patients with a mean blood glucose <7 mmol/l within the first 24 hours of treatment as compared to controls (95.4% versus 67.4%, $p < 0.0001$). Infarct growth was, however, also significantly larger in the IIT group (29.7 ml versus 10.8 ml, $p = 0.04$). There was no difference between the two groups in terms of functional outcome, mortality after 3 months and the occurrence of severe adverse events. Hypoglycemia defined as a blood glucose <3 mmol/l occurred only in the IIT group (5 patients, 5.7%; 8 episodes; all asymptomatic). When hypoglycemia was defined as a blood glucose of <3.6 mmol/l, the frequency of this event was 34.5% in the IIT group versus 1.1% in controls.

Although data on ischemic stroke and ICH patients in particular are scarce, in light of those results intensive insulin treatment cannot be recommended for the clinical routine.

REFERENCES

1. Stratton, R.J., M. Elia, Deprivation linked to malnutrition risk and mortality in hospital. *Br J Nutr*, 2006;**96**(5):870–6.
2. Martineau, J., *et al.*, Malnutrition determined by the patient-generated subjective global assessment is associated with poor outcomes in acute stroke patients. *Clin Nutr*, 2005;**24**(6):1073–7.
3. Davis, J.P., *et al.*, Impact of premorbid undernutrition on outcome in stroke patients. *Stroke*, 2004;**35**(8):1930–4.
4. FOOD-Trial-Collaboration, Poor nutritional status on admission predicts poor outcomes after stroke: observational data from the FOOD trial. *Stroke*, 2003;**34**(6):1450–6.
5. Davalos, A., *et al.*, Effect of malnutrition after acute stroke on clinical outcome. *Stroke*, 1996;**27**(6):1028–32.
6. Axelsson, K., *et al.*, Nutritional status in patients with acute stroke. *Acta Med Scand*, 1988;**224**(3):217–24.
7. Finestone, H.M., *et al.*, Prolonged length of stay and reduced functional improvement rate in malnourished stroke rehabilitation patients. *Arch Phys Med Rehabil*, 1996;**77**(4):340–5.
8. Perry, L., S. McLaren, An exploration of nutrition and eating disabilities in relation to quality of life at 6 months post-stroke. *Health Soc Care Community*, 2004;**12**(4):288–97.
9. Stratton, R.J., *et al.*, 'Malnutrition Universal Screening Tool' predicts mortality and length of hospital stay in acutely ill elderly. *Br J Nutr*, 2006;**95**(2):325–30.
10. Finestone, H.M., *et al.*, Measuring longitudinally the metabolic demands of stroke patients: resting energy expenditure is not elevated. *Stroke*, 2003;**34**(2):502–7.
11. Weekes, E., M. Elia, Resting energy expenditure and body composition following cerebro-vascular accident. *Clin Nutr*, 1992;**11**(1):18–22.
12. Chalela, J.A., *et al.*, Acute stroke patients are being underfed: a nitrogen balance study. *Neurocrit Care*, 2004;**1**(3):331–4.

13. Bardutzky, J., *et al.*, Energy demand in patients with stroke who are sedated and receiving mechanical ventilation. *J Neurosurg*, 2004;**100**(2):266–71.
14. Bruder, N., *et al.*, Influence of body temperature, with or without sedation, on energy expenditure in severe head-injured patients. *Crit Care Med*, 1998;**26**(3):568–72.
15. Moore, R., M.P. Najarian, C.W. Konvolinka, Measured energy expenditure in severe head trauma. *J Trauma*, 1989;**29**(12):1633–6.
16. Bardutzky, J., *et al.*, Energy expenditure in ischemic stroke patients treated with moderate hypothermia. *Intensive Care Med*, 2004;**30**(1):151–4.
17. Dennis, M.S., S.C. Lewis, C. Warlow, Routine oral nutritional supplementation for stroke patients in hospital (FOOD): a multicentre randomised controlled trial. *Lancet*, 2005;**365**(9461):755–63.
18. Gariballa, S.E., *et al.*, A randomized, controlled, single-blind trial of nutritional supplementation after acute stroke. *JPEN J Parenter Enteral Nutr*, 1998;**22**(5):315–19.
19. Williams, L.S., *et al.*, Effects of admission hyperglycemia on mortality and costs in acute ischemic stroke. *Neurology*, 2002;**59**(1):67–71.
20. Milne, A.C., A. Avenell, J. Potter, Oral protein and energy supplementation in older people: a systematic review of randomized trials. *Nestle Nutr Workshop Ser Clin Perform Programme*, 2005;**10**:103–20; discussion 120–5.
21. Stratton, R.J., *et al.*, Enteral nutritional support in prevention and treatment of pressure ulcers: a systematic review and meta-analysis. *Ageing Res Rev*, 2005;**4**(3):422–50.
22. Lewis, S.J., *et al.*, Early enteral feeding versus 'nil by mouth' after gastrointestinal surgery: systematic review and meta-analysis of controlled trials. *BMJ*, 2001;**323**(7316):773–6.
23. Marik, P. E., G. P. Zaloga, Early enteral nutrition in acutely ill patients: a systematic review. *Crit Care Med*, 2001;**29**(12):2264–70.
24. Blackmer, J., Tube feeding in stroke patients: a medical and ethical perspective. *Can J Neurol Sci*, 2001;**28**(2):101–6.
25. Dennis, M.S., S.C. Lewis, C. Warlow, Effect of timing and method of enteral tube feeding for dysphagic stroke patients (FOOD): a multicentre randomised controlled trial. *Lancet*, 2005;**365**(9461):764–72.
26. Singh, S., S. Hamdy, Dysphagia in stroke patients. *Postgrad Med J*, 2006;**82**(968):383–91.
27. Ekberg, O., *et al.*, Social and psychological burden of dysphagia: its impact on diagnosis and treatment. *Dysphagia*, 2002;**17**(2):139–46.
28. Smithard, D.G., *et al.*, The natural history of dysphagia following a stroke. *Dysphagia*, 1997;**12**(4):188–93.
29. Perry, L., C.P. Love, Screening for dysphagia and aspiration in acute stroke: a systematic review. *Dysphagia*, 2001;**16**(1):7–18.
30. Dziewas, R., *et al.*, Pneumonia in acute stroke patients fed by nasogastric tube. *J Neurol Neurosurg Psychiatry*, 2004;**75**(6):852–6.
31. Mamun, K., J. Lim, Role of nasogastric tube in preventing aspiration pneumonia in patients with dysphagia. *Singapore Med J*, 2005;**46**(11):627–31.
32. Nakajoh, K., *et al.*, Relation between incidence of pneumonia and protective reflexes in post-stroke patients with oral or tube feeding. *J Intern Med*, 2000;**247**(1):39–42.
33. Diener, H.C., N. Putzky, eds. *Leitlinien für Diagnostik und Therapie in der Neurologie*. 4th ed. 2008, Thieme: Stuttgart.
34. Moore, F.A., *et al.*, Early enteral feeding, compared with parenteral, reduces postoperative septic complications. The results of a meta-analysis. *Ann Surg*, 1992;**216**(2):172–83.
35. Nyswonger, G.D., R.H. Helmchen, Early enteral nutrition and length of stay in stroke patients. *J Neurosci Nurs*, 1992;**24**(4):220–3.
36. Heyland, D.K., *et al.*, Canadian clinical practice guidelines for nutrition support in mechanically ventilated, critically ill adult patients. *JPEN J Parenter Enteral Nutr*, 2003;**27**(5):355–73.
37. Kreymann, K.G., *et al.*, ESPEN Guidelines on enteral nutrition: intensive care. *Clin Nutr*, 2006;**25**(2):210–23.
38. Norton, B., *et al.*, A randomised prospective comparison of percutaneous endoscopic gastrostomy and nasogastric tube feeding after acute dysphagic stroke. *BMJ*, 1996;**312**(7022):13–16.
39. Braunschweig, C.L., *et al.*, Enteral compared with parenteral nutrition: a meta-analysis. *Am J Clin Nutr*, 2001;**74**(4):534–42.
40. Kostadima, E., *et al.*, Early gastrostomy reduces the rate of ventilator-associated pneumonia in stroke or head injury patients. *Eur Respir J*, 2005;**26**(1):106–11.
41. Jabbar, A., S.A. McClave, Pre-pyloric versus post-pyloric feeding. *Clin Nutr*, 2005;**24**(5):719–26.
42. Singer, P., *et al.*, ESPEN Guidelines on parenteral nutrition: intensive care. *Clin Nutr*, 2009;**28**(4):387–400.
43. Lipman, T.O., Grains or veins: is enteral nutrition really better than parenteral nutrition? A look at the evidence. *JPEN J Parenter Enteral Nutr*, 1998;**22**(3):167–82.
44. Casaer, M.P., *et al.*, Early versus late parenteral nutrition in critically ill adults. *N Engl J Med*, 2011;**365**(6):506–17.
45. Doig, G.S., *et al.*, Early parenteral nutrition in critically ill patients with short-term relative contraindications to early

enteral nutrition: a randomized controlled trial. *JAMA*, 2013;**309**(20):2130–8.

46. Beisel, W.R., History of nutritional immunology: introduction and overview. *J Nutr*, 1992;**122**(3 Suppl):591–6.
47. Marik, P.E., G.P. Zaloga, Immunonutrition in critically ill patients: a systematic review and analysis of the literature. *Intensive Care Med*, 2008;**34**(11):1980–90.
48. Fogelholm, R., *et al.*, Admission blood glucose and short term survival in primary intracerebral haemorrhage: a population based study. *J Neurol Neurosurg Psychiatry*, 2005;**76**(3):349–53.
49. Broderick, J., *et al.*, Guidelines for the management of spontaneous intracerebral hemorrhage in adults: 2007 update: a guideline from the American Heart Association/American Stroke Association Stroke Council, High Blood Pressure Research Council, and the Quality of Care and Outcomes in Research Interdisciplinary Working Group. *Stroke*, 2007; **38**(6):2001–23.
50. Finfer, S., *et al.*, Intensive versus conventional glucose control in critically ill patients. *N Engl J Med*, 2009;**360**(13):1283–97.
51. Finfer, S., *et al.*, Hypoglycemia and risk of death in critically ill patients. *N Engl J Med*, 2012;**367**(12):1108–18.
52. Oddo, M., *et al.*, Impact of tight glycemic control on cerebral glucose metabolism after severe brain injury: a microdialysis study. *Crit Care Med*, 2008;**36**(12):3233–8.
53. Rosso, C., *et al.*, Intensive versus subcutaneous insulin in patients with hyperacute stroke: results from the randomized INSULINFARCT trial. *Stroke*, 2012;**43**(9):2343–9.

21d

Management of infections in the ICH patient

Edgar Santos and Oliver W. Sakowitz

Description of the problem

The major focus in the treatment of intracerebral hemorrhage (ICH) is on the risk of neurological and cardiovascular deterioration due to mass effects of the clot per se, risk of recurrent or ongoing hemorrhage and the secondary cascades triggered thereby. Approximately 30% of patients with supratentorial ICH and most of the patients with cerebellar and brain stem hemorrhage require sustained critical care, including intubation, which complicates their outcome due to the associated higher risk of nosocomial infections (1,2). Additionally, there is a close relationship between the central nervous system and the immune system that appears to produce systemic suppression of both innate and adaptive immunity in stroke patients (3). As with other, non-hemorrhagic stroke patients their prognosis and final outcome is closely related to the incidence of infectious complications.

During the first 72 hours patients with ICH present with fever more frequently than patients with ischemic stroke. For example, Schwartz and co-workers reported that fever was present in 19% of the patients on admission, but occurred in 91% at least once during the first 72 hours after hospitalization. Fever correlated with worse outcome and with ventricular extension of the hemorrhage (4). Obviously febrile temperatures can have both infectious and non-infectious etiologies. A prompt diagnosis and treatment of infections reduces mortality and length of stay in the ICU (5), but an inappropriate antimicrobial therapy is associated with increased mortality and morbidity for many infectious diseases. It is an ongoing challenge to diagnose infections in ICU patients with a high sensitivity and specificity. A rational use of clinical symptoms, biomarkers, and the adjustment of techniques must be encouraged continuously.

Types of infection

Concomitant infections

Hospital-acquired pneumonia

The occurrence of bacterial pneumonia is associated with higher mortality rates, more severe neurological deficits, and longer hospitalizations (6,7). Nosocomial pneumonia has a reported incidence of 1.5% to 13.0% after acute stroke (8). Pneumonia can occur after aspiration secondary to dysphagia and reduced level of consciousness (9). Risk factors in ICH patients are age > 60 years, surgery, decrease in gastric pH, cardiopulmonary resuscitation, continuous sedation, re-intubation, presence of a nasogastric tube, reduced cough reflex, and immobilization (10). Prevention strategies are based on the general infection prevention principles applied to ICU patients. Hospital staff should be trained to follow the hygiene measures and isolation and cleaning principles. They should have expertise in identifying dysphagia.

Critical Care of the Stroke Patient, ed. Stefan Schwab, Daniel Hanley, and A. David Mendelow. Published by Cambridge University Press.

Oral feeding should be stopped if the patient is unable to swallow small amounts of water, and cannot cough by command. There is no 'gold-standard' for detecting dysphagia, but a simple protocol to explore lower cranial nerve function can be useful. Nasogastric or duodenal feeding reduces the risk of aspiration pneumonia. Percutaneous endoscopic gastrostomy (PEG) is recommended for long-term feeding, but early PEG catheter placement has no significant advantage over nasogastric feeding in preventing pneumonia (11). Other risk factors can be reduced by respiratory physiotherapy and mobilization.

According to the American Thoracic Society and Infectious Disease Society of America (12), a sputum culture from the lower respiratory tract should be collected in all patients before initiation of antimicrobial therapy, whereby empirical therapy should not be delayed in critically ill patients. Early, appropriate, broad-spectrum antimicrobial therapy that covers multidrug resistant (MDR) pathogens and uses agents that the patient has not recently received should be prescribed at adequate doses for all patients with suspected hospital acquired pneumonia. Changing to narrow spectrum or oral therapy should be considered once the results of cultures and the patient's clinical response are known. There is still much discussion on how the therapy should be guided (13), either by severity, time to clinical response, and the pathogenic organism or just the time to clinical response and not the pathogen involved. In the last case, patients should be treated for at least 72 hours after the clinical response. Clinical response usually takes 2–3 days; non-responding patients should be evaluated for extrapulmonary sites of infection, possible MDR pathogens, complications of pneumonia and its therapy (13).

Ventilator-associated pneumonia (VAP)

VAP is a consequence of intubation and 48 hours or more of positive pressure mechanical ventilation. This is related to decreased clearance of secretions, a dry open mouth, and microaspiration of secretions. Neuromuscular blockade is sometimes used in ICH patients. It is associated with a higher risk of pneumonia and sepsis (14). VAP occurs in 9–27% of all intubated patients with a mortality of up to 20% (10).

The use of antibiotics to prevent VAP is controversial, and the American Thoracic Society guidelines do not recommend antibiotic use without signs of infection. However, some studies have found that selective decontamination of the digestive system with oral or IV antibiotics may decrease the risk of VAP (15). Ventilator-related strategies are the use of non-invasive ventilation and fewer re-intubations, semi-recumbent positioning, continuous clearing of secretions, and hygiene precautions with ventilator use (10).

Urinary tract infections (UTI)

In the general medical population, the risk of contracting a UTI is 3–10% per day of catheterization, approaching 100% after 30 days (16). UTI do not seem to impact patient outcome as severely as other types of infections; nevertheless, it is of concern that hospitalized patients with stroke are at a particularly high risk of developing UTI. Urinary retention is very common in the acute phase of stroke patients requiring the use of urinary catheters. However, even non-catheterized patients have more than double the odds when compared with the general medical and surgical populations (17). Risk factors include the duration of urinary catheter use, female gender, obesity, length of stay in ICU, and poor cognitive function (10,18). Catheter-associated UTI is also the leading cause of secondary nosocomial bloodstream infections. Catheters should only be placed in patients with stroke who require them for strict monitoring of fluid status due to a concurrent medical condition or in those with acute bladder obstruction (19). Strategies to reduce the use of catheterization are likely to have more impact on the incidence of this type of infection than any other recommendation (20). The use of prophylactic antibiotics to prevent UTI after stroke is unclear (19).

A UTI is diagnosed in catheterized patients or in patients whose catheter has been removed within the previous 48 hours presenting with symptoms or signs compatible with a UTI with no other identified source of infection along with $\geq 10^3$ colony-forming units/ml of ≥ 1 bacterial species in a single catheter urine specimen

(19). Catheter-associated UTI are often polymicrobial and caused by MDR uropathogens, so urine cultures should be obtained prior to treatment to confirm that the empiric regimen provides appropriate coverage and the catheter should be replaced. Empirical antibiotic treatment should be based on the information available, including the urine gram stain, sensitivity of pathogens isolated in the same hospital, and previous urine culture results. In general, 7 days is the recommended duration of antibiotic treatment in those patients with a clinical response, and 10 to 14 days for those with a delayed response. The possibility of fungal infections (e.g. Candida species) should be considered in patients with no response. They represent 10–15% of nosocomial UTIs.

Bloodborne infection

Catheter-related sepsis. The use of central venous catheters is important for most ICH patients. The most important risk factors for infection are long-term catheter use, number of catheters, number of lumens, and the use of parenteral nutrition. Strategies for prevention start with considering the necessity of the catheter, the correct insertion technique, and constant evaluation of its necessity in order to remove the catheter as soon as possible. The use of prophylactic antibiotics is not recommended, with the exception of high-risk patients, for example, with a history of recurrent catheter-related infections and in patients with prosthetic heart valves (10).

Sepsis. In ICH patients, the treatment of both sepsis, defined as infection plus systemic manifestations of infection including systemic inflammatory response, enhanced coagulation, and impaired fibrinolysis, and septic shock, defined as sepsis-induced hypotension that is refractory to a fluid challenge, does not differ from that in other patients. The prompt timing and appropriateness of therapy are crucial for the outcome. For that reason it is important to detect the systemic inflammatory response syndrome (SIRS) early. SIRS is defined by the constellation of fever or hypothermia, tachycardia, tachypnea, and leukocytosis, leukopenia, or the presence of immature neutrophils. Sepsis is present in many patients during their stay in ICU, but its variability in presentations among patients makes it sometimes difficult to identify. There is still no single sensitive and specific test. Procalcitonin and C-reactive protein have been identified as potential diagnostic tools (21).

Among all ICU patients with sepsis, the best practical predictor of outcome is the number of organ systems with sepsis-induced dysfunction, adding 10–15% mortality rate per organ system (22).

An organized and methodological approach applied by trained physicians and nurses as soon as possible is believed to play a central role in reducing mortality and morbidity (cf. 'International guideline for management of severe sepsis and septic shock' is encouraged (23)).

Two blood cultures should be obtained from different sources, as well as other potential sites of infections before initiating antimicrobial therapy without delaying appropriate treatment. Empirical treatment should not be used for more than 3–5 days and treatment should be reviewed daily and adjusted as soon as the susceptibility profile is known. The total length of treatment is typically 7–10 days, but some exceptions are warranted in slow-response patients.

ICH-related infection

There are some special situations in which the etiology of ICH in itself is associated with a higher risk of infection due to hematological and/or immunological factors. See Table 21d.1 for details.

Immunosuppression in organ donor recipients carries a risk of systemic infections, thrombocytopenia and coagulopathies. Especially patients with either liver transplant rejection or marrow transplantation with

Table 21d.1 Etiologies of ICH associated with an increased risk for infections

Aplastic anemia
Drug abuse
Human immunodeficiency virus
Immunosuppression in liver and kidney recipients
Leukemias and leukemia treatment
Sickle cell disease
Systemic lupus erythematosus
Ulcerative colitis
Vasculitis secondary to CNS infectious disease

platelet counts less than 20000 are at a particularly high risk for ICH. From autopsy studies it has been estimated that more than 15% of patients with leukemia may have ICH (24). History of polycystic kidney disease in renal transplant recipients is also associated with a tenfold increase in the risk for ICH.

Aplastic anemia, a non-malignant hematologic disorder due to marrow failure, can present with neutropenia and thrombocytopenia, predisposing to hemorrhage and bacterial infections. Hemorrhage in acute leukemia is caused by hemorrhagic diathesis, including disseminated intravascular coagulation (DIC), thrombocytopenia, sepsis, leukocytosis, and treatment toxicity. Most patients with acute promyelocytic leukemia (APL) have evidence of DIC by the time of diagnosis. Patients with APL have a higher risk of death during induction therapy compared with patients with other forms of leukemia, most often due to bleeding. From 279 patients enrolled in the APL97 study conducted by the Japan Adult Leukemia Study Group, severe hemorrhage occurred in 18 patients (25). Some forms of leukemia such as chronic lymphocytic leukemia produce immunodeficiency in themselves, in addition to the therapy-related immunosuppression. Preventive strategies based on the degree of neutropenia and prophylactic antibiotics can be given together with the immunosuppressive therapy. Coagulopathy may be temporarily ameliorated by the infusion of platelets, fresh frozen plasma, and cryoprecipitate to cover procedures and decrease the risk of intracerebral hemorrhage (26).

Another situation that predisposes to both stroke, including ICH, and infections is sickle cell disease. The predisposition for infections stems from the impaired splenic function and diminished serum opsonizing activity. Neurological complications occur in more than 25% of the patients. Their relative risk of stroke is 200 to 400 times higher compared with patients without sickle cell disease (27).

Human immunodeficiency virus (HIV)-infected patients can present with intracerebral hemorrhage in the setting of immune-mediated thrombocytopenic purpura, primary cerebral lymphoma, metastatic Kaposi's sarcoma, and cerebral toxoplasmosis or hemophilia (28,29).

ICH can be caused by cerebral vasculitis associated with or secondary to other pathologies such as drug abuse, systemic lupus erythematosus, ulcerative colitis, pregnancy or postpartum period, in which the patient has higher risk of infections. In addition, there are infections such as tuberculosis, fungal infections, shingles, and cytomegalovirus infection that produce vasculitis, which can predispose to intracerebral bleeding requiring simultaneous treatment (30). There are some reported cases of ICH that were followed by intracerebral abscess, but it is not clear which occurred first, one of the possible explanations can be attributed to vasculitis (31,32).

Treatment-related infections

Several neurosurgical interventions have been suggested to address intracerebral hemorrhage and its direct sequelae (e.g. intraventricular extension, acute and chronic hydrocephalus). While the available evidence for their benefit will be addressed elsewhere in this volume, this chapter will highlight infection complications of these measures.

The most common infections secondary to neurosurgical interventions in order of likelihood are skin and soft tissue infections, meningitis, ventriculitis, cerebritis, brain abscess, subdural empyema, osteomyelitis, secondary systemic sepsis, endocarditis, and intra-abdominal abscess formation (5).

Meningitis, ventriculitis

External ventricle drainages are used very commonly in ICH patients and they are the gold-standard for measuring intracranial pressure (ICP). They are used as a temporary cerebrospinal fluid (CSF) drainage system in patients with hydrocephalus (e.g. obstructive hydrocephalus in ICH patients with intraventricular blood), and/or as a rapid therapeutic measure to drain CSD in patients with high ICP. ICP monitoring can also be accomplished using other techniques, including intraparenchymal fiberoptic catheters, subarachnoid bolts, epidural devices, and subdural catheters (33). They are very useful, but all of them bring a higher risk of bacterial colonization (up to 19% in intraventricular catheters) (34) and infection (rates from 0–27%) (14,35). Reported risk factors for infections in patients who have those devices include long-term monitoring, (for example, ventricular catheterization for more than 5 days), intracranial hypertension, irrigation of the system, CSF leaks, and concurrent non-CNS infections.

S. epidermidis, which occur in 70% of the cases of ventricular meningitis, *S. aureus*, Streptococci and gram-negative organisms are the most common agents in patients with ICP monitors and EVDs (5).

There is no evidence that changing catheters prophylactically at regular intervals would reduce the incidence of infection (5). The routine use of prophylactic antibiotics for ICP monitors and EVD is not warranted. It does not reduce the CNS infection rate and is associated with more resistant pathogens in subsequent infections (33,36). The use of antibiotic-coated EVDs or complete shunt systems is a promising new avenue, which has been adopted by many neurosurgeons as an option for patients at high risk of shunt infection. For a general recommendation of these products further exploration and testing is necessary.

For diagnosis in patients with ICH, who are frequently sedated, and in whom neurological exploration can be limited, the use of laboratory parameters plays an important role: CSF glucose, increased CSF protein, CSF pleocytosis and corrected cell number, CSF cultures, gram stains, and the clinical exam whenever possible (fever, signs of meningeal irritation, reduced level of consciousness, and photo- and phonophobia) (5). The use of CRP and procalcitonin can also be helpful in ascertaining a precise diagnosis (5,37).

The first-generation cephalosporin cefazolin is effective against all Staphylococci. Vancomycin can be a good alternative, especially when the patient is allergic to penicillin, but side effects should be considered.

Abscess and empyema

Brain abscess formation and empyema are rare complications in ICH patients. The same surgical principles as in other purulent infections can be applied. Prompt evacuation and asservation of specimens for further microbiologic work-up should be attempted whenever the suspicion of abscess or empyema occurs (as indicated by imaging studies or obvious clinical signs such as open purulent drainage). The route of surgical intervention has to be determined individually (stereotactic drainage or open surgery). Further treatment involves the identification of the causative organism and appropriate antibiotic administration. Postoperative abscesses are addressed with drainage, surgery, or both, as dictated by the clinical situation (38).

Prophylactic antibiotic treatment in non-immunocompromised patients with craniotomies and/or CSF diversion is controversial (39,40).

Treatment of infectious complications

Modifiable risk factors

The treatment of nosocomial infections starts with their prevention. A number of risk factors in the ICU are modifiable. Table 21d.2 summarizes these measures.

Patients with ICH are often critically ill and dependent. In these cases one has to constantly remind oneself

Table 21d.2 Modifiable risk factors in the ICU

Modifiable risk factors in the hospital environment (10)	Note
Air and water filtration systems	Caution should be taken in any ICU that plumbing, water, and air-filtration systems are monitored at regular intervals
Hand hygiene	Extremely cost-effective
Isolation measures	Gown and glove use may improve overall compliance with isolation precautions
Patient decolonization or prevention of colonization	Controversial
Patient room hygiene	Patient rooms may harbor significant pathogens long after the source patient was moved
Patient screening	Surveillance cultures to detect MRSA and VRE have shown significant success in decreasing the rate of colonization and infection with these organisms

of the potentially avoidable iatrogenic causes and spread of infections. Skin integrity is compromised by peripheral and central venous access devices, arterial lines as well as postoperative wounds; ventilator use predisposes to pneumonia. Underlying medical conditions may predispose patients to infectious complications, for example, immunosupressive therapy. Potentially modifiable risk factors are related to nutrition, health care personnel, and the hospital environment. Daily multidisciplinary rounds with discussion of the prevention protocols for mechanical ventilators, central lines, and urinary catheters, and periodic reminders of infection prevention policies can help reduce infection rates (10).

General principles of infection management

Appropriate cultures of the suspected source, ideally obtained before initiation of antibiotics, allow for future de-escalation of antibiotics, or the decision to discontinue antibiotics. A non-judicious plan and use of prophylactic antibiotics when unnecessary can increase pathogen resistance. Rationalization of antibiotic use plays an important role especially in the ICU, because infections with resistant pathogens are more frequent (41). Non-infectious possibilities should be considered and eliminated to avoid unnecessary treatment with antibiotics.

Antibiotic treatment

A full discussion on antibiotic selection and strategies is beyond the scope of this chapter. The suggested antibiotics shown in Table 21d.3 have been collected from contemporary sources; most importantly, every institution should develop standards and guidelines for infectious control according to the spectrum of

Table 21d.3 A summary of antibiotic strategies

Infection	Agent	Treatment
Pneumonia in patients at risk for infection with MDR pathogens (13)	*P. aeruginosa, K. pneumoniae, Acinetobacter* spp. and MRSA	Ideally two antibiotics are used. One of the following three options: Cefepime 2 g q12h or Ceftazidime 2 g q8h or Piperacillin/ Tazobactam 4.5 g q6h or Meropenem 1 g q8h or Imipenem 500 mg q6h, plus one of the following two options: Vancomycin 1 g q12h (15 mg/kg q12h) or Linezolid 600 mg q12h
Pneumonia with no known risk factors for MDR pathogens, and early onset (5 days) (13)	Antibiotic-sensitive, aerobic, enteric, gram-negative bacilli (*Enterobacter* spp., *E. coli, Klebsiella* spp., *Proteus* spp. and *Serratia marcescens*) community pathogens such as *Haemophilus influenzae* and *Streptococcus pneumoniae* and methicillin-sensitive *S. aureus*	Ideally two antibiotics are used. One of the following three options: Ceftriaxone 1 g q24h or Cefotaxine 2 g q8h or Ampicillin/ Sulbactam 3 g q6h, plus one of the following two options: Azithromycin 500 mg q24h or Levofloxacin 750 mg q24h. Optionally a quinolone monotherapy can be used: Moxifloxacin 400 mg q24h
Post OP meningitis (42)	Mainly *S. aureus, S. epidermidis*	Empirical therapy with Vancomycin 1 g q12h plus either Cefepime 2 g q12h or Ceftazidime 2 g q8h or Meropenem 1 g q8h. Prophylaxis with Cefazolin 1–2 g IV or Vancomycin 1 g IV
Sepsis (43)	Most likely pathogens depending on the suspected site of origin	If no origin is known: Piperacillin/ Tazobactam 4.5 g q6h or Meropenem 1–2 g q8h plus Vancomycin 1 g q12h plus Tobramycin 7 mg/kg q24h

Table 21d.3 (cont.)

Infection	Agent	Treatment
Shunt infections (44)	Mainly *S. aureus* and *S. epidermidis*, but also Gram-negative bacteria, *Streptococci*, *Diphtheroid*, anaerobes and mixed cultures	Empirical therapy similar to post OP meningitis
Skin and soft tissue (44)	*S. aureus*, *Streptococcus* spp, Gram-negatives, anaerobic species	Ceftriaxone 1 g q24h or Clindamycin 600 mg q6h plus Metronidazole 500 mg q8h or Ertapenem 1 g q24h or Ampicillin/ Sulbactam 3 g q6h or Moxifloxacin 400 mg q24h or Ciprofloxacin 400 mg q12h plus Metronidazole 500 mg q8h or Tigecycline monotherapy 50 mg q12h (after 100 mg loading dose) Any of the above (except Tigecycline) plus Vancomycin 1 g q12h (15 mg/kg q12h) or Linezolid 600 mg q12h
UTI patients with evidence of pyelonephritis or urosepsis (44)	Often polymicrobial	Gentamicin 2 mg/kg q12h plus broader spectrum antibiotics: Piperacillin/ Tazobactam 4.5 g q6h or Meropenem 1 g q8h or Imipenem 500 mg q6h or Ciprofloxacin 400 mg q12h or Levofloxacin 500 mg q24h or Ertapenem 1 g q24h or Ampicillin/Sulbactam 3 g q6h or Ceftriaxone 1 g q24h or Ampicillin 2 g q4h
UTI patients with mild-to-moderate illness without alterations in mental status or hemodynamic status (44)	Often polymicrobial	Urinary fluoroquinolone (Ciprofloxacin 250 mg PO q12h or Levofloxacin 250 mg PO q24h) Broad-spectrum Cephalosporin (Ceftriaxone 1 g q24h or Cefepime)
UTI with Gram stain gram-positive cocci in Gram stain (44)	Enterococci or staphylococci	Vancomycin 1 g q12h (15 mg/kg q12h)

infections occurring and the pathogens involved. Resistance patterns must be followed in order to avoid the increasing incidence of multidrug-resistant strains.

Summary

The most common infections in the ICU are pneumonia, urinary tract infections, blood stream infections, and sepsis (35,45,46). In ICH patients, general measures including fever control and prevention of aspiration pneumonia and bedsores are the same as for patients with ischemic stroke (47). In adults with acute stroke, the use of prophylactic antibiotics is controversial and does not seem to reduce mortality (48).

REFERENCES

1. Gujjar AR, Deibert E, Manno EM, Duff S, Diringer MN. Mechanical ventilation for ischemic stroke and intracerebral hemorrhage: indications, timing, and outcome. *Neurology*. 1998;**51**(2):447–51.
2. Ohwaki K, Yano E, Nagashima H, Nakagomi T, Tamura A. Impact of infection on length of intensive care unit stay after intracerebral hemorrhage. *Neurocrit Care*. 2008;**8**(2):271–5.

3. Offner H, Vandenbark AA, Hurn PD. Effect of experimental stroke on peripheral immunity: CNS ischemia induces profound immunosuppression. *Neuroscience.* 2009;**158**(3):1098–111.
4. Schwarz S, Häfner K, Aschoff A, Schwab S. Incidence and prognostic significance of fever following intracerebral hemorrhage. *Neurology.* 2000;**54**(2):354–61.
5. Beer R, Lackner P, Pfausler B, Schmutzhard E. Nosocomial ventriculitis and meningitis in neurocritical care patients. *J. Neurol.* 2008;**255**(11):1617–24.
6. Davenport RJ, Dennis MS, Wellwood I, Warlow CP. Complications after acute stroke. *Stroke.* 1996;**27**(3):415–20.
7. Johnston KC, Li JY, Lyden PD, *et al.* Medical and neurological complications of ischemic stroke: experience from the RANTTAS trial. RANTTAS Investigators. *Stroke.* 1998;**29**(2):447–53.
8. Roth EJ, Lovell L, Harvey RL, *et al.* Incidence of and risk factors for medical complications during stroke rehabilitation. *Stroke.* 2001;**32**(2):523–9.
9. Riquelme R, Torres A, El-Ebiary M, *et al.* Community-acquired pneumonia in the elderly: A multivariate analysis of risk and prognostic factors. *Am. J. Respir. Crit. Care Med.* 1996;**154**(5):1450–5.
10. Barsanti MC, Woeltje KF. Infection prevention in the intensive care unit. *Infect. Dis. Clin. North Am.* 2009;**23**(3):703–25.
11. Dennis MS, Lewis SC, Warlow C. Effect of timing and method of enteral tube feeding for dysphagic stroke patients (FOOD): a multicentre randomised controlled trial. *Lancet.* 2005;**365**(9461):764–72.
12. Levy MM, Baylor MS, Bernard GR, *et al.* Clinical issues and research in respiratory failure from severe acute respiratory syndrome. *Am. J. Respir. Crit. Care Med.* 2005;**171**(5):518–26.
13. Carey W, Cleveland Clinic Foundation. *Current clinical medicine.* Premium ed. Philadelphia PA: Saunders/Elsevier; 2009.
14. Broderick J, Connolly S, Feldmann E, *et al.* Guidelines for the management of spontaneous intracerebral hemorrhage in adults: 2007 update: a guideline from the American Heart Association/American Stroke Association Stroke Council, High Blood Pressure Research Council, and the Quality of Care and Outcomes in Research Interdisciplinary Working Group. *Circulation.* 2007;**116**(16):e391–413.
15. Liberati A, D'Amico R, Pifferi, Torri V, Brazzi L. Antibiotic prophylaxis to reduce respiratory tract infections and mortality in adults receiving intensive care. *Cochrane Database Syst. Rev.* 2004;(**1**):CD000022.
16. Gould CV, Umscheid CA, Agarwal RK, Kuntz G, Pegues DA. Guideline for prevention of catheter-associated urinary tract infections 2009. *Infect. Control Hosp. Epidemiol.* 2010;**31**(4):319–26.
17. Ersoz M, Ulusoy H, Oktar MA, Akyuz M. Urinary tract infection and bacteriurua in stroke patients. *Am. J. Phys. Med. Rehabil.* 2007;**86**(9):734–41.
18. Stott D, Falconer A, Miller H, Tilston J, Langhorne P. Urinary tract infection after stroke. *QJM.* 2009;**102**(4):243–9.
19. Poisson SN, Johnston SC, Josephson SA. Urinary tract infections complicating stroke: mechanisms, consequences, and possible solutions. *Stroke.* 2010;**41**(4):e180–e184.
20. Hooton TM, Bradley SF, Cardenas DD, *et al.* Diagnosis, prevention, and treatment of catheter-associated urinary tract infection in adults: 2009 International Clinical Practice Guidelines from the Infectious Diseases Society of America. *Clin. Infect. Dis.* 2010;**50**(5):625–63.
21. Martin JB, Wheeler AP. Approach to the patient with sepsis. *Clin. Chest Med.* 2009;**30**(1):1–16, vii.
22. Martin GS, Mannino DM, Eaton S, Moss M. The epidemiology of sepsis in the United States from 1979 through 2000. *N. Engl. J. Med.* 2003;**348**(16):1546–54.
23. Dellinger RP, Levy MM, Carlet JM, *et al.* Surviving Sepsis Campaign: international guidelines for management of severe sepsis and septic shock: 2008. *Crit. Care Med.* 2008;**36**(1):296–327.
24. Graus F, Rogers LR, Posner JB. Cerebrovascular complications in patients with cancer. *Medicine* (Baltimore). 1985;**64**(1):16–35.
25. Yanada M, Matsushita T, Asou N, *et al.* Severe hemorrhagic complications during remission induction therapy for acute promyelocytic leukemia: incidence, risk factors, and influence on outcome. *Eur. J. Haematol.* 2007;**78**(3):213–19.
26. Zivković SA, Abdel-Hamid H. Neurologic manifestations of transplant complications. *Neurol Clin.* 2010;**28**(1):235–51.
27. Hoffman R. *Hematology: basic principles and practice.* Philadelphia, PA: Churchill Livingstone; 2005.
28. Bradley W. *Neurology in clinical practice.* Boston: Butterworth-Heinemann; 2000.
29. Castrillero EC. Intracranial hematoma in a patient with AIDS. *CMAJ.* 2005;**172**(10):1297.
30. Jain R, Deveikis J, Hickenbottom S, Mukherji SK. Varicella-zoster vasculitis presenting with intracranial hemorrhage. *AJNR Am. J. Neuroradiol.* 2003;**24**(5):971–4.
31. Dashti SR, Baharvahdat H, Sauvageau E, *et al.* Brain abscess formation at the site of intracerebral hemorrhage

secondary to central nervous system vasculitis. *Neurosurg. FOCUS*. 2008 6;**24**(6):E12.

32. Thomas SG, Moorthy RK, Rajshekhar V. Brain abscess in a non-penetrating traumatic intracerebral hematoma: case report and review of literature. *Neurol. India*. 2009;**57**(1):73–5.
33. Prabhu V, Kaufman H, Voelker J, *et al.* Prophylactic antibiotics with intracranial pressure monitors and external ventricular drains: a review of the evidence. *Surg. Neurol.* 1999;**52**(3):226–37.
34. Lozier AP, Sciacca RR, Romagnoli MF, Connolly ES. Ventriculostomy-related infections: a critical review of the literature. *Neurosurgery*. 2002;**51**(1):170–81; discussion 181–2.
35. Pinto AN, Melo TP, Lourenço ME, *et al.* Can a clinical classification of stroke predict complications and treatments during hospitalization? *Cerebrovasc. Dis.* 1998;**8**(4):204–9.
36. Stoikes NF, Magnotti LJ, Hodges TM, *et al.* Impact of intracranial pressure monitor prophylaxis on central nervous system infections and bacterial multi-drug resistance. *Surg. Infect. (Larchmt)*. 2008;**9**(5):503–8.
37. Diedler J, Sykora M, Hahn P, *et al.* C-reactive-protein levels associated with infection predict short- and long-term outcome after supratentorial intracerebral hemorrhage. *Cerebrovasc. Dis.* 2009;**27**(3):272–9.
38. Dashti SR, Baharvahdat H, Spetzler RF, *et al.* Operative intracranial infection following craniotomy. *Neurosurg. FOCUS*. 2008 6;**24**(6):E10.
39. Barker FG. Efficacy of prophylactic antibiotics against meningitis after craniotomy: a meta-analysis. *Neurosurgery*. 2007;**60**(5):887–94.
40. Korinek A, Baugnon T, Golmard J, *et al.* Risk factors for adult nosocomial meningitis after craniotomy: role of antibiotic prophylaxis. *Neurosurgery*. 2008;**62** Suppl 2: 532–9.
41. Eggimann P. Infection Control in the ICU. *Chest*. 2001;**120** (6):2059–93.
42. Townsend C. *Sabiston textbook of surgery: the biological basis of modern surgical practice*. Philadelphia: Saunders; 2004.
43. Bope E. *Conn's current therapy 2010*. Philadelphia, PA; London: Saunders; 2010.
44. Mandell G. *Mandell, Douglas, and Bennett's principles and practice of infectious diseases*. Philadelphia, PA: Churchill Livingstone/Elsevier; 2010.
45. Dettenkofer M, Ebner W, Els T, *et al.* Surveillance of nosocomial infections in a neurology intensive care unit. *J. Neurol.* 2001;**248**(11):959–64.
46. Chevret S, Hemmer M, Carlet J, Langer M. Incidence and risk factors of pneumonia acquired in intensive care units. Results from a multicenter prospective study on 996 patients. European Cooperative Group on Nosocomial Pneumonia. *Intensive Care Med.* 1993;**19**(5):256–64.
47. Elliott J, Smith M. The acute management of intracerebral hemorrhage: a clinical review. *Anesth. Analg.* 2010;**110** (5):1419–27.
48. van de Beek D, Wijdicks EFM, Vermeij FH, *et al.* Preventive antibiotics for infections in acute stroke: a systematic review and meta-analysis. *Arch. Neurol.* 2009;**66** (9):1076–81.

Management of cerebral edema in the ICH patient

Neeraj S. Naval and J. Ricardo Carhuapoma

Introduction

Intracerebral hemorrhage (ICH) remains a devastating form of stroke. Our understanding of the physiopathology of processes triggered by this disease has improved significantly over the last decade. Nevertheless, effective interventions that are capable of modifying the natural history of the initial and the secondary injury on brain tissue triggered by the hemorrhage are still lacking. Cerebral edema following ICH has received significant attention as a form of secondary neuronal damage. As we begin to better understand the natural history of this form of edema, interventions with potential to ameliorate its burden on these stroke victims are starting to be identified. However, likely due to its close interrelation to the original hematoma volume, its independent effect on neurological function and recovery following ICH is uncertain at best.

Pathophysiology

Biological events occurring in the periphery of the hematoma following ICH have been the subject of controversy for some years. Initial animal experiments using different models of ICH documented the presence of a rim of ischemia and, in some cases, infarction surrounding the hematoma (1–8). These experiments led to the widely accepted notion of perihematoma cerebral ischemia and they became the rationale for a liberal approach to acute blood pressure control in such stroke patients. Subsequent cerebral blood flow and metabolism studies as well as MRI clinical investigations demonstrated that such perihematoma ischemic condition was far from universal (9–12). Furthermore, these studies demonstrated indirect evidence of perihematoma vasogenic edema, perhaps the result of inflammation, leading to reduced neuronal metabolism. A series of experimental studies have since provided more evidence supporting inflammation as an important component in the process of perihematoma edema development. Microglia and neutrophil infiltration as well as TNF-alpha, IL-1, and free radicals seem to mediate this process (13–18). The expression of these processes also coincides chronologically with the early phases of edema up to its peak. Investigations on the natural history of this form of cerebral edema seem also to suggest that a peak in perihematoma edema volume as large as two to three times the original hematoma volume is reached at approximately 5 days from stroke onset (19–21).

Management

The management of edema in ICH will depend on the clinical effect it has on the neurological condition of the patient. Small hemorrhages with minimal perihematoma edema will likely not require specific interventions to control edema, whereas larger hemorrhages

Critical Care of the Stroke Patient, ed. Stefan Schwab, Daniel Hanley, and A. David Mendelow. Published by Cambridge University Press.

will induce more significant edema volumes leading to intracranial hypertension. This patient group requires a stepwise approach to cerebral edema and elevated ICP. Available treatments include the management of cerebral edema as well as the management of sustained intracranial hypertension due to ICH and perihematomal edema.

Lastly, as it is becoming more evident from studies testing modalities to safely remove parenchymal clots, the ultimate treatment to prevent cerebral edema seems to be minimizing the exposure of brain tissue to blood and its degradation products at the earliest step possible of the disease process.

Emergency management

Acute clinical deterioration that is the result of worsening cerebral edema may present as reduced level of consciousness or signs of cerebral herniation. Prompt implementation of acute interventions in these patients can be life saving and provide the treating team with a time window to institute more long-standing treatments.

Hyperventilation

Intubation and mechanical ventilation is always recommended in instances of acute neurological injury leading to reduced level of consciousness (GCS = or < 8). In addition to the obvious benefits of guaranteeing proper oxygenation, ventilation, and airway protection, hypoxia and hypercarbia can lead to cerebral vasodilation followed by increased cerebral blood volume and further ICP elevation. Hyperventilation to a $PaCO_2$ range of 25–35 mmHg will cause enough vasoconstriction to reduce CBV and ICP for a limited period of time, allowing more permanent therapies to be instituted. It is important to mention that such manipulation of physiological reflexes occurs primarily in viable brain tissue ipsi- and contralateral to the hematoma. Sustained hyperventilation is not only not beneficial but detrimental.

Osmotic therapy

Osmotic therapy aims to create an osmotic gradient between the intracellular/extracellular and intravascular compartments of the brain to shift water between these compartments. The extent to which osmotically active particles remain in the intravascular space is quantified using the reflection coefficient where 1 represents complete impermeability and 0 represents free permeability.

Mannitol: Mannitol is administered at a dose of 1 mg/kg on an as needed basis. Its reflection coefficient is 0.9 and is routinely used in any form of cerebral edema. Traditionally, a serum osmolarity of 310–315 mmol/l is considered therapeutic, although no controlled trials have ever demonstrated this in an objective and systematic manner. The use of mannitol pre-emptively in the absence of intracranial hypertension has not been associated with reduction of mortality or any improvement in functional outcomes (22). Data suggesting the preferential effect of mannitol on the non-infarcted hemisphere in the setting of ischemic stroke raise the concern that multiple doses of mannitol over a prolonged period of time may lead to a reversal of osmotic gradient and potentially worsen brain edema when the blood–brain barrier has been disrupted; alternatively rebound edema is a concern as well while weaning hyperosmolar therapy (23).

23.4% sodium chloride: The use of 23.4% saline has been tested in several studies as an alternative for life-threatening edema and ICP elevation (24,25). Although not tailored to a specific form of cerebral edema, refractory ICP has been shown to respond to this therapy. The ICP reducing effect of 23.4% HTS remains unclear, although hypotheses include rheological effects of this agent facilitating CBF to tissue at risk. It is interesting that the effect on ICP of this agent does not seem to be closely associated to acute elevations in the serum Na concentration, as Qureshi demonstrated (26–28).

Hypertonic saline solutions: Solutions containing 2% and 3% sodium chloride/acetate can be used to allow water translocation into the intravascular space (26–29). The reflection coefficient of Na is 1.0, thus acting as the ‘ideal’ osmotic agent. Continuous infusions of hypertonic saline maintaining a serum Na target of 145–155 mEq/l can be utilized until cerebral edema improves. Clinical trials conducted across a heterogeneous population of brain injured patients (TBI, ICH, SAH, etc.) suggest greater efficacy with equiosmolar doses of hypertonic saline compared to mannitol with greater likelihood of reducing ICP < 20 within an hour of administration and a greater mean decrease in ICP. Whether this benefit with hypertonic saline translates into a difference in clinical outcomes requires further investigation (30). More recent studies have proven that the use of hypertonic saline has been associated with a significant increase in brain oxygenation, and improved cerebral and systemic hemodynamics compared to mannitol (31).

Reported complications of a hypernatremic, hypervolemic hyperosmolar state are several and include hypokalemia, hyperchloremic metabolic acidosis, subdural hematoma, and coagulopathy.

Surgical evacuation

Several systematic attempts to address the efficacy of favorably modifying outcomes with open craniotomy and hematoma evacuation have been conducted. Different methodologies in these clinical trials make generalizations difficult; however, evidence of uniform positive impact following surgical intervention is lacking (32–34). Alternatives to open craniotomy will therefore be discussed in the following sections.

Hemicraniectomy

While well studied in the setting of ischemic stroke, with a meta-analysis of three randomized clinical trials showing a statistically significant benefit of early (< 48 h) hemicraniectomy, this intervention has not been studied in a well-designed clinical trial in the setting of hemorrhagic stroke. In an analysis of 12 patients, hemicraniectomy was life saving in over 90% of patients that survived to discharge, with over 50% of the survivors having a good functional outcome on outpatient follow-up (35). Of note, half the patients with ICH volume > 60 cc exhibited a good functional outcome. Another analysis of 23 patients that underwent hemicraniectomy with durotomy for putaminal ICH (2), only three of whom did so on an emergent basis secondary to clinical signs of cerebral herniation, showed an association with a hospital mortality of only 13% with good 3-month functional outcomes in 65% of the survivors (35). Patients with ICH volume < 30 cc were more likely to have a good outcome compared to patients with larger ICH. This may suggest some potential benefit of early hemicraniectomy in the setting of ICH but identification of the patient population that would benefit from this procedure based on age, admission GCS, ICH volume and clot location, and analyzing the optimal timing for the procedure warrants further investigation.

Hematoma removal using minimally invasive techniques

Clot evacuation combining the use of fibrinolysis with clot aspiration has emerged as a promising surgical modality in the acute care of ICH. Clinical trials testing this technique are generating increased interest, particularly given the failure of open evacuation to achieve outcomes superior to medical management. A recently published study by Miller and colleagues using frameless stereotactic aspiration of deep ICHs, followed by local tPA, suggested that this procedure was safe and linked to improved neurologic outcomes, and without increase in the perihematomal edema as reported by these investigators (36). Barrett *et al.* (37) and Carhuapoma *et al.* (38) found similar results when studying the interaction between hemorrhage volume and perihematomal edema in a convenient cohort of ICH patients using thrombolysis and MIS. A meta-analysis conducted by Zhou and coworkers suggests that patients with ICH may benefit more from MIS than other treatment options, particularly if they are between 30 and 80 years of age, with a superficial hematoma, GCS equal to or greater than 9, hematoma volume 25–40 cc, and treated within 72 hours from ictus (39).

More recently, as a result of the Minimally Invasive Surgery in the Treatment of Intracerebral Hemorrhage Evacuation (MISTIE) clinical trial, more evidence supporting the impact of hematoma removal on perihematomal edema has been obtained (40). MISTIE II is a prospective randomized controlled trial testing the safety of tPA thrombolysis and MIS in the treatment of ICH. Early results from this trial demonstrate a significant and graded effect of hematoma removal on edema volume at the end of treatment, such as it was suggested by previous investigators in early case control reports (unpublished data).

Conclusions

Targeted treatment of cerebral edema following ICH remains elusive. Current available therapies are nonspecific and have not evolved significantly over the last two decades. There is a need for studies assessing the natural history of this form of edema as well as its physiopathology as it evolves in the acute setting of this disease. Also, a better understanding of the independent influence of this form of edema on the survival and neurological outcome of these strokes victims is needed to properly test future therapies. MISTIE and other clinical trials are providing information that will lead to a better understanding of perihematomal edema. Such knowledge should be utilized for the design and execution of future clinical trials for the treatment of this form of cerebral edema.

REFERENCES

1. Ropper AH, Zervas NT. Cerebral blood flow after experimental basal ganglia hemorrhage. *Ann Neurol.* 1982;**11**(3):266–71.
2. Nath FP, Jenkins A, Mendelow AD, Graham DI, Teasdale GM. Early hemodynamic changes in experimental intracerebral hemorrhage. *J Neurosurg.* 1986;**65**(5):697–703.
3. Sinar EJ, Mendelow AD, Graham DI, Teasdale GM. Experimental intracerebral hemorrhage: effects of a temporary mass lesion. *J Neurosurg.* 1987;**66**(4):568–76.
4. Kingman TA, Mendelow AD, Graham DI, Teasdale GM. Experimental intracerebral mass: description of model, intracranial pressure changes and neuropathology. *J Neuropathol Exp Neurol.* 1988;**47**(2):128–37.
5. Bullock R, Brock-Utne J, vanDellen J, Blake G. Intracerebral hemorrhage in a primate model: effect on regional cerebral blood flow. *Surg Neurol.* 1988;**29**(2):101–7.
6. Nehls DG, Mendelow AD, Graham DI, Sinar EJ, Teasdale GM. Experimental intracerebral hemorrhage: progression of hemodynamic changes after production of a spontaneous mass lesion. *Neurosurgery.* 1988;**23**(4):439–44.
7. Nehls DG, Mendelow DA, Graham DI, Teasdale GM. Experimental intracerebral hemorrhage: early removal of a spontaneous mass lesion improves late outcome. *Neurosurgery.* 1990;**27**(5):674–82, discussion 682.
8. Yang GY, Betz AL, Chenevert TL, Brunberg JA, Hoff JT. Experimental intracerebral hemorrhage: relationship between brain edema, blood flow, and blood-brain barrier permeability in rats. *J Neurosurg.* 1994;**81**(1):93–102.
9. Carhuapoma JR, Wang PY, Beauchamp NJ, *et al.* Diffusion-weighted MRI and proton MR spectroscopic imaging in the study of secondary neuronal injury after intracerebral hemorrhage. *Stroke.* 2000;**31**(3):726–32.
10. Zazulia AR, Diringer MN, Videen TO, *et al.* Hypoperfusion without ischemia surrounding acute intracerebral hemorrhage. *J Cereb Blood Flow Metab.* 2001;**21**(7):804–10.
11. Mayer SA, Lignelli A, Fink ME, *et al.* Perilesional blood flow and edema formation in acute intracerebral hemorrhage: a SPECT study. *Stroke.* 1998;**29**(9):1791–8.
12. Kidwell CS, Saver JL, Mattiello J, *et al.* Diffusion-perfusion MR evaluation of perihematomal injury in hyperacute intracerebral hemorrhage. *Neurology.* 2001;**57**(9):1611–17.
13. Castillo J, Dávalos A, Alvarez-Sabín J, *et al.* Molecular signatures of brain injury after intracerebral hemorrhage. *Neurology.* 2002;**58**(4):624–9.
14. Leira R, Dávalos A, Silva Y, *et al.* Early neurologic deterioration in intracerebral hemorrhage: predictors and associated factors. *Neurology.* 2004;**63**(3):461–7.
15. Silva Y, Leira R, Tejada J, *et al.* Molecular signatures of vascular injury are associated with early growth of intracerebral hemorrhage. *Stroke.* 2005;**36**(1):86–91.
16. Xi G, Hua Y, Keep RF, Younger JG, Hoff JT. Systemic complement depletion diminishes perihematomal brain edema in rats. *Stroke.* 2001;**32**(1):162–7.
17. Peeling J, Yan HJ, Corbett D, Xue M, Del Bigio MR. Effect of FK-506 on inflammation and behavioral outcome following intracerebral hemorrhage in rats. *Exp Neurol.* 2001;**167**(2):341–7.
18. Masada T, Hua Y, Xi G, *et al.* Attenuation of intracerebral hemorrhage and thrombin-induced brain edema by overexpression of interleukin-1 receptor antagonist. *J Neurosurg.* 2001;**95**(4):680–6.
19. Olivot JM, Mlynash M, Kleinman JT, *et al.* MRI profile of the perihematomal region in acute intracerebral hemorrhage. *Stroke.* 2010;**41**(11):2681–3.
20. Venkatasubramanian C, Mlynash M, Finley-Caulfield A, *et al.* Natural history of perihematomal edema after

intracerebral hemorrhage measured by serial magnetic resonance imaging. *Stroke*. 2010;**42**(1):73–80.

21. Carhuapoma JR, Hanley DF, Banerjee M, Beauchamp NJ. Brain edema after human cerebral hemorrhage: a magnetic resonance imaging volumetric analysis. *J Neurosurg Anesthesiol*. 2003;**15**(3):230–3.
22. Misra UK, Kalita J, Ranjan P, Mandal SK. Mannitol in intracerebral hemorrhage: a randomized controlled study. *J Neurol Sci*. 2005;**234**(1–2):41–5.
23. Videen TO, Zazulia AR, Manno EM, *et al*. Mannitol bolus preferentially shrinks non-infarcted brain in patients with ischemic stroke. *Neurology*. 2001;**57**(11):2120–2.
24. Koenig MA, Bryan M, Lewin JL, *et al*. Reversal of transtentorial herniation with hypertonic saline. *Neurology*. 2008;**70**(13):1023–9.
25. Nakagawa K, Chang CWJ, Koenig MA, Yu M, Tokumaru S. Treatment of refractory intracranial hypertension with 23.4% saline in children with severe traumatic brain injury. *J Clin Anesth*. 2012;**24**(4):318–23.
26. Qureshi AI, Suarez JI, Bhardwaj A. Malignant cerebral edema in patients with hypertensive intracerebral hemorrhage associated with hypertonic saline infusion: a rebound phenomenon? *J Neurosurg Anesthesiol*. 1998;**10**(3):188–92.
27. Qureshi AI, Wilson DA, Traystman RJ. Treatment of elevated intracranial pressure in experimental intracerebral hemorrhage: comparison between mannitol and hypertonic saline. *Neurosurgery*. 1999;**44**(5):1055–63, discussion 1063–4.
28. Qureshi AI, Suarez JI. Use of hypertonic saline solutions in treatment of cerebral edema and intracranial hypertension. *Crit Care Med*. 2000;**28**(9):3301–13.
29. Suarez JI, Qureshi AI, Parekh PD, *et al*. Administration of hypertonic (3%) sodium chloride/acetate in hyponatremic patients with symptomatic vasospasm following subarachnoid hemorrhage. *J Neurosurg Anesthesiol*. 1999;**11**(3):178–84.
30. Kamel H, Navi BB, Nakagawa K, Hemphill JC, Ko NU. Hypertonic saline versus mannitol for the treatment of elevated intracranial pressure: a meta-analysis of randomized clinical trials. *Crit Care Med*. 2011;**39**(3):554–9.
31. Oddo M, Levine JM, Frangos S, *et al*. Effect of mannitol and hypertonic saline on cerebral oxygenation in patients with severe traumatic brain injury and refractory intracranial hypertension. *J Neurol Neurosurg Psychiatr*. 2009;**80**(8):916–20.
32. Fayad PB, Awad IA. Surgery for intracerebral hemorrhage. *Neurology*. 1998;**51**(3 Suppl 3):S69–73.
33. Prasad K, Mendelow AD, Gregson B. Surgery for primary supratentorial intracerebral haemorrhage. *Cochrane Database Syst Rev*. 2008;(**4**):CD000200.
34. Mitchell P, Gregson BA, Vindlacheruvu RR, Mendelow AD. Surgical options in ICH including decompressive craniectomy. *J Neurol Sci*. 2007;**261**(1–2):89–98.
35. Murthy JMK, Chowdary GVS, Murthy TVR K, Bhasha PSA, Naryanan TJ. Decompressive craniectomy with clot evacuation in large hemispheric hypertensive intracerebral hemorrhage. *Neurocrit Care*. 2005;**2**(3):258–62.
36. Miller CM, Vespa PM, McArthur DL, Hirt D, Etchepare M. Frameless stereotactic aspiration and thrombolysis of deep intracerebral hemorrhage is associated with reduced levels of extracellular cerebral glutamate and unchanged lactate pyruvate ratios. *Neurocrit Care*. 2007;**6**(1):22–9.
37. Barrett RJ, Hussain R, Coplin WM, *et al*. Frameless stereotactic aspiration and thrombolysis of spontaneous intracerebral hemorrhage. *Neurocrit Care*. 2005;**3**(3):237–45.
38. Carhuapoma JR, Barrett RJ, Keyl PM, Hanley DF, Johnson RR. Stereotactic aspiration-thrombolysis of intracerebral hemorrhage and its impact on perihematoma brain edema. *Neurocrit Care*. 2008;**8**(3):322–9.
39. Zhou X, Chen J, Li Q, *et al*. Minimally invasive surgery for spontaneous supratentorial intracerebral hemorrhage: A meta-analysis of randomized controlled trials. *Stroke*. 2012 Sep 18.
40. Dey M, Stadnik A, Awad IA. Thrombolytic evacuation of intracerebral and intraventricular hemorrhage. *Curr Cardiol Rep*. 2012 Sep 4.

22a

Surgery for spontaneous intracerebral hemorrhage

A. David Mendelow, Barbara A. Gregson, and Patrick Mitchell

Intracerebral hemorrhage (ICH) is not a homogeneous condition and neither is its response to surgical removal. In some situations surgical removal is clearly indicated. Early presentation and hemorrhage in relatively non-eloquent areas that compromise function in other areas via mass effect argue for surgical removal. Post-operative hematomas that inevitably follow about 3% (61/1806) of craniotomies (1) present early and, when significant, are removed. Hematomas that expand while the patient is on the neurosurgical ward are another example of an acute presentation (of expansion) and are commonly removed. Early intervention may save brain in the penumbra of functionally impaired but potentially viable tissue that surrounds the clot immediately following the ictus. Cerebellar hematomas are inclined to cause secondary hydrocephalus which, where significant, is treated. The clot in the cerebellum may compromise brain stem function via mass effect which is also commonly treated by surgical removal.

Late presentation and hemorrhages in the thalamus or brain stem argue for non-surgical treatments.

In practice most cases lie between these extremes. For them simple mechanistic arguments or personal observations do not adequately inform surgical decision making. There have been many attempts to discover whether surgical evacuation of the majority of intracerebral hemorrhages is beneficial or not. The results of this effort have been mixed, an important exception being for aneurysmal ICH which the Heiskanen prospective randomized controlled trial (2) showed to be better treated surgically.

There are also technical considerations: deep seated and basal ganglia hematomas are difficult to access via craniotomy and lend themselves to minimal intervention techniques. By contrast, superficial hematomas (particularly those reaching the cortical surface) are accessed easily by craniotomy that allows more direct hemostasis than do minimal access techniques.

More than a dozen prospective randomized controlled trials have been performed for supratentorial non-aneurysmal ICH, and several are ongoing both for spontaneous and traumatic ICH. These have helped to narrow down the clinical and radiological criteria that will select appropriate patients for surgery and improve their outcome. There can be little reliance on intuitive reasoning because so few patients do well on the one hand. Also, on the other, the 'treatment limiting decision', made in many hospitals, becomes a self-fulfilling prophesy (3) that inevitably leads to mortality. Many patients therefore die because of the withdrawal of treatment. Intuitive reasoning may therefore be misleading with supratentorial ICH.

In the first Surgical Trial in Intracerebral Haemorrhage (STICH) (4) 1033 patients from 87 centers around the world were randomized to early surgery or initial conservative treatment within 72 hours of ictus. These were patients with supratentorial

Critical Care of the Stroke Patient, ed. Stefan Schwab, Daniel Hanley, and A. David Mendelow. Published by Cambridge University Press.

spontaneous ICH who were operated upon within 24 hours of randomization. Standardized clinical trial methodology was used in a parallel group design with intention-to-treat analysis. A prognosis-based eight point Glasgow Outcome Scale by postal questionnaire at 6 months was used as the primary outcome measure. The result was a non-significant trend towards benefit from surgery with favorable outcomes in 26% of 468 patients randomized to early surgery and in 24% of 496 randomized to initial conservative treatment.

The STICH II trial randomized 601 patients with lobar supratentorial spontaneous hematomas to early surgery (within 48 hours of ictus) or initial conservative treatment (5). One hundred and seventy four (59%) of 297 patients in the early surgery group had an unfavorable outcome versus 178 (62%) of 286 patients in the initial conservative treatment group (absolute difference 3.7% [95% CI 4.3–11.6], odds ratio 0.86 [0.62–1.20]; p = 0.367). Patients with a Glasgow Coma Score of between 9 and 12 responded best to early surgery although this group of patients represents only a small percentage of all patients with ICH.

These findings are presented, with those of the other 15 published trials, in meta-analysis in Figure 22a.1. Overall there appears to be a marginal advantage to surgery with the odds of death and disability reduced (odds ratio 0.74 (95% CI 0.64–0.86)). This meta-analysis represents the summation of the results from 3367 patients that have been randomized over the period of the last half a century. The simple interpretation of these results is that for the type of cases enrolled in the trials, surgery is marginally beneficial, but we believe this to be inappropriately reductive.

Subgroup analysis

Patients enrolled in these trials had heterogeneous ICHs. Data suggest that the overall result may represent the average of some groups with significant benefit from surgery and some with harm. A number of

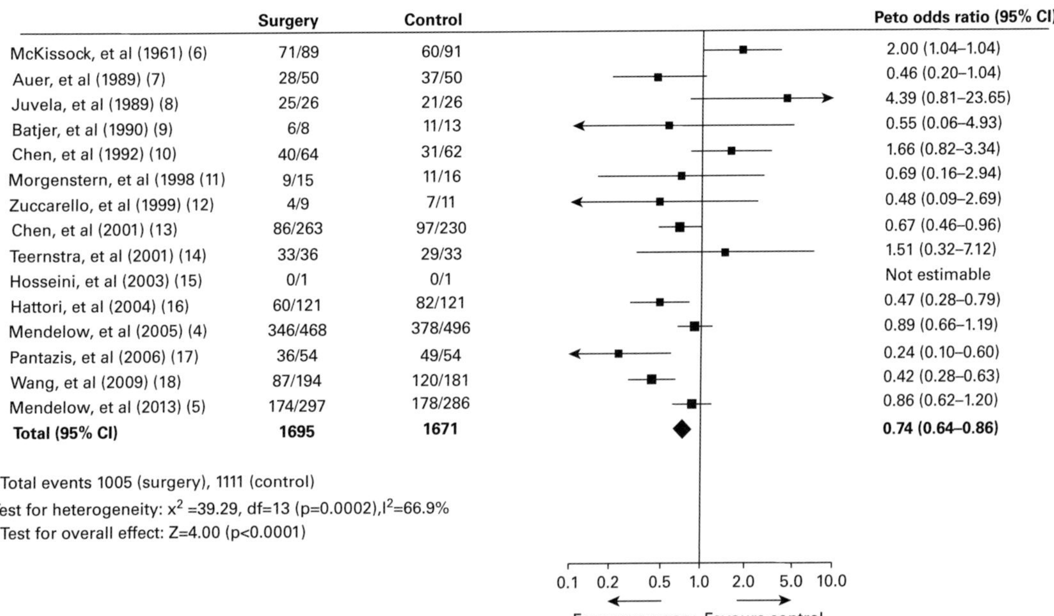

Fig. 22a.1 Meta-analysis of 15 prospective randomized controlled trials of surgery compared with conservative treatment. 1a = death; 1b= death and disability (4–18) (Reprinted with permission from reference (5)).

hypotheses were pre-specified in the largest of these trials: the STICH trials (4,5). These were published in the original papers and a few trends were identified. The trials were not powered for subgroup analysis and none of these pre-specified subgroups demonstrated a statistically significant benefit from early surgery (Fig. 22a.2). However, of all the pre-specified comparisons, superficial lobar hematomas appeared to fare best with early surgery. There was a trend for patients in coma (GCS<9) to have a worse outcome with early surgery. These observations have triggered several ongoing initiatives that have resulted in pooling of raw data from those trials that have been able to submit their original data (19). Together with the post-hoc analyses (vide infra) these observations led to the STICH II trial that focused on these subgroups.

The post-hoc analysis of the STICH data and meta-analysis of original data from some of these trials has confirmed the mechanistic argument and common experience that superficial hematomas fare better with surgery (Fig. 22a.3). Such lobar clots do not have ventricular hemorrhage or hydrocephalus and lend themselves to craniotomy. By contrast, deep-seated hematomas lend themselves to minimally invasive techniques and intra-cavity and intra-ventricular thrombolysis. These techniques are described in Chapters 25 and 26 and are the concepts behind the MISTIE III and CLEAR III trials respectively. The role of craniotomy for superficial hematomas is discussed in this chapter and craniotomy was the dominant technique in the STICH II trial. The STICH II trial was randomizing patients with lobar hematomas within

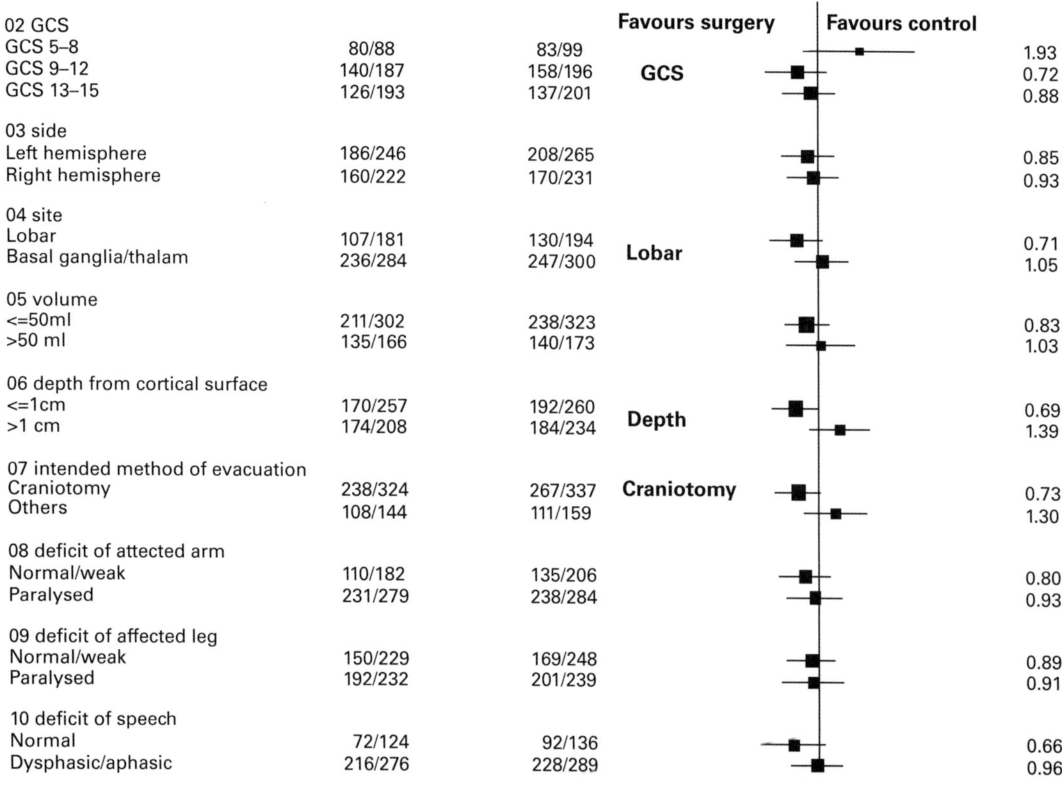

Fig. 22a.2 Forest plot of pre-specified subgroups in the STICH trial.

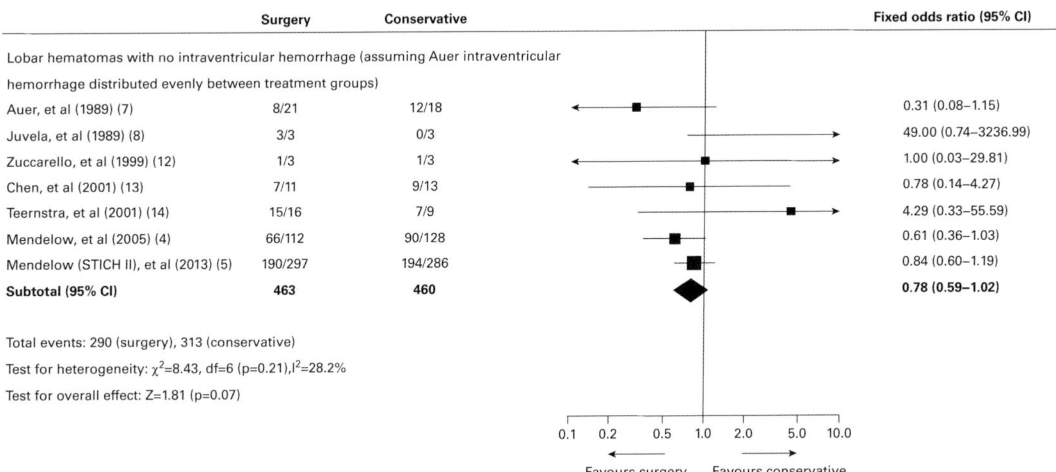

Fig. 22a.3 Meta-analysis of the results of surgery for lobar ICH with no IVH. (Reprinted with permission from Mendelow *et al.* (5)).

10 mm of the cortical surface to early surgery (within 48 hours) or to initial conservative treatment. Patients with ventricular hemorrhage or hydrocephalus were excluded.

The *time is brain* concept familiar from ischemic stroke also applies to ICH. Ischemic brain damage (IBD) has been demonstrated in brain tissue surrounding ICH (20,21). Some ICH patients may have a penumbra of functionally impaired but potentially viable tissue around their clots. If these patients could be targeted for early surgery, outcome would be expected to improve. Trials have emphasized early surgery rather than any surgery but have not recruited significant numbers in under 4 hours from the onset of symptoms. To date no trials have attempted to randomize patients after the sort of cerebral blood flow (CBF) imaging that would be needed to identify such a penumbra (PET scanning; SPECT; Cold Xenon CT). Such trials are very complex and expensive as has proven to be the case with the second large EC-IC bypass trial (22,23) that utilizes 'misery perfusion' identified on PET scanning as the inclusion criterion for randomization to bypass or not. Future trials of surgery for supratentorial ICH may well also have to utilize such CBF measurement in the selection of patients.

Coagulopathies with ICH

Any clotting disorder should be reversed immediately because many intracerebral hematomas increase in size as a result of further bleeding especially during the first 24 hours (24,25). Some patients are already on warfarin or antiplatelet therapy so that they effectively have a coagulopathy at the time of the hemorrhage. The appropriate therapy should be given and, in the case of warfarin, vitamin K, fresh frozen plasma, and prothrombin complex concentrate (PCC Beriplex®) should be given immediately to correct the INR to within normal limits. This should be done whether or not surgery is undertaken. If platelet function has been affected by antiplatelet therapy, then platelet transfusions or platelet-rich plasma should be given at the start of surgery.

Craniotomy for ICH

The ubiquitous availability of craniotomy makes it the most widespread and practical surgical technique for the removal of a supratentorial ICH. Almost all neurosurgical units around the world can offer immediate craniotomy for these lesions. The skin incision can either be linear or using a conventional flap. Flap placement is straightforward and image guidance surgery (IGS) can be used for more accurate placement over the most superficial part of the clot. This limits the cortical damage that might otherwise be necessary to get to the clot. An alternative is to create a slightly larger craniotomy and to use intra-operative ultrasound as the form of image guidance. The Brain Lab Image Guidance system utilizes intra-operative 3D ultrasound to update the position of the clot or any residual clot once the surgeon feels that the whole clot has been removed. Using these IGS techniques, complete clot removal with minimal damage to surrounding brain can be achieved.

If the ICP is high and the brain immediately starts to herniate once the first dural incision is made, then aspiration of the ICH with a Dandy type cannula will reduce the pressure and facilitate safer dural opening even if only a few milliliters are removed.

There are various retraction systems that can be used once the clot has been entered. Suction will be used to evacuate the clot under vision, often with the operating microscope. Bleeding vessels should be coagulated with bipolar coagulation using non-stick forceps. Again, several different types are available. It is better not to use hemostatic agents until all vessels have been coagulated because placing of hemostats allows more clot to accumulate beneath whichever material is used. Then a peri-cavity new hematoma may form. Therefore, good coagulation of all vessels is the preferred method of hemostasis. This is best achieved with the operating microscope because of the excellent lighting and magnification that it allows.

If there is clot tucked away under eloquent cortex, then the endoscope can be utilized. Several different types of angled endoscopes can be safely deployed into the cavity while the microscope remains in situ. This is best achieved with a pneumatic robotic arm (Storz) that holds the endoscope absolutely rigid within the operating microscope's field. Once hemostasis has been achieved, then hemostatic materials can be used to line the cavity to prevent later re-hemorrhage as for example can take place if there is a surge in blood pressure during emergence from anesthesia or postoperatively. There are a wide variety of topical hemostatic materials including Surgicel®, Fibrillar® GelatiCel®, and Floseal®. These are easily applied to the lining of the evacuated clot after careful coagulation of all bleeding vessels but they are not a substitute for careful hemostasis with bipolar coagulation. When used after such coagulation, then they add to the value of craniotomy because they cannot be used with the minimal invasive techniques.

Sometimes an unexpected lesion will be encountered such as a metastatic tumor or AVM. If possible, such lesions should be removed although the finding of a surprise AVM makes decision making difficult because the arterial feeding anatomy is unknown. If hemostasis has been achieved, then it may be wiser **not** to try to remove a previously unrecognized AVM unless intra-operative angiography can be immediately performed. If such angiography reveals that it is technically safe and possible to continue to remove the AVM, then it should indeed be removed. If there are large inaccessible feeders, then it may be wiser to close the wound if hemostasis is satisfactory. Under such circumstances embolization and a 'second look' procedure is a reasonable, and perhaps safer, way forward.

If, after clot removal, the brain is very swollen, then secondary clots should be suspected. They can be diagnosed with intra-operative ultrasound and should be dealt with before closing the dura. If, on the other hand, there is no residual clot, then the bone flap can be removed. Such decompressive craniectomy has not been proven as effective with ICH (26) but may seem appropriate if there is severe brain swelling (27). Such decompression will be ineffective if a small image-guided flap has been cut. Then the choice would be to enlarge the craniectomy and/or post-operative ventilation in critical care with sedation and ICP monitoring. If the ICP remains low, delayed reversal of sedation would be sensible, but if not, further CT imaging will determine if there is residual clot. Occasionally large residual clots will be found and return to theatre may be required.

Trials

The Surgical Trial in **Lobar** Intracerebral Haemorrhage (STICH II) has focused on patients with spontaneous superficial supratententorial ICH that have a better prognosis than those in the first STICH trial. The inclusion and exclusion criteria for STICH II were derived as a result of detailed analysis of the STICH CT scans. There was intraventricular hemorrhage (IVH) present in 42% of the patients who had assessable scans. These patients have a much poorer prognosis. When patients with IVH or deep-seated non-lobar ICH were removed from the STICH trial there were only 223 patients with superficial lobar ICH and no intraventricular hemorrhage or hydrocephalus. These patients had a 49% favorable outcome with early surgery compared with only 37% in the initial conservative treatment group. Furthermore analysis of the prognosis-based modified Rankin score for this subgroup showed a significant benefit from early surgery compared with initial conservative treatment in this post hoc identified sub group of patients with ICH (p = 0.013). The aim of the STICH II trial is to randomize this sub group of patients to even earlier surgery (within 48 hours of ictus and surgery to be performed within 12 hours of randomization). So the maximum time to operation from ictus was 60 hours in STICH II while within the first STICH trial this maximum time was 96 hours.

STICH II randomized 601 patients with superficial lobar spontaneous supratentorial ICH with no IVH or hydrocephalus to early surgery or to initial conservative treatment. The characteristics of these randomized patients are shown in Figure 22a.4. These data show that the median age of patients randomized was 65. The median volumes and depths from the cortical surface are shown in Figure 22a.5. Mortality at 6 months was reduced from 24% to 18% with early surgery but this and the ordinal analysis of the primary outcome was not quite statistically significant: Figure 22a.6 (p = 0.07). The MISTIE III and CLEAR III trials address a different group of patients with ICH and IVH. In these two trials catheter drainage of the clot and the ventricles

	Early surgery group (n=305)	Initial conservative treatment group (n=292)
Age (years)		
Median (IQR; range)	65 (55 to 74; 17 to 90)	65 (56 to 74; 23 to 94)
Mean (SD)	63·9 (13·0)	63·9 (13·7)
<60	105 (34%)	106 (36%)
60–69	89 (29%)	70 (24%)
≥70	111 (36%)	116 (40%)
Sex		
Male	174 (57%)	166 (57%)
Female	131 (43%)	126 (43%)
Preintracerebral haemorrhage Rankin*		
0	240 (80%)	236 (81%)
1	41 (14%)	37 (13%)
2	17 (6%)	11 (4%)
3	2 (<1%)	5 (2%)
4	1 (<1%)	2 (<1%)
Preintracerebral haemorrhage mobility*†		
Able to walk 200 m	283 (94%)	275 (95%)
Able to walk indoors	17 (6%)	13 (4%)
Unable to walk	1 (<1%)	2 (<1%)
Glasgow Coma Score, eye		
2	26 (9%)	27 (9%)
3	69 (23%)	65 (22%)
4	210 (69%)	200 (68%)
Glasgow Coma Score, verbal		
1	40 (13%)	44 (15%)
2	36 (12%)	25 (9%)
3	37 (12%)	35 (12%)
4	93 (30%)	96 (33%)
5	99 (32%)	92 (32%)
Glasgow Coma Score, motor		
5	83 (27%)	71 (24%)
6	222 (73%)	221 (76%)
Glasgow Coma Score, total		
8	12 (4%)	4 (1%)
9	9 (3%)	15 (5%)
10	23 (8%)	21 (7%)
11	32 (10%)	32 (11%)
12	32 (10%)	34 (12%)
13	46 (15%)	43 (15%)
14	70 (23%)	68 (23%)
15	81 (27%)	75 (26%)

Fig 22a.4 The two groups in the STICH II trial.

	Early surgery group (n = 305)	Initial conservative treatment group (n = 292)
Volume (ML)		
Median (IQR; range)	38 (24 – 54; 10 – 100)	36 (22 – 58; 10 – 100)
Mean (SD)	41.4 (21.2)	41.0 (22.9)
Depth (mm)		
Median (IQR; range)	1(0 – 2; 0 – 10)	1(0 – 2; 0 – 10)
Mean (SD)	1.6 (2.4)	1.6 (2.5)
Side of haemorrhage*		
Left	158 (52%)	149 (51%)
Right	147 (48%)	142 (49%)

Fig. 22a.5 Characteristics of the two groups in the STICH II trial.

respectively is assisted with the use of thrombolytic agents that liquefy the clot and prevent the catheters from clotting off. These trials are described in detail in Chapters 25 and 26.

Conclusions

Factors that argue for surgical removal of spontaneous ICH include early presentation, superficial hemorrhage and hemorrhage in relatively non-eloquent areas that compromise function in the penumbra or other areas via mass effect. The best results for early surgery appear

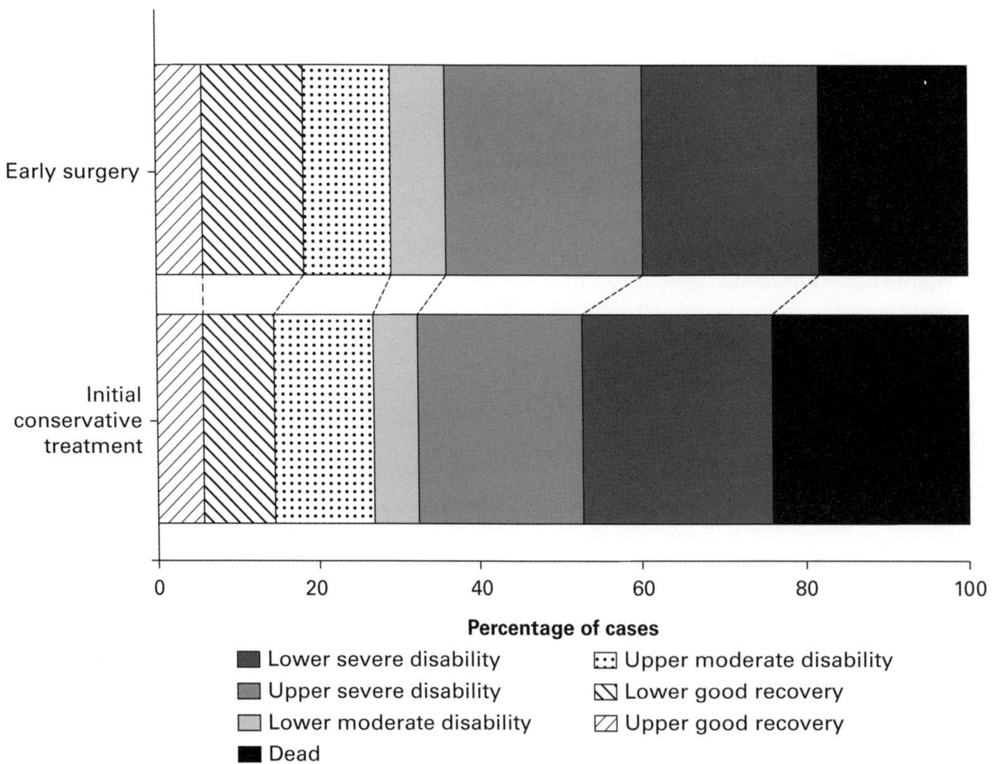

Fig. 22a.6 Glasgow Outcome Scale at 6 months for STICH II patients. (See plate section for color version).

to be in patients with a Glasgow Coma Score of between 9 and 12 at presentation. These observations are based on mechanism and surgeon opinion but trial sub-group analyses tend to support them. To date trial data suggest a marginal benefit for surgery. Ongoing research (including the STICH II, MISTIE III, and CLEAR III trials) seeks greater benefits in more selected patient groups.

REFERENCES

1. Palmer JD, Sparrow OC, *et al.* Postoperative hematoma: a 5-year survey and identification of avoidable risk factors. *Neurosurgery* 1994;**35**(6):1061–4; discussion 1064–5.
2. Heiskanen O, Poranen A, *et al.* Acute surgery for intracerebral haematomas caused by rupture of an intracranial arterial aneurysm. A prospective randomized study. *Acta Neurochir* 1988;**90**(3–4):81–3.
3. Hemphill JC III, White DB. Clinical nihilism in neuroemergencies. *Emerg Med Clin North Am* 2009;**27**(1):27–37.
4. Mendelow AD, Gregson BA, *et al.* Early surgery versus initial conservative treatment in patients with spontaneous supratentorial intracerebral haematomas in the International Surgical Trial in Intracerebral Haemorrhage (STICH): a randomised trial. *Lancet* 2005;**365**(9457):387–97.
5. Mendelow AD, Gregson BA, *et al.* Early surgery versus initial conservative treatment in patients with spontaneous supratentorial lobar intracerebral haematomas (STICH II): a randomised trial. *Lancet.* 2013;**382**(9890):397–408.
6. McKissock W, Richardson A, *et al.* Primary intracerebral haemorrhage: a controlled trial of surgical and conservative treatment in 180 unselected cases. *Lancet* 1961;**2**:221–6.
7. Auer LM, Deinsberger W, *et al.* Endoscopic surgery versus medical treatment for spontaneous intracerebral hematoma: a randomized study. *J Neurosurg* 1989;**70**(4):530–5.
8. Juvela S, Heiskanen O, *et al.* The treatment of spontaneous intracerebral hemorrhage. A prospective randomized trial of surgical and conservative treatment. *J Neurosurg* 1989;**70**:755–8.
9. Batjer HH, Reisch JS, *et al.* Failure of surgery to improve outcome in hypertensive putaminal hemorrhage. A prospective randomized trial. *Arch Neurol* 1990;**47**(10):1103–6.
10. Chen X, Yang H, *et al.* A prospective randomised trial of surgical and conservative treatment for hypertensive intracerebral haemorrhage. *Acta Acad Med Shanghai* 1992;**19**:237–40.
11. Morgenstern LB, Frankowski RF, *et al.* Surgical treatment for intracerebral hemorrhage (STICH): a single-center, randomized clinical trial. *Neurology* 1998;**51**(5):1359–63.
12. Zuccarello M, Brott T, *et al.* Early surgical treatment for supratentorial intracerebral hemorrhage: a randomized feasibility study. *Stroke* 1999;**30**(9):1829–33.
13. Chen X-C, Wu J-S, *et al.* The randomized multicentric prospective controlled trial in the standardized treatment of hypertensive intracerebral hematomas: The comparison of surgical therapeutic outcomes with conservative therapy. *Chinese J Clin Neurosci* 2001;**4**:365–8.
14. Teernstra OPM, Evers SMAA, *et al.* Stereotactic treatment of intracerebral hematoma by means of a plasminogen activator: a multicenter randomized controlled trial (SICHPA). *Stroke* 2003;**34**:968–74.
15. Hosseini H, Leguerinel C, *et al.* Stereotactic aspiration of deep intracerebral hematomas under computed tomographic control: a multicentric prospective randomised trial. *Cerebrovasular Dis* 2003;**16**S:57.
16. Hattori N, Katayama Y, *et al.* Impact of stereotactic hematoma evacuation on activities of daily living during the chronic period following spontaneous putaminal hemorrhage: a randomised study. *J Neurosurg* 2004;**101**:417–20.
17. Pantazis G, Tsitsopoulos P, *et al.* Early surgical treatment vs conservative management for spontaneous supratentorial intracerebral hematomas: A prospective randomized study. *Surg Neurol* 2006;**66**(5):492–501.
18. Wang WZ, Jiang B, *et al.* Minimally invasive craniopuncture therapy vs. conservative treatment for spontaneous intracerebral hemorrhage: results from a randomized clinical trial in China. *Int J Stroke* 2009;**4**(1):11–16.
19. Gregson BA, Broderick JP, *et al.* Individual patient data subgroup meta-analysis of surgery for spontaneous supratentorial intracerebral hemorrhage. *Stroke.* 2012;**43**(6):1496–504.
20. Mendelow AD, Bullock R, *et al.* Intracranial haemorrhage induced at arterial pressure in the rat. Part 2: Short term changes in local cerebral blood flow measured by autoradiography. *Neurol Res* 1984;**6**(4):189–93.
21. Siddique MS, Fernandes HM, *et al.* Reversible ischemia around intracerebral hemorrhage: a single-photon emission computerized tomography study. *J Neurosurg* 2002;**96**(4):736–41.

22. Adams HP Jr., Powers WJ, *et al.* Preview of a new trial of extracranial-to-intracranial arterial anastomosis: the carotid occlusion surgery study. *Neurosurg Clin N Am* 2001;**12** (3):613–24.
23. Powers WJ, Clarke WR, *et al. Results of the Carotid Occlusion Surgery Study (COSS). International Stroke Conference.* Los Angeles. 2011.
24. Broderick JP, Brott TG, *et al.* Ultra-early evaluation of intracerebral hemorrhage. *J Neurosurg* 1990;**72**(2):195–9.
25. Broderick JP, Diringer MN, *et al.* Determinants of intracerebral hemorrhage growth: an exploratory analysis. *Stroke* 2007;**38**(3):1072–5.
26. Mitchell P, Gregson BA, *et al.* Surgical options in ICH including decompressive craniectomy. *J Neurol Sci* 2007;**261**(1–2):89–98.
27. Fung C, Murek M, *et al.* Decompressive hemicraniectomy in patients with supratentorial intracerebral hemorrhage. *Stroke* 2012;**43**:3207–11.

22b

Minimally invasive treatment options for spontaneous intracerebral hemorrhage

Andrew Losiniecki and Mario Zuccarello

Introduction

Spontaneous intracerebral hemorrhage (SICH) remains a major cause a death and disability with an incidence ranging from 13–35 per 100 000 population [1–4]. The high prevalence of mortality and severity of morbidity associated with current management of SICH is high in comparison with other types of stroke, making identification of potential surgical candidates that may benefit from surgical evacuation an area of focus. For roughly 50 years, studies [5–7] comparing medical to surgical management have been conducted and as of yet a definitive answer remains elusive as to which patients would benefit from a particular intervention. This elusiveness is in part due to a changing paradigm for what constitutes best medical management as well as determining when these become futile and a more invasive therapy is required. The advent of minimally invasive (MIS) techniques has provided a surgical option that would seem to carry less risk than traditional open craniotomy techniques.

The management of SICH can be simplified into two main pathways: medical and surgical. Until recently surgical intervention had been undertaken only when patients were no longer able to be managed medically. With worsening of neurologic symptoms or if increased poorly controlled intracranial pressure was noted it was at this point that surgical options were considered. Outcomes of patients undergoing surgery during these circumstances is usually poor with significant risk of morbidity and mortality [6,7].

Stereotactic evacuation of SICH provides a seemingly quick, MIS approach to this difficult problem (Fig. 22b.1). Minimizing collateral injury during stereotactic evacuation may improve patient outcomes in those patients who would benefit from the removal of clot burden. It is just this point, identifying those patients who would benefit from SICH evacuation, that continues to confound to this date. Although guidelines for management of SICH have been created, very little Class I data exists [8] and is certainly lacking in the MIS arena.

Minimally invasive/stereotactic evacuation of ICH

The idea of using a MIS technique to aid in evacuation of ICH is not new. For almost 40 years various techniques have been studied to evacuate SICH while attempting to minimize cortical injury associated with brain retraction that is necessary to reach the clot. Initially these techniques included insertion of a cannula and an Archimedes screw aspirator to aid in the break-up of the blood clot and evacuation of SICH. Initial results were disappointing, however, with a mortality rate over 80%, exceeding that of the rates known for the medical management group [9]. Technical advances included insertion of a modified nucleotome [10], a

Critical Care of the Stroke Patient, ed. Stefan Schwab, Daniel Hanley, and A. David Mendelow. Published by Cambridge University Press.

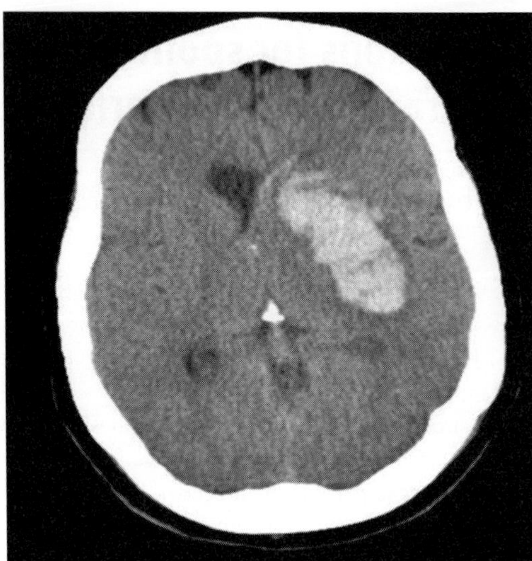

Fig. 22b.1 Non-contrast head CT demonstrating left-sided deep ICH that would be a candidate for MIS evacuation to avoid damage to the overlying un-injured brain.

double track aspiration system [11] and ultrasonic aspirator [12], and a water jet irrigating system [13] among others. All of these techniques had a similar goal which was to extract as much of the clot as possible through a small cortical opening with avoidance of damaging the surrounding brain. The SICH breakdown products such as hemoglobin, bilirubin, hemin and $FeCl_2$ have been shown to cause the edema and inflammation associated with SICH that lead to the high morbidity and poor outcomes associated with this condition [14].

The widespread availability of imaging modalities like CT and MRI have provided the motivation to improve MIS techniques that take advantage of these points that improve lesion location and quantification while addressing the SICH much earlier. The early MIS results had mixed results when compared to traditional open surgical evacuation and best medical management patient groups. The landmark study by Morgenstern *et al.* [7] was the first study that attempted to prospectively randomize patients between surgical and medical management of SICH but did not provide a clear treatment plan. Mendelow *et al.* [6] expanded on the initial study to include multiple centers and increase the number of patients. A conclusion drawn from this study was that all non-craniotomy techniques had worse outcome over conservative management but these data did not reach statistical significance. Many of the patients chosen to have MIS evacuations in this study were those with deep-seated lesions that were poor open surgical candidates, seemingly destined to do poorly [15]. Peresedov *et al.* [16] reported an improvement in overall mortality from 42.5% to 21.9% when a MIS stereotactic approach was utilized, but this was a retrospective evaluation of data and did not take into account long-term functional outcome.

Stereotactic image guidance has provided a major advance for improving the efficacy of MIS techniques for SICH evacuation. One key to the success of MIS techniques lies in the accuracy of clot localization. Techniques for localization first included ultrasound then advanced to use CT scans and finally MRI with potential intra-operative use to improve precision of localization. Systems available today allow for either CT or MR imaging of the brain to serve as the 3D localization map for SICH evacuation. The accuracy of the systems in use today allow for accuracy in placement of evacuation tools that were not available in the past. It is now possible to know within a few millimeters the location of the catheter or aspirator tip even deep within the brain tissue.

The theoretical advantages of minimally invasive techniques are significant. Use of local anesthesia, shorter operating time and less damage to normal surrounding brain can be favorable to those options available from the traditional craniotomy techniques. It is important to consider that although the etiology of most SICHs are small vessel-related, a vascular study such as CTA or MRA may be needed to identify a structural lesion such as an aneurysm or arteriovenous malformation as the cause of the ICH. Anatomical knowledge of hemorrhage patterns that are indicative of a middle cerebral artery aneurysm (ICH near the sylvian fissure) or dural arteriovenous fistula (ICH near the junction of the sigmoid and transverse sinus) as examples should not be overlooked.

Once the ICH has been accurately localized and an underlying structural lesion has been ruled out the next step involves evacuation of the ICH, for which various techniques are available and others still under study. The ideal technique is quick, done with minimal trauma to surrounding tissues, while allowing for assessment of complete hematoma removal, and provides a means for verification of hemostasis after the evacuation has been completed.

Endoscopic techniques have been described for ICH evacuation and consist of insertion of an endoscope through a burr-hole directly into the ICH cavity and evacuation of contents under direct visualization. The trajectory and planning of the burr-hole placement can be simplified with use of stereotactic guidance. The placement of the entry point and planned trajectory is dependent on ICH location with all attempts made to avoid eloquent tissue and known vascular structures, including but not limited to cortical arteries and veins. Endoscopic techniques have been described using a lavage and then suction of the ICH and have been reported to evacuate nearly 90% of clot burden [15]. A randomized study of 100 patients associated with this technique suggested prolonged survival for the surgical group especially apparent in those patients with large (> 50 cc) ICHs. Patients younger than 60 with lobar hemorrhages showed a significant benefit over best medical management in quality of life assessments in this endoscopic population [15]. An additional study by Prasad *et al.* [17] supporting further investigation of MIS (endoscopic techniques) demonstrated that endoscopic evacuated lesions showed improved outcomes when compared to traditional open evacuation. In experienced hands endoscopic evacuation also has the benefit of being quick, having been shown to have a time to evacuation that was completed in the 1 hour range [18].

Stereotactic aspiration of ICH utilizes an ideology similar to that of endoscopic evacuation but instead of direct visualization, an aspirating needle is placed into the middle of the hemorrhage cavity. As the availability of intra-operative MRIS increases their role for evaluating the effect of SICH, evacuation will become more defined. The real-time images (Fig. 22b.2) that intra-operative CT provides will allow for improved evacuation of SICH while providing evidence of hemostasis.

Once the ICH clot is evacuated, a drain can be placed directly into the ICH cavity to encourage further drainage. If a CT scan of the head still shows residual clot, an injection of a thrombolytic agent [19] has been shown to provide additional evacuation. The injection of a thrombolytic agent into an ICH would seem to be counterintuitive to maintenance of hemostasis but studies have shown rebleeding rates in the range of those encountered in traditional open craniotomy [20].

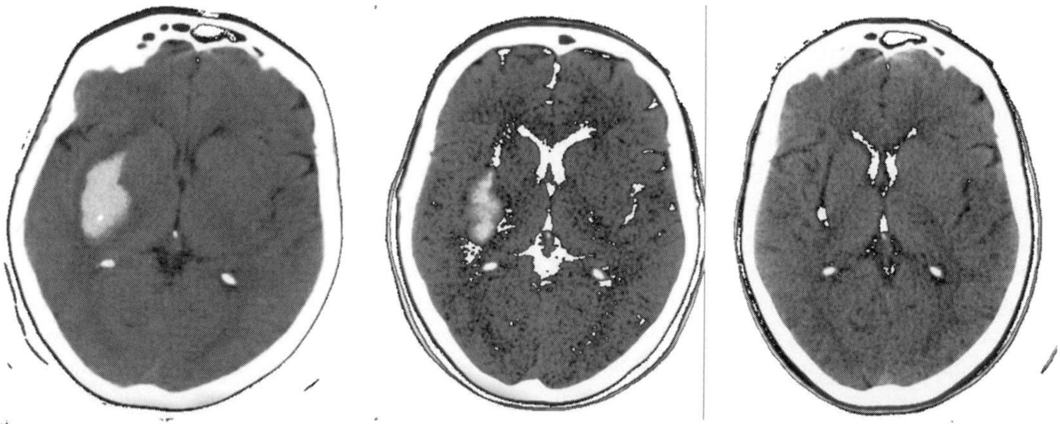

Fig. 22b.2 Time-lapsed CT images of stereotactic aspiration of a right-sided basal ganglia ICH. Pre-treatment images located on the far left, immediate post-op in the middle, and 2 days post-op on the far right. Images show near complete clot evacuation.

The initial studies involving injection of thrombolytic agents utilized urokinase which is no longer available in the U.S. More recent studies have shown tPA to be a viable alternative [21–23]. Currently the Minimally Invasive Surgery plus tPA for Intracerebral Hemorrhage Evacuation (MISTIE) trial funded by the National Institute of Health is underway and hopes to better answer this question. The MISTIE trial is a randomized study that examines minimally invasive (stereotactic) surgery and use of rtPA for ICH extraction in comparison to best medical management. The surgical arm involves the stereotactic placement of a catheter into the center of the SICH clot and infusion of tPA to aid in clot dissolution and evacuation.

Complications of the MIS techniques are similar to those of traditional craniotomies with some important differences. Endoscopic evacuation of ICH carries a rebleeding risk of roughly 3% [18] which is in the reported rate of rebleeding for traditional open craniotomy [24–26]. The use of indwelling catheter into the ICH cavity would seem to increase the risk of infection and questions regarding prophylactic use of antibiotics need to be researched for this scenario. The use of tPA as mentioned above introduces a risk of rebleeding not inherently present for traditional craniotomy but does not appear to reach clinical significance. When using tPA it must be noted that studies have shown that aspiration earlier than 6 hours shows an increase in rebleeding with a rate of nearly 40% if done within the first 4 hours; of note these studies did not include a thrombolytic agent [27,28]. Taking this information with the described maximal surgical benefit appearing to occur no later than 12 to 24 hours post hemorrhage [28,29] would provide an ideal but short window for evacuation in the 6–24 hour range.

Limited surgical field can prove to be challenging. It should go without saying but neurosurgeons not familiar with the MIS technique and apparatus should avoid this approach until a level of comfort exists. Discovering a structural lesion at the time of the evacuation, such as an aneurysm or arteriovenous malformation, will require conversion to a traditional open craniotomy. It is this scenario that requires one to thoughtfully place the burr-hole with a bailout plan for conversion to open craniotomy always being a consideration.

Although unable to provide statistical significance in regards to patient outcome, studies have suggested that minimally invasive techniques, especially endoscopic techniques, are more cost-effective than traditional open craniotomy techniques while entailing shorter ICU stays [18].

Conclusion

Stereotactic MIS evacuation of SICH may be the future in their management; however, with the data available today it is reasonable to proceed with medical management of ICH at least initially. On the failure of medical management either with progression of neurological deficits and/or increasing intracranial pressures, surgical evacuation of ICH should be considered. The goal of surgical evacuation is to remove the blood clot, with the aim of reducing further damage to the brain, and so improving the patient's chances of survival and maximizing functional outcome.

Stereotactic surgical techniques for evacuation of ICH exist and provide an alternative to traditional open surgical evacuation. Standard craniotomy utilized to evacuate ICH appears relatively ineffective or may be even worse than medical treatment in certain instances. The less invasive techniques including stereotactic evacuation may improve the chances of making a meaningful recovery as they are able to avoid injury to surrounding areas of uninjured brain. The numbers of available trials comparing medical management to minimally invasive techniques are limited, but as the use of intra-operative imaging increases they need to be further studied. Currently available trials also looked at routine rather than selective use of surgery in patients who most likely may benefit. As our imaging techniques continue to advance and become more available in the community setting, minimally invasive evacuation may prove not only to be available earlier but also to be a better long-term technique than traditional open craniotomy for treatment of ICH.

Many questions remain in regards to patient selection, timing of evacuation and which modality is the most effective for clot evacuation. Lesion size and location are also important variables that need further study before definitive recommendations can be made as to the appropriate method of treatment. Future areas of exploration may include the use of high-frequency ultrasonic aspiration and potentially radio-surgical techniques or an as-of-yet to be determined modality for dissolution of the blood clot related to SICH.

REFERENCES

1. Fogelholm R, Nuutila M, Vuorela AL. Primary intracerebral hemorrhage in the Jyväskylä region, central Finland, 1985–89: incidence, case fatality rate and functional outcome. *J Neurol Neurosurg Psychiatry.* 1992;**55**:546–52.
2. Giroud M, Gras P, Chadan N, *et al.* Cerebral hemorrhage in a French prospective population study. *J Neurol Neurosurg Psychiatry.* 1991;**54**:595–8.
3. Nilsson OG, Lindgren A, Stohl N. Incidence of intracerebral and subarachnoid hemorrhage in Southern Sweden. *J Neurol Neurosurg Psychiatry.* 2000;**69**:601–7.
4. Ojemann RG, Heros RC. Spontaneous brain hemorrhage. *Stroke.* 1983;**14**:468–75.
5. McKissock W, Richardson A, Taylor J. Primary intracerebral haemorrhage: a controlled trial of surgical and conservative treatment in 180 unselected cases. *Lancet.* 1961;**278**:221–6.
6. Mendelow AD, Gregson BA, Fernandes HM, *et al.* Early surgery versus initial conservative treatment in patients with spontaneous supratentorial intracerebral haematomas in the International Surgical Trial in Intracerebral Haemorrhage (STICH): a randomised trial. *Lancet.* 2005;**365**:387–97.
7. Morgenstern LB, Frankowski RF, Shedden P, Pasteur W, Grotta JC. Surgical treatment for intracerebral hemorrhage (STICH): a single center, randomized clinical trial. *Neurology.* 1998;**51**(5):1359–63.
8. Broderick J, Connolly S, Feldmann E, *et al.* Guidelines for the management of spontaneous intracerebral hemorrhage in adults: 2007 update: a guideline from the American Heart Association/American Stroke Association Stroke Council, High Blood Pressure Research Council, and the Quality of Care and Outcomes in Research Interdisciplinary Working Group. *Circulation.* 2007;**116** (16):e391–413.
9. Broseta J, Gonzalez-Darder J, Barcia-Salorio JL. Stereotactic evacuation of intracerebral hematomas. *Appl Neurophysiol.* 1982;**45**:443–8.
10. Nguyen JP, Decq P, Brugieres P, *et al.* A technique for stereotactic aspiration of deep intracerebral hematomas under computed tomographic control using a new device. *Neurosurgery.* 1992;**31**:330–4.
11. Tanikawa T, Amano K, Kawamura H, *et al.* CT-guided stereotactic surgery for evacuation of hypertensive intracerebral hematoma. *Appl Neurophysiol.* 1985;**48**:431–9.
12. Donauer E, Faubert C. Management of spontaneous intracerebral and cerebellar hemorrhage. In: Kaufman HH, ed. *Intracerebral Hematomas.* New York, NY: Raven Press; 1992: 211–27.
13. Mukai H, Yamashita J, Kitamura A, Ito H. Stereotactic aqua-stream and aspirator in the treatment of intracerebral hematoma: an experimental study. *Stereotact Funct Neurosurg.* 1991;**57**(4):221–7.
14. Huang FP, Xi G, Keep RF, *et al.* Brain edema after experimental intracerebral hemorrhage: role of hemoglobin degradation products. *J Neurosurg.* 2002;**96**(2):287–93.
15. Auer LM, Deinsberger W, Niederkorn K, *et al.* Endoscopic surgery versus medical treatment for spontaneous intracerebral hematoma: a randomized study. *J Neurosurg.* 1989;**70**:530–5.
16. Peresedov VV. Strategy, technology, and techniques of surgical treatment of supratentorial intracerebral hematomas. *Comput Aided Surg* 1999;**4**:51–63.
17. Prasad K, Browman G, Srivasta A, *et al.* Surgery in primary supratentorial intracerebral hematoma: a meta-analysis of randomized trials. *Acta Neurol Scand* 1997;**95**:103–10.
18. Cho DY, Chen CC, Cheng CS, Lee WY, Tso M. Endoscopic surgery for spontaneous basal ganglia hemorrhage: comparing endoscopic surgery, sterotactic aspiration, and craniotomy in noncomatose patients. *Surgical Neurology* 2006;(**65**):547–56.
19. Zuccarello M, Brott T, Derex L, *et al.* Early surgical treatment for supratentorial intracerebral hemorrhage: a randomized feasibility study. *Stroke.* 1999;**30**:1833–9.
20. Fujii Y, Tanaka R, Takeuchi S, Koike T, Minakawa T, Sasaki O. Hematoma enlargement in spontaneous intracerebral hemorrhage. *J Neurosurg.* 1994;**80**:51–7.
21. Lippitz BE, Mayfrank L, Spetzger U, *et al.* Lysis of basal ganglia haematoma with recombinant tissue plasminogen activator (rtPA) after stereotactic aspiration: initial results. *Acta Neurochir (Wien).* 1994;**127**:157–60.
22. Schaller C, Rohde V, Meyer B, Hassler W. Stereotactic puncture and lysis of spontaneous intracerebral hemorrhage using recombinant tissue plasminogen activator. *Neurosurgery.* 1995;**36**:328–33.
23. Vespa P, McArthur D, Miller C, *et al.* Frameless stereotactic aspiration and thrombolysis of deep intracerebral

hemorrhage is associated with reduction of hemorrhage volume and neurological improvement. *Neurocrit Care.* 2005;**2**(3):274–81.

24. Broderick JP, Brott T, Zuccarello M. Management of intracerebral hemorrhage. In: Batjer HH, ed. *Cerebrovascular Disease.* Philadelphia, PA: Lippincott-Raven; 1997: 611–27.
25. Kanaya H, Kuroda K. Development in neurosurgical approaches to hypertensive intracerebral hemorrhage in Japan. In: Kaufman HH, ed. *Intracerebral Hematomas.* New York, NY: Raven Press; 1992: 197–210.
26. Kaufman HH. Stereotactic aspiration with fibrinolytic and mechanical assistance. In: Kaufman HH, ed. *Intracerebral Hematoma.* New York, NY: Raven Press; 1992: 182–5.
27. Niizuma H, Shimizu Y, Yonemitsu T, Nakasato N, Suzuki J. Results of stereotactic aspiration in 175 cases of putaminal hemorrhage. *Neurosurgery.* 1989;**24**:814–19.
28. Morgenstern LB, Frankowski RF, Shedden P, Pasteur W, Grotta JC. Surgical treatment for intracerebral hemorrhage (STICH): a single center, randomized clinical trial. *Neurology.* 1998;**51**(5):1359–63.
29. Lee JI, Nam do H, Kim JS, *et al.* Stereotactic aspiration of intracerebral hematoma: significance of surgical timing and hematoma volume reduction. *J Clin Neurosci.* 2003;**10**(4):439–43.

Image-guided endoscopic evacuation of spontaneous intracerebral hemorrhage

Justin A. Dye, Daniel T. Nagasawa, Joshua R. Dusick, Winward Choy, Isaac Yang, Paul M. Vespa, and Neil A. Martin

Spontaneous intracerebral hemorrhage (sICH) has an annual prevalence of approximately 10–30 cases per 100 000 individuals, constituting a significant source of worldwide morbidity and mortality [1–4]. Within the United States alone, nearly 70 000 cases occur each year, resulting in more than $8 billion in total healthcare costs [5–8]. Risk factors for sICH include hypertension, male gender, African American or Hispanic race, and age; with a particular increase in incidence after 55 years [6,9–11]. As the United States' population continues to age, the occurrence of sICH is anticipated to double by 2050, representing a significant healthcare issue [10].

Causes of intracerebral hemorrhage include cerebral amyloid angiopathy, aneurysmal rupture, vascular malformations, trauma, tumors, and hemorrhagic stroke. Yet despite best diagnostic efforts, the etiology of spontaneous ICH often remains unknown until lesion tissue can be examined postmortem [12,13].

Hemorrhagic stroke is the most fatal category of infarct, with a 35% mortality rate within 1 week of the initial bleeding and 50% mortality during the first month. Additionally, only 10% of patients within the first 4 weeks respond with significant recovery to allow for a quality of life consistent with independent living [14–20]. As such, there has been much debate regarding the ideal treatment strategy to optimize patient outcomes and minimize healthcare costs [21–23].

While historical management of sICH included monitoring the patient's condition and considering surgical intervention only if they demonstrated clinical deterioration, modern theories advocate a more proactive approach to prevent the onset of secondary injury which may lead to better outcomes. Neurosurgical intervention is believed to aid in inhibiting active bleeding, prevent rebleeding, reduce mass effect on nearby vital structures, and minimize secondary damage. Given the potential for improved outcomes with hematoma evacuation and the shortcomings of the open craniotomy, the utilization of minimally invasive techniques, particularly endoscopic evacuation procedures, has been a topic of interest with encouraging results.

In this book chapter, we focus on modern minimally invasive techniques for the treatment of sICH, with an emphasis on stereotactic image-guided endoscopic evacuation of intracerebral hematomas which has emerged as a promising endeavor. In addition, we detail issues related to pre-operative medical management, ideal timing of surgery, and post-operative patient management. Overall, the utilization of endoscopic evacuations of sICH may allow for lower morbidity and mortality, decreased operative time, decreased blood loss, increased evacuation rates, and improved recovery for patients. However, appropriate patient selection and ideal surgical timing still necessitate further investigation in order to improve neurosurgical efforts and optimize patient outcomes.

Critical Care of the Stroke Patient, ed. Stefan Schwab, Daniel Hanley, and A. David Mendelow. Published by Cambridge University Press.

Treatment of sICH

The traditional approach of 'watchful waiting' for the treatment of sICH relied on the concept that for a stable hematoma, the vast majority of the brain injury occurs with the initial insult, and therefore evacuation would not improve outcome. However, recent studies suggest that intracerebral hematomas can also cause secondary brain damage resulting from elevated intracranial pressures, disruptions in regional blood flow, and cytotoxic effects of blood degradation products [24–40]. Subsequently, modern theories advocate a more proactive approach to prevent the onset of secondary injury which may lead to better outcomes [24].

Neurosurgical intervention is believed to aid in inhibiting active bleeding, prevent rebleeding, reduce mass effect on nearby vital structures, and minimize secondary damage [24–40]. Current interventional management for sICH includes craniotomy with surgical evacuation, bedside catheter drainage with rt-PA, and endoscopic evacuation [16,22,41]. Yet the exact role and optimal timing of surgical treatments have remained a topic of much controversy throughout the years [42–44]. In 1939, McKissock [45] published the first randomized trial evaluating the role of surgical intervention for sICH and concluded that there was no added benefit with surgery. However, with the advancements in neuroimaging and improvements in neurosurgical techniques, 13 other trials have evaluated this topic with mixed findings. [21,22,24,27,44,46–53] In 2005, Mendelow and colleagues [16, 22] published iSTICH (International Surgical Trial in Intracerebral Haemorrhage), their multicenter, international randomized trial demonstrating that early (< 24 hours) surgical intervention did not produce any benefits in morbidity or mortality as compared to conventional medical management. However, this study may have been limited by its subjective inclusion criteria, treatment crossover, and lack of consistency regarding surgical techniques [16]. Anik *et al.* reported similar findings in their 2011 meta-analysis. However, while this study concluded that there was no significant difference in overall morbidity or mortality between surgical and medical treatments for sICH, subgroup analysis did demonstrate improved surgical outcomes for those with hematoma volumes greater than 40 ml, those who received surgical intervention within 24 hours, and those with initial Glasgow Coma Scale (GCS) scores ≥ 6 [54]. In a more recent study, Gregson *et al.* [24] reported in 2012 on subgroup analysis of eight studies (2186 cases) evaluating spontaneous supratentorial ICH. This meta-analysis determined that there was improved clinical outcome if surgery was conducted within 8 hours of the inciting bleed, the hematoma volume was between 20 and 50 cc, the GCS was between 9 and 12, or the patient was between 50 and 69 years of age. In addition, they indicated that overall, there was no evidence to suggest that hematomas located in the basal ganglia or thalamus may benefit from traditional surgical techniques. However, they stated that modern methods of minimally invasive procedures may still be advantageous for these subpopulations [24,41,51,55].

The inability of conventional surgical evacuations to produce significant improvements in patient outcomes may be attributed to innate qualities of the procedures themselves. While traditional open craniotomy is effective in hematoma volume reduction, the process often results in injury to adjacent healthy tissue overlying and surrounding the lesion [16]. Thus, given the potential for improved outcomes with hematoma evacuation and the shortcomings of the open craniotomy, the utilization of minimally invasive techniques, particularly endoscopic evacuation procedures, have been a topic of interest with encouraging results [27,41,50,56,57].

Minimally invasive approaches

Vespa and colleagues [58] reported in 2005, describing the utilization of frameless stereotactic catheter aspiration with the application of t-PA, demonstrating a mean hematoma volume reduction of 77% and patient improvements in NIH stroke scale scores. This technique, however, may take several days to achieve substantial hematoma evacuation.

Another minimally invasive technique involves image-guided keyhole evacuation [59,60], which has yielded average volume reductions of 97.5% and improved clinical outcomes [60]. Yet while this strategy produces more immediate results with greater clot removal than bedside catheter drainage, it still necessitates a fair degree of cortical exposure, manipulation, and retraction.

Thus, the utilization of image-guided endoscopic evacuation of spontaneous ICH has emerged as a promising endeavor over the course of the past few decades [16]. This technique was first reported by Auer *et al.* [30,61] in 1985. Then in 1989, Auer and colleagues [27] described the results of their randomized controlled trial including 100 patients with sICH in which half underwent ultrasound-guided endoscopic evacuation and the remainder were treated conservatively with medical management. They concluded that their endoscopic evacuations demonstrated lower mortality rates (30% versus 70% in those managed medically) and reduced morbidity (40% with no or minimal deficits versus 25% in those managed medically). Interestingly, surgical patients with lesions less than 50 cc had a greater clinical recovery but similar mortality as compared with those treated medically. Conversely, those with larger lesions had lower post-operative mortality rates, but similar functional recoveries. Later, Prasad and colleagues [42, 62] reported that endoscopic evacuations resulted in decreased mortality and increased functional independence in patients younger than 60 years. Cho *et al.* [42] reported on 90 patients with basal ganglia hemorrhages in 2006 with findings to suggest that both stereotactic aspiration and endoscopic surgery confer lower morbidity and mortality as compared to traditional craniotomy. Furthermore, their study found that endoscopic evacuation had the advantage of decreased delay in hematoma evacuation from the time of initial patient presentation when compared to stereotactic aspiration. In their study using image-guided endoscopic evacuation of sICH, Miller *et al.* [16] reported a mean hematoma volume reduction of 80%, with a 90-day mortality rate of less than half that of the patients treated medically. More recently, Kuo and colleagues [28] reported on 68 patients treated with endoscopic evacuation demonstrating a 6% mortality rate, 4% morbidity, and overall hematoma reduction of 93%. In fact, recent literature has demonstrated evacuation rates ranging from 84 to 99% given modern advancements in technique and instrumentation [28,30,42,63–66]. Similarly, Nagasaka *et al.* [30] reported on 43 patients treated with either neuroendoscopic procedures or microsurgical craniotomy revealing that the endoscopic group demonstrated improved evacuation rates (99% vs. 96%) and increased 7-day GCS (12 vs. 9).

Endoscopic techniques can also be used to treat sICH with intraventricular extension. Chen and colleagues [67] evaluated the benefits of endoscopic evacuation in thalamic hemorrhages, which constitute approximately 10–15% of all ICH [67–69]. Given their proximity to the ventricular system, thalamic hematomas are prone to intraventricular bleeding and subsequent acute hydrocephalus. While external ventricular drains (EVD) may be beneficial for temporary hydrocephalus relief, they cannot prevent shunt-dependent hydrocephalus. In fact, approximately two-thirds of all thalamic ICH patients eventually require shunt placement [67,70]. In their study, Chen *et al.* achieved a decrease in shunt-dependent hydrocephalus from 90% (EVD group) to 48% (endoscopic evacuation group) in this patient population after endoscopic evacuation. They attributed their success to expeditious evacuation of intraventricular blood and prompt reduction of ventricular dilatation and intracranial pressure. As the volume of intraventricular blood is one of the strongest prognostic factors for these patients, rapid evacuation is paramount [67,71]. Yet despite its benefits of decreased hydrocephalus and shorter ICU stays, the endoscopic group did not experience improvements in mortality compared with those treated with EVDs [67].

While there is still no consensus for the treatment of patients with sICH, the authors have developed a protocol which includes perioperative management in a neurointensive care unit as well as stereotactic CT-guided endoscopic evacuation. This protocol is part of an ongoing multi-center trial known as Intraoperative CT guided Endoscopic Surgery for ICH (ICES), which receives funding from a NIH SPOTRIAS grant. The rest of this chapter will describe the pre-operative, intra-operative, and post-operative management guidelines gained from this experience.

Pre-operative medical management

Initial evaluation

In the current protocol patients undergo a full neurologic history and physical exam performed by a member of the neurosurgical team. Diagnosis of intracerebral hemorrhage is made based on this evaluation and initial CT or MRI of the brain. Patients are first admitted to the neuro-ICU and undergo standard neurocritical care for ICH. Patient and family discussion is held, consent is obtained, and randomization occurs into the study protocol. Key inclusion criteria for this study include age 18–80 years, spontaneous supratentorial hemorrhage, ICH volume ≤ 20 cc, GCS 5 to ≤ 14, NIHSS score ≤ 6, symptom onset less than 12 hours prior to initial CT scan, stable clot size based on a stability scan with an interval of at least 6 hours, SBP <200 mmHG sustained for 6 hours, and intention to start surgery within 48 hours after initial CT scan.

Correction of coagulopathies

According to recommendations reported in 2010 by the American Heart Association [72], patients with severe coagulation factor deficiencies should receive necessary replacement of clotting factors, and those with severe thrombocytopenia should be given sufficient platelet replacement. Patients on oral anticoagulants with an elevated INR should have vitamin K-dependent factors replenished and warfarin withheld. In the current protocol, patients do not proceed to the OR until INR has been corrected to < 1.3 and platelets are > 100 000. Additionally, any patient on daily antiplatelet therapy receives one dose of DDAVP (0.3 mcg/kg) and one unit of platelets.

Management of blood pressure

While there remains a lack of indisputable evidence to support the utility of stringent blood pressure control, the following management is recommended until ongoing trials are able to more clearly elucidate this topic. In patients with systolic blood pressure (SBP) 150–220 mmHg, acute decrease to 140 mmHg is likely safe. If SBP is greater than 200 or mean arterial pressure (MAP) is greater than 150, aggressive blood pressure reduction should be pursued with continuous intravenous infusions. If SBP is greater than 180 mmHg or MAP is greater than 130 mmHg with the likelihood of increased intracranial pressure (ICP), blood pressure may be decreased using intravenous medications either intermittently or continuously, although cerebral perfusion pressure should remain above 60 mmHg. A more modest reduction in blood pressure may be considered if there is no suggestion of elevated ICP [72]. At UCLA, it has been our experience that outcomes are optimal when maintaining a SBP of 100–140 during the entire peri-operative period.

Neuroimaging

Active bleeding may last for hours following initial sICH presentation, contributes to a large proportion of early decreases in neurological function, and is predictive of increased morbidity and mortality [72–76]. As such, appropriate neuroimaging to monitor the stability of the potentially expanding lesion is essential. Not surprisingly, the sooner the first imaging is completed following the inciting incident, the more likely additional neuroimaging will demonstrate lesion enlargement [72,75,77,78]. In fact, for those with CT imaging completed within 3 hours of sICH onset, 28–38% demonstrated lesion expansion of greater than 30% on subsequent findings [72,73,76].

In the current protocol, the initial CT of the brain is used both to diagnose the ICH and to calculate the volume of the hematoma using the formula (length × width × height)/2 (Fig. 22c.1). Length and width are measured on the CT slice with the largest area of ICH. To calculate the height of the hematoma without coronal reconstructions the number of slices containing the hematoma on axial imaging is multiplied by the slice thickness in centimeters (e.g. 6 slices × 0.5 cm = 3 cm). In order to more accurately determine the volume of the hematoma, the first and last slices where the hematoma is seen are not counted when measuring the height. A repeat non-contrast CT scan is completed no earlier than 6 hours after the initial scan. This stability scan includes a 1 mm/cut CT angiogram which both evaluates for any

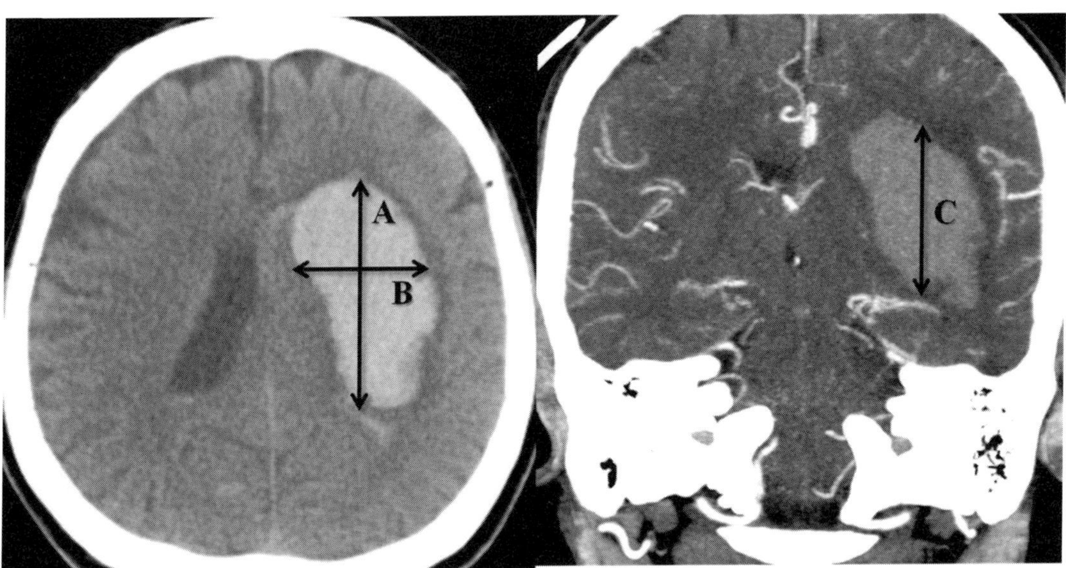

Fig. 22c.1 The formula (A x B x C)/2 is used to calculate the hematoma volume using the initial head CT.

underlying vascular malformation and is also used intraoperatively for neuronavigation. If the repeat scan shows enlargement of the ICH, another CT scan is completed 6 hours later to evaluate for stability. It is important to note that any evidence of an underlying vascular malformation or ongoing hematoma expansion is a contraindication to the endoscopic approach.

Timing of surgery

Although it is generally believed that a certain interval should be waited prior to surgical evacuation to prevent rebleeding, the precise timing has yet to be established [42, 57]. Clinical studies have described results for surgical procedures ranging from within 4 hours following symptom onset up to 96 hours [22,44,47,49,72]. Morgenstern and colleagues [23,54] reported that postoperative rebleeding occurred in 40% of patients who received surgical intervention within 4 hours and in 12% of those evacuated within 12 hours. Pantazis *et al.* [49,54] found similar results, reporting a 22% rebleeding rate for those operated on within 3–5 hours and 9% for those within 6–8 hours. Although some caution against early removal of the tamponade effect reinforced by the hematoma [23,24], others advocate that intervention within 7 hours may be advantageous [23,30,47,79], as the lesion is believed to reach its maximum volume within approximately 6 hours [54,78]. Similarly, the American Heart Association suggests minimally invasive evacuation ideally within 12 hours [2,30], although some randomized trials of surgical interventions have produced mixed results regarding this time window [44,47,49,72]. However, literature does suggest that the rebleeding rate is actually rather low for endoscopic evacuations (0–3.3%) as compared to that of the traditional craniotomy technique utilized in many of these studies (5–10%) [28,30,42]. While there remains a lack of consensus regarding the optimal window for evacuation, current ongoing trials may help to elucidate this ambiguity [24,41,80,81].

As part of the inclusion criteria in the current protocol, there must be an intention to start surgery within 48 hours after the initial CT scan. Furthermore, patients do not proceed to the OR earlier than 6–8 hours given the need for medical optimization and the time interval for the stability CT scan. In our current series of 41 patients who underwent endoscopic evacuation of sICH we did not find a significant difference in outcome between patients who underwent early surgery versus late surgery (< 12 hours vs. > 12 hours or < 24 hours vs. > 24 hours). While one of the goals of this protocol is timely evacuation of the hematoma in order to prevent secondary injury, it is also important to note that each of these patients is initially admitted to the neuro-ICU and treated medically prior to proceeding to the OR. We believe this approach decreases the risk of intra-operative complications and poor outcomes.

Surgical technique

While allowing for decreased surgical time and healthy tissue preservation compared to traditional craniotomy [2,65], the endoscopic approach unfortunately also confers a limited surgical exposure [64,65,82]. Yet the practice of utilizing an endoscope for the evacuation of sICH has evolved throughout the years, and while initial attempts focused on visually-directed endoscopic manipulation, we are now capable of exploiting the benefits of stereotactic guidance [42,83,84].

In the author's technique, after the patient's head is fixed in the Mayfield headholder, the cranial landmarks are registered to the pre-operative thin-cut CT imaging to permit for frameless neuronavigation. This allows the surgeon to accurately identify the ideal entry point and trajectory for optimal bleed evacuation along the long axis of the hematoma.

For anteriorly positioned basal ganglia hemorrhages, we advocate the frontal approach with the burr hole in the supraorbital bone just lateral to the frontal sinus. Given the commonly elongated, ovoid shape of these lesions, this approach allows for access to the long axis of the hematoma, optimizes total volume evacuation, and minimizes the necessity for endoscopic manipulation that may result in injury to adjacent parenchyma. For anterior basal ganglia hemorrhages that are more spherical in shape, the middle frontal gyrus approach may be employed, which utilizes an entry point over the coronal suture. Spontaneous ICH in the posterior basal ganglia or thalamic regions may be best evacuated using a parieto-occipital approach. Superficial lobar hematomas are often drained using an entry point directly over the lesion in the area where the hematoma comes closest to the surface (Fig. 22c.2). Of note, our experience has been one of difficultly when evacuating hematomas with volumes less than 20 cc, regardless of their location. However, the surgical decision on whether to evacuate these sICHs is not based upon lesion size, but rather clinical findings related to severe focal deficits which correlate with the location of the hematoma.

Once the ideal entry point and trajectory are determined and cortical access is acquired, the endoscope (with obturator in place) should be advanced to a depth two-thirds of the way along the long axis of the hematoma using stereotactic guidance. With the endoscope sheath held securely in place by a Mitaka robotic arm (Mitaka Optical Co., Ltd, Tokyo, Japan), the obturator is then removed and regulated wall suction is attached. Reduction of the distal portion of the hematoma allows adjacent elements to collapse into the suction tip, minimizing the need to adjust the angle of instrumentation which may damage sensitive nearby structures. It also prevents premature collapse of the cavity necessitating inflation methods to access residual blood products [28]. Once maximal hematoma evacuation has been achieved at this depth, the sheath should then be withdrawn to a point one-third of the length of the lesion's long axis and suction reinitiated until maximal evacuation has been achieved (Fig. 22c.3).

Regulated wall suction is attached to a side port of the endoscope sheath and the surgeon is able to control how much suction is applied to the hematoma by placing a thumb over the open end of the sheath (Fig. 22c.4). Suction begins at 50 Torr and increases by 50 Torr until the hematoma begins to be removed. 100–200 Torr appears to be the safest and most effective pressure. The hematoma is collected and the amount recorded in a Luken trap.

While the main function of the evacuation is to reduce the mass effect on surrounding tissue, there remains a lack of evidence to indicate to what extent residual hematoma may impact neurological recovery once the brain has been decompressed. Although these remaining blood degradation products may confer a neurotoxic effect, aggressive evacuation may cause more immediate injury to vital structures and

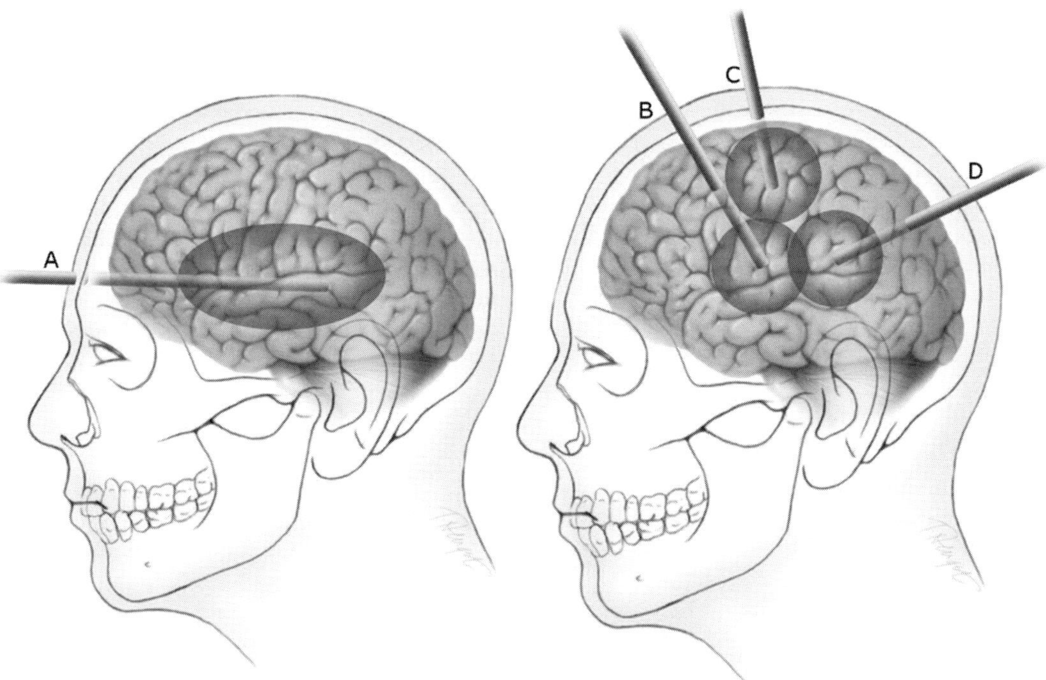

Fig. 22c.2 Hematomas in different locations are approached with different trajectories. A = Supraorbital approach; B = Middle frontal gyrus approach; C = Superficial lobar approach; D = Parietoccipital approach.

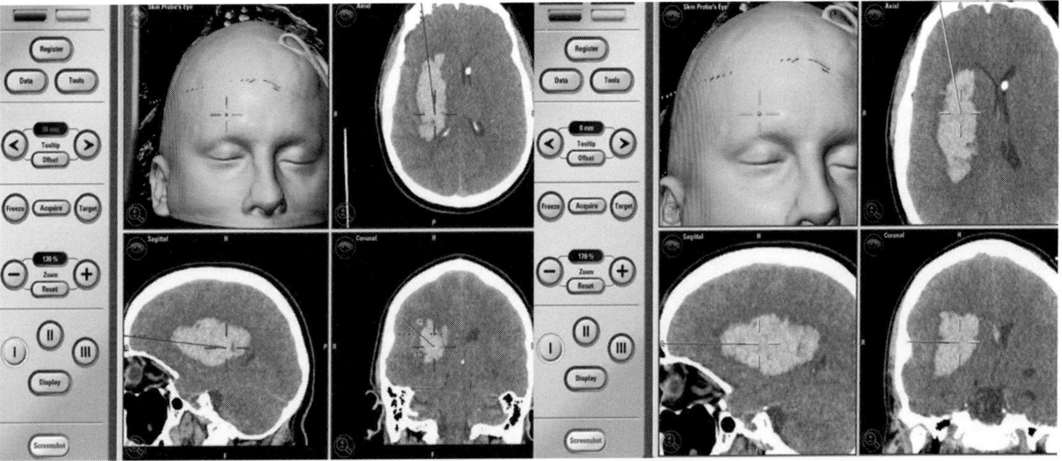

Fig. 22c.3 Using the stereotactic neuronavigation system the endoscope sheath is guided to suction point #1 which is two-thirds of the way along the long axis of the hematoma (left). It is then withdrawn to suction point #2 which is one-third of the way along the long axis of the hematoma (right).

intra-operative hemorrhage during manipulations. Thus, the authors advocate that after 75–85% of the volume has been removed (as determined by the pre-operative imaging calculations compared to what is collected in the Luken trap), evacuation should be stopped.

Given the advantages of the current technique with stereotactic guidance, the endoscope camera is only inserted once adequate hematoma evacuation has been achieved for monitoring of hemostasis during continuous irrigation. Hemostasis usually occurs after 15–30 min of continuous irrigation through the endoscope. We have found that one dose of intravenous DDAVP at 0.3 mcg/kg may shorten this time period. Once hemostasis has been achieved, the camera and sheath are withdrawn together to assess for adequate hemostasis along the endoscopic tract. In rare cases of active bleeding that is refractory to continuous irrigation and intravenous DDAVP, endoscopic monopolar or bipolar electocautery is applied for direct coagulation. Figure 22c.5 shows two intra-operative endoscopic views.

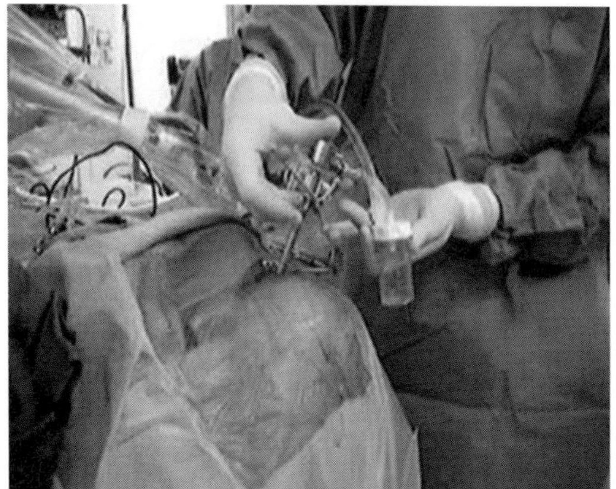

Fig. 22c.4 The endoscope sheath is held securely in place with a hydraulic arm and the hematoma is collected in a Luken trap.

Variations in endoscopic technique

Kuo *et al.* documented their surgical technique with endoscope-assisted hematoma evacuations of supratentorial intracerebral hemorrhage utilizing a transparent sheath [28]. For their strategy, a stylet with a transparent sheath measuring 10 mm in external diameter and of variable length (ranging from 5 to 15 cm) was placed through the corridor created by a small corticotomy. The stylet was then removed and in place, a 4 mm rod-lens endoscope with irrigation capability was introduced into the transparent sheath. The use of a transparent sheath compared to traditional opaque or metal sheaths was noted to provide

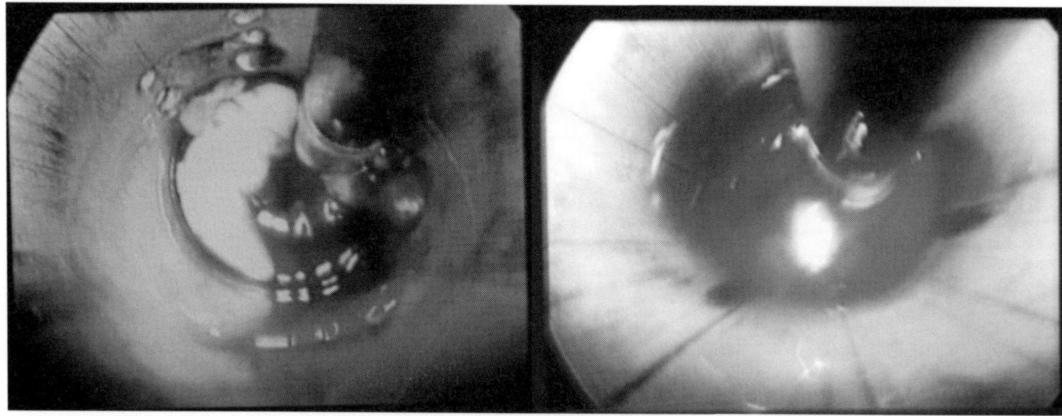

Fig. 22c.5 Intraoperative endoscopic views of a spontaneous intracerebral hemorrhage are shown. (See plate section for color version).

improved visualization of the surgical field. Sixty-eight patients were included in this retrospective study, comprising 35 putaminal ICH, 24 thalamic ICH, and 9 subcortical ICH [28]. Overall median hematoma evacuation rate was 93%. Detectable intra-operative bleeding was present in 30% of patients, with rebleeding noted in 1.5%. Overall morbidity and mortality was 4.4% and 5.9%, respectively. Average blood loss was 65 ml, and mean duration of surgery was 85 minutes. With regards to functional status, mean GCS score pre-operatively was 7.1 for all patients, and 1 week post-operative and 6 months post-operative GCS scores were 11.0 and 11.6, respectively [28]. Zhu and colleagues [85]. utilized a similar technique and found that, compared to traditional craniotomies, the evacuation rate using the endoscopic approach was significantly greater, with a reduced rate of infection. Mortality rates, however, did not differ between groups.

In 2010, Lin *et al.* [32] described their application of three-dimensional reconstructed CT scans during their endoscopic evacuations as a simple, economic, and accurate means of targeting their lesion of interest with an average preparation time of 15 minutes. After the optimal trajectory was determined for access to the hematoma, a steel sheath was inserted via the burr hole opening and positioning confirmed with ultrasound. Their average evacuation rate for all patients was 82%, with an average Glasgow Outcome Scale score of 3.5 at 3 months follow-up for their 11 patients studied with hypertensive putaminal hemorrhages who had an average GCS of 8.6 pre-operatively. In fact, ten patients regained consciousness within 7 days of surgery, and there were no surgery-associated morbidities.

Post-operative management

Following completion of the surgery, a head CT is required to assess the quality of the evacuation and decompression. This may be done either in the operating room if a portable CT scanner is available, or within 1 hour post-operatively in the radiology suite. Subsequent surveillance imaging, either a CT or MRI scan, should be completed on post-operative days one, seven, and additionally as clinically indicated to evaluate for rebleeding.

Patients are re-admitted to the neuro-intensive care unit and systolic blood pressure is maintained between 100 and 140 mmHg. Daily labs are followed, sodium is kept within normal limits and any coagulopathy is corrected.

Conclusion

The UCLA experience with endoscopic evacuation of sICH includes 41 patients over a 9-year interval. During this time period our aspiration technique advanced from direct endoscopic visualization to the current technique of stereotactic guidance for hematoma evacuation at two specific locations. This technique relies on careful pre-operative planning and intra-operative stereotactic guidance rather than direct endoscopic visualization of the hematoma. This approach allows the surgeon to access the long axis of the hematoma, providing excellent reduction in ICH volume while minimizing manipulation of the endoscope sheath. Overall, post-operative sICH volumes were found to be reduced by nearly 70%, with greater than 50% reduction in approximately 80% of patients (Fig. 22c.6). While our series, with an overall average ICH score of two, would be expected to display a mortality of 26%, our 12% 30-day mortality represents a considerable improvement in patient survival [23]. Thirty-day morbidities included one incident of rebleeding (2.4%), an ipsilateral stroke (2.4%) and a subdural hematoma (2.4%). In our series, there was a trend towards increased ICH evacuation volumes (81% versus 58.5%, $p = 0.08$) and improved clinical outcomes with the transition to our current stereotactic guidance aspiration technique.

The utilization of endoscopic evacuation of sICH may allow for lower morbidity and mortality, decreased operative time, decreased blood loss, increased evacuation rates, and improved recovery for patients [28]. However, while operations performed on patients who are deeply comatose with severe irreversible brain damage may be lifesaving, they likely will not

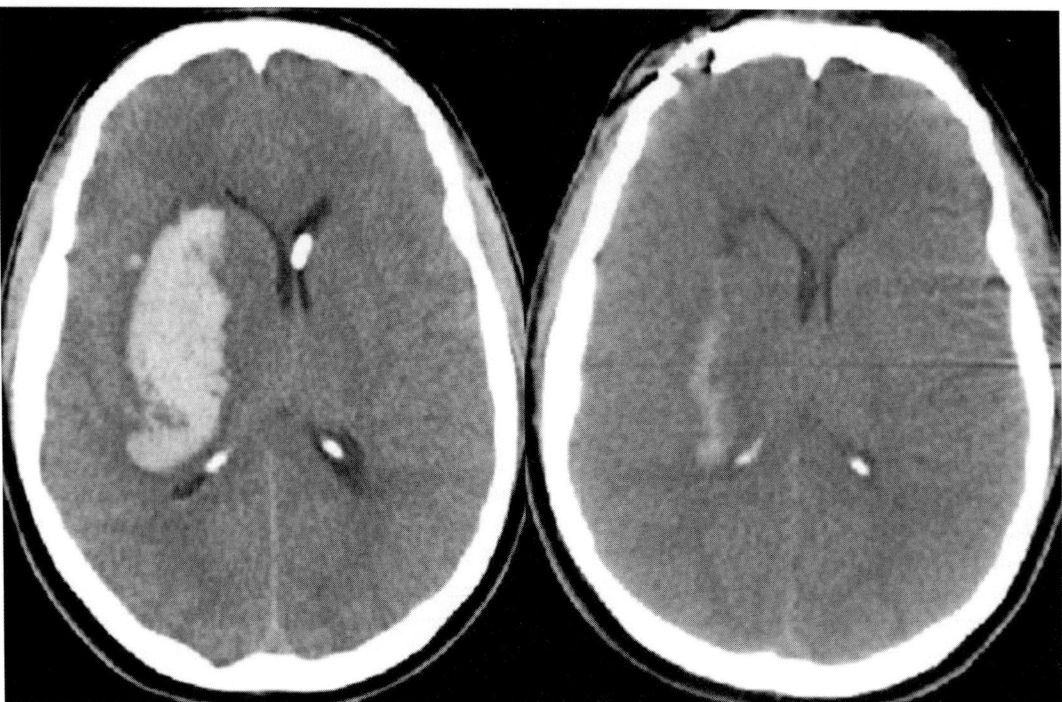

Fig. 22c.6 Non-contrast CT scans are shown before (left) and after (right) endoscopic evacuation.

afford much functional improvement and can be a costly endeavor [27,42,86,87]. As such, appropriate patient selection and ideal surgical timing still necessitate further investigation in order to improve neurosurgical efforts and optimize patient outcomes.

REFERENCES

1. Daverat, P., *et al.*, Death and functional outcome after spontaneous intracerebral hemorrhage. A prospective study of 166 cases using multivariate analysis. *Stroke*, 1991;**22**(1):1–6.
2. Broderick, J., *et al.*, Guidelines for the management of spontaneous intracerebral hemorrhage in adults: 2007 update: a guideline from the American Heart Association/American Stroke Association Stroke Council, High Blood Pressure Research Council, and the Quality of Care and Outcomes in Research Interdisciplinary Working Group. *Stroke*, 2007;**38**(6):2001–23.
3. Flaherty, M.L., Anticoagulant-associated intracerebral hemorrhage. *Semin Neurol*, 2010;**30**(5):565–72.
4. Furlan, A.J., J.P. Whisnant, L.R. Elveback, The decreasing incidence of primary intracerebral hemorrhage: a population study. *Annals Neurol*, 1979;**5**(4):367–73.
5. Brown, R.D., *et al.*, Stroke incidence, prevalence, and survival: secular trends in Rochester, Minnesota, through 1989. *Stroke*, 1996;**27**(3):373–80.
6. Flaherty, M.L., *et al.*, Racial variations in location and risk of intracerebral hemorrhage. *Stroke*, 2005;**36**(5):934–7.
7. Kissela, B., *et al.*, Stroke in a biracial population: the excess burden of stroke among blacks. *Stroke* 2004;**35**(2):426–31.
8. Taylor, T., *et al.*, Lifetime cost of stroke in the United States. *Stroke*, 1996;**27**(9):1459–66.
9. Hinton, D.R., E. Dolan, and A.A. Sima, The value of histopathological examination of surgically removed blood clot in determining the etiology of spontaneous intracerebral hemorrhage. *Stroke*, 1984;**15**(3):517–20.
10. Labovitz, D.L., *et al.*, The incidence of deep and lobar intracerebral hemorrhage in whites, blacks, and Hispanics. *Neurology*, 2005;**65**(4):518–22.

11. Woo, D., *et al.*, Effect of untreated hypertension on hemorrhagic stroke. *Stroke*, 2004;**35**(7):1703–8.
12. Cordonnier, C., *et al.*, Radiological investigation of spontaneous intracerebral hemorrhage: systematic review and trinational survey. *Stroke*, 2010;**41**(4):685–90.
13. Knudsen, K.A., *et al.*, Clinical diagnosis of cerebral amyloid angiopathy: validation of the Boston criteria. *Neurology*, 2001;**56**(4):537–9.
14. Broderick, J.P., *et al.*, Intracerebral hemorrhage more than twice as common as subarachnoid hemorrhage. *J Neurosurgery*, 1993;**78**(2):188–91.
15. Sacco, S., *et al.*, Incidence and 10-year survival of intracerebral hemorrhage in a population-based registry. *Stroke*, 2009;**40**(2):394–9.
16. Miller, C.M., *et al.*, Image-guided endoscopic evacuation of spontaneous intracerebral hemorrhage. *Surg Neurol*, 2008;**69**(5):441–6; discussion 446.
17. Counsell, C., *et al.*, Primary Intracerebral Hemorrhage in the Oxfordshire Community Stroke Project. 2. Prognosis. *Cerebrovasc Dis*, 1995;**5**(1):26–34.
18. Douglas, M.A., A.F. Haerer, Long-term prognosis of hypertensive intracerebral hemorrhage. *Stroke*, 1982;**13**(4):488–91.
19. Helweg-Larsen, S., *et al.*, Prognosis for patients treated conservatively for spontaneous intracerebral hematomas. *Stroke*, 1984;**15**(6):1045–8.
20. Kojima, S., *et al.*, Prognosis and disability of stroke patients after 5 years in Akita, Japan. *Stroke*, 1990;**21**(1):72–7.
21. Batjer, H.H., *et al.*, Failure of surgery to improve outcome in hypertensive putaminal hemorrhage. A prospective randomized trial. *Arch Neurol*, 1990;**47**(10):1103–6.
22. Mendelow, A.D., *et al.*, Early surgery versus initial conservative treatment in patients with spontaneous supratentorial intracerebral haematomas in the International Surgical Trial in Intracerebral Haemorrhage (STICH): a randomised trial. *Lancet*, 2005;**365**(9457):387–97.
23. Morgenstern, L.B., *et al.*, Rebleeding leads to poor outcome in ultra-early craniotomy for intracerebral hemorrhage. *Neurology*, 2001;**56**(10):1294–9.
24. Gregson, B.A., *et al.*, Individual patient data subgroup meta-analysis of surgery for spontaneous supratentorial intracerebral hemorrhage. *Stroke*, 2012;**43**(6):1496–504.
25. Suzuki, J., T. Ebina, Sequential changes in tissue surrounding ICH, in Pia HW, Langmaid C, Zierski J (eds). *Spontaneous Intracerebral Hematomas. Advances in Diagnosis and Therapy*. 1980, Berlin: Spinger-Verlag.
26. Mendelow, A.D., Bullock, F.P. Nath, Experimental intracerebral haemorrhage: intracranial pressure changes and cerebral blood flow, in Miller JD, Teasdale GM, Rowan JO, *et al.* (eds). *Intracranial Pressure VI*. 1986, Berlin: Springer-Verlag. 515–20.
27. Auer, L.M., *et al.*, Endoscopic surgery versus medical treatment for spontaneous intracerebral hematoma: a randomized study. *J Neurosurg*, 1989;**70**(4):530–5.
28. Kuo, L.T., *et al.*, Early endoscope-assisted hematoma evacuation in patients with supratentorial intracerebral hemorrhage: case selection, surgical technique, and long-term results. *Neurosurg Focus*, 2011;**30**(4):E9.
29. Zuo, Y., *et al.*, Gross-total hematoma removal of hypertensive basal ganglia hemorrhages: a long-term follow-up. *J Neurol Sci*, 2009;**287**(1–2):100–4.
30. Nagasaka, T., *et al.*, Early recovery and better evacuation rate in neuroendoscopic surgery for spontaneous intracerebral hemorrhage using a multifunctional cannula: preliminary study in comparison with craniotomy. *J Stroke Cerebrovasc Dis* 2011;**20**(3):208–13.
31. Juttler, E., and T. Steiner, Treatment and prevention of spontaneous intracerebral hemorrhage: comparison of EUSI and AHA/ASA recommendations. *Expert Rev Neurotherapeutics*, 2007;**7**(10):1401–16.
32. Lin, H.L., *et al.*, Endoscopic evacuation of hypertensive putaminal hemorrhage guided by the 3D reconstructed CT scan: a preliminary report. *Clin Neurol Neurosurg*, 2010;**112**(10):892–6.
33. Kwak, R., S. Kadoya, T. Suzuki, Factors affecting the prognosis in thalamic hemorrhage. *Stroke*, 1983;**14**(4):493–500.
34. Mendelow, A.D., Mechanisms of ischemic brain damage with intracerebral hemorrhage. *Stroke*, 1993;**24**(12 Suppl): I115–17; discussion 118–19.
35. Jenkins, A., *et al.*, Experimental intracerebral haematoma: the role of blood constituents in early ischaemia. *Br J Neurosurg*, 1990;**4**(1):45–51.
36. Liu, Z.H., *et al.*, Evacuation of hypertensive intracerebral hematoma by a stereotactic technique. *Stereotactic and Functional Neurosurg*, 1990;**54**–5:451–2.
37. Muiz, A.J., *et al.*, Spontaneous intracerebral hemorrhage in northeast Malaysian patients: a four-year study. *Neuroepidemiology*, 2003;**22**(3):184–95.
38. Nehls, D.G., *et al.*, Experimental intracerebral hemorrhage: early removal of a spontaneous mass lesion improves late outcome. *Neurosurgery*, 1990;**27**(5):674–82; discussion 682.
39. Takasugi, S., S. Ueda, K. Matsumoto, Chronological changes in spontaneous intracerebral hematoma – an experimental and clinical study. *Stroke*, 1985;**16**(4):651–8.
40. Ropper, A.H., N.T. Zervas, Cerebral blood flow after experimental basal ganglia hemorrhage. *Annals Neurol*, 1982;**11**(3):266–71.

41. Morgan, T., *et al.*, Preliminary findings of the minimally-invasive surgery plus rtPA for intracerebral hemorrhage evacuation (MISTIE) clinical trial. *Acta Neurochirurgica*. Supp, 2008;**105**:147–51.
42. Cho, D.Y., *et al.*, Endoscopic surgery for spontaneous basal ganglia hemorrhage: comparing endoscopic surgery, stereotactic aspiration, and craniotomy in noncomatose patients. *Surg Neurol*, 2006;**65**(6):547–55; discussion 555–6.
43. Lee, J.I., *et al.*, Stereotactic aspiration of intracerebral haematoma: significance of surgical timing and haematoma volume reduction. *J Clin Neurosci*, 2003;**10**(4):439–43.
44. Morgenstern, L.B., *et al.*, Surgical treatment for intracerebral hemorrhage (STICH): a single-center, randomized clinical trial. *Neurology*, 1998;**51**(5):1359–63.
45. McKissock, W., Parasagittal meningioma of pre-natal origin. *Proc Royal Soc Med*, 1939;**32**(3):221–2.
46. Juvela, S., *et al.*, The treatment of spontaneous intracerebral hemorrhage. A prospective randomized trial of surgical and conservative treatment. *J Neurosurg*, 1989;**70**(5):755–8.
47. Zuccarello, M., *et al.*, Early surgical treatment for supratentorial intracerebral hemorrhage: a randomized feasibility study. *Stroke*, 1999;**30**(9):1833–9.
48. Teernstra, O.P., *et al.*, Stereotactic treatment of intracerebral hematoma by means of a plasminogen activator: a multicenter randomized controlled trial (SICHPA). *Stroke*, 2003;**34**(4):968–74.
49. Pantazis, G., *et al.*, Early surgical treatment vs conservative management for spontaneous supratentorial intracerebral hematomas: A prospective randomized study. *Surg Neurol*, 2006;**66**(5):492–501; discussion 501–2.
50. Hattori, N., *et al.*, Impact of stereotactic hematoma evacuation on activities of daily living during the chronic period following spontaneous putaminal hemorrhage: a randomized study. *J Neurosurg*, 2004;**101**(3):417–20.
51. Wang, W.Z., *et al.*, Minimally invasive craniopuncture therapy vs. conservative treatment for spontaneous intracerebral hemorrhage: results from a randomized clinical trial in China. *Int J Stroke*, 2009;**4**(1):11–16.
52. Chen, X., H. Yang, Z. Cheng, A prospective randomised trial of surgical and conservative treatment of hypertensive intracerebral haemorrhage. *Acta Acad Shanghai Med*, 1992;**19**:237–240.
53. Hosseini, H., *et al.*, Stereotactic aspiration of deep intracerebral hematomas under computed tomographic control: a multicentric prospective randomised trial. *Cerebrovasc Dis*, 2003;**16**s:57.
54. Anik, I., *et al.*, Meta-analyses of intracerebral hematoma treatment. *Turkish Neurosurg*, 2011;**21**(1):6–14.
55. Zhou, H., *et al.*, Minimally invasive stereotactic puncture and thrombolysis therapy improves long-term outcome after acute intracerebral hemorrhage. *J Neurol*, 2011;**258**(4):661–9.
56. Miller, C.M., *et al.*, Frameless stereotactic aspiration and thrombolysis of deep intracerebral hemorrhage is associated with reduced levels of extracellular cerebral glutamate and unchanged lactate pyruvate ratios. *Neurocrit Care*, 2007;**6**(1):22–9.
57. Niizuma, H., *et al.*, Results of stereotactic aspiration in cases of putaminal hemorrhage. *Neurosurgery*, 1989;**24**(6):814–19.
58. Vespa, P., *et al.*, Frameless stereotactic aspiration and thrombolysis of deep intracerebral hemorrhage is associated with reduction of hemorrhage volume and neurological improvement. *Neurocrit Care*, 2005; **2**(3):274–81.
59. Carvi, Y.N.M., *et al.*, Evaluation of invasiveness and efficacy of 2 different keyhole approaches to large basal ganglia hematomas. *Surg Neurol*, 2005;**64**(3):253–9; discussion 260.
60. Barlas, O., *et al.*, Image-guided keyhole evacuation of spontaneous supratentorial intracerebral hemorrhage. *Minimally Invasive Neurosurg*, 2009;**52**(2):62–8.
61. Auer, L.M., Endoscopic evacuation of intracerebral haemorrhage. High-tech surgical treatment – a new approach to the problem? *Acta Neurochirurgica*, 1985;**74**(3–4):124–8.
62. Prasad, K., *et al.*, Surgery in primary supratentorial intracerebral hematoma: a meta-analysis of randomized trials. *Acta Neurologica Scandinavica*, 1997;**95**(2):103–10.
63. Hsieh, P.C., *et al.*, Endoscopic evacuation of putaminal hemorrhage: how to improve the efficiency of hematoma evacuation. *Surg Neurol*, 2005;**64**(2):147–53; discussion 153.
64. Nagasaka, T., *et al.*, Inflation-deflation method for endoscopic evacuation of intracerebral haematoma. *Acta Neurochirurgica*, 2008;**150**(7):685–90; discussion 690.
65. Nagasaka, T., *et al.*, Balanced irrigation-suction technique with a multifunctional suction cannula and its application for intraoperative hemorrhage in endoscopic evacuation of intracerebral hematomas: technical note. *Neurosurgery*, 2009;**65**(4):E826–7; discussion E827.
66. Nishihara, T., *et al.*, Newly developed endoscopic instruments for the removal of intracerebral hematoma. *Neurocrit Care*, 2005;**2**(1):67–74.
67. Chen, C.C., *et al.*, Endoscopic surgery for intraventricular hemorrhage (IVH) caused by thalamic hemorrhage: comparisons of endoscopic surgery and external

ventricular drainage (EVD) surgery. *World Neurosurg*, 2011;**75**(2):264–8.

68. Arboix, A., *et al.*, Site of bleeding and early outcome in primary intracerebral hemorrhage. *Acta Neurologica Scandinavica*, 2002;**105**(4):282–8.
69. Steinke, W., *et al.*, Thalamic stroke. Presentation and prognosis of infarcts and hemorrhages. *Arch Neurol*, 1992;**49** (7):703–10.
70. Miller, C., G. Tsivgoulis, P. Nakaji, Predictors of ventriculoperitoneal shunting after spontaneous intraparenchymal hemorrhage. *Neurocrit Care*, 2008;**8**(2):235–40.
71. Nishikawa, T., *et al.*, A priority treatment of the intraventricular hemorrhage (IVH) should be performed in the patients suffering intracerebral hemorrhage with large IVH. *Clin Neurol Neurosurg*, 2009;**111**(5):450–3.
72. Morgenstern, L.B., *et al.*, Guidelines for the management of spontaneous intracerebral hemorrhage: a guideline for healthcare professionals from the American Heart Association/American Stroke Association. *Stroke*, 2010;**41**(9):2108–29.
73. Brott, T., *et al.*, Early hemorrhage growth in patients with intracerebral hemorrhage. *Stroke*, 1997;**28**(1):1–5.
74. Leira, R., *et al.*, Early neurologic deterioration in intracerebral hemorrhage: predictors and associated factors. *Neurology*, 2004;**63**(3):461–7.
75. Cucchiara, B., *et al.*, Hematoma growth in oral anticoagulant related intracerebral hemorrhage. *Stroke*, 2008;**39**(11): 2993–6.
76. Davis, S.M., *et al.*, Hematoma growth is a determinant of mortality and poor outcome after intracerebral hemorrhage. *Neurology*, 2006;**66**(8):1175–81.
77. Kazui, S., *et al.*, Predisposing factors to enlargement of spontaneous intracerebral hematoma. *Stroke*, 1997;**28**(12): 2370–5.
78. Fujii, Y., *et al.*, Multivariate analysis of predictors of hematoma enlargement in spontaneous intracerebral hemorrhage. *Stroke*, 1998;**29**(6):1160–6.
79. Kaneko, M., *et al.*, Long-term evaluation of ultra-early operation for hypertensive intracerebral hemorrhage in 100 cases. *J Neurosurg*, 1983;**58**(6):838–42.
80. Mendelow, A.D., *et al.*, Surgical trial in lobar intracerebral haemorrhage (STICH II) protocol. *Trials*, 2011;**12**:124.
81. Morgan, T., *et al.*, Preliminary report of the clot lysis evaluating accelerated resolution of intraventricular hemorrhage (CLEAR-IVH) clinical trial. *Acta Neurochirurgica. Supp*, 2008;**105**:217–20.
82. Bakshi, A., A.K. Banerji, Neuroendoscope-assisted evacuation of large intracerebral hematomas: introduction of a new, minimally invasive technique. Preliminary report. *Neurosurg Focus*, 2004;**16**(6):e9.
83. Lin, C.Y., M.C. Yang, S.H. Liou, Estimating the costs of cerebrovascular disease for the insured labors under the labor insurance, 1991. *Taiwan J Public Health*, 2001;**20**:34–42.
84. Hellwig, D., *et al.*, Endoscopic stereotaxy – an eight year experience. *Stereotactic and Functional Neurosurg*, 1997;**68**(1–4 Pt 1):90–7.
85. Zhu, H., Z. Wang, W. Shi, Keyhole endoscopic hematoma evacuation in patients. *Turkish Neurosurg*, 2012;**22** (3):294–9.
86. Singh, R.V., C.J. Prusmack, J.J. Morcos, Spontaneous intracerebral hemorrhage: non-arteriovenous malformation, non-aneurysm. *Youmans Neurological Surgery*. 5th ed. in Winn HR (ed). 2003, Philadelphia: Saunders.
87. Hankey, G.J., C. Hon, Surgery for primary intracerebral hemorrhage: is it safe and effective? A systematic review of case series and randomized trials. *Stroke*, 1997;**28**(11): 2126–32.

23

Intraventricular hemorrhage

Wendy C. Ziai and Daniel Hanley

Introduction

Intraventricular hemorrhage (IVH) frequently complicates subarachnoid hemorrhage (SAH) and intracranial hemorrhage (ICH). In both settings, IVH is a significant and independent contributor to morbidity and mortality, yet therapy directed at ameliorating intraventricular clot has been limited (1–6). Mechanisms of IVH-induced brain injury include increased intracranial pressure (ICP) and ischemic encephalopathy by virtue of mass effect from hemorrhage or associated hydrocephalus due to ventricular outflow obstruction. More recently, direct toxicity of blood products within the ventricle has been implicated in mechanisms by which IVH exerts deleterious effects (7).

We review the topic intraventricular hemorrhage, articulating the scope of the problem, standard and investigational therapies, management issues, and relevant questions for future research.

Epidemiology

Brain hemorrhage is the stroke subtype with the highest morbidity and mortality. Respectively, ICH and SAH account for about 15% and 5% of the 750 000 strokes occurring yearly in the United States, totaling more than 45 000 patients per year (8–10). Approximately 45% of spontaneous ICH and 25% of aneurysmal SAH extend into the ventricles (8,10–12). For patients with both ICH and significant IVH, the expected mortality is 50–80% (13,14). Patients with severe IVH are twice as likely to have poor outcomes (a modified Rankin scale [mRS] score of 4–6 at hospital discharge) and nearly three times more likely to die than their cohorts without IVH (7).

Risk factors for IVH in association with ICH include older age, higher baseline ICH volume, mean arterial pressure (MAP) values greater than 120 mmHg, and deep subcortical location of primary ICH in close proximity to ventricles (13).

Definition and IVH subtypes

IVH is the occurrence of bleeding into any part of the ventricular system in the brain. IVH can range from mild layering of the blood in the posterior horn of the lateral ventricle to complete casting of all the ventricles. Primary IVH, with a reported incidence of 3–7% is confined to the ventricular system and ependymal lining of the ventricle, and originates from either an intraventricular source or a lesion within the ventricular wall (e.g. intraventricular trauma, aneurysm, vascular malformation or tumor usually involving the choroid plexus (1)). Dural arteriovenous malformations have rarely been described in association with primary IVH with the explanation that retrograde venous drainage creates backflow into subependymal veins causing their rupture (15). Secondary IVH is the result of

Critical Care of the Stroke Patient, ed. Stefan Schwab, Daniel Hanley, and A. David Mendelow. Published by Cambridge University Press.

Table 23.1 Etiologies of intraventricular hemorrhage

Primary IVH
Head trauma
Insertion/removal of a ventricular catheter
Intraventricular vascular malformation, aneurysm, tumor
Bleeding diathesis
Moyamoya disease
Choroid plexus vascular malformation
Secondary IVH
Extension of intracerebral hematoma or subarachnoid hemorrhage caused by:
Hypertension
Cerebral aneurysm
Head trauma
Arteriovenous malformation
Vasculitis
Coagulation disorder
Hemorrhagic transformation of an ischemic infarct
Tumor
Extension of a germinal matrix hematoma (premature infants)

Adapted from Andrews CO, Engelhard HH. 2001 (16).

extension of an intracerebral hemorrhage or subarachnoid hemorrhage into the ventricular system (Table 23.1).

Pathophysiology

Within the first week of hemorrhage onset, the intraventricular clot is solid and there is CSF circulation of blood and blood degredation products to the basal cisterns and subarachnoid space. In the absence of any underlying vascular lesion, vascular rupture into the ventricle from parenchymal ICH may occur by two proposed pathogenic mechanisms. Although lacking photographic evidence, Gordon described erosion of the ventricular wall under the ventricular hemorrhage, and distention of regional subependymal vessels with some vessels occluded by thrombus (17). It is not clear, however, if ependymal erosion is the primary event or occurs secondary to the presence of intraventricular blood (18). Small hemorrhagic infarcts in the parenchyma at the ventricular edge with presumed secondary rupture through the ependyma have also been described (18).

IVH contributes to morbidity by causing acute obstructive hydrocephalus, which elevates intracranial pressure (ICP) and decreases cerebral perfusion pressure and, if severe enough, results in brain herniation. Controlling ICP as with an external ventricular drain (EVD), however, does not usually result in immediate mental status improvement (19). Thus, direct mass effect of IVH may be a significant pathophysiologic factor independent of ICP elevation. Cerebral ischemia, and the toxic effects of ventricular blood on adjacent periventricular brain tissue, including hippocampus, diencephalon, and brainstem may also play an important role (20). Vasospasm due to CSF circulation of blood into the basal cisterns may contribute to the role of inflammation (21). The primary treatment for IVH with hydrocephalus, an EVD may also worsen edema and inflammation when complicated by bacterial meningitis. Finally, permanent occlusion and scarring of arachnoid granulations where CSF is absorbed results in delayed communicating hydrocephalus, which necessitates permanent CSF shunt placement in 30–60% and is associated with impaired cognition, gait, balance, and urinary continence (22–25).

Prognostication in IVH

IVH volume is a surrogate for IVH severity and larger volumes correlate with worse prognosis. This relationship was originally described by Tuhrim, who developed a model in which IVH volume contributed significantly to 30-day outcome prediction when controlling for the presence or absence of hydrocephalus and size of associated ICH, thus establishing IVH volume as an independent prognostic factor of poor outcome, together with Glasgow coma scale (GCS) score (Fig. 23.1)(26). Patients with IVH in addition to ICH have lower initial GCS and larger ICH volume. Number of ventricles containing blood, and blood in the fourth ventricle also contribute to poorer outcome. In a series of patients with supratentorial ICH and IVH,

Table 23.2 IVH score

Component	Points
GCS score	
≥ 13	0
9–12	1
≤ 8	2
ICH volume (ml)	
< 30	0
≥ 30	1
≥ 60	2
Hydrocephalus	
Absent	0
Moderate	1
Severe	2
Age	
< 70	0
≥ 70	1
Total	0–7

GCS: Glasgow Coma Scale; ICH: intracerebral hemorrhage. Thirty-day mortality for scores of 2,3,4,5 and 6 were 9.1%, 14.3%, 46.2%, 75% and 100% respectively (31).

Young *et al.* (27) demonstrated that patients with more than 20 cc of interventricular blood in general had poor outcome. Another study examining patients with large IVH found that the etiology of the IVH was more important in predicting outcome than the volume of IVH (28).

Anatomic factors related to hydrocephalus may also be important. Both third and fourth hemorrhagic ventricular dilation were reported as significant predictors of long-term poor outcome in separate studies (29,30). Stein *et al.* developed an IVH score for prediction of 30-day mortality in patients treated with external ventricular drainage (EVD) (31). Independent predictors of outcome were ICH volume > 60 ml, severe hydrocephalus, GCS ≤ 8 and age ≥ 70 years (Table 23.2). This score performed favorably when compared to other prognostic models for ICH especially for prediction of 30-day mortality and functional outcome at 6 months (32). ICH scoring tools which performed best were those that included the quantification of IVH or grading of hydrocephalus.

Expansion of IVH in the first 24 hours has been identified as a predictor of death or severe disability (14, 33). In the FAST trial (recombinant activated factor VII-rFVIIa), IVH growth, by 24 hours, defined as an increase in IVH volume of > 2 ml, occurred in 17%

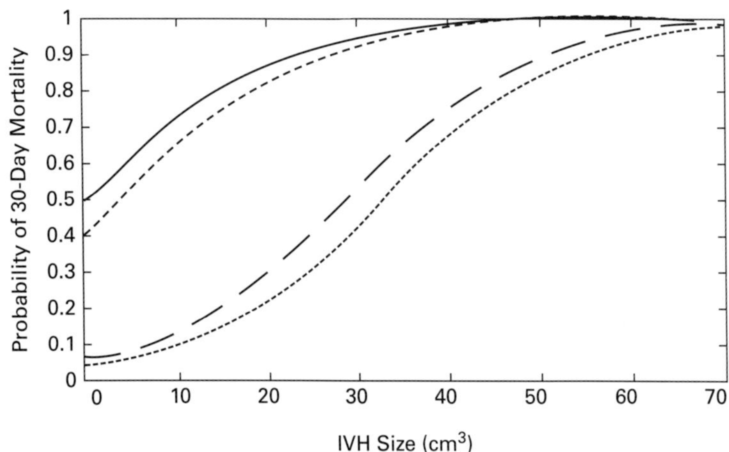

Fig. 23.1. Effect of increasing IVH volume on predicted 30-day mortality. Lines represent specific disease severity groupings. In this model, IVH volume accounts for > 50% of mortality independent of GCS or initial ICH size. Adapted from: Turhim S *et al.* 1999 (26).

and 10% of placebo- and rFVIIa-treated patients, respectively (14). Risk factors for IVH growth included baseline MAP greater than 120 mmHg, larger baseline ICH volume, IVH present at baseline, shorter time from symptom onset to baseline CT scan, and treatment with rFVIIa (versus placebo). Early IVH growth was also found to be an independent predictor of death or severe disability among other factors (older age, lower baseline GCS, larger baseline ICH volume, IVH present at baseline or 24 hours, and treatment with rFVIIa).

IVH in patients with aneurysmal SAH is associated with greater likelihood of clinical deterioration, higher frequency of symptomatic vasospasm and cerebral infarction, higher likelihood of hydrocephalus and fever at day eight, and shunt-dependent chronic hydrocephalus (34). SAH patients with IVH have significant cognitive deficits compared to those without IVH on neuropsychological testing (35). IVH in association with blunt TBI reflects the severity of the head injury and is associated with poor outcome; only half of patients are independent at 6 month follow-up (36). A better outcome can be expected if only the lateral ventricles are involved and there is no associated extra-axial or intracerebral hemorrhage.

Grading IVH

Several scoring systems have been developed for calculating the amount and hence severity of IVH. Software dependent volumetric analysis is expected to become a clinically accessible tool in the near future.

The Graeb scale (Table 23.3) (1) is the most commonly reported scale in adults and has a reported significant correlation with short-term outcome (Glasgow Outcome Score at 1 month) (37). In patients with ICH volume < 60 cc, a Graeb score ≥ 6 is associated with acute hydrocephalus and a Graeb score ≤ 5 is associated with GCS ≥ 12 on admission.

The modified Graeb scale (mGS) expanded the original Graeb scale with estimated IVH volume divided into quartiles and extra points given for expansion of separate ventricle compartments (Table 23.3) (38). It is currently used in the CLEAR IVH clinical trial. Agreement between operators for measurement of the mGS appears to be high (Interclass Correlation Coefficient > 0.94, 95% CI: [0.93, 0.95]) and correlation between the mGS and IVH volume (by computerized volumetry) was strong (R = 0.81, 95% CI: [0.77, 0.85]). Baseline mGS was found to be predictive of mRS at 180 days (area under receiving operating characteristic curve 0.74, 95% confidence interval, 0.57–0.91); each unit increase in the mGS led to a 12% increase in the odds of a poor outcome.

The IVH score (IVHS) uses a similar concept, and can be converted to IVH volume in ml using a logarithmic transformation (39). The IVHS is similar to the Graeb score with respect to assigning a number to each lateral ventricle based on amount of blood and adding one point for presence of hydrocephalus. One point was given for up to one-third filling of the ventricle with blood, 2 points for one-third to two-thirds filled with blood, and 3 points for a ventricle mostly or completely filled with blood. The third and fourth ventricles were each assigned a score of 0 for no blood and 1 for partial or complete filling with blood. The final formula for calculating the IVHS is:

IVHS = 3 × (RV + LV) + III + IV + 3 × H, where RV = right ventricle, LV = left ventricle, III = third ventricle, IV = fourth ventricle, and H = hydrocephalus score. The IVHS ranges from 0–23.

The formula for converting the IVHS to volume is: IVH volume (ml) = $e^{IVHS/5}$. One can also use a reference card (Table 23.3). The addition of IVH volume to ICH volume (using ABC/2 method) to produce total hemorrhage volume improved upon the predictive power for poor outcome and mortality over both the Graeb score and the ICH score (40). The IVHS remains to be prospectively validated.

The LeRoux scale (41) was developed for evaluating traumatic IVH. Although fairly simple, when compared with the IVH and Graeb scores in a series of 73 primary ICH patients with IVH, it predicted outcome relatively well and with similarly good accuracy when assessed at admission and within 6 days after hemorrhage (42).

Table 23.3 IVH scales

Graeb scale (maximum total score = 12)(1)
Lateral ventricles (each one scored separately)
1 = trace of blood or mild bleeding
2 = less than half of the ventricle filled with blood
3 = more than half of the ventricle filled with blood
4 = ventricle filled with blood and expanded
Third and fourth ventricles (each one scored separately)
1 = blood present, ventricle size normal
2 = ventricle filled with blood and expanded

Modified Graeb scale (maximum total score = 32)(37)

	Scores for each ventricle							
% of blood	R ant tip	R lateral	R post tip	L ant tip	L lateral	L post tip	IIIrd	IVth
None	0	0	0	0	0	0	0	0
≤ 25%	1	1	1	1	1	1	2	2
> 25% to ≤ 50%	1	2	1	1	2	1	2	2
> 50% to ≤ 75%	2	3	2	2	3	2	4	4
> 75% to 100%	2	4	2	2	4	2	4	4
Expanded	+1	+1	+1	+1	+1	+1	+1	+1

IVH score: reference card for converting IVH score to IVH volume (39)

IVH score	IVH volume (ml)	IVH score	IVH volume (ml)
1	1 .2	13	13.5
2	1 .5	14	16.4
3	1 .8	15	20.1
4	2.2	16	24.5
5	2.7	17	30.0
6	3.3	18	36.6
7	4.1	19	44.7
8	5.0	20	54.6
9	6.0	21	66.7
10	7.4	22	81.5
11	9.0	23	99.5
12	11.0		

Le Roux scale (each ventricle graded separately, and the scores summed) (36). Score range: 1–16.
1 = trace of blood
2 = less than half of the ventricle filled with blood
3 = more than half of the ventricle filled with blood
4 = ventricle filled with blood and expanded

Conventional therapy

The standard of care for management of IVH causing obstructive hydrocephalus remains placement of an EVD for cerebral spinal fluid (CSF) diversion and ICP control. The EVD also assists with removal of some ventricular blood breakdown products which may contribute to chemical meningitis (43).

Hydrocephalus occurs in 20–40% of all IVH patients (44). The clinical benefit of external ventricular drainage (EVD) is debated (45) despite the knowledge that obstructive hydrocephalus on admission CT is an independent predictor of increased in-hospital and 30-day mortality (44, 46) and also of 6 month neurologic outcome for caudate ICH (47). In the STICH trial (Surgical Treatment for ICH), favorable outcomes were less frequent when IVH was present and significantly lower when hydrocephalus was also present (48).

Indications for EVD in IVH

Although ICP is possibly managed medically with sedation and osmotic diuretics, such management is often insufficient to reduce ICP. Precise diagnosis and management in almost all settings call for EVD placement (49). An analysis of an IVH cohort from a large prospective randomized study of thrombolysis for IVH demonstrated that continuous drainage of CSF contributes to the normalization of ICP and that higher ICP (> 30 mmHg) was an independent predictor of morbidity and mortality (50). Huttner found that long-term outcomes in patients with pure ganglionic ICH were not different from those with IVH and EVD treatment, suggesting that drainage of CSF was beneficial (51). In another systematic review of 23 retrospective studies of IVH in the setting of ICH and SAH, the placement of an EVD improved mortality, but not morbidity of IVH (52). The case fatality rate was 78% in conservatively treated patients (n = 176) vs. 58% with EVD (n = 118); unfavorable outcome (modified Rankin score 4 or 5) was not different: 90% vs. 89% respectively). These findings suggest that EVD assists with control of ICP, lowering early mortality, but has little impact on morbidity, perhaps due to underlying damage from associated cerebral ischemia, and the toxic effects of ventricular blood on adjacent periventricular brain tissue, including hippocampus, diencephalon and brainstem. EVD does not alter the rate of blood clot resolution (53) and therefore fails to decrease the degree and incidence of communicating hydrocephalus. Moreover, catheter occlusions occur frequently in the setting of large IVH volume and can result in poor ICP control. Catheter occlusions also require repeated catheter removals and insertions, thus increasing the risks of hemorrhage and infection (54). The precise thresholds for insertion of EVD after IVH have not been clarified, but it is generally agreed that the presence of hydrocephalus and deteriorating neurologic condition are an indication for placing an EVD. It is unclear whether an EVD is beneficial in anticipation of potential ventricular obstruction in patients with good neurologic condition, or to enhance clearance of obstructive IVH. Similarly, the precise target(s) for placement of EVD(s) has not been systematically investigated.

Investigational therapies

The natural history of IVH is for radiographically observed blood to gradually disappear over a period of 2–3 weeks although IVH may persist for many months after onset. Naff *et al.* (55) showed that blood clot resolution in CSF follows first-order kinetics. An EVD does not immediately clear the ventricular clot and is sometimes not effective by itself due to obstruction of the catheter by blood. The EVD may even potentially slow the rate of IVH clearance by removing the tissue plasminogen activator (tPA) released from the clot into the CSF. The injection of thrombolytic agents into the ventricular space has therefore evolved in response to the problems of catheter obstruction and slow IVH clearance, and has been shown to be safe and effective in animal studies (56–58), and in small clinical case series (59–63). In experimental studies thrombolytic-mediated removal of clot facilitates blood clot removal and improves hydrocephalus and inflammation (64–66). A systematic review of four randomized and eight observational studies comparing EVD alone (n = 149) and EVD combined with intranventricular fibrinolysis (IVF) (n = 167) in the setting of severe IVH due to spontaneous supratentorial ICH found that overall mortality risk decreased from 46.7% in the EVD alone group to 22.7% in the EVD+IVF group (overall pooled Peto OR of 0.32 [95% CI, 0.19 to 0.5])(67). IVF was also associated with an increase in good functional outcome and with no difference between the two groups in terms of shunt dependence or complications. This result was highly significant with urokinase, but not with recombinant tissue-type plasminogen activator (tPA) suggesting that the therapeutic effect may be different for the two thrombolytics. These findings are consistent with an earlier systematic review of 16 retrospective studies including 201 patients with severe IVH (Graeb score ≥ 7) secondary to ICH in which therapy with EVD and IVF (n = 33) was associated with a mortality rate of 9% and a much lower risk for unfavorable outcome (22%), as compared to patients treated with EVD alone (n = 75) (mortality 56%; poor outcome: 87%)(52). A Cochrane review of 10 independent studies (eight case series or retrospective studies, one quasi-randomized study, one randomized study with a biased control group) using intraventricular thrombolytic agents found anecdotal evidence supporting safety and possible therapeutic value (68). More recently, Staykov *et al.* performed a systematic review of 23 studies (1993–2010) involving 436 patients with ICH and IVH (69). They reported a mortality rate of 53% (n = 133) for EVD alone and 16% (n = 212) for EVD plus thrombolysis, compared to 71% (n = 91) in conservatively treated patients. Unfavorable outcome was not as low in the IVF group (45% vs. 70% EVD alone vs. 86% conservative treatment), compared to the other systematic reviews, but still suggested significant potential benefit from IVF. All of these reviews are limited by the nature of comparison with historical groups and most available data originates from small and mainly low-quality non-randomized studies.

Intraventricular thrombolysis is a rational therapy, with some data supporting its safety. A prospective placebo controlled randomized trial is still needed to provide convincing evidence to recommend routine use in clinical practice. The Phase II clinical trial of Clot Lysis Evaluating Accelerated Resolution of IVH (CLEAR-IVH) was completed in March 2008 (70) and preliminary results show that low-dose rt-PA for the treatment of ICH with IVH has an acceptable safety profile compared to placebo and prior historical controls (71). The ongoing Phase III CLEAR-IVH trial is expected to finish recruitment in June 2014, with trial completion 1 year later. A total of 500 patients with primary or secondary IVH causing obstructive hydrocephalus are planned to be randomized (1:1) to IVF with rt-PA or placebo (http://www.cleariii.com).

Strategies to improve fibrinolytic drug delivery

Ongoing experience with fibrinolytic therapy has led to further insight on how to optimize the delivery of fibrinolytic agents to maximize intraventricular clot resolution. Historically doses up to 8 mg of rt-PA in a single bolus have been reported, although findings of the the Intraventricular Hemorrhage Thrombolysis Safety Trial, which randomized 48 patients with severe IVH to treatment with 3 mg rt-PA vs. placebo, suggested that a 3 mg bolus dose may be associated with a higher than acceptable symptomatic bleeding rate (23% vs. 5% in placebo-treated patients) (55). One study assessing dose response found that patients treated with high-dose IVF (4 mg alteplase every 12 hours, maximum 20 mg) and low-dose IVF (1 mg alteplase every 8 hours, maximum 12 mg) had similar IVH clearance from the third and fourth ventricles and a similar safety profile (one case of asymptomatic ventricular bleeding in the high-dose group) (72). The total clot half-life was significantly longer in the low-dose group by approximately 1 day, but outcomes at 3 months were not different between groups. Evaluation of even lower doses in the dose finding studies of the CLEAR-IVH trials did report a dose response relationship (73). In this study 64 patients with IVH+EVD were randomized to placebo or 0.3 mg, 1 mg, or 3 mg of rt-PA twice daily. Twelve subregions of the ventricles were scored from 0 to 4. Effect of dose on IVH clearance to 50% of baseline score was compared by survival analysis for all regions combined and by subregion. IVH clearance to 50% occurred faster across all regions with increasing rt-PA dose and was quickest in the midline ventricles, followed by the anterior half of the lateral ventricles and slowest in the posterior half of the lateral ventricles. The regional difference is probably due to increasing drug exposure with greater proximity of IVH to the EVD. Once the midline ventricles are open, rt-PA is diverted away from the posterolateral ventricles, potentially limiting the effectiveness of subsequent doses of intraventricular rt-PA for clot regions distant to the EVD. This study could not evaluate the region-dependent effect of rt-PA on clinical outcomes, which must be left to future trials. Clearance of blood from the third and fourth ventricles is believed to be important to alleviate obstructive hydrocephalus faster. There is retrospective evidence that IVF may reduce need for ventriculo-peritoneal shunting (50,60). Another issue is whether distribution or severity of IVH should determine EVD location or rt-PA dose. At this time the dose of intraventricular thrombolytic has been optimized, with 1 mg every 8 hours achieving the most enhanced clearance without increasing hemorrhage risk.

Beyond dosing considerations, factors to consider to potentially improve IVH clot removal are EVD position within the ventricle, laterality of EVD placement relative to side of greatest IVH volume, and use of bilateral or dual EVDs. In an evaluation of all 100 patients from the Clot Lysis Evaluating Accelerated Resolution of Intraventricular Hemorrhage (CLEAR-IVH) phase I + II trials, there was a trend toward more rapid clearance of total IVH through an EVD placed on the side of dominant intraventricular blood compared with an EVD on the side with less blood ($p = 0.09$) (74). In this study, two-thirds of patients had catheters placed on the side with less blood. Clearance of third and fourth ventricular blood was unrelated to EVD laterality. EVD position may be important not only for clot removal, but also to prevent catheter-related hemorrhage in the setting of IVR rt-PA. In a study of 27 patients who received open-label rt-PA for IVH with a median dose of 2 mg, evidence of hemorrhage along the catheter tract (greater than trace blood) was evident in 9/30 EVDs (30%) prior to injection of rt-PA (75). After rt-PA administration, worsening tract hemorrhage (by at least 1 grade) (Fig. 23.2) was seen in 14 out of 30 (46.7 %) of all EVD placements with a significantly higher incidence seen with incorrectly placed EVDs. Correct placement of the EVD was defined as having all fenestrations on the distal end of the EVD fully inside the ventricle, and occurred in 21 out of 30 (70%) EVD placements. Thus EVD position may be a less well recognized factor affecting both IVR thrombolytic safety and efficacy. Studies in which CT was used in all cases to evaluate for EVD-associated intracranial bleeding report rates from 6.5% to 20.7% (76,77). Most of these hematomas are too small to cause neurological deficits and hence are most often asymptomatic, although such patients may have poor neurologic exams to begin with, making it difficult to discover subtle findings. These hemorrhages are, however, far more common than generally suspected. They are most likely attributable to direct vascular trauma, rather than being secondary to rapid drainage of an enlarged ventricular system, because the hematomas are at the pial surface and/or adjacent to the catheter or needle track.

Finally, the strategic placement of more than one catheter into the ventricular clot may improve efficiency of clot removal. Hinson *et al.* showed that, in the setting of very large IVH (> 40 cc) with casting and mass effect, use of bilateral simultaneous EVDs may increase clot resolution with adjunctive thrombolytic therapy (78). In this situation the thrombolytic injection either alternates sides with each dose, or is administered to the side of greatest IVH volume. On the other hand Staykov *et al.* found no difference in clot resolution between the groups treated with one vs. two EVDs in the setting of IVH volume < 40 cc; however, they did find a trend towards a longer EVD duration and higher infection rate in the bilateral EVD group (79). The Staykov study did not include a comparison with single catheter cases, controlling for IVH volume. These studies suggest that while further study is indicated, dual catheters may be useful in the management of very large volume IVH, for trapped ventricles, or for catheter obstruction. Other possible indications yet to be explored are to enhance thrombolytic therapy on the contralateral side, to treat refractory intracranial hypertension or to reduce mass effect from IVH which may precipitate ischemic injury.

To the extent that both the volume of IVH and duration of exposure of CSF to clotted blood contribute to altered consciousness and pathological changes within

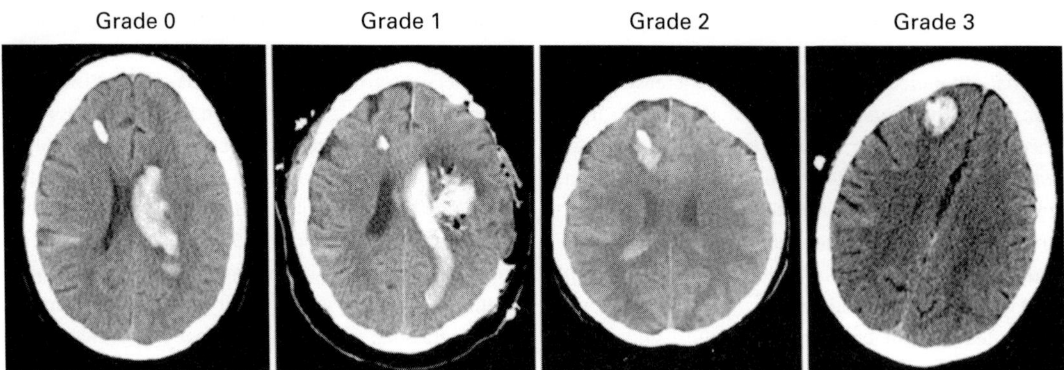

Grade 0: No tract hemorrhage
Grade 1: Trace tract hemorrhage (no mass effect)
Grade 2: Tract hemorrhage with intracerebral hematoma
Grade 3: Massive tract hemorrhage with mass effect

Fig. 23.2. Catheter Tract Hemorrhage Grading Scale (75).

the ventricle, as suggested by experimental studies (58,80), therapies that remove more blood clot faster may have clinical benefit.

Mechanical strategies to improve IVH removal

Several small studies have focused on feasibility and safety of minimally invasive techniques to endoscopically evacuate IVH (81–87). These data include predominantly case series, but also one prospective study with 42 patients and a randomized controlled trial (RCT) with 48 patients (87). The procedure utilizes either flexible or rigid endoscopy via a frontal or rarely occipital approach, either unilateral or bilateral, with aspiration of ventricular blood clot from the lateral, followed by third and fourth ventricles. A variety of irrigation solutions are used, typically Ringers lactate and the use of fibrinolytics (after EVD placement), septotomy or third ventriculostomy have all been described. These studies report relatively rapid removal of IVH although the RCT found no significant difference in mortality rate or outcome at 30 and 90 days between the endoscopic group and the EVD group. Outcome was significantly associated with initial level of consciousness. The need for VP shunting was reduced by half in the endoscopic group and ICU length of stay was significantly shorter compared with the EVD group. A similar size case series of 48 patients treated with endoscopy and compared to 48 historical controls also reported no significant difference in mortality and neurologic outcome, but a significant reduction in shunt-dependent hydrocephalus (86). The endoscopic procedure appears to be relatively uncomplicated although irrigation can cause prolonged intracranial pressure elevations in patients with IVH, which requires further evaluation (88).

Lumbar drainage has been used successfully after clearance of the lower ventricular system to shorten the course of the EVD and treat communicating hydrocephalus (89–91). Huttner *et al.* reported a case series of 16 patients treated with EVD followed by lumbar drainage and compared these to 39 patients treated with EVD alone (89). Patients who received intraventricular fibrinolytic therapy for clot lysis were excluded. In patients who received lumbar drainage, EVD duration was shortened by 4 days on average (16 vs. 12 days), although the total duration of CSF drainage was longer in the EVD + lumbar drain (LD) group (16 days EVD versus 21 days EVD + LD). The need for VP shunting was significantly lower in the EVD + LD group. Combining intraventricular thrombolysis with lumbar drainage may also enhance resolution of IVH. A prospective study of 32 patients with IVH treated with IVR thrombolysis followed by early replacement of the EVD by lumbar drainage, reported on 28 patients who required early LD (after 105 hours EVD duration) (91). At 3 months follow-up only one patient required a VP shunt, suggesting that these sequential procedures may enhance removal of cisternal and lumbar blood breakdown products, reducing development of chronic hydrocephalus. In aneurysmal subarachnoid hemorrhage patients, lumbar drainage may reduce the incidence of vasospasm and delayed ischemic neurologic deficits (92). An ongoing phase III clinical trial of lumbar drainage after SAH (EARLYDRAIN) is anticipated to show if this practice improves clinical outcomes (93).

EVD management

There are several options for managing EVD drainage, depending on the opening pressure and the underlying pathology. In both ICH and SAH, there has been no comparison of intermittent drainage strategies (regularly scheduled intermittent volume, or as needed in response to ICP elevations), versus continuous drainage with the drip chamber set at a particular level (drainage as needed when ICP exceeds that level). Continuous drainage may allow more rapid clearance of ventricular blood, and presumably spasmogenic and irritative contents of bloody CSF, but increases risk of overdrainage during patient suctioning and mobilization (experienced units protocolize temporary clamping of the EVD during those maneuvers). Others have cautioned that overdrainage of CSF at least in SAH could predispose to cerebral vasospasm as well as hydrocephalus (94).

Meningitis/ventriculitis

Incidence of ventriculostomy-related infections has been reported from 0% to 22% (95–99). This frequently necessitates replacement of EVD, prolonged hospital stay, antibiotic related costs and morbidities, and occasionally life-threatening sequelae. Intraventricular hemorrhage is a significant risk factor associated with EVD-related infections, but others in this population include systemic infection, failure to tunnel the catheter, duration of EVD, catheter irrigation, site leaks, and frequency of CSF sampling (100). Many of these factors have not been carefully adjudicated in controlled studies, or even in multivariate analyses. Some studies show an associated risk of infection if the catheter is left in for more than 5 days (101), and a linear correlation between infection rates and duration of catheter and CSF leakage (102). Other studies have shown that EVD duration has no effect on the infection rate (103). Antibiotic prophylaxis, a common practice, may contribute to the development of resistant organisms, or significantly more morbid gram-negative ventriculitis (104). Antibiotic protocols vary widely across centers and commonly include peri-procedural administration with EVD insertion, or continued use for the duration of drainage (101,105). A meta-analysis of randomized clinical trials and observational studies concluded that the use of prophylactic systemic antibiotics throughout the duration of EVD and use of antibiotic-coated EVD appears beneficial in preventing ventriculostomy-related infection (105–109). However, the absolute and relative risk reduction of EVD infections, if any, with antibiotic use has not been carefully assessed and requires further carefully controlled trials. In a prospective, randomized, open-label trial to evaluate infection incidence of antibiotic impregnated (AI) vs. standard EVD catheters, AI catheters were not associated with risk reduction in EVD infection compared to standard catheters (110).

Conclusion

IVH can be a devastating complication associated with ICH, SAH, and TBI, predicting worsened morbidity and mortality. While the pathophysiology of IVH remains incompletely understood, measurement techniques and prognostic models have improved clinical understanding of this condition. Effective management of non-traumatic IVH appears to require therapies that reduce clot volume quickly and minimize the duration and extent of brain tissue exposure to blood products and the subsequent inflammation within the ventricle. CLEAR III is the first randomized, multicenter, double-blinded, placebo-controlled phase III trial assessing the efficacy of intraventricular thrombolytic therapy in IVH patients with an EVD. If the study outcome is positive, it will significantly improve the therapeutic options for acute hemorrhagic stroke treatment. Strategies to improve the efficacy of thrombolytic therapy including EVD positioning within the ventricle, laterality and use of dual catheters are likely to be important considerations. On the horizon are approaches utilizing neuroendoscopy, lumbar drainage and potentially alternative thrombolytic agents. Analysis of ICP control, clot resolution rates, and neurologic outcomes in relation to these approaches and catheter placement strategies will require further clarification in ongoing and future studies.

REFERENCES

1. Graeb DA, Robertson WD, Lapointe JS, Nugent RA, Harrison PB. Computed tomographic diagnosis of intraventricular hemorrhage. Etiology and prognosis. Radiology. 1982;**143**(1):91–6.
2. Little JR, Blomquist GA, Jr., Ethier R. Intraventricular hemorrhage in adults. *Surg Neurol.* 1977;**8**(3):143–9.
3. Pasqualin A, Bazzan A, Cavazzani P, *et al.* Intracranial hematomas following aneurysmal rupture: experience with 309 cases. *Surg Neurol.* 1986;**25**(1):6–17.
4. Ruscalleda J, Peiro A. Prognostic factors in intraparenchymatous hematoma with ventricular hemorrhage. *Neuroradiology.* 1986;**28**(1):34–7.
5. Todo T, Usui M, Takakura K. Treatment of severe intraventricular hemorrhage by intraventricular infusion of urokinase. *J Neurosurg.* 1991;**74**(1):81–6.
6. Mayfrank L, Hutter BO, Kohorst Y, *et al.* Influence of intraventricular hemorrhage on outcome after rupture of intracranial aneurysm. *Neurosurg Rev.* 2001;**24**(4):185–91.
7. Hallevi H, Walker KC, Kasam M, *et al.* Inflammatory response to intraventricular hemorrhage: time course, magnitude and effect of t-PA. *J Neurol Sci.* 2012;**15;**315 (1–2):93–5.
8. Brott T, Thalinger K, Hertzberg V. Hypertension as a risk factor for spontaneous intracerebral hemorrhage. *Stroke,* 1986:**17**(6):1078–83.
9. Broderick JP, *et al.* Intracerebral hemorrhage more than twice as common as subarachnoid hemorrhage. *J Neurosurg.* 1993;**78**(2):188–91.
10. Woo D, *et al.* Effect of untreated hypertension on hemorrhagic stroke. *Stroke.* 2004;**35**(7):1703–8.
11. Daverat P, Castel JP, Dartigues JF, Orgogozo JM. Death and functional outcome after spontaneous intracerebral hemorrhage. A prospective study of 166 cases using multivariate analysis. *Stroke.* 1991;**22**(1):1–6.
12. Mohr G, *et al.* Intraventricular hemorrhage from ruptured aneurysm. Retrospective analysis of 91 cases. *J Neurosurg.* 1983;**58**(4):482–7.
13. Coplin WM, *et al.* A cohort study of the safety and feasibility of intraventricular urokinase for nonaneurysmal spontaneous intraventricular hemorrhage. *Stroke.* 1998;**29**(8):1573–9.
14. Steiner T, *et al.* Dynamics of intraventricular hemorrhage in patients with spontaneous intracerebral hemorrhage: risk factors, clinical impact, and effect of hemostatic therapy with recombinant activated factor VII. *Neurosurgery.* 2006;**59**(4):767–73; discussion 773–4.
15. Irie F, Fujimoto S, Uda K, *et al.* Primary intraventricular hemorrhage from dural arteriovenous fistula. *J Neurol Sci.* 2003;**215**(1–2):115–18.
16. Andrews CO, Engelhard HH. Fibrinolytic therapy in intraventricular hemorrhage. *Ann Pharmacother.* 2001;**35**(11): 1435–48.
17. Gordon A. Primary ventricular hemorrhage: further contribution to a characteristic symptom group. *Arch Neurol Psychiatr.* 1938;**39**:1272–6.
18. Gates PC, Barnett HJ, Vinters HV, Simonsen RL, Siu K. Primary intraventricular hemorrhage in adults. *Stroke.* 1986;**17**(5):872–7.
19. Adams RE, Diringer MN. Response to external ventricular drainage in spontaneous intracerebral hemorrhage with hydrocephalus. *Neurology.* 1998;**50**:519–23.
20. Lee KR, Betz AL, Kim S, Keep RF, Hoff JT. The role of the coagulation cascade in brain edema formation after intracerebral hemorrhage. *Acta Neurochir* 1996; **138**:396–401.
21. Ziai WC, Triantaphyllopoulou A, Razumovsky AY, Hanley DF. Treatment of sympathomimetic induced intraventricular hemorrhage with intraventricular urokinase. *J Stroke Cerebrovasc Dis.* 2003;**12**(6):276–9.
22. Ellington E, Margolis G. Block of arachnoid villus by subarachnoid hemorrhage. *J Neurosurg.* 1969;**30**:651–7.

23. Kibler RF, Couch RSC, Crompton MR. Hydrocephalus in the adult following spontaneous hemorrhage. *Brain.* 1961;**84**:45–61.
24. Huttner HB, Nagel S, Tognoni E, *et al.* Intracerebral hemorrhage with severe ventricular involvement: lumbar drainage for communicating hydrocephalus. *Stroke.* 2007;**38**:183–7.
25. Tung MY, Ong PL, Seow WT, Tan KK. A study on the efficacy of intraventricular urokinase in the treatment of intraventricular haemorrhage. *Br J Neurosurg.* 1998;**12**:234–9.
26. Tuhrim S, Horowitz DR, Sacher M, Godbold JH. Volume of ventricular blood is an important determinant of outcome in supratentorial intracerebral hemorrhage. *Crit Care Med.* 1999;**27**(3):617–21.
27. Young WB, Lee KP, Pessin MS, *et al.* Prognostic significance of ventricular blood in supratentorial hemorrhage: a volumetric study. *Neurology.* 1990;**40**(4):616–19.
28. Roos YB, Hasan D, Vermeulen M. Outcome in patients with large intraventricular haemorrhages: a volumetric study. *J Neurol Neurosurg Psychiatry.* 1995;**58**(5):622–4.
29. Shapiro SA, Campbell RL, Scully T. Hemorrhagic dilation of the fourth ventricle: an ominous predictor. *J Neurosurg.* 1994;**80**(5):805–9.
30. Ozdemir O, Calisaneller T, Hasturk A, *et al.* Prognostic significance of third ventricle dilation in spontaneous intracerebral hemorrhage: a preliminary clinical study. *Neurol Res.* 2008;**30**(4):406–10.
31. Stein M, Luecke M, Preuss M, *et al.* Spontaneous intracerebral hemorrhage with ventricular extension and the grading of obstructive hydrocephalus: the prediction of outcome of a special life-threatening entity. *Neurosurgery.* 2010;**67**(5):1243–1251; discussion 1252.
32. Stein M, Luecke M, Preuss M, *et al.* The prediction of 30-day mortality and functional outcome in spontaneous intracerebral hemorrhage with secondary ventricular hemorrhage: a score comparison. *Acta Neurochir Suppl.* 2011;**112**:9–11.
33. Broderick JP, Diringer MN, Hill MD, *et al.* Determinants of intracerebral hemorrhage growth: an exploratory analysis. *Stroke.* 2007;**38**(3):1072–5.
34. Rosen DS, Macdonald RL, Huo D, *et al.* Intraventricular hemorrhage from ruptured aneurysm: clinical characteristics, complications, and outcomes in a large, prospective, multicenter study population. *J Neurosurg.* 2007;**107**(2): 261–5.
35. Hutter BO, Kreitschmann-Andermahr I, Gilsbach JM. Cognitive deficits in the acute stage after subarachnoid hemorrhage. *Neurosurgery.* 1998;**43**(5):1054–65.
36. LeRoux PD, Haglund MM, Newell DW, Grady MS, Winn HR. Intraventricular hemorrhage in blunt head trauma: an analysis of 43 cases. *Neurosurgery.* 1992;**31**(4):678–84; discussion 84–5.
37. Ruscalleda J, Peiro A. Prognostic factors in intraparenchymatous hematoma with ventricular hemorrhage. *Neuroradiology.* 1986;**28**(1):34–7.
38. Morgan TC, Dawson J, Spengler D, *et al.* The modified Graeb score: an enhanced tool for intraventricular hemorrhage measurement and prediction of functional outcome. *Stroke.* 2013;**44**(3):635–41.
39. Hallevi H, Dar NS, Barreto AD, *et al.* The IVH score: a novel tool for estimating intraventricular hemorrhage volume: clinical and research implications. *Crit Care Med.* 2009;**37** (3):969–74, e1.
40. Hemphill JC 3rd, Bonovich DC, Besmertis L, Manley GT, Johnston SC. The ICH score: a simple, reliable grading scale for intracerebral hemorrhage. *Stroke.* 2001;**32** (4):891–7.
41. LeRoux PD, Haglund MM, Newell DW, Grady MS, Winn HR. Intraventricular hemorrhage in blunt head trauma: an analysis of 43 cases. *Neurosurgery.* 1992;**31**(4):678–84; discussion 84–5.
42. Hwang BY, Bruce SS, Appelboom G, *et al.* Evaluation of intraventricular hemorrhage assessment methods for predicting outcome following intracerebral hemorrhage. *J Neurosurg.* 2012;**116**(1):185–92.
43. Hallevi H, Walker KC, Kasam M, *et al.* Inflammatory response to intraventricular hemorrhage: time course, magnitude and effect of t-PA. *J Neurol Sci.* 2012;**315** (1–2):93–5.
44. Diringer MN, Edwards DF, Zazulia AR. Hydrocephalus: a previously unrecognized predictor of poor outcome from supratentorial intracerebral hemorrhage. *Stroke.* 1998;**29** (7):1352–7.
45. Adams RE, Diringer MN. Response to external ventricular drainage in spontaneous intracerebral hemorrhage with hydrocephalus. *Neurology.* 1998;**50**(2):519–23.
46. Phan TG, Koh M, Vierkant RA, Wijdicks EF. Hydrocephalus is a determinant of early mortality in putaminal hemorrhage. *Stroke.* 2000;**31**(9):2157–62.
47. Liliang PC, Liang CL, Lu CH, *et al.* Hypertensive caudate hemorrhage prognostic predictor, outcome, and role of external ventricular drainage. *Stroke.* 2001;**32**(5):1195–200.

48. Bhattathiri PS, Gregson B, Prasad KS, Mendelow AD. Intraventricular hemorrhage and hydrocephalus after spontaneous intracerebral hemorrhage: results from the STICH trial. *Acta Neurochir Suppl.* 2006;**96**:65–8.
49. Ronning P, Sorteberg W, Nakstad P, Russell D, Helseth E. Aspects of intracerebral hematomas - an update. *Acta Neurol Scand.* 2008;**118**(6):347–61.
50. Ziai WC, Melnychuk E, Thompson CB, *et al.* Occurrence and impact of intracranial pressure elevation during treatment of severe intraventricular hemorrhage. *Crit Care Med.* 2012;**40**(5):1601–8.
51. Huttner HB, Kohrmann M, Berger C, Georgiadis D, Schwab S. Influence of intraventricular hemorrhage and occlusive hydrocephalus on the long-term outcome of treated patients with basal ganglia hemorrhage: a case-control study. *J Neurosurg.* 2006;**105**(3):412–17.
52. Nieuwkamp DJ, de Gans K, Rinkel GJ, Algra A. Treatment and outcome of severe intraventricular extension in patients with subarachnoid or intracerebral hemorrhage: a systematic review of the literature. *J Neurol.* 2000;**247**(2): 117–21.
53. Naff NJ, Williams MA, Rigamonti D, Keyl PM, Hanley DF. Blood clot resolution in human cerebrospinal fluid: evidence of first-order kinetics. *Neurosurgery.* 2001;**49**(3):614–19; discussion 619–21.
54. Carhuapoma JR. Thrombolytic therapy after intraventricular hemorrhage: do we know enough? *J Neurol Sci.* 2002;**202**(1–2):1–3.
55. Naff NJ, Hanley DF, Keyl PM, *et al.* Intraventricular thrombolysis speeds blood clot resolution: results of a pilot, prospective, randomized, double-blind, controlled trial. *Neurosurgery.* 2004;**54**(3):577–83; discussion 83–4.
56. Pang D, Sclabassi RJ, Horton JA. Lysis of intraventricular blood clot with urokinase in a canine model: Part 2. In vivo safety study of intraventricular urokinase. *Neurosurgery.* 1986;**19**(4):547–52.
57. Pang D, Sclabassi RJ, Horton JA. Lysis of intraventricular blood clot with urokinase in a canine model: Part 3. Effects of intraventricular urokinase on clot lysis and posthemorrhagic hydrocephalus. *Neurosurgery.* 1986;**19**(4):553–72.
58. Pang D, Sclabassi RJ, Horton JA. Lysis of intraventricular blood clot with urokinase in a canine model: Part 1. Canine intraventricular blood cast model. *Neurosurgery.* 1986;**19**(4):540–6.
59. Shen PH, Matsuoka Y, Kawajiri K, *et al.* Treatment of intraventricular hemorrhage using urokinase. *Neurol Med Chir (Tokyo).* 1990;**30**(5):329–33.
60. Huttner HB, Tognoni E, Bardutzky J, *et al.* Influence of intraventricular fibrinolytic therapy with rt-PA on the long-term outcome of treated patients with spontaneous basal ganglia hemorrhage: a case-control study. *Eur J Neurol.* 2008;**15**(4):342–9.
61. Vereecken KK, Van Havenbergh T, De Beuckelaar W, Parizel PM, Jorens PG. Treatment of intraventricular hemorrhage with intraventricular administration of recombinant tissue plasminogen activator A clinical study of 18 cases. *Clin Neurol Neurosurg.* 2006;**108**(5):451–5.
62. Kumar K, Demeria DD, Verma A. Recombinant tissue plasminogen activator in the treatment of intraventricular hemorrhage secondary to periventricular arteriovenous malformation before surgery: case report. *Neurosurgery.* 2003; **52**(4):964–8; discussion 968–9.
63. Findlay JM, Weir BK, Stollery DE. Lysis of intraventricular hematoma with tissue plasminogen activator. Case report. *J Neurosurg.* 1991;**74**(5):803–7.
64. Wagner KR, Xi G, Hua Y, *et al.* Ultra-early clot aspiration after lysis with tissue plasminogen activator in a porcine model of intracerebral hemorrhage: edema reduction and blood-brain barrier protection. *J Neurosurg.* 1999;**90** (3):491–8.
65. Mayfrank L, Kim Y, Kissler J, *et al.* Morphological changes following experimental intraventricular haemorrhage and intraventricular fibrinolytic treatment with recombinant tissue plasminogen activator. *Acta Neuropathol.* 2000;**100** (5):561–7.
66. Narayan RK, Narayan TM, Katz DA, *et al.* Lysis of intracranial hematomas with urokinase in a rabbit model. *J Neurosurg.* 1985;**62**(4):580–6.
67. Gaberel T, Magheru C, Parienti JJ, *et al.* Intraventricular fibrinolysis versus external ventricular drainage alone in intraventricular hemorrhage: a meta-analysis. *Stroke.* 2011;**42**(10):2776–81.
68. Lapointe M, Haines S. Fibrinolytic therapy for intraventricular hemorrhage in adults. *Cochrane Database Syst Rev.* 2002(3):CD003692.
69. Staykov D, Bardutzky J, Huttner HB, Schwab S. Intraventricular fibrinolysis for intracerebral hemorrhage with severe ventricular involvement. *Neurocrit Care.* 2011;**15**(1):194–209.
70. Hanley D. Final results CLEAR-IVH Trial: clot lysis, safety and 30 day functional outcomes. In: *European stroke conference*, Nice, France, 13–16th May 2008.
71. Morgan T, Awad I, Keyl P, Lane K, Hanley D. Preliminary report of the clot lysis evaluating accelerated resolution of

intraventricular hemorrhage (CLEAR-IVH) clinical trial. *Acta Neurochir Suppl.* 2008;**105**:217–20.

72. Staykov D, Wagner I, Volbers B, *et al.* Dose effect of intraventricular fibrinolysis in ventricular hemorrhage. *Stroke.* 2011;**42**(7):2061–4.
73. Webb AJ, Ullman NL, Mann S, *et al.* Resolution of intraventricular hemorrhage varies by ventricular region and dose of intraventricular thrombolytic: the Clot Lysis: Evaluating Accelerated Resolution of IVH (CLEAR IVH) program. *Stroke.* 2012;**43**(6):1666–8.
74. Jaffe J, Melnychuk E, Muschelli J, *et al.* Ventricular catheter location and the clearance of intraventricular hemorrhage. *Neurosurgery.* 2012;**70**(5):1258–63; discussion 1263–4.
75. Jackson DA, Patel AV, Darracott RM, *et al.* Safety of intraventricular hemorrhage (IVH) thrombolysis based on CT localization of external ventricular drain (EVD) fenestrations and analysis of EVD tract hemorrhage. *Neurocrit Care.* 2012 Apr 28.
76. Wiesmann M, Mayer TE. Intracranial bleeding rates associated with two methods of external ventricular drainage. *J Clin Neurosci.* 2001;**8**(2):126–8.
77. Ehtisham A, Taylor S, Bayless L, Klein MW, Janzen JM. Placement of external ventricular drains and intracranial pressure monitors by neurointensivists. *Neurocrit Care.* 2009;**10**(2):241–7.
78. Hinson HE, Melnychuk E, Muschelli J, *et al.* Drainage efficiency with dual versus single catheters in severe intraventricular hemorrhage. *Neurocrit Care.* Jun 17.
79. Staykov D, Huttner HB, Lunkenheimer J, *et al.* Single versus bilateral external ventricular drainage for intraventricular fibrinolysis in severe ventricular haemorrhage. *J Neurol Neurosurg Psychiatry.* 2010;**81**(1):105–8.
80. Mayfrank L, Kissler J, Raoofi R, *et al.* Ventricular dilatation in experimental intraventricular hemorrhage in pigs. Characterization of cerebrospinal fluid dynamics and the effects of fibrinolytic treatment. *Stroke.* 1997;**28**(1):141–8.
81. Longatti PL, Martinuzzi A, Fiorindi A, *et al.* Neuroendoscopic management of intraventricular hemorrhage. *Stroke.* 2004;**35**:e35–e38.
82. Longatti P, Fiorindi A, Martinuzzi A. Neuroendoscopic aspiration of hematocephalus totalis: technical note. *Neurosurgery* 2005; **57** (Suppl 4):E409.
83. Yadav YR, Mukerji G, Shenoy R, *et al.* Endoscopic management of hypertensive intraventricular haemorrhage with obstructive hydrocephalus. *BMC Neurol* 2007;**7**:1.
84. Zhang Z, Li X, Liu Y, *et al.* Application of neuroendoscopy in the treatment of intraventricular hemorrhage. *Cerebrovasc Dis* 2007;**24**:91–6.
85. Hamada H, Hayashi N, Kurimoto M, *et al.* Neuroendoscopic removal of intraventricular hemorrhage combined with hydrocephalus. *Minim Invasive Neurosurg* 2008;**51**:345–9.
86. Basaldella L, Marton E, Fiorindi A, *et al.* External ventricular drainage alone versus endoscopic surgery for severe intraventricular hemorrhage: a comparative retrospective analysis on outcome and shunt dependency. *Neurosurg Focus* 2012; **32**:E4.
87. Chen CC, Liu CL, Tung YN, *et al.* Endoscopic surgery for intraventricular hemorrhage (IVH) caused by thalamic hemorrhage: comparisons of endoscopic surgery and external ventricular drainage (EVD) surgery. *World Neurosurg* 2011;**75**:264–8.
88. Trnovec S, Halatsch ME, Putz M, *et al.* Irrigation can cause prolonged intracranial pressure elevations during endoscopic treatment of intraventricular haematomas. *Br J Neurosurg* 2012;**26**:247–51.
89. Huttner HB, Nagel S, Tognoni E, *et al.* Intracerebral hemorrhage with severe ventricular involvement: lumbar drainage for communicating hydrocephalus. *Stroke* 2007;**38**:183–7.
90. Huttner HB, Schwab S, Bardutzky J. Lumbar drainage for communicating hydrocephalus after ICH with ventricular hemorrhage. *Neurocrit Care* 2006;**5**:193–6.
91. Staykov D, Huttner HB, Struffert T, *et al.* Intraventricular fibrinolysis and lumbar drainage for ventricular hemorrhage. *Stroke* 2009;**40**:3275–80.
92. Al-Tamimi YZ, Bhargava D, Feltbower RG, *et al.* Lumbar drainage of cerebrospinal fluid after aneurysmal subarachnoid hemorrhage: a prospective, randomized, controlled trial (LUMAS). *Stroke.* 2012;**43**:677–82.
93. Bardutzky J, Witsch J, Juttler E, *et al.* EARLYDRAIN – outcome after early lumbar CSF-drainage in aneurysmal subarachnoid hemorrhage: study protocol for a randomized controlled trial. *Trials.* 2011;**12**:203.
94. Kasuya H, Shimizu T, Kagawa M. The effect of continuous drainage of cerebrospinal fluid in patients with subarachnoid hemorrhage: a retrospective analysis of 108 patients. *Neurosurgery.* 1991;**28**(1):56–9.
95. Holloway KL, Barnes T, Choi S, *et al.* Ventriculostomy infections: the effect of monitoring duration and catheter exchange in 584 patients. *J Neurosurg.* 1996;**85**(3):419–24.
96. Chan KH, Mann KS. Prolonged therapeutic external ventricular drainage: a prospective study. *Neurosurgery.* 1988;**23**(4):436–8.
97. Kanter RK, Weiner LB. Ventriculostomy-related infections. *N Engl J Med.* 1984;**311**(15):987.

98. Park P, Garton HJ, Kocan MJ, Thompson BG. Risk of infection with prolonged ventricular catheterization. *Neurosurgery.* 2004;**55**(3):594–9; discussion 599–601.
99. Dasic D, Hanna SJ, Bojanic S, Kerr RS. External ventricular drain infection: the effect of a strict protocol on infection rates and a review of the literature. *Br J Neurosurg.* 2006;**20**(5):296–300.
100. Hoefnagel D, Dammers R, Ter Laak-Poort MP, Avezaat CJ. Risk factors for infections related to external ventricular drainage. *Acta Neurochir (Wien).* 2008;**150**(3):209–14; discussion 214.
101. Beer R, Lackner P, Pfausler B, Schmutzhard E. Nosocomial ventriculitis and meningitis in neurocritical care patients. *J Neurol.* 2008;**255**(11):1617–24.
102. Lyke KE, Obasanjo OO, Williams MA, *et al.* Ventriculitis complicating use of intraventricular catheters in adult neurosurgical patients. *Clin Infect Dis.* 2001;**33**(12):2028–33.
103. Korinek AM, Reina M, Boch AL, *et al.* Prevention of external ventricular drain-related ventriculitis. *Acta Neurochir (Wien).* 2005;**147**(1):39–45; discussion 46.
104. Ortiz R, Lee K. Nosocomial infections in neurocritical care. *Curr Neurol Neurosci Rep.* 2006;**6**(6):525–30.
105. Lucey MA, Myburgh JA. Antibiotic prophylaxis for external ventricular drains in neurosurgical patients: an audit of compliance with a clinical management protocol. *Crit Care Resusc.* 2003;**5**(3):182–5.
106. Wong GK, Poon WS, Lyon D, Wai S. Cefepime vs. Ampicillin/Sulbactam and Aztreonam as antibiotic prophylaxis in neurosurgical patients with external ventricular drain: result of a prospective randomized controlled clinical trial. *J Clin Pharm Ther.* 2006;**31**(3):231–5.
107. Sonabend AM, Korenfeld Y, Crisman C, *et al.* Prevention of ventriculostomy-related infections with prophylactic antibiotics and antibiotic-coated external ventricular drains: a systematic review. *Neurosurgery* 2011;**68**(4): 996–1005.
108. Pfausler B, Spiss H, Beer R, *et al.* Treatment of staphylococcal ventriculitis associated with external cerebrospinal fluid drains: a prospective randomized trial of intravenous compared with intraventricular vancomycin therapy. *J Neurosurg.* 2003;**98**(5):1040–4.
109. Pons VG, Denlinger SL, Guglielmo BJ, *et al.* Ceftizoxime versus vancomycin and gentamicin in neurosurgical prophylaxis: a randomized, prospective, blinded clinical study. *Neurosurgery.* 1993;**33**(3):416–22; discussion 422–3.
110. Pople I, Poon W, Assaker R, *et al.* Comparison of infection rate with the use of antibiotic-impregnated vs standard extraventricular drainage devices: a prospective, randomized controlled trial. *Neurosurgery.* 2012;**71**(1): 6–13.

Interventions for cerebellar hemorrhage

Jens Witsch and Eric Jüttler

Introduction

Spontaneous cerebellar hemorrhages (SCH) demand special consideration among the different types of intracerebral hemorrhages (ICH) due to the anatomical proximity of the cerebellum to the brain stem. Concerning its volume the cerebellum fills the largest part of the posterior fossa. Its upper surface is located immediately next to the occipital lobes of the cerebrum, separated only by the tentorium. The lower surface comprises the back of the fourth ventricle and borders the pons and medulla oblongata.

Thus, secondary complications such as compression of the brain stem and blockage of the fourth ventricle by an expanding hematoma may affect vital brain functions or cause obstructive hydrocephalus early in the course of the disease, which consequently may require emergency interventions. Thus rapid diagnosis is crucial.

This chapter deals with the symptomatic treatment of SCH and the treatment of its early complications. Surgical treatment options will be depicted briefly. The final part of this chapter contains an overview of all available studies as well as case series of severe cerebellar hemorrhage with a focus on clinical outcome.

For the diagnosis and treatment of other entities that might cause a cerebellar hemorrhage (i.e. AV-malformation, aneurysms), please refer to the corresponding chapters of this book ('AV-malformation' and 'SAH'). Likewise epidural and subdural hematomas of the posterior fossa are not described here (see 'Vascular disease syndromes associated with TBI').

Epidemiology and risk factors

Incidence

Cerebellar hemorrhages comprise approximately 10% of all intracranial hemorrhages, about 15% of cerebellar strokes, but up to 40% of severe and space-occupying strokes. In larger population-based studies incidence rates for cerebellar hemorrhage of 3–4/100 000 inhabitants per year were found [1–5]. Unlike in other ICH subtypes incidence rates seem not to vary significantly between different races and sexes [1].

Predisposing factors

Data investigating risk factors specifically for cerebellar hemorrhage are very rare and risk factors are currently believed to be identical with risk factors for spontaneous cerebral hemorrhage in general. Age seems to be the most important unmodifiable risk factor, the peak incidence of the disease occurring in the sixth, seventh, and eighth decade of life. As for other stroke subtypes the most frequent modifiable predisposing factor for non-traumatic cerebellar hemorrhage is arterial hypertension which is present in at least half of all cases [2,6,7]. Coagulation disorders including oral anticoagulation

Critical Care of the Stroke Patient, ed. Stefan Schwab, Daniel Hanley, and A. David Mendelow. Published by Cambridge University Press.

are also predisposing, especially when coinciding with arterial hypertension. Furthermore, vascular malformation and malignancies have been found to be a frequently underlying cause in cerebellar hemorrhage and should therefore not be overlooked [8,9]. The etiological role and importance of amyloid angiopathy – well established in supratentorial hematomas – is unclear in cerebellar hemorrhage. Intraventricular hemorrhage seems to be more frequent in cerebellar hematomas, because within the cerebellum the hematoma tends to rupture into the ventricular system. There is a slight propensity for the hemorrhages to occur in the left hemisphere [10–14].

Clinical manifestations of cerebellar hemorrhage

As in cerebellar infarction clinical symptoms and signs are often unspecific in cerebellar hemorrhage. Although clinical signs are more severe and deterioration in consciousness occurs earlier and more frequently in cerebellar hemorrhage compared with cerebellar infarction, cerebellar infarction may be accompanied with additional brain stem infarct, which may then mimic the space-occupying effect caused by a hematoma. Indeed, the few studies available in this field show that a distinctive clinical syndrome specific for cerebellar hemorrhage or allowing hemorrhage to be differentiated from infarction does not exist [15]. In addition, adequate scoring systems could not be identified up to now and the ones that exist have been shown to be inefficient [16]. As a result, early imaging is mandatory.

Unspecific symptoms

Typically in cerebellar hemorrhage symptoms develop rapidly, but may also develop over one and even up to several hours. Coma at symptom onset is rare. Initially several patients notice a sudden occipital headache accompanied by other unspecific symptoms such as vomiting and dizziness due to rupture of blood into the CSF [17]. Headache, sometimes accompanied by meningism, seems to be more common in cerebellar ICH than in cerebellar infarct due to the affection of the meninges [18]. As unspecific symptoms they are not very helpful to the physician in differential diagnosis, but may rather serve as warning signs (see 'Ischemic stroke', and 'Cerebellar stroke').

Cerebellar signs

Some authors claim that cerebellar signs are slightly less frequent in cerebellar bleeding than ischemia but that knowledge remains to be reproduced in studies including larger numbers of patients [19]. However, it is usually later in the course of cerebellar hemorrhage that cerebellar signs occur: gait or trunk ataxia, vertigo, nystagmus, dysmetria, dysarthria, and ipsilateral gaze palsy, sometimes accompanied by cranial nerve abnormalities [7]. Limb ataxia can be mistaken for weakness either by the patient or by the physician. Hemiparesis is very rare in patients presenting with a cerebellar hematoma unless there is displacement of the brain stem at the time of presentation. All these signs may not occur at all or only several hours after disease onset. Table 24.1 gives an overview of the most frequent initial signs and symptoms at ictus described in larger case series in the literature. Table 24.2 provides an overview of the neurologic findings in patients who were awake on admission.

Deterioration in the level of consciousness – either due to direct compression of the brain stem or to secondary elevated intracranial pressure caused by

Table 24.1 Symptoms and signs in cerebellar hemorrhage at onset (given as % of patients).

Symptom	St Louis *et al.* 1998 (n = 72)	Mezzadri *et al.* 1993 (n = 50)	Ott *et al.* 1972 (n = 44)
Vomiting	81	26	95
Headache	67	46	73
Dizziness/ vertigo	60	40	55
Staggering	56	na	30
Dysarthria	42	12	32
Drowsiness	42	ns	na
Confusion	11	2	na

na = not applicable

Table 24.2 Neurologic findings in non-comatose patients with cerebellar hemorrhage on admission (given as % of patients).

Neurologic findings	St Louis *et al.* 1998 (n = 72)	Ott *et al.* 1972 (n = 38)
Anisocoria	14	0
Pin-point pupils/ miosis	6	30
Nystagmus	33	51
Altered corneal reflex	13	30
Gaze palsy	na	54
Facial paresis	18	61
Dysarthria	25	ns
Ataxia (gait/ truncal/limb)	44	78
(New) hemiparesis	11	0

na = not applicable

hydrocephalus – is very common and predominantly occurs within 24 hours afterwards. However, deterioration of consciousness to coma may also occur early after symptom onset or may develop quite suddenly at any time after the ictus and requires close clinical monitoring. In several retrospective case series it was reported that a considerable number of patients were admitted to the hospital in a comatose state or deteriorated to coma within a few hours after admission. The percentage of initially comatose patients varies between approximately 20% to 30% [10,20,21].

Diagnosis

Neurological examination

A complete neurological examination should be carried out whenever this is allowed by the medical state of the patient. As pointed out above, patients often display a rather unspecific constellation of symptoms (headache, vomiting, dizziness) and making a diagnosis solely on clinical observations is difficult and often incorrect [22]. At this early stage of the diagnostic process it is sufficient to have cerebellar bleeding among the differential diagnoses [23]. However, in the awake and cooperative patient, systematically paying attention to cerebellar signs can help the diagnosis: gait ataxia may be the first cerebellar symptom and may be missed if the patient is not explicitly asked to walk. Although rather uncommon during the first phase after ictus further cerebellar signs should be looked for: tremor, dysmetria, nystagmus, dysarthria. Furthermore, affection of cranial nerves can be present. Therefore, one ought to look for signs like subtle ipsilateral facial palsy or absent corneal reflex.

In case the diagnosis is suspected, computed tomography (CT)-imaging should be given priority among the diagnostic examinations and unnecessary delay should be avoided since clinical diagnosis alone always bears a high degree of inaccuracy in this entity.

Scales

The **Glasgow Coma Scale (GCS)** score has been shown to correlate with 30-day survival in patients suffering from a supratentorial ICH. In patients with a cerebellar hematoma, in which alteration of consciousness is often present, the GCS is also an important clinical tool, but reliable clinical data to predict outcome or to trigger therapeutic intervention are almost lacking.

In ICH patients in general the National Institute of Health Stroke Scale (NIHSS) [24–26], the Scandinavian Stroke Scale [27,28], and the Unified Neurological Stroke Scale [29] are all being used, but their value in clinical monitoring of patients with cerebellar ICH remains uncertain. The 'ICH score' might be of interest in the clinical evaluation of patients with cerebellar bleeding, 'infratentorial origin of ICH' constituting one of its five components, 'GCS score', 'ICH volume', 'presence of IVH' and 'age' being the other [30]. Because all these clinical scales have their strengths and limitations a prospective clinical outcome study is needed to investigate their predictive value in cerebellar hemorrhage and/or establish ideal grading scales to enable rational treatment approaches in these patients [31]. Currently no scale can be recommended.

Neuroimaging

As pointed out above, neuroimaging is indispensable for the establishment of the diagnosis (see Fig. 24.1).

CT and magnetic resonance imaging (MRI) both allow the detection of blood in the cerebellum and accompanying hydrocephalus with high accuracy and high specificity (i.e. distinction of another cerebellar or brain stem process possible, especially cerebellar ischemia) [32]. When the hematoma is visible, usually a non-contrast CT scan will suffice in the acute phase. Whenever possible without time delay, MRI may be used instead of CT. In this case imaging should include T2*-weighted sequences in order to depict blood in the acute phase. MRI has the advantage that rarer causes of cerebellar hemorrhage such as low-flow vascular malformations including cavernomas are clearly detectable [33]. The same is true for hemorrhages secondary to tumors. When evaluating the imaging material attention should be paid to hematoma size, location (especially extension into the vermis), presence of hydrocephalus, quadrigeminal cistern obliteration, intraventricular blood, brain stem compression or distortion, and signs of upward or downward herniation [8].

Vascular imaging

Vascular imaging modalities for further diagnostic evaluation in cerebellar hemorrhage include CT angiography (CTA), MR angiography (MRA), and conventional or digital subtraction angiography (DSA).

The locations of most cerebellar hematomas are compatible with the diagnosis of a hypertensive hemorrhage. Vice versa, there is no location of a cerebellar hematoma that does exclude another underlying cause. In other words hardly any information can be extracted from the non-contrast CT scan about possible underlying pathologies such as vascular malformations or malignancies. Thus as a practical rule in elderly patients with

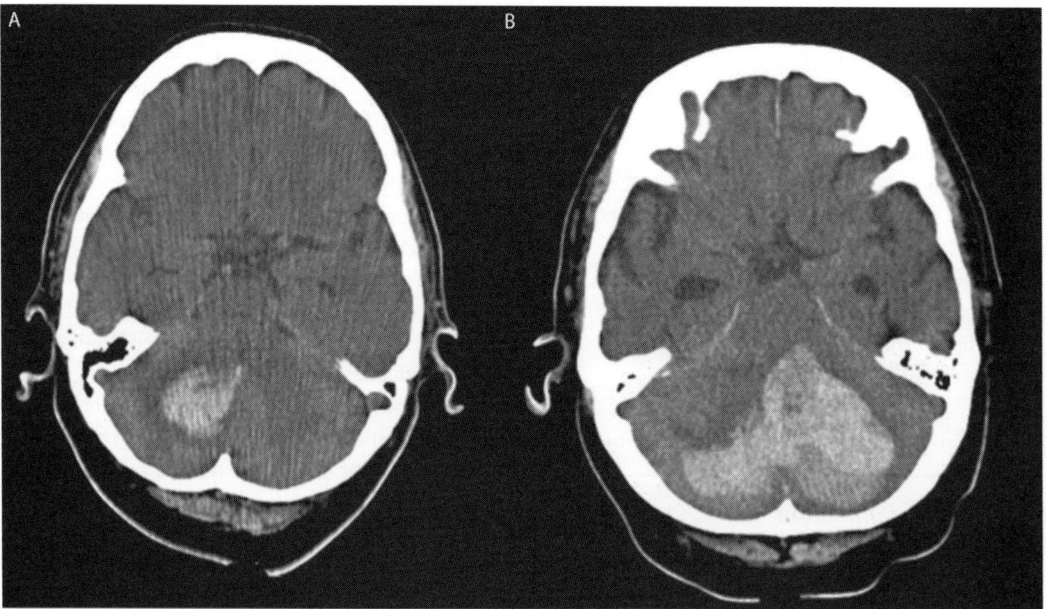

Fig. 24.1 A: CT scan of a right hemispheric cerebellar hematoma in a 51-year-old patient with history of headache and dysarthria 30 minutes before admission. On admission she was drowsy, but orientated (GCS 13). B: CT scan of a 78-year-old patient who was last seen healthy 2 hours before admission. 20 minutes before admission he was found comatose (GCS score 3), brain stem reflexes were absent, and Babinski sign were positive on both sides. CT scan shows massive cerebellar hematoma involving both hemispheres.

a known history of hypertension further imaging studies are not necessarily needed, at least not in the acute phase. In young patients or in patients without history of arterial hypertension conventional imaging should be supplemented with MRA, CTA, and/or DSA. Of these CTA is usually the imaging method of choice in patients with a cerebellar hemorrhage that are candidates for emergency surgery and are likely to have an intracranial bleeding due to a secondary cause. CTA is also indicated in most high-flow vascular malformations, such as most arteriovenous malformations (AVM) and aneurysms [34]. However, DSA remains the gold standard in patients with AVM or aneurysm. The consideration to carry out DSA in a patient should always include the question if this diagnostic measure may lead to a consequence since it entails a higher peri-procedural risk than CTA or MRA.

Other tests

In all patients with hemorrhagic strokes coagulation parameters, at least including INR, partial thromboplastin time, and platelet count should be determined. This should be done for diagnostic reasons and in case surgery is considered as a treatment option.

One should refrain from performing a lumbar puncture as a diagnostic measure because of the risk of herniation in case of elevated intracranial pressure. In the case of rupture of the bleeding into the ventricular system, cerebrospinal fluid (CSF) will be found to contain macroscopically visible blood, but usually the procedure does not contribute diagnostic information beyond imaging studies.

Complications

The most important and life-threatening complications in the acute phase are brain stem compression and the development of hydrocephalus. The latter may be the consequence of compression of the fourth ventricle and/or the aqueduct, but may also be caused by malresorption due to intraventricular blood.

Compression of the fourth ventricle is frequently seen on initial CT scans due to the mass effect originating from the cerebellar hematoma [35]. Although many studies have found an association between size and location of the bleeding and the degree of hydrocephalus, fourth ventricular narrowing and hematoma size are not necessarily correlated. No hydrocephalus may be present despite a hematoma diameter exceeding 4 cm; conversely the appearance of a pronounced hydrocephalus can be associated with only a minor hemorrhage. Development of hydrocephalus mainly seems to depend on hematoma location: a vermian clot will usually lead to hydrocephalus, a bleeding lateral of the vermis in most cases [36,37]. Another criterion for predicting the development of a hydrocephalus is obliteration of the quadrigeminal cistern. Extravasation of blood into the ventricles may also lead to obstruction of CSF flow and may thus cause hydrocephalus, even in patients with small hematomas [38]. Figure 24.2 demonstrates an example of a cerebellar hemorrhage in which compression of the fourth ventricle and IVH lead to hydrocephalus.

Involvement of the brain stem is often a catastrophic scenario and immediately life-threatening. The brain stem is usually affected by the direct mass effect of the cerebellar blood clot. Sometimes also additional bleeding occurs in the brain stem itself. The challenge for the clinician arises from the time course by which the clinical picture develops. A slow sequence of events – comprising a slow decline of level of consciousness, sixth nerve palsy, hemiparesis, and further brain stem signs – that could aid recognizing the complication unfortunately occurs rarely. Usually there is a rapid decline of consciousness or the patient is already in coma on admission. The fact that the clinical picture usually does not help to detect the underlying pathological process has given rise to many ideas and numerous studies that tried to identify factors predicting brain stem involvement and the course of the disease (see below).

Treatment

Before describing conservative and surgical management, the indication for one or the other treatment approach shall be discussed. Since the first reported successful surgical intervention in a 12-year-old boy with cerebellar hemorrhage in 1906 [39] the indication to perform surgery in these patients has been controversial

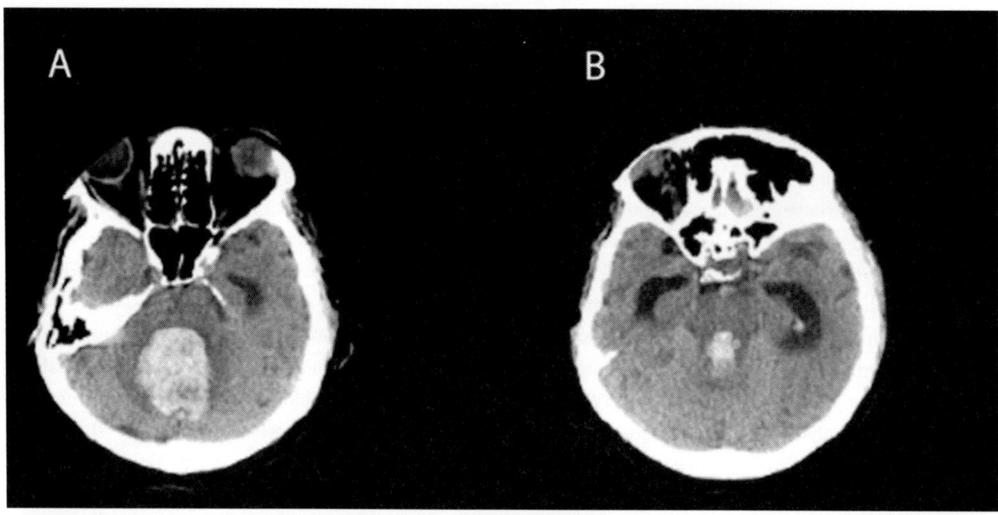

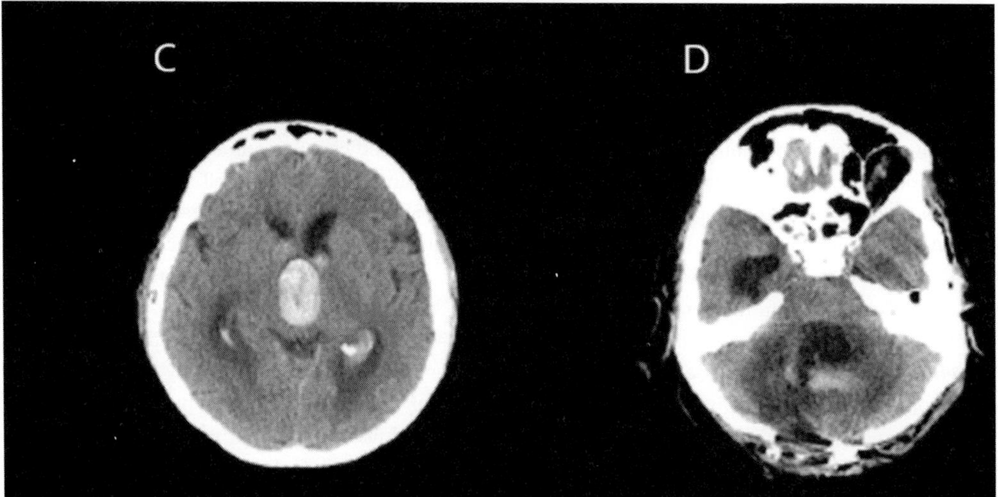

Fig. 24.2 CT scan showing a midline cerebellar hemorrhage with rupture into the ventricular system in a 60-year-old patient. A–C: Blood can be seen in the fourth and third ventricles, which are both obstructed, and in the lateral ventricles. The temporal horns of the lateral ventricles are clearly dilated. D: Postoperative scan after craniotomy and removal of the hematoma.

[7,9,40,41]. Many authors believe that a surgical approach by hematoma evacuation and/or decompression of the posterior fossa is the only treatment option improving survival in acute cerebellar hemorrhage [42,43]. However, there is neither a clear consensus concerning the indication for surgical intervention, nor concerning the type of intervention, nor timing and sequence of possible therapeutic measures among neurosurgeons and among neurointensivists. Considerations guiding decision making whether to operate in supratentorial ICH may not necessarily be useful in infratentorial ICH [44–46]. In addition, unlike for supratentorial hemorrhage, there are few studies, among them many case reports or small case series, very few prospective studies, no large trials, and no randomized controlled trials available that may help to create evidence-based recommendations [9,47,48]. Moreover, in most instances these studies were conducted in only one center and, as a result, are hardly comparable due to patient selection, lacking control groups, different treatment protocols, surgical techniques as well as medical measures, none of which is standardized. In addition, many neurosurgeons feel that surgery is necessary in a patient with a deteriorating state of consciousness, which might be the reason for a bias towards surgery in many studies [49]. Furthermore, one may assume that there is a publication bias for cases that were treated successfully.

In these studies the following factors have been suggested to predict poor outcome:

1. Decreased GCS score of the patient on admission [9,47,48,50–52].
2. Presence and evolution of clinical brain stem signs [53–55].
3. Increased hematoma size on CT [10,36,41,48,55–57].
4. Midline hematoma location on CT [8].
5. Presence of hydrocephalus on initial CT [8,10,56,58].
6. Compression of fourth ventricle or brain stem involvement on CT [10,38,47,50].
7. Presence of intraventricular blood on CT [47].
8. A secondary cause of hemorrhage [59].

Despite all the above-mentioned limitations some practical conclusions may be deduced from the data provided in the literature. The clinical state of the patient, especially the level of consciousness and brain stem signs, on admission, is probably the most important factor for treatment decisions. The most common surgical approach in patients deteriorating and with large hematomas is decompressive surgery in combination with hematoma evacuation. Patients in coma on admission in whom brain stem reflexes are preserved will usually also undergo surgery. Patients who have been in a coma for several hours on admission and in whom brain stem reflexes are absent are usually not operated and treated conservatively.

This approach requires close observation, ideally on a neurological intensive care unit. An alert patient with a GCS score of 14 or 15 and a small hematoma on CT or MRI may initially be treated on a stroke unit. Repeated neuroimaging should be done at least 24 hours after the ictus or immediately in case of clinical deterioration [35].

A therapeutic scheme that has gained much acceptance was rendered by Kobayashi *et al.* [48]. The treatment algorithm was based on the retrospective analysis of 52 patients. This algorithm is mainly based on the patients' GCS score and the hematoma size on CT. It was subsequently tested prospectively in a second group of 49 patients.

1. Patients with GCS scores of 14 or 15 and with a hematoma of less than 40 mm in maximum diameter are treated conservatively.
2. For patients with GCS scores of 13 or less and with a hematoma of 40 mm or more in diameter, hematoma evacuation plus decompressive suboccipital craniectomy should be the treatment of choice.
3. For the patient whose brain stem reflexes are entirely lost, with flaccid tetraplegia, or whose general condition is poor, intensive therapy is not indicated.

Using hematoma size alone as the discriminating factor between surgical and non-surgical patients was advocated by Little *et al.* [36], which still forms the basis of the current American and European guidelines for intracerebral hemorrhage [44]. In a series of only 10 patients those with a hematoma diameter of less than 3 cm had a benign course without surgery, whereas those with a hematoma diameter of more than 3 cm were operated on. Meanwhile other investigators found that also patients with large hematomas may have a benign clinical course and good outcomes without surgery, on the other hand patients with small hematomas may require surgery due to its unfavorable location or may have a poor outcome irrespective of treatment due to complications such as IVH, additional brain stem hemorrhage, malignant concomitant diseases, or others [21,37,38,60,61]. This discrepancy illustrates that single clinical studies are insufficient and that large-scale prospective trials are needed in order to find appropriate treatment algorithms for all patients.

General treatment

Medical treatment of cerebellar hemorrhage does not essentially differ from treatment of supratentorial ICH (see 'Intracranial hemorrhage', and 'Medical therapy'). Its main goals are cardiovascular, metabolic and respiratory stabilization of the acute and critically ill patient.

This includes referring the patient to a specialized center, admission on a stroke unit or neurointensive care unit, monitoring basic vital functions and providing prophylaxis of complications, especially aspiration pneumonia, gastric ulcer, and deep venous thrombosis/ pulmonary embolism [44].

Intubation

Many patients with cerebellar hemorrhages are comatose on admission or deteriorate early. Low GCS scores or absent protecting reflexes often demand early intubation. Because the necessity of ventilation is an independent predictor of an unfavorable long-term outcome in these patients [10], it is always demanding for the physician, whom to intubate and what is the most appropriate time to do that, especially in patients with an intermediate GCS score or in patients whose state of consciousness slowly deteriorates. Other predictors for outcome which are mentioned below may help to guide this decision.

Blood pressure

Special attention should be paid to blood pressure control. It has been shown that aggressive treatment of elevated blood pressure in the acute phase after hemorrhagic stroke is not beneficial. Given the high prevalence of patients with pre-existing hypertension in spontaneous cerebellar hemorrhage elevated blood pressure should be treated with particular caution. Because guidelines derived from randomized controlled trials are lacking, the following rules might be considered. These recommendations do not differ from the treatment of supratentorial spontaneous cerebral hemorrhages. In all patients in whom reduction of blood pressure is not indicated or contraindicated for other reasons (i.e. mainly cardiac reasons) blood pressure should not be reduced by more than 20% of the initial value. Guidelines by the European Stroke Organisation are comparatively more aggressive than those by the American Heart Association. In patients with a known history of hypertension, blood pressure should only be treated when the systolic value exceeds 180 mmHg, in patients without history of hypertension blood pressure should be treated when the systolic value exceeds 160 mmHg with target values of 170 mmHg and 150 mmHg, respectively. It is recommended to monitor cerebral perfusion pressure, which should be kept > 60 mmHg [44,62].

Increased intracranial pressure (ICP)

Because of the immediate effect of the hematoma in the narrow posterior fossa and the high incidence of hydrocephalus in patients with cerebellar bleeding, therapy of increased intracranial pressure is an important element of medical management of these patients in the ICU (for details please refer to 'ICP' and ''Antiedema therapy'). The purpose of ICP-lowering therapy is to minimize damage to brain tissue caused either by direct compression or by secondary ischemia. Therefore, the modern concept of ICP-lowering therapy consists of two strategies, the first is primarily mechanistic, the second is CPP-oriented. Both largely overlap and do not exclude each other. Primary measures include elevation of the head by 15 to 30° and analgosedation. Further interventions include hyperventilation, osmotherapy, administration of buffers, and/or administration of barbiturates. Most of these measures have been shown to be effective in reducing ICP, although most have only short-term effects, but none of them has been shown to have a beneficial effect on long-term outcome, either in patients with cerebellar hemorrhages, in patients with cerebral hemorrhages in general, or in stroke patients in general [63–66]. Some of these strategies, however, should be used with special care, because their effects, apart from being unproven or ineffective, may have serious side effects or may even be detrimental. Barbiturates for example, although capable of decreasing ICP, do this at the cost of lowering CPP and cerebral oxygen pressure as well [67]. Thus, they should only be applied as a bridging therapy in patients where more promising therapies such as surgical interventions are planned or as a last treatment option after all other therapies have failed.

Surgical treatment

Patients with acute cerebellar hematomas can rapidly deteriorate to coma and death due to local mass effect and compression of the brain stem. This puts an emphasis on mechanical thinking and the role of surgery in these patients. The purpose of surgical intervention is to release CSF from within the skull, remove the hematoma, and/or create space within the posterior fossa, thereby secondarily diminishing pressure on the brain stem that is exerted by an expanding hematoma or by supratentorial brain structures in the case of obstructive hydrocephalus. This can be achieved by insertion of a ventricular drain, evacuation of the hematoma, and/or suboccipital decompressive surgery (or a combination of these), respectively. Few studies include different surgical approaches that will be mentioned shortly (for further details on surgical techniques of hematoma removal in cerebral hemorrhage please refer to 'Decompressive surgery' and 'Management of ventricular drains').

Ventricular drainage

Ventricular drainage via insertion of an extraventricular drain (EVD) is a neurosurgical standard procedure, an effective measure to reduce intracranial pressure originating from obstructive hydrocephalus, and can be done bedside. In addition to CSF drainage it allows drainage of blood in case of accompanying intraventricular hemorrhage, which may be combined with intraventricular clot lysis. It is usually employed together with decompressive surgery. Few studies have investigated the outcome in patients treated with EVD placement only. Patients in these studies are subject to selection bias, adequate control groups are lacking, and results are heterogeneous [19,37,47,52,68,69]. Therefore, definitive recommendations using an EVD alone in patients with obstructive hydrocephalus due to a cerebellar hematoma cannot be given. Apart from other risks inherent to EVD catheter placement the surgeon has to be aware of possibly inducing upward herniation. Upward herniation designates an inverse herniation of parts of the posterior fossa through the tentorium in a caudal to cranial direction. This can occur when the pressure accumulating in the posterior fossa is suddenly relieved by supratentorial EVD. Although mentioned in several case reports in the literature, most experienced neurosurgeons agree that this is a rare and very uncommon complication, but may occur in patients when mass effect of the cerebellar hematoma and pronounced hydrocephalus is visible on neuroimaging. To avoid this EVD should be combined with suboccipital decompressive craniectomy in these cases. Alternatively to EVD placement third ventriculostomy can be used [70,71].

Suboccipital craniotomy and craniectomy

Surgical approaches to a cerebellar hematoma comprise craniectomies and craniotomies ('burr hole' or 'key hole' craniotomy). Besides removal of blood, craniectomy has the purpose of creating space outside the skull for residual blood and accompanying edema and relieving the pressure exerted on the tissue underneath, and comprises one of the standard techniques in neurosurgical departments. The chosen anatomical approach to the cerebellum for craniotomy and craniectomy mainly depends on the size and location of the blood clot and whether displacement of the fourth ventricle or brain stem is present. Midline suboccipital craniectomy will be preferred when it is the goal to gain access to the vermis or both cerebellar hemispheres. Paramedian suboccipital craniectomy will be preferred when the clot is located exclusively or predominantly in one hemisphere. Small craniotomies with subsequent CT-guided aspiration of the hematoma can be carried out in case the hematoma is located closely or adjacent to the skull. Theoretically, a burr-hole approach is less invasive and may have fewer side effects, on the other hand a large craniectomy may create more space. Few studies have compared these different surgical techniques in patients with a cerebellar hemorrhage. Tamaki *et al.* compared large suboccipital craniectomy with minimally invasive small paramedian suboccipital craniectomy. No differences were found in the two groups ('large craniectomy' n = 21; 'mini craniectomy' n = 25) concerning postoperative outcome. However, operating time was shorter and patients were less likely to require blood transfusions and had less postoperative liquorrhea when treated with 'mini craniectomy' [72]. Another study in 23 patients with spontaneous cerebellar hemorrhage investigated the efficacy of a small 3-cm-keyhole craniotomy demonstrating satisfactory results; however, the technique was not directly compared with standard surgical approaches [73].

Table 24.3 Mortality rates in cerebellar hemorrhage. Data based on 67 studies including 1843 patients. Studies were included in this analysis only if they clearly distinguished between surviving and deceased patients. 37.3% of all patients died. The mortality rate was 42.6% and 32% for the medical and the surgical group respectively.

All patients with cerebellar hemorrhage (N, (%))		Conservative therapy (N, (%))		Hematoma evacuation and/or decompressive surgery, with or without EVD (N, (%))		EVD alone (N, (%))	
died	survived	died	survived	died	survived	died	survived
435 (37.3)	730 (62.7)	185 (42.6)	249 (57.4)	192 (32)	408 (68)	54 (43.2)	71 (56.8)

Prognosis

The following data are based on an extensive literature review including 67 publications on cerebellar hemorrhage, where at least an abstract providing relevant data was available in English or German. These report on 1843 patients. In addition, there are few case reports or small case series from the pre-CT era between 1937 and 1955 or written in French, Spanish, or Japanese. Some of these abstracts were not available in English so they are not included in this analysis [74–87]. Most of these studies are retrospective and monocentre studies and are always subject to a high selection bias, especially when comparing surgical and conservative treatment, thereby limiting the reliability of these available data, which must be interpreted very carefully, especially in terms of generalizability.

Mortality

Results are given in Table 24.3. There is a clear discrepancy between older studies, especially those without the diagnostic help of CT or MRI, and recent studies concerning mortality rates in cerebellar hemorrhage irrespective of treatment. In older studies very high overall mortality rates are reported ranging from 58% to 90% [7,15,23,88,89]. In more recent studies mortality rates between 27% and 48% are reported [10,37,48,55,90,91]. Only few studies have assessed outcome more than 3 months after the ictus [10,37,40,48,50,55,69]. In the study by Lui *et al.* including 26 patients, overall mortality was 35% (follow-up 6 months to 4 years) [55]. Dolderer *et al.* report a higher overall mortality rate of 48% (mean time to follow-up 4 years) [10].

Mortality rates in surgically treated patients are heterogeneous. In the study by Dolderer *et al.* mortality rate after surgery was higher (64%) than overall mortality [10]. Most studies, however, report lower mortality rates after surgery. Lui *et al.* 27%, Kobayashi *et al.* 19%, Dammann *et al.* 25% [48,51,55]. Brain stem compression before surgery seems to be a strong predictor for poor outcome in these patients. Waidhauser *et al.* found a strong discrepancy in mortality between those patients with brain stem compression and those without, with mortality rates of 57% and 9%, respectively [69]. Unfortunately, there are no larger studies or case series evaluating mortality after external ventricular drainage alone.

In patients undergoing medical management Kobayashi *et al.* reported a mortality rate of 0%. In other studies mortality rates of 25% [69], 28% [37], and 39% [10] are reported. Again, brain stem compression seems to be a most strong predictor for increased mortality. In the cohort of Waidhauser *et al.* mortality rate in these patients was 100% [69].

When interpreting these numbers one needs to be aware of potential patient selection bias, publication bias, diagnostic difficulties (particularly before the introduction of CT), and procedural and semantic inaccuracies inherent in the studies that have provided the analyzed data.

Outcome in survivors

Table 24.4 demonstrates the pooled patient data from eight studies that included 223 patients giving outcome data of surviving patients after cerebellar hemorrhage and either used comparable clinical outcome scales (usually the Glasgow Outcome Scale or the modified

Table 24.4 Outcome in survivors of cerebellar hemorrhage according to treatment.

	All patients with cerebellar hemorrhage (N, (%))			Conservative therapy (N, (%))			Hematoma evacuation and/or decompressive surgery, with or without EVD (N, (%))			EVD alone (N, (%))		
Disability of survivors	none to mild	moderate	severe	none to mild	moderate	severe	none to mild	moderate	severe	none to mild	moderate	severe
Total patients available: 223	129 (57.8)	37 (16.6)	57 (25.6)	50 (94.3)	2 (3.8)	1 (1.9)	71 (44.1)	35 (21.7)	55 (34.2)	8 (88.9)	0 (0)	1 (11.1)

Rankin Scale) or described outcome precisely enough that made allocation to one of the three outcome categories possible [6,10,48,51,53,55,72,92]. 57.8% of surviving patients had no or mild disability. This was more than twice as high among patients that were managed medically or by EVD alone than in the surgical group (94.3% vs. 88.9% vs. 44.1%, respectively).

About one quarter of all patients were severely disabled, again with a large difference between the treatment groups (1.9% after conservative treatment, 11.1% after EVD alone, and 34.2% after surgical treatment).

The higher percentage of patients with unfavorable outcome among surgically treated patients in turn most likely reflects the selection of patients that undergo surgery, i.e. surgically treated patients usually had more severe strokes, more often a deteriorating state of consciousness or coma on admission. Therefore, again, these data must be interpreted with caution. Nevertheless, these numbers may help to estimate the prognosis and thereby be one piece in the process of decision making.

In this context it must be noted that these data also question the current belief reflected in international guidelines that outcome in survivors of cerebellar hemorrhage is usually good. It is surprising that European as well as American recommendations claim that 'surprisingly good results have been reported with surgical evacuation of cerebellar hematomas' and 'nonrandomized studies showing that patients with cerebellar ICH larger than 3 cm in diameter or those with brain stem compression or hydrocephalus had good outcomes whereas similar patients managed medically did poorly', and give comparatively clear recommendations such as 'ventricular drainage and evacuation of the hematoma should be considered if hydrocephalus occurs or if hematomas are > 2–3 cm in diameter (level C evidence)' and 'patients with cerebellar hemorrhage who are deteriorating neurologically or who have brain stem compression and/or hydrocephalus from ventricular obstruction should undergo surgical removal of the hemorrhage as soon as possible (Class I, level of evidence B)' [44].

In fact, it is currently unclear which factors predict a poor outcome (hydrocephalus, location of the hematoma, additional brain stem infarct, additional intraventricular bleeding, size of the hematoma…). As a result, also the best medical and surgical approaches are currently unclear and, until data from large prospective studies or randomised trials are available, lie in the hands of the treating physicians, their personal experience, and their personal beliefs.

REFERENCES

1. Flaherty ML, Woo D, Haverbusch M, *et al.* Racial variations in location and risk of intracerebral hemorrhage. *Stroke* 2005;**36**:934–7.
2. Dinsdale HB. Spontaneous hemorrhage in the posterior fossa. A study of primary cerebellar and pontine hemorrhages with observations on their pathogenesis. *Arch Neurol* 1964;**10**:200–17.
3. McCormick WF, Rosenfield DB. Massive brain hemorrhage: a review of 144 cases and an examination of their causes. *Stroke* 1973;**4**:946–54.
4. Inagawa T, Ohbayashi N, Takechi A, Shibukawa M, Yahara K. Primary intracerebral hemorrhage in Izumo City, Japan: incidence rates and outcome in relation to the site of hemorrhage. *Neurosurgery* 2003;**53**:1283–97; discussion 1297–8.
5. Sypert GWA, Lvord EC J. Cerebellar infarction. A clinicopathological study. *Arch Neurol* 1975;**32**:357–63.
6. Freeman JW, Kennedy RM, Petty SS. Prognosis of nonoperated cerebellar hemorrhage. *Ann Neurol* 1978;**4**:389–90.
7. Ott KH, Kase CS, Ojemann RG, Mohr JP. Cerebellar hemorrhage: diagnosis and treatment. A review of 56 cases. *Arch Neurol* 1974;**31**:160–7.
8. St Louis EK, Wijdicks EF, Li H. Predicting neurologic deterioration in patients with cerebellar hematomas. *Neurology* 1998;**51**:1364–9.
9. Kirollos RW, Tyagi AK, Ross SA, van Hille PT, Marks PV. Management of spontaneous cerebellar hematomas: a prospective treatment protocol. *Neurosurgery* 2001;**49**:1378–86; discussion 1386–7.
10. Dolderer S, Kallenberg K, Aschoff A, Schwab S, Schwarz S. Long-term outcome after spontaneous cerebellar haemorrhage. *Eur Neurol* 2004;**52**:112–19.
11. Itoh Y, Yamada M, Hayakawa M, Otomo E, Miyatake T. Cerebral amyloid angiopathy: a significant cause of cerebellar as well as lobar cerebral hemorrhage in the elderly. *J Neurol Sci* 1993;**116**:135–41.
12. Cuny E, Loiseau H, Rivel J, Vital C, Castel JP. Amyloid angiopathy-related cerebellar hemorrhage. *Surg Neurol* 1996;**46**:235–9.

13. Wattendorff AR, Bots GT, Went LN, Endtz LJ. Familial cerebral amyloid angiopathy presenting as recurrent cerebral haemorrhage. *J Neurol Sci* 1982;**55**:121–35.
14. Yamada M. Cerebral amyloid angiopathy: an overview. *Neuropathology* 2000;**20**:8–22.
15. McKissock W, Richardson A, Walsh L. Spontaneous cerebellar hemorrhage: a study of 34 consecutive cases treated surgically. *Brain* 1960;**83**:1–9.
16. Weir CJ, Murray GD, Adams FG, *et al.* Poor accuracy of stroke scoring systems for differential clinical diagnosis of intracranial haemorrhage and infarction. *Lancet* 1994;**344**:999–1002.
17. Mohr JP, Caplan LR, Melski JW, *et al.* The Harvard Cooperative Stroke Registry: a prospective registry. *Neurology* 1978;**28**:754–62.
18. Melo TP, Pinto AN, Ferro JM. Headache in intracerebral hematomas. *Neurology* 1996;**47**:494–500.
19. Hojer C, Bewermeyer M, Huber M, *et al.* Kleinhirninfarkte und Kleinhirnblutungen. Eine vergleichende, retrospektive Studie an 78 Patienten. *Akt Neurol* 1991;**18**:88–94.
20. Melamed N, Satya-Murti S. Cerebellar hemorrhage. A review and reappraisal of benign cases. *Arch Neurol* 1984;**41**:425–8.
21. Dunne JW, Chakera T, Kermode S. Cerebellar haemorrhage-diagnosis and treatment: a study of 75 consecutive cases. *Q J Med* 1987;**64**:739–54.
22. Rosenberg GA, Kaufman DM. Cerebellar hemorrhage: reliability of clinical evaluation. *Stroke* 1976;**7**:332–6.
23. Fisher CM, Picard EH, Polak A, Dalal P, Pojemann RG. Acute hypertensive cerebellar hemorrhage: Diagnosis and surgical treatment. *J Nerv Ment Dis* 1965;**140**:38–57.
24. Brott T, Adams HP, Jr., Olinger CP, *et al.* Measurements of acute cerebral infarction: a clinical examination scale. *Stroke* 1989;**20**:864–70.
25. Goldstein LB, Bertels C, Davis JN. Interrater reliability of the NIH stroke scale. *Arch Neurol* 1989;**46**:660–2.
26. Brott T, Marler JR, Olinger CP, *et al.* Measurements of acute cerebral infarction: lesion size by computed tomography. *Stroke* 1989;**20**:871–5.
27. Multicenter trial of hemodilution in ischemic stroke-background and study protocol. Scandinavian Stroke Study Group. *Stroke* 1985;**16**:885–90.
28. Lindenstrøm E, Boysen G, Waage Christiansen L, à Rogvi Hansen B, Würtzen Nielsen P. Reliability of Scandinavian Neurological Stroke Scale. *Cerebrovasc Dis* 1991;**1**:103–7.
29. Orgogozo JM, Asplund K, Boysen G. A unified form for neurological scoring of hemispheric stroke with motor impairment. *Stroke* 1992;**23**:1678–9.
30. Hemphill JC, 3rd, Bonovich DC, Besmertis L, Manley GT, Johnston SC. The ICH score: a simple, reliable grading scale for intracerebral hemorrhage. *Stroke* 2001;**32**:891–7.
31. Hwang BY, Appelboom G, Kellner CP, *et al.* Clinical grading scales in intracerebral hemorrhage. *Neurocrit Care* 2010;**13**:141–51.
32. Muller HR, Wuthrich R, Wiggli U, Hunig R, Elke M. The contribution of computerized axial tomography to the diagnosis of cerebellar and pontine hematomas. *Stroke* 1975;**6**:467–75.
33. George B, Celis-Lopez M, Kato T, Lot G. Arteriovenous malformations of the posterior fossa. *Acta Neurochir (Wien)* 1992;**116**:119–27.
34. Uysal E, Yanbuloglu B, Erturk M, Kilinc BM, Basak M. Spiral CT angiography in diagnosis of cerebral aneurysms of cases with acute subarachnoid hemorrhage. *Diagn Interv Radiol* 2005;**11**:77–82.
35. Elkind MS, Mohr JP. Cerebellar hemorrhage. *New Horiz* 1997;**5**:352–8.
36. Little JR, Tubman DE, Ethier R. Cerebellar hemorrhage in adults. Diagnosis by computerized tomography. *J Neurosurg* 1978;**48**:575–9.
37. van der Hoop RG, Vermeulen M, van Gijn J. Cerebellar hemorrhage: diagnosis and treatment. *Surg Neurol* 1988;**29**:6–10.
38. Taneda M, Hayakawa T, Mogami H. Primary cerebellar hemorrhage. Quadrigeminal cistern obliteration on CT scans as a predictor of outcome. *J Neurosurg* 1987;**67**:545–52.
39. Ballance H. A case of traumatic haemorrhage into the left lateral lobe of the cerebellum treated by operation with recovery. *Surg Gyn Obstet* 1906: 223–35.
40. Salvati M, Cervoni L, Raco A, Delfini R. Spontaneous cerebellar hemorrhage: clinical remarks on 50 cases. *Surg Neurol* 2001;**55**:156–61; discussion 161.
41. Cohen ZR, Ram Z, Knoller N, Peles E, Hadani M. Management and outcome of non-traumatic cerebellar haemorrhage. *Cerebrovasc Dis* 2002;**14**:207–13.
42. Sypert GW. Cerebellar hemorrhage and infarction. *Compr Ther* 1977;**3**:42–7.
43. Arseni C, Oprescu I. Cerebellar hematomas. *J Neurosurg* 1959;**16**:503–7.
44. Steiner T, Kaste M, Forsting M, *et al.* Recommendations for the management of intracranial haemorrhage-part I: spontaneous intracerebral haemorrhage. The European Stroke Initiative Writing Committee and the Writing Committee for the EUSI Executive Committee. *Cerebrovasc Dis* 2006;**22**:294–316.

45. Mathew P, Teasdale G, Bannan A, Oluoch-Olunya D. Neurosurgical management of cerebellar haematoma and infarct. *J Neurol Neurosurg Psychiatry* 1995;**59**:287–92.
46. Mendelow AD, Unterberg A. Surgical treatment of intracerebral haemorrhage. *Curr Opin Crit Care* 2007;**13**:169–74.
47. Donauer E, Loew F, Faubert C, Alesch F, Schaan M. Prognostic factors in the treatment of cerebellar haemorrhage. *Acta Neurochir (Wien)* 1994;**131**:59–66.
48. Kobayashi S, Sato A, Kageyama Y, *et al.* Treatment of hypertensive cerebellar hemorrhage – surgical or conservative management? *Neurosurgery* 1994;**34**:246–50; discussion 250–1.
49. Wijdicks EF, St Louis EK, Atkinson JD, Li H. Clinician's biases toward surgery in cerebellar hematomas: an analysis of decision-making in 94 patients. *Cerebrovasc Dis* 2000;**10**:93–6.
50. van Loon J, Van Calenbergh F, Goffin J, Plets C. Controversies in the management of spontaneous cerebellar haemorrhage. A consecutive series of 49 cases and review of the literature. *Acta Neurochir (Wien)* 1993;**122**:187–93.
51. Dammann P, Asgari S, Bassiouni H, *et al.* Spontaneous cerebellar hemorrhage: experience with 57 surgically treated patients and review of the literature. *Neurosurg Rev* 2010;**34** (1):77–86.
52. Firsching R, Huber M, Frowein RA. Cerebellar haemorrhage: management and prognosis. *Neurosurg Rev* 1991;**14**:191–4.
53. Brennan RW, Bergland RM. Acute cerebellar hemorrhage. Analysis of clinical findings and outcome in 12 cases. *Neurology* 1977;**27**:527–32.
54. Auer LM, Auer T, Sayama I. Indications for surgical treatment of cerebellar haemorrhage and infarction. *Acta Neurochir (Wien)* 1986;**79**:74–9.
55. Lui TN, Fairholm DJ, Shu TF, *et al.* Surgical treatment of spontaneous cerebellar hemorrhage. *Surg Neurol* 1985;**23**:555–8.
56. Mezzadri JJ, Otero JM, Ottino CA. Management of 50 spontaneous cerebellar haemorrhages. Importance of obstructive hydrocephalus. *Acta Neurochir (Wien)* 1993;**122**:39–44.
57. Zieger A, Vonofakos D, Steudel WI, Dusterbehn G. Nontraumatic intracerebellar hematomas: prognostic value of volumetric evaluation by computed tomography. *Surg Neurol* 1984;**22**:491–4.
58. Shenkin HA, Zavala M. Cerebellar strokes: mortality, surgical indications, and results of ventricular drainage. *Lancet* 1982;**2**:429–32.
59. Hill MD, Silver FL. Epidemiologic predictors of 30-day survival in cerebellar hemorrhage. *J Stroke Cerebrovasc Dis* 2001;**10**:118–21.
60. Heros RC. Cerebellar hemorrhage and infarction. *Stroke* 1982;**13**:106–9.
61. Bogousslavsky J, Regli F, Jeanrenaud X. Benign outcome in unoperated large cerebellar haemorrhage. Report of 2 cases. *Acta Neurochir (Wien)* 1984;**73**:59–65.
62. Morgenstern LB, Hemphill JC, 3rd, Anderson C, *et al.* Guidelines for the management of spontaneous intracerebral hemorrhage: a guideline for healthcare professionals from the American Heart Association/American Stroke Association. *Stroke* 2010;**41**:2108–29.
63. Christensen MS, Brodersen P, Olesen J, Paulson OB. Cerebral apoplexy (stroke) treated with or without prolonged artificial hyperventilation. 2. Cerebrospinal fluid acid-base balance and intracranial pressure. *Stroke* 1973;**4**:620–31.
64. Bereczki D, Liu M, do Prado GF, Fekete I. Mannitol for acute stroke. *Stroke* 2008;**39**:512–13.
65. Schwarz S, Schwab S, Bertram M, Aschoff A, Hacke W. Effects of hypertonic saline hydroxyethyl starch solution and mannitol in patients with increased intracranial pressure after stroke. *Stroke* 1998;**29**:1550–5.
66. Wolf AL, Levi L, Marmarou A, *et al.* Effect of THAM upon outcome in severe head injury: a randomized prospective clinical trial. *J Neurosurg* 1993;**78**:54–9.
67. Steiner T, Pilz J, Schellinger P, *et al.* Multimodal online monitoring in middle cerebral artery territory stroke. *Stroke* 2001;**32**:2500–6.
68. Greenberg J, Skubick D, Shenkin H. Acute hydrocephalus in cerebellar infarct and hemorrhage. *Neurology* 1979;**29**:409–13.
69. Waidhauser E, Hamburger C, Marguth F. Neurosurgical management of cerebellar hemorrhage. *Neurosurg Rev* 1990;**13**:211–17.
70. Gurol ME, St Louis EK. Treatment of cerebellar masses. *Curr Treat Options Neurol* 2008;**10**:138–50.
71. Roux FE, Boetto S, Tremoulet M. Third ventriculocisternostomy in cerebellar haematomas. *Acta Neurochir (Wien)* 2002;**144**:337–42.
72. Tamaki T, Kitamura T, Node Y, Teramoto A. Paramedian suboccipital mini-craniectomy for evacuation of spontaneous cerebellar hemorrhage. *Neurol Med Chir (Tokyo)* 2004;**44**:578–82; discussion 583.
73. Tokimura H, Tajitsu K, Taniguchi A, *et al.* Efficacy and safety of key hole craniotomy for the evacuation of spontaneous cerebellar hemorrhage. *Neurol Med Chir (Tokyo)* 2010;**50**:367–72.
74. Guillaume J, Rogé R, Janny P. *Les hématomes spontanés du cervelet: étude clinique et thérapeutique.* Presse Méd 1949;57.
75. Siris JH, Beller AJ. Spontaneous intracerebellar hemorrhaage; surgical treatment. *Surg Clin N Amer* 1948;**28**:412–15.

76. Dickmann GH, Zimmann L. Hemorragia intracerebelosa espontanea. Tratamiento quirurgico. *Rev Asoc Méd Argent* 1949;**63**:356–8.

77. Ferey D. A new case of recent, spontaneous intra-cerebellar hematoma. *Rev Otoneuro-ophtalmol* 1950;**22**:577–8.

78. Ferey D. Le traitement chirurgical des hématomes intracérébraux et intracérébelleux: a propos de 33 cas operés. *Rev Neurol* 1950;**83**.

79. Gross SW. Posterior fossa hematomas. *J Mt Sinai Hosp N Y* 1955;**22**:286–9.

80. Ferrari M, Arana Iniguez R, Nin R, Etorena O. Spontaneous cerebellar hematoma cured surgically. *An Fac Med Univ Repub Montev Urug* 1953;**38**:179–84.

81. Werden DH. Spontaneous intracerebral and cerebellar hematoma: report of six cases with operative treatment. *Bull Los Angel Neuro Soc* 1951;**16**:174–84.

82. Obrador S, Anastasia JV, Boixadós JR. Un caso de hematoma espontaneo del cerebelo. *Rev Clín Esp* 1952;**44**:199–201.

83. Den Hartog Jager WA. Apoplexia cerebelli. *Ned T Geneesk* 1951;**95**:2533–7.

84. Friedman JM. *Bull Los Angeles Neurol Soc* 1941;**6**:135.

85. Hamby WB. Gross intracerebral hematomas: Report of 16 surgically treated cases. *New York J Med* 1945;**45**:866–75.

86. LeBeau, M. Hématomes spontanés chroniques du cervelet opérés et guéris. *Rev Neurol* 1947;**79**:42–4.

87. Guillaume J. Syndrome hypertension intracrannienne aiguè par hématome intracérébelleux: Découverte operatoire d'ún hémangiome origine de l'hemorragie. *Rev Neurol* 1943;**75**:246.

88. Norris JW, Eisen AA, Branch CL. Problems in cerebellar hemorrhage and infarction. *Neurology* 1969;**19**:1043–50.

89. Rey-Bellet J. Cerebellar hemorrhage, a clinico-pathological study. *Neurology* 1960;**10**:217–22.

90. Da Pian R, Bazzan A, Pasqualin A. Surgical versus medical treatment of spontaneous posterior fossa haematomas: a cooperative study on 205 cases. *Neurol Res* 1984;**6**:145–51.

91. Flaherty ML, Haverbusch M, Sekar P, *et al.* Long-term mortality after intracerebral hemorrhage. *Neurology* 2006;**66**:1182–6.

92. Yanaka K, Meguro K, Fujita K, Narushima K, Nose T. Immediate surgery reduces mortality in deeply comatose patients with spontaneous cerebellar hemorrhage. *Neurol Med Chir (Tokyo)* 2000;**40**:295–9; discussion 299–300.

25

Interventions for brainstem hemorrhage

Berk Orakcioglu and Andreas W. Unterberg

Introduction

Intracerebral hemorrhage (ICH) accounts for up to 20% of all strokes in western civilized countries. Out of these hematomas approximately 6–10% can be subdivided into brainstem hematomas (1). Brainstem bleedings have been historically divided into hematomas and hemorrhage. Hematomas were identified as secondary bleedings related to a vascular anomaly, whereas hemorrhages were understood to be of primary cause in patients suffering arterial hypertension. When diagnosis of primary pontine hemorrhage (PPH), the most common type of brainstem hemorrhage, depended on autopsy, it was considered a fatal neurological disease. Meanwhile it has been understood that brainstem hematomas were more likely to result in an acceptable neurological outcome than such lesions that were classified as brainstem hemorrhage. With intensified treatment regimens that were developed in neuro-intensive care in the past two decades this rather devastating subtype of 'cerebral stroke' gained more attention. However, it is of major importance to classify these lesions immediately in order to enhance or abort diagnostic and treatment measures.

Etiology

Focal subependymal brainstem hematoma (1), and diffuse tegmentobasilar hypertensive hemorrhage (2) must be carefully distinguished (2). Mangiardi *et al.* (2) suggested a generally still accepted classification in 1988 (Fig. 25.1).

Hematomas are thought to be locally expanding bleeds that arise from vascular anomalies, such as cavernous malformations (CM), developmental venous anomalies (DVA), and arterio-venous malformations (AVM). Hematomas related to vascular lesion will mostly be limited in size as the expanding mass is sufficient to cause autodestruction of the primary lesion, i.e. CM or AVM. This explains why they present with lesser clinical severity. Furthermore, they rather displace than destroy brain tissue. Mainly cranial nerve deficits and signs of obstructive hydrocephalus lead to the diagnosis of brainstem hematoma. Before the era of CT and MRI therapeutic strategies were developed according to the initial presentation of the patient, realizing that mildly impaired GCS and focal deficits can be reversed with appropriate treatments. It was understood that an initial comatose state will lead to death in about 90% of cases. In rare cases brainstem hematomas may be related to glial tumors, or manifestations of tumor metastases.

Hemorrhages of the brainstem are related to arterial hypertension and originate from intraparenchymal midpontine branches of the basilar artery. Only in rare cases with smaller hemorrhages the originating vessels are perforators from long circumferential vessels that enter the tegmentum laterally. Hemorrhage is a diffuse extravasation of blood into the cerebral tissue that interrupts neural structures and thereby causes a large primary defect. Infarctions after basilar artery occlusion may also provoke secondary hemorrhage into the brainstem and go along with a very poor prognosis.

Critical Care of the Stroke Patient, ed. Stefan Schwab, Daniel Hanley, and A. David Mendelow. Published by Cambridge University Press.

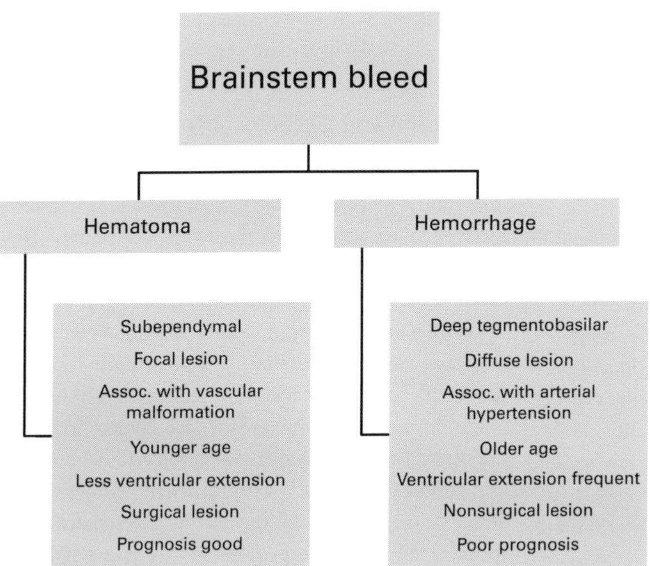

Fig 25.1 Classification schematic diagram.

Anatomical and radiological considerations

Almost all hemorrhages in the brainstem originate from the pons. They may involve neighboring structures such as the midbrain, medulla oblongata, the fourth ventricle or cerebellar regions. Most arteriopathic brainstem hemorrhages are localized in the paramedian pons. One vital structure of the paramedian pons among others is the reticular formation. Direct hemorrhage-induced reticular formation damage explains immediate and irreversible loss of consciousness in the majority of the arteriopathic brainstem hemorrhages. Previous publications have classified PPH into four different types: massive paramedian pontine, bilateral tegmental, basal tegmental, and small unilateral tegmental. The survival rates of these subtypes were 7.1%, 14.3%, 26.1% and 94.1%, respectively (3). Patients suspected for any kind of stroke will routinely undergo an initial CT scan or stroke MRI in selected stroke centers. Patients with massive PPH can be straightforwardly identified with CT. As the prognosis of patients with an early comatose state is poor per se, usually no further diagnostic measures will be undertaken. In those who initially presented with cranial nerve deficits, signs of hydrocephalus and an initial GCS > 5 should be investigated with stroke MRI and digital subtraction angiography (DSA) in selected cases. These methods may identify vascular anomalies in patients that were primarily thought to have undergone a brainstem hemorrhage. However, in the early stage after the bleed even advanced MRI sequences involving FLAIR (fluid attenuated inversion recovery), gradient-echo, diffusion, and susceptibility weighted sequences will often confirm the diagnosis of hemorrhage or hematoma. If patients survive, MRI or DSA should be repeated in the subacute and chronic stage (2–8 weeks) after onset of clinical symptoms. Due to degradation of hemoglobin and liquefaction of the blood the space-occupying effect will diminish and the previously occult underlying vascular pathology may become visible.

Prognostic considerations

In clinical practice, early prediction of the prognosis is the mainstay for stroke physicians in any subtype of cerebrovascular disease. The early recognition of predicting factors will help determine the extent of intensive care, diagnostic measures, and therapeutic approaches. In 1988 Mangiardi *et al.* reported that hematoma size was the main prognostic factor as lesions measuring more than 10 cc usually had a fatal outcome

(2). Others reported case fatality rates in PPH of 60.7% defining death within 7 days as being related to PPH. With increasing size of the hemorrhage the likelihood of intraventricular rupture into the fourth ventricle is high and may cause hydrocephalus with increased intracranial pressure which will add to the morbidity and mortality if left untreated. Once neighboring structures like the cerebellum and midbrain are additionally involved prognosis will be worse.

A previous CT-based study showed that a lateral tegmental extension of the hemorrhage was associated with a favorable prognosis (4). The authors of this study confirmed the finding that large, especially paramedian hemorrhages predict high mortality (93% of cases). Furthermore, that a transverse diameter of the hemorrhage of greater than 20 mm represents a reliable prognostic predictor of very poor outcome. In conclusion from these data the most predictive variables are: 1) clinical symptoms, 2) descriptive CT parameters, and 3) size of the hemorrhage.

Treatment

The large variety of onset symptoms from mild cranial nerve deficits to deep coma and death certainly encompasses multiple aspects of emergency care. Cornerstones of primary care of ICH of any kind should be applied. They comprise: 1) the establishment of a distinct diagnosis and bleeding source, 2) the initiation of primary emergency care covering vital functions, 3) consideration of specific neuro-intensive aspects such as extended monitoring and management of intracranial pressure (ICP), 4) specific treatments to limit hematoma/hemorrhage growth including blood pressure control, reversal of anticoagulation and coagulopathies, and 5) finally evaluation of surgical options.

Intensive care

There are no data available on the general principles of intensive care of brainstem hemorrhage patients. However, it is assumed that basic concepts, such as the effect of mechanical ventilation on intracranial pressure or sedative/analgesic strategies do not differ significantly from patients with other acute brain injuries. In the following, general treatment approaches are discussed.

Ventilation and tracheostomy

Approximately one third of patients with hemorrhagic stroke must be ventilated (5). Indications for intubation and ventilation are vigilance due to the localization of the bleeding and/or space-occupying effect, a loss of protective reflexes, or a neurosurgical intervention such as the removal of the bleeding or the installation of ventricular drainage. General guidelines on ventilation strategies specifically in patients with ICH and brainstem hemorrhage do not exist from prospective clinical trials. An important aspect is the increase of intracranial pressure in a subset of patients with obstructive hydrocephalus. Some concepts, such as the use of a ventilator PEEP (positive end expiratory pressure) were examined in relation to their impact on the ICP. It was found that a high PEEP does not significantly increase in ICP (6). The negative effect on the cerebral perfusion pressure (CPP) by the global hemodynamic impairment due to the PEEP was compensated for by adjusting the mean arterial pressure (MAP). Increased ICP is therefore no contraindication to apply PEEP.

An early tracheostomy ($\leq$ 10 days) in patients with cerebral insults may be related to moderate survival advantage (7). In addition, early tracheostomized patients could be weaned faster from mechanical ventilation. Tracheotomy may improve patients with brainstem hemorrhage, which cannot be extubated within 10 days after onset. In this case, patients should be identified with a risk of prolonged mechanical ventilation as early as possible in the ICU. However, controversies remain between neuro-intensivists of different cultures as to whether or not early tracheostomy really should be considered in prognostically poor patients or is better left untreated.

Sedation

Adequate sedation is one of the basic measures in patients with either critically increased ICP or local effects of brainstem compression, and adequate pain management may often be the key to a normalization in the context of a stress reaction and high blood pressure. The downsides of sedation are reduced neurological assessability and an increased risk for complications associated with sedation. The need for sedation should be closely scrutinized and re-evaluated after defined periods.

ICP-lowering regimen

Patients with brainstem hemorrhage may suffer because of the space-occupying effects of the bleeding, due to the formation of a perifocal edema, or by hematocephalus and subsequent critical increases in ICP. Medical treatment of increased ICP mostly represents a short-lasting measure until more invasive measures such as the removal of the bleeding or the establishment of ventricular drainage. However, surgical removal of brainstem hemorrhage is no longer counted as a true option, whereas brainstem hematomas which originate from vascular malformations pose a formidable challenge for surgeons. Brainstem hemorrhage without any initial obstruction of cerebrospinal fluid pathways may profit from osmodiuretic agents like mannitol or hypertonic saline. By building an effective osmotic gradient, water is displaced from the interstitial brain tissue into the vascular system. This effect counteracts the development of perifocal edema around the hemorrhage. Suitable dosing for the acute treatment is 15–20% mannitol solution (0.25 to 1 g/kg as a bolus) or hypertonic saline (100 ml of 10% sodium chloride). If necessary, the medication can be repeated within 3–6 hours, depending on the neurological status, the fluid balance and serum osmolality. The latter is increased by repeated doses of mannitol and should reach maximum values of 300–320 mosmol/liter. The value of osmotherapy remains controversial. Important and common side effects are kidney failure and electrolyte disturbances.

Hemorrhage surgery

Except for distinct exceptions there is no indication for brainstem hemorrhage open surgery. Brainstem hemorrhages do not occur in predisposed 'cavities' as for example in cavernoma-related hematomas. They disrupt brainstem tissue and because of that no surgical plane can be identified. In cases of relatively small brainstem hemorrhages with consecutive obstructive hydrocephalus the treatment of hydrocephalus is mandatory.

Treatment of hydrocephalus

The external ventricular drain (EVD) is the main method for the treatment of acute hydrocephalus. Particularly in the acute setting, a temporary obstruction of CSF pathways can be treated very effectively.

In addition to the standard EVD systems with a simple catheter, which can either be used for drainage of cerebrospinal fluid or in the closed state for ICP monitoring, there are now external drains available that can simultaneously measure the ICP and drain CSF. EVD standard systems are used most often. Depending on the adjustment of the drip chamber in relation to the foramen of Monro the amount of CSF outflow will be regulated. If necessary, the drainage amount can be increased to up to 40 ml/h to achieve a rapid reduction in intracranial pressure.

It remains of utmost prognostic importance if patients' consciousness rapidly increases after the placement of an EVD and early drainage. If increased ICP is suspected due to brainstem hemorrhage on the one hand, but early CSF drainage fails to improve patients' neurological situation, thereafter prognosis is poor with a very high likelihood.

Hematoma surgery

As briefly mentioned above, the advent of refined diagnostic tools (i.e. diffusion tensor imaging, tractography etc.) and surgical approaches brought along more aggressive and safer surgical treatments in brainstem hematoma.

It has been understood that brainstem hematomas originate from vascular disorders of different kinds. Patients either suffer from previous cranial nerve deficits that worsen during the event of hematoma formation or hematoma formation with concomitant deficits may be the first ever experienced incidence.

The adequate management of brainstem hematomas remains a matter of discussion. Acute surgery for hematoma evacuation and removal of the causative lesion (if existing) is advocated by some authors (8). Other authors propose a more conservative approach, with elective surgery only in patients surviving the acute post-hemorrhagic phase and in whom the source of bleeding could be identified neuroradiologically (9,10). However, even advanced MRI does not allow differentiation between cavernoma and arteriopathic hematoma in the acute post-hemorrhagic state.

Cavernoma surgery

Cavernous malformations of the brain are defined as hamartomatous vascular lesions with specific characteristics. Macroscopically they appear as well-circumscribed lesions with a reddish purple, multilobulated appearance resembling a mulberry (11). Microscopically they can be clearly distinguished from other vascular malformations due to specific features. It is well known that brainstem cavernomas have a much higher bleeding rate compared to supratentorial cavernomas (12). In fact, the annual bleeding risk of brainstem cavernomas ranges around 5% in larger studies (12,13). Most hematomas related to supratentorial cavernomas will remain clinically silent; however, permanent neurological deficits are much more likely to occur in the brainstem. This fact needs to be considered if previously conservatively treated patients with known brainstem cavernomas rebleed and clinically worsen. Early surgery to the hematoma may be considered in these cases even if patients are comatose initially. Otherwise a delayed surgical policy is recommended because hematoma degradation will allow easier removal and MRI may point out the vascular malformation more precisely without exaggerating susceptibility effects. In Figure 25.2 a large right-sided paramedian pontine cavernoma with blood levels within the cavity is demonstrated. The susceptibility insensitive T1- and T2-weighted MRI sequences clearly show the extension of the hematoma cavity to the fourth ventricle

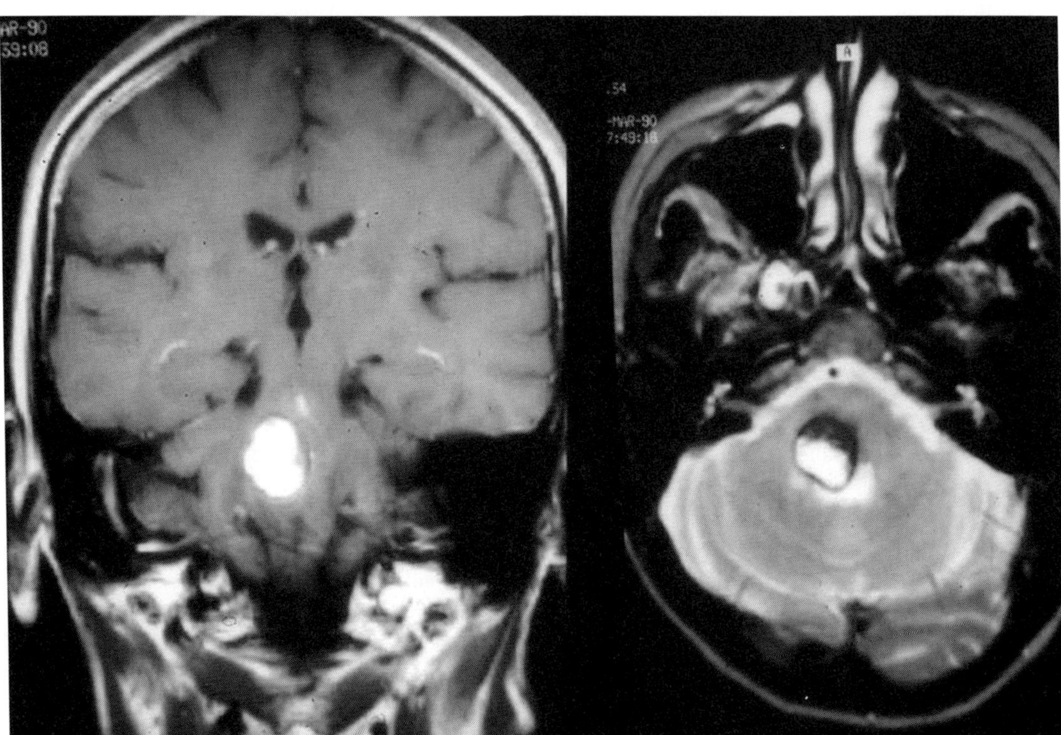

Fig. 25.2 Right-sided paramedian pontine cavernoma with blood levels within the cavity.

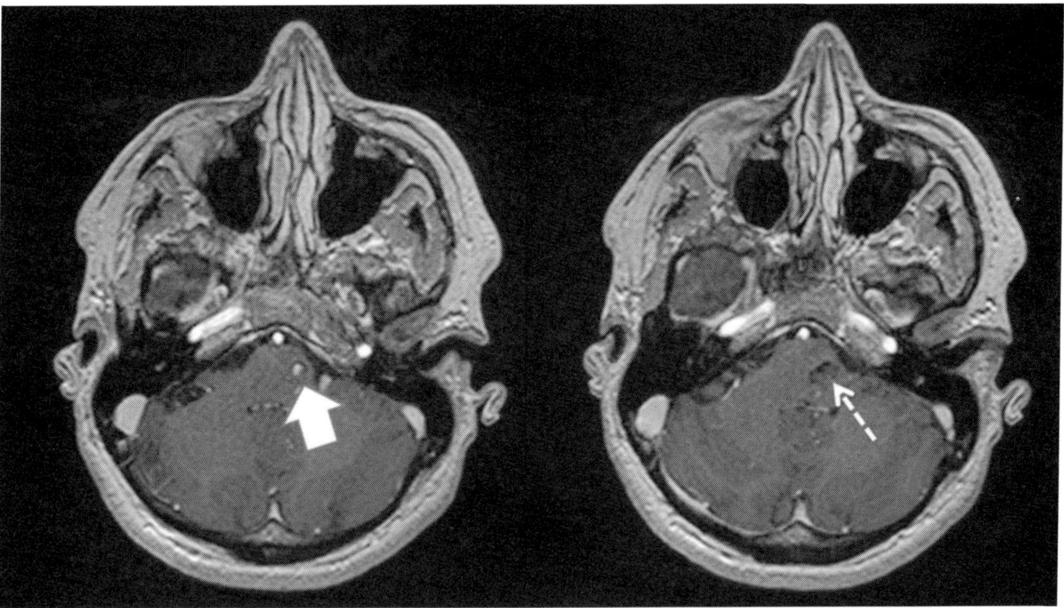

Fig. 25.3 Associated developmental venous anomaly (solid arrow) next to a cavernous malformation (dashed arrow) in the pontomedullary junction.

without intraventricular components in the chronic stage after onset. Patients alike are excellent candidates for sophisticated neurosurgery and complete removal of the underlying lesion. However, if accompanying developmental venous anomalies (DVA) are encountered (Fig. 25.3), surgical removal of a brainstem cavernoma must be undertaken without resection of the DVA.

Other surgical approaches to brainstem hemorrhages are known but remain with unproven evidence of efficacy and therefore are not further discussed in this chapter (14).

REFERENCES

1. Freytag E. Fatal hypertensive intracerebral haematomas: a survey of the pathological anatomy of 393 cases. *J. Neurol. Neurosurg. Psychiatr.* 1968;**31**(6):616–20.
2. Mangiardi JR, Epstein FJ. Brainstem haematomas: review of the literature and presentation of five new cases. *J. Neurol. Neurosurg. Psychiatr.* 1988;**51**(7):966–76.
3. Chung CS, Park CH. Primary pontine hemorrhage: a new CT classification. *Neurology.* 1992;**42**(4):830–4.
4. Dziewas R, Kremer M, Lüdemann P, *et al.* The prognostic impact of clinical and CT parameters in patients with pontine hemorrhage. *Cerebrovasc. Dis.* 2003;**16**(3):224–9.
5. Gujjar AR, Deibert E, Manno EM, Duff S, Diringer MN. Mechanical ventilation for ischemic stroke and intracerebral hemorrhage: indications, timing, and outcome. *Neurology.* 1998;**51**(2):447–51.
6. Georgiadis D, Schwarz S, Baumgartner RW, Veltkamp R, Schwab S. Influence of positive end-expiratory pressure on intracranial pressure and cerebral perfusion pressure in patients with acute stroke. *Stroke.* 2001;**32**(9):2088–92.
7. Scales DC, Thiruchelvam D, Kiss A, Redelmeier DA. The effect of tracheostomy timing during critical illness on long-term survival. *Crit. Care Med.* 2008;**36**(9):2547–57.
8. Konovalov AN, Spallone A, Makhmudov UB, Kukhlajeva JA, Ozerova VI. Surgical management of hematomas of the brain stem. *J. Neurosurg.* 1990;**73**(2):181–6.
9. Porter RW, Detwiler PW, Spetzler RF, *et al.* Cavernous malformations of the brainstem: experience with 100 patients. *J. Neurosurg.* 1999;**90**(1):50–8.
10. Samii M, Eghbal R, Carvalho GA, Matthies C. Surgical management of brainstem cavernomas. *J. Neurosurg.* 2001;**95**(5):825–32.

11. Voigt K, Yaşargil MG. Cerebral cavernous haemangiomas or cavernomas. Incidence, pathology, localization, diagnosis, clinical features and treatment. Review of the literature and report of an unusual case. *Neurochirurgia (Stuttg).* 1976;**19**(2):59–68.
12. Aiba T, Tanaka R, Koike T, *et al.* Natural history of intracranial cavernous malformations. *J. Neurosurg.* 1995;**83**(1): 56–9.
13. Labauge P, Brunereau L, Lévy C, Laberge S, Houtteville JP. The natural history of familial cerebral cavernomas: a retrospective MRI study of 40 patients. *Neuroradiology.* 2000;**42**(5):327–32.
14. Takimoto H, Iwaisako K, Kubo S, *et al.* Transaqueductal aspiration of pontine hemorrhage with the aid of a neuroendoscope. *Technical Note. J. Neurosurg.* 2003;**98**(4): 917–19.

SECTION 5

Critical Care of Arteriovenous Malformations

Surgery for arteriovenous malformations

A. David Mendelow, Anil Gholkar, Raghu Vindlacheruvu, and Patrick Mitchell

There are two main roles for surgery in the treatment of cerebral arteriovenous malformations (AVMs). Firstly, there is the prophylactic removal of a source of hemorrhage and secondly, the removal of hemorrhage caused by an AVM at which time the AVM itself is removed. These two circumstances are entirely different and the response time may also have to be different.

With prophylactic surgical excision, the decision-making process has to be considered carefully in relation to the natural history, in relation to the risks and benefits of embolization, and in relation to the risks and benefits of stereoradiosurgery, as well as to the various combinations of these treatments. The decision-making process in prophylactic treatment is thus complex and it will be considered later in this chapter.

The first section therefore deals with the technical aspects of surgery and the best intuitive indications and methods for surgical excision.

Surgical techniques

Operative excision has the advantage of immediate removal of the risk of hemorrhage from the AVM. This is an advantage it has over stereoradiosurgery. A disadvantage is the risk of post-operative hemorrhage which is about 4% in most craniotomy series (1), although this is dependent upon the size and Spetzler grading of the AVM (2). Larger lesions have a higher post-operative hemorrhage rate, while the smaller lesions have a lower post-operative hemorrhage rate.

The key to successful surgical excision depends upon accurate anatomical localization of the lesion. Sometimes, the lesion is visible on the cortical surface and the craniotomy is strategically placed over the lesion to give sufficient access to arterial feeders which have to be occluded. Accurate placement of craniotomy is dependent on good pre-operative planning with angiography and appropriate imaging. Modern image guidance techniques (e.g. Brain Lab®) make this type of planning easier, particularly in inexperienced hands. The pre-operative angiogram will display the main feeding arteries which should be approached initially to avoid excessive hemorrhage. With large AVMs, the risk of blood loss intra-operatively is much higher and occlusion of the main feeding arteries initially will reduce the total amount of hemorrhage.

Pre-operative planning: Examination of the angiogram and scans is essential prior to undertaking any surgical procedure. It is important to assess all the arterial feeders, the nidus of the AVM and the venous drainage. Some AVMs may be associated with intra- and pre-nidal aneurysms. These will need to be considered during surgical planning. Some arterial feeders will be easily accessible and may even lie on the cortical surface, thus making pre-operative embolization unnecessary. By contrast, deep inaccessible arterial feeders should be occluded with pre-operative

Critical Care of the Stroke Patient, ed. Stefan Schwab, Daniel Hanley, and A. David Mendelow. Published by Cambridge University Press.

embolization, thus minimizing intra-operative blood loss. Pre-operative embolization may be performed as a staged procedure or just prior to surgery. The goal of embolization is to occlude inaccessible feeders and reduce the size of the nidus. Embolization carries with it the risk of dissection and stroke. These risks need to be balanced against the advantages of embolization, so that small superficial AVMs may be easily removed without the risk of embolization. The newer embolic agents such as Onyx are relatively soft and can be manipulated easily during surgery: it is malleable and easily cut with delicate micro-instruments.

Pre-operative image guidance should be undertaken and can be updated with 3-D ultrasound acquired intra-operatively (Brain Lab®). If the arterial feeders and draining veins are clearly identified pre-operatively, then the operative plan will be easier to execute. It is also useful to draw the margins of the AVM using the pre-operative imaging phase so that the intra-operative image injection into the operating microscope will allow the margins of the AVM to be clearly identified as the dissection proceeds.

Initial incision and approach: The initial skin flap should be placed to avoid major venous sinuses and to allow access to arterial feeders at an early stage. This may mean making a flap that is larger than would be required just to excise the AVM. For example, with un-embolized middle cerebral arterial feeders, access to the Sylvian fissure may be required before approaching the AVM itself. Failure to provide such access will prevent temporary clipping of major arterial feeders if they have not been occluded with pre-operative embolization. It may not always be possible to embolize such feeders, particularly if they arise with the lenticulo-striate branches of the middle cerebral artery. If the inaccessible feeders have all been embolized successfully and if the AVM is relatively small and superficial, image guidance allows a small linear incision and a small craniotomy just sufficient to reach all the perimeter of the AVM. Taking into account the above considerations, the craniotomy is performed and the dura opened. Care should be taken with the dural opening because large draining veins may be attached to it. The dural flap should be created with this in mind. Large draining veins should not be occluded until all the arterial feeders have been identified and occluded and the complete perimeter of the AVM dissected. After opening the dura, the edge of the malformation is identified and normal cortex should be easily visible. The arachnoid at this junction should be opened and a tissue plane between the AVM and normal cortex developed. This tissue plane is extended on each side to separate the AVM from the normal brain. Each large arterial feeder is occluded with a titanium micro-clip proximally (Ligaclip®) and bipolar coagulation distally. Non-stick bipolar forceps render the whole process much easier and various types are available. The 'Iso-cool®' bipolar forceps (Codman) are disposable. Self-irrigating bipolar forceps are a useful addition to the surgical armamentarium (3). The main draining veins should be avoided and should not be occluded until the AVM has been completely isolated. In this way the AVM and its coils are excised with a pedicle of venous drainage which is finally occluded at the main draining sinus or cortical vein using a large titanium clip that can be removed if it is noted that the AVM swells. Such swelling after venous clip application indicates that some of the arterial feeders have not been properly occluded and the clip should be removed. In some circumstances, access to the AVM will be blocked by a large number of superficial cortical draining veins which make surgical excision impossible. This situation should not be encountered if careful pre-operative planning is undertaken. Where there are such veins that form a curtain that hides the nidus of the AVM and its arterial feeders, other strategies will have to be considered. There is often a plane of gliotic brain around the nidus. If this is associated with liquid hematoma, it also facilitates dissection.

Techniques to minimize blood loss: Pre-operative preparation with beta-blockers, calcium antagonists, dexamethasone, and ranitidine all help with neuroprotection and maintain a relatively low normal blood pressure. Having a low intra-operative and post-operative blood pressure minimizes blood loss more efficiently than other techniques. Pre-operative embolization of inaccessible feeders is one of the keys to minimizing intra-operative blood loss and careful planning together with the neuroradiologist is the best way to minimize this. The use of the 'Cell Save®' equipment allows intra-operative autologous blood transfusion. This is particularly the case with larger AVMs where blood loss can otherwise be a problem.

Sites that make surgery more hazardous: An AVM that extends from the cortical surface through the corpus callosum with deep draining veins presents a formidable operative challenge. It is for this reason that the Spetzler Martin grading system (2) adds one point for deep venous drainage. Because of the proximity of the internal capsule to the basal ganglia and thalamus, lesions in these areas are also best avoided with open surgery. Similarly, lesions that occupy the internal capsule are likely, with surgical excision, to lead to a hemiparesis or hemiplegia. The Spetzler Martin grading system also adds one point for eloquence. Eloquent areas include the motor cortex and the banks of the left Sylvian fissure because of the increased focal neurological disability associated with excision. Brainstem AVMs present a particularly hazardous situation, because access is difficult in the event of massive arterial bleeding and because preservation of essential arteries and perforators becomes difficult or even impossible, if blood loss is overwhelming. Cerebellar AVMs that remain behind the fourth ventricle can be removed but surgery should not be undertaken if the cerebellar AVM extends into any part of the brainstem. Although there is usually no functioning brain within the nidus, access to the nidus is what may cause brain damage: surfacing lesions are therefore a more attractive surgical prospect.

Other technology that helps the surgeon: Perioperative angiography with a mobile digital subtraction angiogram image intensifier allows a check angiogram to be performed on the operating table after the AVM has been removed. This ensures complete removal of the lesion. If residual AVM is still evident, then immediate further surgery ensures 100% excision and obliteration of the AVM. The disadvantages of peroperative angiography are that it is time consuming and the image quality from mobile units is generally poorer than that available for fixed angiographic installations. More recently, per-operative angiography has been supplanted by intra-operative image guidance. Such image guidance can use CT, MRI or ultrasound. Image guidance not only helps with the initial exposure of the AVM but is also invaluable in defining the limits of the lesion as it is excised. Because of brain shift intra-operatively, re-registration with peroperative imaging adds additional precision. However, intra-operative CT and MRI are also very time-consuming and expensive. 3-D ultrasound with color-coded Doppler allows re-registration and assessment of any residual AVM. Most image guidance systems will offer intraoperative 3-D ultrasound (Brain Lab®) and some have dedicated 3-D acquisition (Sono wand ®). Modern Doppler ultrasound is highly sensitive to flowing blood even in small vessels and it takes familiarity with the system to tell residual AVM from normal vasculature.

Post-operative management: Even with successful and complete excision of the AVM, there will be juxta-nidal collaterals which are very thin-walled and accustomed to a low perfusion pressure (4). On removal of the AVM and its A-V shunting effect, local perfusion pressure rises. Any elevation of the BP postoperatively puts stress on these juxta-nidal vessels and post-operative hemorrhage may occur. This phenomenon has also been known as the Normal Perfusion Pressure Breakthrough Phenomenon (NPPBP) (5). It is best prevented by maintaining a low normal post-operative and emergence blood pressure with a slow and gradual recovery from anesthesia. Once again the pre-operative use of beta-blockers and calcium antagonists helps facilitate this low and normal blood pressure. The larger the AVM, the more important it is to avoid NPPBP. Intravenous barbiturates may be given prior to extubation for two reasons: as anticonvulsants and also to maintain low blood pressure. If a hematoma does develop, then the patient may mount a Cushing response that would tend to push the blood pressure up. The intensivist and the surgeon must be aware of this and have a low threshold for post-operative CT scanning and/or intracranial pressure monitoring.

Early post-operative DSA confirms cure, allows for chemical thrombo-embolic prophylaxis and, in the event of post-operative ICH, alters the surgical strategy and complexity – simple clot evacuation compared with identification and complex resection of residual nidus.

Results and decision making

Results of surgical excision for small superficial AVMs: As an example of the utility, efficacy, and safety of surgical excision, our results in Spetzler grade 1 and 2 lesions are presented in Fig 26.1. In the small lesions the cure rate is high and instantaneous while morbidity and mortality is very low. In some cases with small superficial lesions direct surgery without any other treatment modality is sufficient.

Results of surgical excision for large AVMs: The morbidity and mortality rise with increasing Spetzler Martin grade and the elimination rate drops. Knowing the risks of intervention for the different Spetzler grades, together with the particular treatment modality and/or their combination/s, allows the treatment risks to be compared with the natural history related to the life expectancy. This is the critical issue when offering treatment to patients with AVMs. This should be recognized as the total treatment risk.

Similar arguments should be made for embolization and Gamma Knife treatment risks. With multimodality treatment the total treatment risk needs to be known so that the patient can evaluate this against the residual lifetime risk of hemorrhage (vide infra).

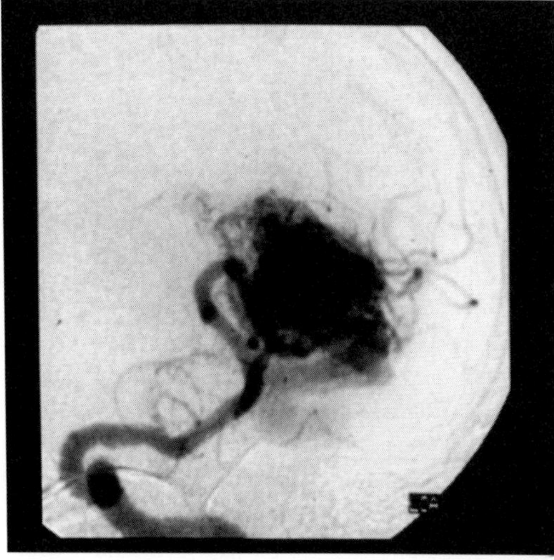

Fig. 26.1 Grade III AVM (eloquent) with a large overlying draining vein that would limit surgical access.

Residual lifetime risk: So, for an elderly patient or for a patient with a known disease with a limited life expectancy, the residual lifetime risk of hemorrhage is small. For a ruptured AVM the risk of hemorrhage is approximately 6% in the first year and 3% per year thereafter. A patient with a 2-year life expectancy therefore has a 9% risk of hemorrhage in their residual life (residual lifetime risk). This is what should be balanced against the total treatment risk.

Vindelacheruvu (6) extracted data from three natural history studies in which there were 124 episodes of recurrent hemorrhages for 416 patients with a total of 1515 patient years of follow-up: 8.2% annual risk of hemorrhage (excluding the index hemorrhage).

Balancing the residual lifetime risk against the total treatment risk: This can be a difficult concept for the patient to grasp. The residual lifetime risk is a long-term risk that is the accumulation of annual risks of hemorrhage. This is lower for unruptured AVMs than it is for ruptured AVMs: about 1% per year. So a patient with a 10-year life expectancy with an unruptured AVM has a residual lifetime risk of only about 10%. By contrast, a fit patient in their twenties with a ruptured AVM will have a very high residual lifetime risk (certainly close to 100%). This has been incorporated into the risk analysis method reported by Kondziolka *et al.* (7). The life expectancy of the patient is therefore very important and the benefit of intervention can be balanced against the life expectancy by calculating the years gained or lost by intervention. In this way, AVMs can be divided into small, medium, and large according to the Spetzler Martin grading system. If each of these three sizes is plotted against years gained or lost, the benefit of intervention can be calculated (6) (Figs. 26.2–7).

So, for example, with a large unruptured AVM, intervention at any age will result in a loss of life years compared with the natural history. It can be seen that in any type of large unruptured AVM the loss of life years is considerable, particularly for deep and eloquent lesions where a 20-year-old would lose about 15 life years compared with the natural

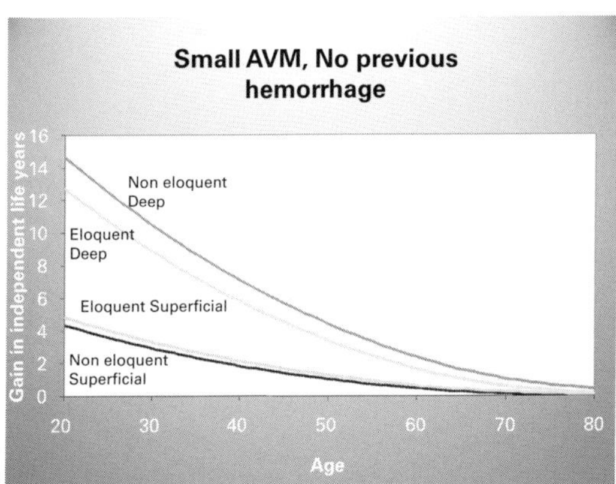

Fig. 26.2 The gain in independent life years (free of disability) in years (Y axis) plotted against age at intervention (X axis) for small (<3 cm) AVMs that are non-eloquent and deep, eloquent and deep, eloquent and superficial, and non-eloquent and superficial. (Life expectancy calculated from 2001 UK census and interventional outcomes calculated from literature review by R Vindelacheruvu 2010(6)). (See plate section for color version).

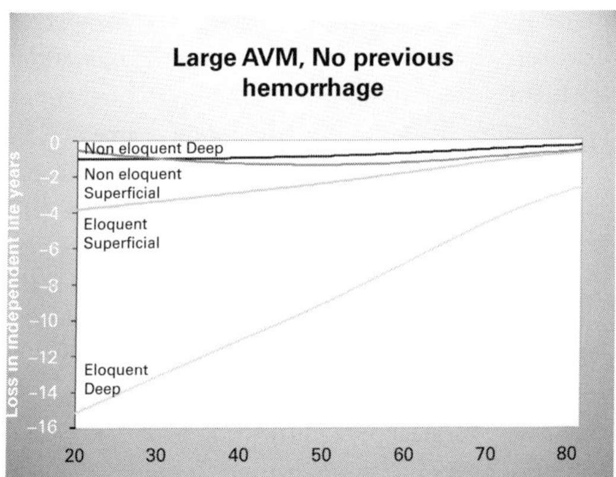

Fig. 26.4 The loss in independent life years plotted against age for large (>6 cm) unruptured AVMs in the same four categories. (See plate section for color version).

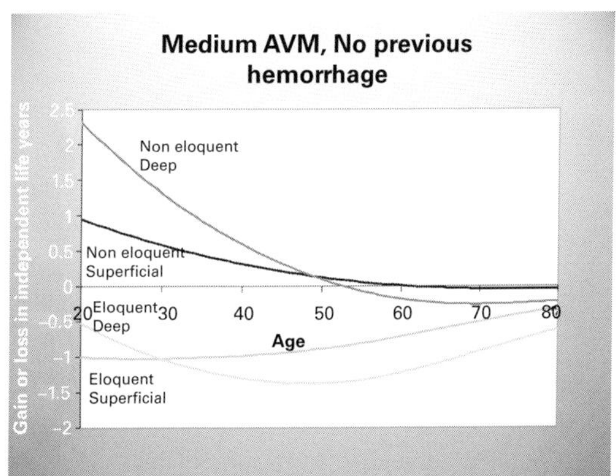

Fig. 26.3 The gain or loss in independent life years plotted against age for medium (3 to 6 cm) unruptured AVMs in the same four categories. (See plate section for color version).

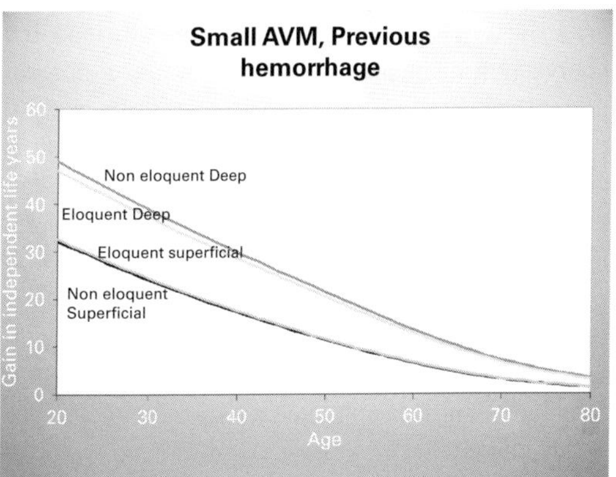

Fig. 26.5 The gain in independent life years plotted against age for small (<3 cm) ruptured AVMs in the same four categories. (See plate section for color version).

history. This type of analysis appears to have such obvious implications for decision making that it would be difficult to randomize such a patient in the ARUBA trial (8,9). Apart from this one category (large unruptured AVMs), younger patients are more likely to gain from earlier intervention.

Unruptured AVMs: Sometimes there is a clear advantage in excising or treating a small, easily accessible AVM in a young person. By contrast, a deep-seated unruptured lesion in an elderly person with co-morbidity will lend itself to non-interventional treatment. For those cases between these extremes there is a zone of uncertainty that will vary from doctor to doctor. Randomizing patients in these zones of uncertainty is the objective of the ARUBA trial. Equipoise will vary but

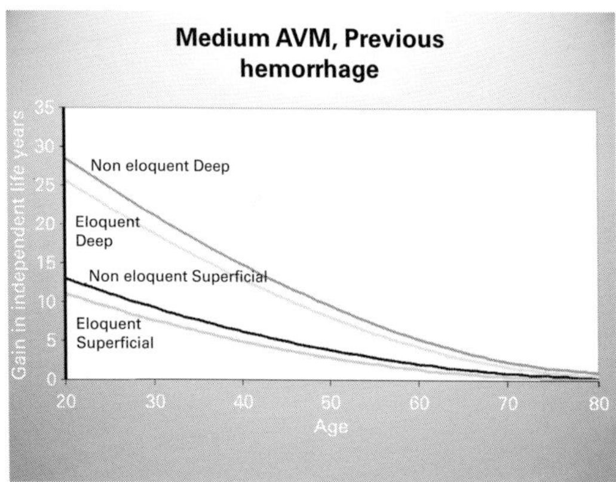

Fig. 26.6 The gain in independent life years plotted against age for medium (3 to 6 cm) ruptured AVMs in the same four categories. (See plate section for color version).

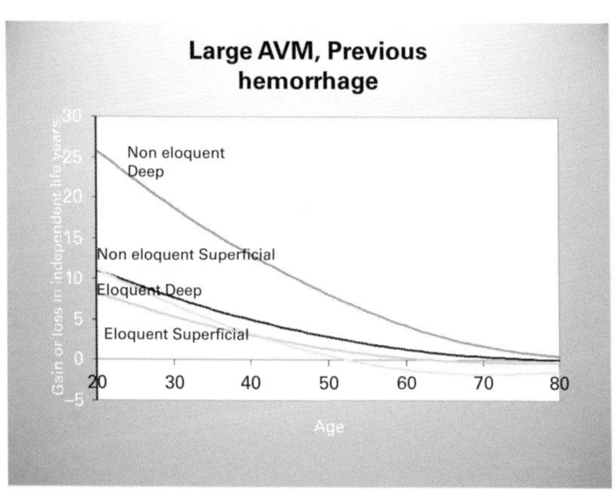

Fig. 26.7 The gain or loss in independent life years plotted against age for large (>6 cm) ruptured AVMs in the same four categories. (See plate section for color version).

should ensure a sufficiently wide range of patients to make the ARUBA trial result meaningful, provided that intervention maintains the goal of complete elimination of the AVM. If partial elimination occurs in many of the patients randomized to intervention, then the trial will inevitably be biased against intervention. Hopefully this will not occur and the investigators will only randomize those patients in whom there is the prospect of complete elimination of the AVM. The ARUBA trial has been stopped and the preliminary short-term results reveal a higher morbidity and mortality in the treated group than in the untreated group (10). Follow-up needs to continue for at least one decade to see if the untreated patients bleed at a rate that would exceed the treated group.

Surgical excision with associated intracerebral hemorrhage (ICH)

When an intracerebral hemorrhage occurs without a known underlying AVM, the intra-operative discovery of the abnormal coils of an AVM is disconcerting because severe bleeding may follow and the surgeon will not be aware of the anatomy of the malformation. Pre-operative angiography reduces but does not eliminate this risk. Increasingly, patients undergoing surgical evacuation of an ICH will have had a CT angiogram, so the accidental discovery of an AVM within or adjacent to an AVM is becoming rarer. About 5% of all ICHs are due to an AVM so unexpected discovery will take place in about 1 in 20 operations for ICH in which angiograms are not routinely done pre-operatively. Also, the presentation may be so urgent, with tentorial herniation and a fixed dilated pupil, that immediate surgery becomes the life-saving priority even though an AVM is expected. Such emergency surgery should make use of pre-operative mannitol, the ‘Cell Saver®’ system (Haemonetics) and adequate blood transfusion facilities because brain swelling and blood loss are the main challenges of such neurosurgical procedures.

If the ICH is small or not thought to require immediate surgery, then careful angiography and planning can be undertaken within a more relaxed time frame. A delayed and more elective approach leads to certain considerations. Firstly, the patient’s condition needs careful monitoring in a neurocritical-care environment because re-bleeding, clot expansion, hydrocephalus, and brain edema may occur in the hours, days, and weeks that follow the initial bleed. Were any of these to occur, then surgery would become more urgent.

Secondly, the clot itself creates space that can be utilized by the surgeon to aid dissection or retraction of undamaged brain. The surgical planning and approach may be different because of the clot. Also, the clot itself and the yellowish brown discoloration of the affected brain will help the surgeon to identify the AVM, which often lies in the wall of such a clot. Because clots absorb with time, the elective surgery should not be delayed for too long because the dissection planes may be lost as the clot absorbs. In general, elective surgery of an AVM with an associated clot should be undertaken within 3 months of the hemorrhage. During this period, embolization of inaccessible arterial feeders can be planned to minimize intra-operative blood loss.

The objective of treatment of the AVM should be complete excision. Failure to completely obliterate the AVM leaves the patient at risk of further hemorrhage. There is increasing evidence that partial treatment increases this risk several fold. However, one recent large series from Finland (11) suggests that partial treatment may reduce the annual risk of hemorrhage. This experience may, however, reflect a highly selected group of patients in the hands of a very experienced team that achieved complete obliteration in the majority of their patients (11). Most authors agree that surgery should not be embarked upon unless it is considered feasible to achieve full elimination of the lesion.

REFERENCES

1. Palmer JD, Sparrow O, *et al.* Postoperative hematoma: A 5-year survey and identification of avoidable risk factors. *Neurosurgery* 1994;**35**(6):1061–5.
2. Spetzler RF, Martin NA. A proposed grading system for arteriovenous malformations. *J Neurosurg* 1986;**65**:476–83.
3. Rhoton ALJ. Operative techniques and instrumentation for neurosurgery. *Neurosurgery* 2003;**53**(4):907–33.
4. Sato S, Kodama N, *et al.* Perinidal dilated capillary networks in cerebral arteriovenous malformations. *Neurosurgery* 2004;**54**(1):163–8; discussion 168–70.
5. Spetzler RF, Hargraves RW, *et al.* Relationship of perfusion pressure and size to risk of hemorrhage from arteriovenous malformations. *J Neurosurg* 1992;**76**(6):918–23.
6. Vindelacheruvu R. Haemorrhage from cerebrovascular lesions. *Neurosurgery.* 2010. Cambridge, Cambridge. MD.
7. Kondziolka D, McLaughlin MR, *et al.* Simple risk predictions for arteriovenous malformation hemorrhage. *Neurosurgery* 1995;**37**(5):851–5.
8. Stapf C, Mohr JP. Unruptured brain arteriovenous malformations should be treated conservatively; Yes. *Stroke* 2007;**38**:3308–9.
9. Mohr JP, Moskowitz AJ, *et al.* The ARUBA trial: current status, future hopes. *Stroke* 2010;**41**(8):e537–40.
10. Mohr JP, Stapf C, *et al.* Preliminary results of the ARUBA trial. *European Stroke Congress.* H. M. London. 2013.
11. Laakso A, Dashti R, *et al.* Long-term excess mortality in 623 patients with brain arteriovenous malformations. *Neurosurgery* 2008;**63**:244–53.

27

Radiation therapy for arteriovenous malformations

Oliver Ganslandt, Sabine Semrau, and Reiner Fietkau

Introduction

Arteriovenous malformations (AVMs) account only for 1–2% of all strokes (1). These vascular lesions of the brain consist of abnormal dilated arteries and veins in which arterial blood flow is shunted directly into the venous system bypassing a capillary system, resulting in high-flow lesions prone to rupture. The estimated detection rate of AVMs has been reported to be 1 per 100 000 person/year (2). AVMs are congenital lesions with a tendency to enlarge with age developing to medium- and high-flow high-pressure lesions. Therefore a lifelong risk for hemorrhage exists with an annual risk of 2–4%; however, in deep-seated AVMs with deep venous drainage the risk accumulates to more than 8% (3). Each hemorrhage has a mortality of 10% and risk of neurological deficits of 30–50% (4).

The next most common presentation is seizure, which occurs in 20–25% of cases (5). Seizures can be either focal or generalized and may be an indicator of the location of the lesion. Other presentations include headaches in 15% of patients, focal neurological deficit in fewer than 5% of cases, and pulsatile tinnitus. There is a 20% risk for the development of seizures within 20 years after diagnosis of an AVM (6). Headaches, cerebral ischemia due to steal phenomena or elevated intracranial pressure are rare symptoms of AVMs.

The treatment of AVMs aims consequently at eliminating the risk of hemorrhage, which can only be achieved by complete obliteration. Over the last decades endovascular surgery and stereotactic radiotherapy (SRT) and radiosurgery (SRS) emerged as new and minimally invasive techniques in the treatment of AVMs that can be used either in conjunction or as an alternative to microsurgery, which is still considered the gold standard in the treatment of AVMs as it is the only method that virtually eliminates the risk of future hemorrhage (7). However, there may be reasons not to operate on an AVM and for these instances the option of SRT and SRS are valuable and established methods. This chapter highlights the role of modern radiotherapy in the treatment of AVMs.

Indications

The indications of choosing an alternative treatment to microsurgery are ruled by risk assessment of possible complications, morbidity, and mortality of a given treatment. Initially reserved for inoperable AVMs, the indications have been liberalized in many centers and radiosurgery is now considered by some proponents as an appropriate therapeutic option for respectable AVMs. One should keep in mind that each of these treatment modalities is associated with risks, and each has distinct advantages and disadvantages. The primary advantages of microsurgical resection are the high cure rates and immediate elimination of the risk of hemorrhage. The primary advantages of radiosurgery are its non-invasive character and the absence of the

Critical Care of the Stroke Patient, ed. Stefan Schwab, Daniel Hanley, and A. David Mendelow. Published by Cambridge University Press.

Table 27.1 The Spetzler–Martin grading system for arteriovenous malformations (7).

Size of lesion	
Small (< 3 cm)	1 point
Medium (3–6 cm)	2 points
Large (> 6 cm)	3 points
Location	
Non-eloquent site	0 points
Eloquent site*	1 point
Pattern of venous drainage	
Superficial only	0 points
Any deep	1 point

*Sensorimotor, language, or visual cortex, hypothalamus or thalamus; internal capsule; brainstem; cerebellar peduncles; or cerebellar nuclei.

Table 27.2 Volumetric evaluation for AVMs. Reproduced with permission (11).

Diameter (cm)	Radius (cm)	Volume (ccm)*
1	0.5	0.52
2	1	4.17
2.5	1.25	8.18
3	1.5	14.13
3.5	1.75	22.44
4	2	33.5
5	2.5	65.41

*Assuming purely spherical volumes.

risks of a craniotomy and specific risks related to the individual AVM. These risks, however, vary from lesion to lesion and range from nearly no risk to an unacceptably high risk (Spetzler–Martin grade 5–6). To assess the risk of an individual AVM the Spetzler–Martin grading system has become widely accepted as an accurate method to predict patient outcomes after resection of AVMs (Table 27.1). It was designed to preoperatively assess the surgical risk from a large collection of cases in the author's series and has over time proven to be a valid measure for planning a treatment in AVMs (7).

Although the Spetzler–Martin grading system is generally considered an accurate method to predict patient outcomes after microsurgery, it may be less effective in predicting radiosurgical outcomes (8). The system fails to take into account a number of prognostic factors that have been associated with successful radiosurgery, such as radiation dose, AVM volume, specific location, and patient age (9). In addition, the nature, complications, and patient selection criteria of the two treatment modalities markedly differ. Despite these issues, the Spetzler–Martin grading system is easy to use and has been shown to be relatively predictive of radiosurgical outcome in a number of studies (10). It has been debated if the Spetzler–Martin scale is applicable for radiosurgery and endovascular treatment as the complications of these types of treatment differ from those of surgery. For this reason the Pittsburgh radiosurgery-based AVM grading scale has been proposed that includes target volume, age, and location to calculate the effective risk. There are other predictive scales that measure the factors leading to obliteration of the AVM like the K-index (12) and the obliteration prediction index (13).

There is consensus that AVMs that are good candidates for SRS are small deep-seated lesions, located in eloquent brain areas, the basal ganglia or the brainstem. The ideal target volume should be no larger than 10 ccm or have a maximum diameter < 3 cm (14). Assuming purely spherical volumes, the maximum diameter, which can be treated ideally with SRS, is 2.75 cm (see Table 27.2).

Spetzler–Martin grade I and II AVMs should be considered for microsurgery as complication rates are low and an excellent outcome has been reported in the literature (15). For larger AVMs, that cannot be treated with SRS because their volume exceeds the dose restrictions, treatment becomes more difficult and the outcome of these patients gets worse. These cases should be treated in a stroke center in which a multidisciplinary expert team consisting of cerebrovascular practitioners interacts effectively on a day-to-day basis (16). One of the treatment options in large AVMs is hypofractionated stereotactic radiotherapy or staged radiosurgery. Considering the natural history of AVMs the option 'no therapy' is a very rational and reasonable approach in some patients.

The indication for radiosurgery of AVMs has long been debated for questions regarding superior outcome of each modality, cost effectiveness, and complication rate (17,18). To date there seems consensus that small deep-seated AVMs which are located in eloquent brain areas or located in the brainstem are better treated with radiosurgery (11).

Technical considerations

Presently there are a number of different radiosurgery systems on the market that are designed to deliver a high dose to a small target volume in a single fraction. The most prominent machines are the Gamma Knife (Elekta), the Cyber Knife (Accuray) and the Novalis (BrainLAB). The two latter systems are also capable of fractionated stereotactic radiotherapy (SRT) and body stereotaxy. It is also possible to treat AVMs using a multi-leaf collimator as an add-on in conjunction with a standard LINAC. Only limited and biased data are currently available that show no superiority of a given system, although differences exist regarding conformity indices of the different systems (19). Clinical outcome and survival rates of the main indications for SRS do not differ between the systems (20,21).

Among many factors that influence the obliteration after radiosurgery, like location, age and size, there is a strong correlation between dose and obliteration success. The rate of AVM obliteration from radiosurgery depends on the marginal dose administered with a dose–response curve that reaches a maximum of approximately 88%. The marginal dose delivered to the AVM nidus should encompass 20 Gy to achieve best results. Higher doses lead to increased neurotoxicity and complications without better obliteration results (22).

Results

The efficacy of SRS and SRT is relatively uniform when compared across institutions using varied techniques and energy sources. The goal of radiosurgery is to obliterate the AVM, prevent re-hemorrhage, improve seizure control, and relieve headaches. The results from patient series have been published (1971 through to the present), and radiosurgery has been found to be a safe and effective treatment for specific AVMs. However, all studies lack enough power to make up for class one or two data in terms of evidence-based medicine. Radiosurgery leads to complete AVM obliteration (elimination of the hemorrhage risk) in about 80% of patients within 2–3 years, a result that is stratified by AVM size. Smaller AVMs (< 10 ccm) respond better because more radiation can be delivered safely (23). Angiography is still the standard to confirm complete obliteration.

A very intriguing alternative to radiosurgery has been introduced with the concept of hyofractionated conformal stereotactic radiotherapy (HCSRT). The idea behind this scheme is to use the biological benefits of fractionation for the normal tissue and the precision of stereotactic radiosurgery with fairly high dose per fraction applied in a few sessions. Various radiation schedules have been reported, using the technique of HCSRT (24,25). The choice of dose per fraction, number of fractions, and total dose differ between publications. In a recent publication from Sweden an obliteration rate of 92.5% was reported using a protocol of 35 Gy in five fractions (26). Other authors communicated a 3-year actuarial obliteration rate of 53% when using 35 Gy in four fractions (27). Of concern is a reported increase in hemorrhage in HCSRT patients of 8.5% in one publication (25); other reports, however, do not confirm this observation (Fig. 27.1).

Complications

Complications of SRS and SRT after treatment of AVMs are: rebleeding, radiation induced lesion (e.g. necrosis, edema, and cyst formation), and occurrence of new neurological deficits. The probability of adverse effects is a function of dose and treatment volume. Postoperative morbidity leading to permanent deficits is observed in 0.4–20.6% of patients in the current literature (28,29,30). Two factors have been shown to be predictive of permanent injury: AVM location and the volume of tissue receiving radiation in excess of 12 Gy (29).

Embolization and SRS

The concept of embolization followed by radiosurgery has been advocated as a useful therapy to reduce nidus

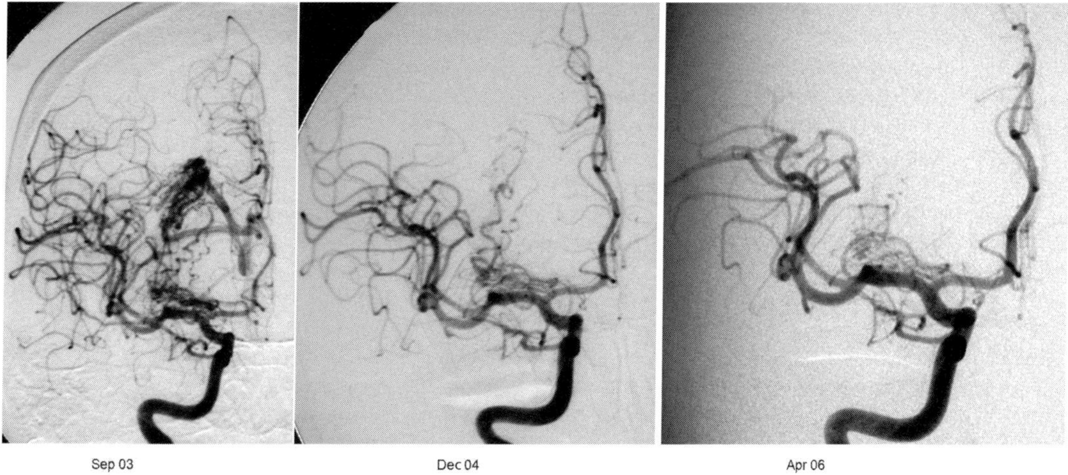

Fig. 27.1 Obliteration of an AVM near the basal ganglia after LINAC radiosurgery with a dose of 20 Gy to the 90% isodose. Note a second AVM near the right ICA that was treated later.

size and, therefore, the radiosurgical target volume, as well as to reduce the risk for hemorrhage while awaiting the delayed, radiosurgically induced AVM obliteration. In many cases embolization does not reduce the treatment target volume but rather decreases the density within a fixed volume and therefore is of limited benefit in the overall treatment plan for larger AVMs (11). Unfortunately, there is even growing evidence that embolization prior to radiosurgery actually decreases the success of obliteration (31).

Conclusions

After thorough review of the literature, it is apparent that AVMs that are difficult to treat by surgery are also difficult targets for radiosurgery. Thus, a team of physicians, including microvascular surgeons, radiosurgeons, and endovascular surgeons, is needed to assess each case individually. The treating physicians must have a clear understanding of the natural history of the disorder and the factors that influence that natural history. Furthermore, the physician must understand the risks and benefits of all therapeutic options to determine whether to treat a particular AVM and which therapeutic strategy is best for an individual patient. Essentially, AVM volume and location are the central factors in selecting the most appropriate treatment modality. For large AVMs, the utility of pretreatment embolization remains unclear. Fractionated schemes for these lesions need greater evaluation. Stereotactic radiotherapy, embolization, and microsurgery are not competitive treatment options for AVMs but rather complementary alternatives that should be offered by an experienced stroke center.

REFERENCES

1. Furlan AJ, Whisnant JP, Elveback LR: The decreasing incidence of primary intracerebral hemorrhage: a population study. *Ann Neurol* 1979;**5**:367–73.
2. Al-Shahi R, Warlow C: A systematic review of the frequency and prognosis of arteriovenous malformations of the brain in adults. *Brain* 2001;**124**:1900–26.
3. Stapf C, Mast H, Sciacca RR, *et al.*: Predictors of hemorrhage in patients with untreated brain arteriovenous malformation. *Neurology* 2006;**66**:1350–5.

4. Hartmann A, Mast H, Mohr JP, *et al.*: Morbidity of intracranial hemorrhage in patients with cerebral arteriovenous malformation. *Stroke* 1998;**29**:931–4.
5. Brown RD, Jr., Wiebers DO, Forbes G, *et al.*: The natural history of unruptured intracranial arteriovenous malformations. *J Neurosurg* 1988;**68**:352–7.
6. Crawford PM, West CR, Chadwick DW, Shaw MD: Arteriovenous malformations of the brain: natural history in unoperated patients. *J Neurol Neurosurg Psychiatry* 1986;**49**:1–10.
7. Spetzler RF, Martin NA: A proposed grading system for arteriovenous malformations. *J Neurosurg* 1986;**65**:476–83.
8. Pollock BE, Flickinger JC, Lunsford LD, Bissonette DJ, Kondziolka D: Hemorrhage risk after stereotactic radiosurgery of cerebral arteriovenous malformations. *Neurosurgery* 1996;**38**:652–9; discussion 659–61.
9. Meder JF, Oppenheim C, Blustajn J, *et al.*: Cerebral arteriovenous malformations: the value of radiologic parameters in predicting response to radiosurgery. *Am J Neuroradiol* 1997;**18**:1473–83.
10. Andrade-Souza YM, Zadeh G, Ramani M, *et al.*: Testing the radiosurgery-based arteriovenous malformation score and the modified Spetzler-Martin grading system to predict radiosurgical outcome. *J Neurosurg* 2005;**103**:642–8.
11. Stieg PE, Friedlander RM, Loeffler JS, Alexander EI: Arteriovenous malfomation: indications for stereotactic radiosurgery, in Howard MAI (ed): *Clinical Neurosurgery*. Philadelphia, Lippincott Williams & Wilkins, 2000: 242–8.
12. Karlsson B, Lindquist C, Steiner L: Prediction of obliteration after gamma knife surgery for cerebral arteriovenous malformations. *Neurosurgery* 1997;**40**:425–30; discussion 430–1.
13. Schwartz M, Sixel K, Young C, *et al.*: Prediction of obliteration of arteriovenous malformations after radiosurgery: the obliteration prediction index. *Can J Neurol Sci* 1997;**24**:106–9.
14. Lunsford LD, Kondziolka D, Flickinger JC, *et al.*: Stereotactic radiosurgery for arteriovenous malformations of the brain. *J Neurosurg* 1991;**75**:512–24.
15. Ogilvy CS, Stieg PE, Awad I, *et al.*: AHA Scientific Statement: Recommendations for the management of intracranial arteriovenous malformations: a statement for healthcare professionals from a special writing group of the Stroke Council, American Stroke Association. *Stroke* 2001;**32**:1458–71.
16. Batjer HH: Treatment decisions in brain AVMs, in Grady MS (ed): *Clinical Neurosurgery*. Seattle, The Congress of Neurological Surgeons, 1998: 319–25.
17. Nussbaum ES, Heros RC, Camarata PJ: Surgical treatment of intracranial arteriovenous malformations with an analysis of cost-effectiveness. *Clin Neurosurg* 1995;**42**:348–69.
18. Pikus HJ, Beach ML, Harbaugh RE: Microsurgical treatment of arteriovenous malformations: analysis and comparison with stereotactic radiosurgery. *J Neurosurg* 1998;**88**:641–6.
19. Schoonbeek A, Monshouwer R, Hanssens P, *et al.*: Intracranial radiosurgery in the Netherlands. A planning comparison of available systems with regard to physical aspects and workload. *Technol Cancer Res Treat* 2010;**9**:279–90.
20. Orio P, Stelzer KJ, Goodkin R, Douglas JG: Treatment of arteriovenous malformations with linear accelerator-based radiosurgery compared with Gamma Knife surgery. *J Neurosurg* 2006;105 Suppl:58–66.
21. Wowra B, Muacevic A, Tonn JC: Quality of radiosurgery for single brain metastases with respect to treatment technology: a matched-pair analysis. *J Neurooncol* 2009;**94**:69–77.
22. Flickinger JC, Kondziolka D, Maitz AH, Lunsford LD: An analysis of the dose-response for arteriovenous malformation radiosurgery and other factors affecting obliteration. *Radiother Oncol* 2002;**63**:347–54.
23. Flickinger JC, Pollock BE, Kondziolka D, Lunsford LD: A dose-response analysis of arteriovenous malformation obliteration after radiosurgery. *Int J Radiat Oncol Biol Phys* 1996;**36**:873–9.
24. Veznedaroglu E, Andrews DW, Benitez RP, *et al.*: Fractionated stereotactic radiotherapy for the treatment of large arteriovenous malformations with or without previous partial embolization. *Neurosurgery* 2008;62 Suppl **2**:763–75.
25. Zabel-du Bois A, Milker-Zabel S, Huber P, Schlegel W, Debus J: Linac-based radiosurgery or hypofractionated stereotactic radiotherapy in the treatment of large cerebral arteriovenous malformations. *Int J Radiat Oncol Biol Phys* 2006;**64**:1049–54.
26. Lindvall P, Bergstrom P, Blomquist M, Bergenheim AT: Radiation schedules in relation to obliteration and complications in hypofractionated conformal stereotactic radiotherapy of arteriovenous malformations. *Stereotact Funct Neurosurg* 2010;**88**:24–8.
27. Aoyama H, Shirato H, Nishioka T, *et al.*: Treatment outcome of single or hypofractionated single-isocentric stereotactic irradiation (STI) using a linear accelerator for intracranial arteriovenous malformation. *Radiother Oncol* 2001;**59**:323–8.
28. Bollet MA, Anxionnat R, Buchheit I, *et al.*: Efficacy and morbidity of arc-therapy radiosurgery for cerebral arteriovenous malformations: a comparison with the

natural history. *Int J Radiat Oncol Biol Phys* 2004;**58**:1353–63.

29. Flickinger JC, Kondziolka D, Lunsford LD, *et al.*: Development of a model to predict permanent symptomatic postradiosurgery injury for arteriovenous malformation patients. Arteriovenous Malformation Radiosurgery Study Group. *Int J Radiat Oncol Biol Phys* 2000;**46**:1143–8.
30. Gobin YP, Laurent A, Merienne L, *et al.*: Treatment of brain arteriovenous malformations by embolization and radiosurgery. *J Neurosurg* 1996;**85**:19–28.
31. Andrade-Souza YM, Ramani M, Scora D, *et al.*: Embolization before radiosurgery reduces the obliteration rate of arteriovenous malformations. *Neurosurgery* 2007;**60**:443–51; discussion 451–2.

28

Management of cavernous angiomas of the brain

Mahua Dey and Issam A. Awad

Introduction and lesion definition

Cerebral cavernous malformation (CCM) also known as cavernoma, cavernous angioma, and cavernous hemangioma, is a vascular lesion found primarily in the central nervous system, and less frequently elsewhere in the body. The lesions, which may affect any brain region or the spinal cord, consist of clusters of dilated vascular sinusoids of varying size, filled with blood or thrombus at different stages of organization, giving it the gross appearance of a mulberry (Figs. 28.1–2). They grow by a process of vascular cavern proliferation in the setting of repetitive intralesional hemorrhages (1). Lesions typically exhibit hallmarks of previous perilesional hemorrhage, including gliosis and hemosiderin deposit (1). Patients harboring CCMs are predisposed to a lifetime risk of focal neurologic deficits related to hemorrhage or lesion proliferation and epilepsy (2). Hemorrhage from CCM lesion is less likely apoplectic than with higher flow arteriovenous anomalies (3–5); however, at times it can be life threatening (6). The CCM may present as solitary pathology, or often in association with other vascular lesions.

Capillary malformations and CCMs: Capillary vascular malformations, also known as capillary telangiectases, are vascular malformations that consist of a collection of dilated capillaries with normal intervening brain parenchyma (7). Most commonly described in the pons, they are typically an incidental finding at autopsy, although in some cases, symptomatic capillary malformations have been revealed on MR images as indistinct patches of punctate contrast enhancement (Fig. 28.3) (8–10). Capillary malformations may also be found in association with more clinically overt lesions, such as CCMs or venous malformations. Microscopically, the vessel walls of capillary malformations appear similar to those of normal capillaries, lined with a single layer of vascular endothelium. While both capillary telangiectases and CCMs represent dilated capillaries, the presence of hemorrhage (identifiable on MR imaging or histopathological examination) has been the cardinal difference traditionally distinguishing CCMs from capillary malformations in the clinical setting.

The association of CCMs and capillary malformations in the same patient has been recognized for many years, with Wyburn-Mason having noted as early as 1943 that 'cavernous angioma develops from telangiectases and both may occur in the same case . . . hence it seems that there is no justification for dividing cavernous angiomata from telangiectases' (11). This was confirmed in more recent studies (12), but the exact prevalence of this association remains uncertain, in view of diagnostic insensitivity of classic imaging modalities for non-hemorrhagic capillary ectasia. More recently, however, transgenic animal models of CCM disease have demonstrated non-hemorrhagic capillary ectasia, as the apparent early stage of CCM development (13). And recent imaging advances in man, with susceptibility weighted MR sequences, are revealing a greater lesion burden in familial cases of CCM disease than was noted with conventional and

Critical Care of the Stroke Patient, ed. Stefan Schwab, Daniel Hanley, and A. David Mendelow. Published by Cambridge University Press.

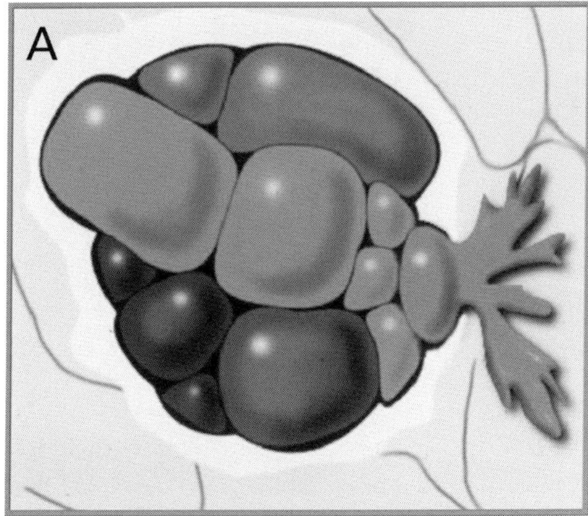

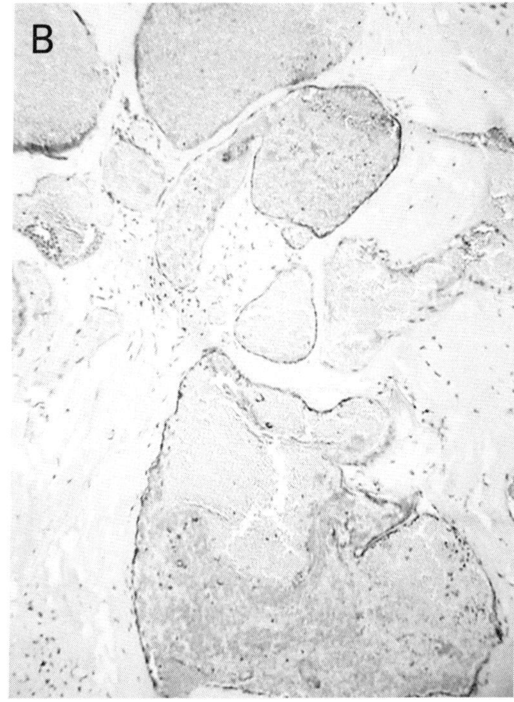

Fig. 28.1. (A) Artist's illustration of cavernous malformation, with cavern proliferation and hemorrhage. (B) Histologic appearance of CCM, with blood-filled thin-walled caverns of various sizes, lined by endothelium (immunopositivity for von Willebrand Factor shown). Intervavernous matrix comprises an amorphous structure devoid of smooth muscle, elastic lamella or mature blood vessel wall angioarchitecture.

gradient echo MR sequences (Fig. 28.4), with many of the tinier lesions possibly representing capillary ectasia, precursors of more mature CCM lesions (14,15).

'Capillary telangiectasiae' (capillary malformations) should not be confused with micro-arteriovenous malformations of hereditary hemorrhagic telangiectasia (Osler-Weber-Rendu disease), the latter affecting brain, skin, mucosa, and lungs in association with gene loci unrelated to CCM disease and lesions of different histology than CCM (16).

Cerebral venous malformations and CCMs: The most common cerebrovascular malformation is the venous malformation, also known as venous angioma or developmental venous anomaly (DVA). This lesion rarely bleeds, except in association with a CCM (17, 18). The DVA is composed of abnormally enlarged venous channels separated by normal neural parenchyma. The anomaly reflects regional venous dysmorphism, arranged in a radial pattern extending from a dilated central venous trunk, and there is paucity of other normal venous drainage in the region of the anomaly (19). Sporadic non-familial CCMs are often associated with a DVA, detected on contrast enhanced T1-weighted MR sequences (Fig. 28.4), while multifocal CCMs associated with autosomal dominant inheritance and the three gene loci of CCM disease are not typically associated with DVA (Fig. 28.5) (17,20).

Mixed lesions and the spectrum of angiographically occult vascular malformations: Despite the apparently distinct clinical, imaging, and pathological profiles of the various cerebral vascular malformations, some CCM lesions exhibit mixed or transitional features, implying related pathobiological mechanisms (10,21–24). Portions of CCMs may, like arteriovenous or venous malformations, exhibit partial or complete mature vessel wall elements, and many CCMs appear

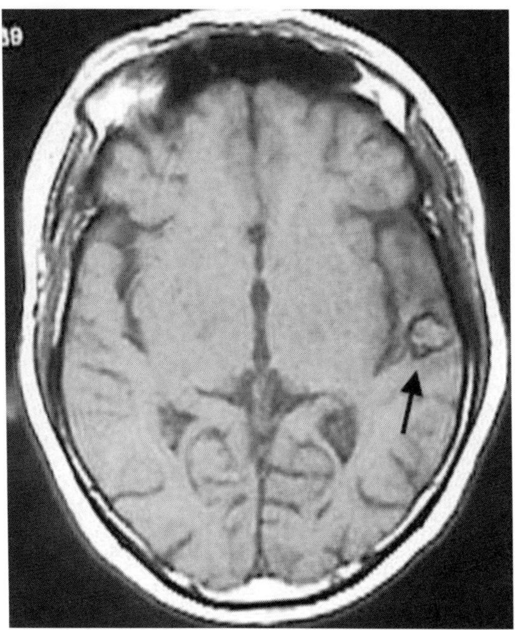

Fig. 28.2 Left temporal lobe CCM shown by T1-weighted MRI. Note popcorn like appearance, representing multiple caverns, surrounded by a thin ring of hypointensity, representing hemosiderin stain. Patient presented with partial complex seizures. In view of eloquent lesion location, lesionectomy was performed without additional resection of adjacent tissue. The patient has been lesion free, but continues anticonvulsant medications.

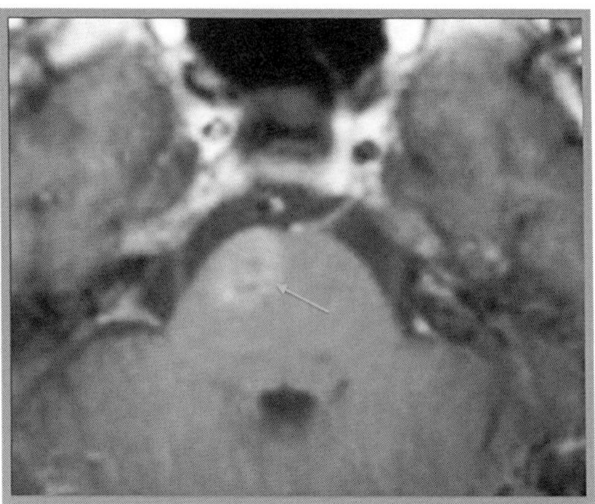

Fig. 28.3 T1 MRI appearance of pontine capillary malformation (telangiectasia), with punctate contrast enhancement shown. There is no signal of bleeding, and no 'blooming' effect on gradient echo sequences (not shown).

to arise in close proximity to DVAs or capillary malformations as noted above. Various cerebrovascular malformations may be associated with skin lesions in rare syndromatic settings, as with hereditary hemorrhagic telangiectasia (Osler-Weber-Rendu disease noted above) and encephalofacial angioma (Sturge-Weber disease). The skin lesions that occur infrequently in association with familial CCMs have been characterized as hyperkeratotic angioma (25), but their precise prevalence and clinical significance have not been well studied.

Epidemiology

Cerebral cavernous malformations (CCM) are a common vascular anomaly affecting more than 0.5% of the population (5) and account for 5% to 13% of all vascular malformations (26,27). In 60% to 80% cases CCMs are sporadic solitary lesions (Figs. 28.2, 28.6–8). On rare occasions they occur as focal clusters of lesions near a developmental venous anomaly (Fig. 28.5) or lesions in previously irradiated brain region. The remaining cases manifest an autosomal dominant inheritance pattern and variable clinical expression, and typically involve multifocal lesions scattered throughout the brain in a volume distribution (5), some of which may only be revealed by gradient-echo MR, or other specialized imaging techniques (Fig. 28.4). Three distinct gene foci on chromosomes 7q, 7p, and 3q have each been linked to familial CCM (28). The identified proteins encoded by CCM genes interact with the endothelial cytoskeleton during angiogenesis, and are expressed in neural tissue, potentially explaining the occurrence of these lesions in the central nervous system (28,29). The prevalence of multifocal CCM lesions approaches 100% in adults with genotyped familial case, imaged with gradient echo or susceptibility weighed MR sequences (26,30–36). Hispanic Americans of Mexican descent have a higher predilection for familial CCMs (33,34,37), related to a

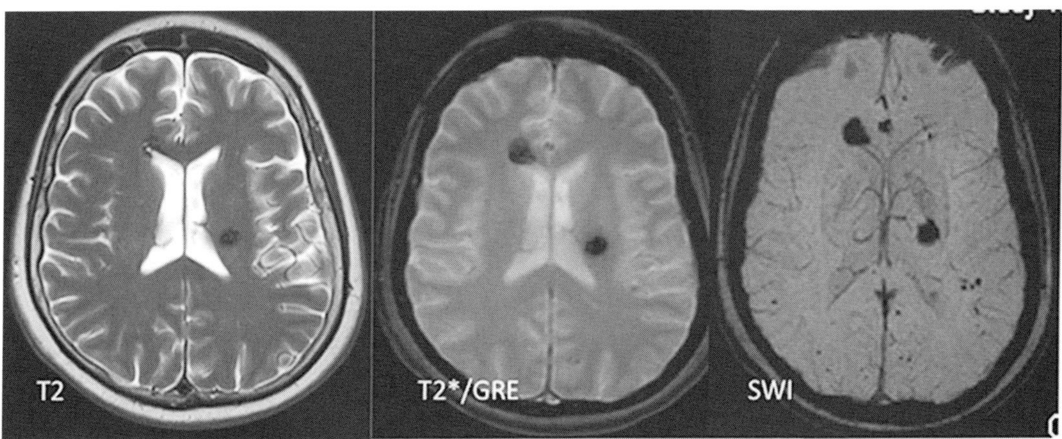

Fig. 28.4 MRI appearance of multifocal CCM (familial type). Left, T2-weighted MR showing typical lesions with popcorn like appearance surrounded by hemosiderin. Middle, T2*/gradient echo images reveal blooming effect of the same lesions, exaggerating the signal of associated hemosiderin. Right, SW images revealing additional lesions not seen on conventional images, showing lesion burden with greater sensitivity.

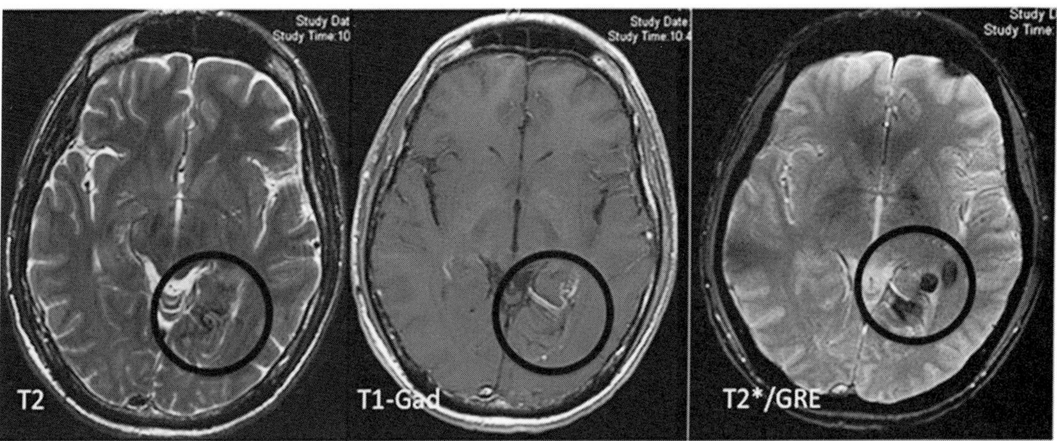

Fig. 28.5 MRI appearance of developmental venous anomaly (DVA) associated with a cluster of CCMs. The patient presented with subtle memory problems and headaches. He has been followed expectantly, without progression of imaging or clinical features during several years. Excision of such cluster of CCMs could be associated with significant morbidity, and potential sacrifice of DVA, with resulting venous infarct or edema.

founder mutation (38), also affecting a large reservoir of patients in the Southwestern United States (20). Another unique founder mutation has recently been described as a cause of CCM in patients of Ashkenazi Jewish heritage (39). In familial clusters of CCMs, successive generations seem to manifest symptoms at earlier ages (31,33,35,40,41).

The majority of studies and all recent large MRI-based analyses demonstrate an equal prevalence of male and female patients with CCMs (4,5,27,42–44). There is a predominance of male patients presenting at <30 years of age, a preponderance of female patients aged 30 to 60 years, and a more equal ratio thereafter (5,45). There is predilection of female patients with middle fossa (extradural) CCMs, a particular variant, and male patients may manifest symptoms at an earlier age than do female patients (5,45).

CCMs have been reported at both extremes of age, but a majority of patients present between the second and fourth decades of life (4,26,36,42,43,46–52). CCMs are less common in the pediatric population (48,49) and account for approximately one-fourth of the patients in published series (43,50,53). Among pediatric patients, there is a bimodal peak of symptomatic presentation, at about 3 and 11 years of age. Patients <40 years old are likely to present with seizures, whereas older patients are more likely to manifest focal neurological deficits (5,54). There is a greater preponderance of hemorrhage and acute neurological deficits as presenting symptoms in children in contrast to that in adult series, accounting for 43% to 78% of symptomatic patients (48,49). Younger children display more active lesion growth compared with the older age group. It has been suggested that pediatric patients have a greater propensity for overt hemorrhage (31,43,46,48,53,55). Data from virtually all clinical series demonstrate that symptomatic lesions are rare in the elderly population.

The CCMs have been reported to range in size from <0.1 to 9 cm (4,26,27,43,50,56). A majority of intracranial CCMs, 64% to 84% of reported CCMs, are supratentorial with lobar preponderance (4,5,26,27,32,42,56). The pons and the cerebellum are the most common infratentorial sites (5,45,56). Other less common intracranial locations include the cerebellopontine angle, pineal gland, middle fossa, cavernous sinus, optic nerve and chiasm, and dura. CCMs are more likely to be part of a mixed lesion than are other vascular malformations, with most frequent association with a venous malformation (12,45). Although a majority of lesions occur in the supratentorial compartment, substantially greater neurological sequelae occur with CCMs in the infratentorial compartment (5,54,56,57). This correlation remains significant even after controlling for lesion size. Angiographically occult brain stem vascular lesions have a high rate of recurrent hemorrhage, up to 69%, and a significant cumulative morbidity (5,54,56,58). They exhibit a characteristic pattern of exacerbations and remission of symptoms (56,57). When a CM is found in conjunction with a venous malformation, the latter is readily angiographically identifiable by its characteristic caput medusae pattern of abnormal venous drainage, whereas the CCM component of the lesion is angiographically occult. Both components of such lesions are generally identifiable on MRI (Fig. 28.5). When lesions exhibit mixed histological features of CCM and AVM or capillary telangiectasia, they are clinically and radiographically indistinguishable from CCMs (12,59). Intracranial CCMs are rarely associated with intraspinal extracerebral soft tissue and visceral hamartomas (60,61) and other central nervous system tumors, such as meningiomas and astrocytomas (44,45,60–62).

Histopathology and pathobiology

Histologic features of CCM include blood-filled sinusoidal spaces (the 'caverns') of various sizes, lined by a single layer of endothelium and separated by a collagenous stroma devoid of elastin, smooth muscle, or other mature vascular wall elements (Fig. 28.1). The endothelial cell layer borders an amorphous collagenous matrix devoid of smooth muscle cells (63). The lesion is not always compact and may include racemose or satellite-like projections into the adjacent brain (64). There are rare reports of disorganized, scattered elastic fibers in lesions that have morphological features consistent with CMs (50). The surrounding parenchyma consistently exhibits evidence of prior microhemorrhage, hemosiderin discoloration, and hemosiderin-filled macrophages. Within the lesion, hyalinization, thrombosis with varying degrees of organization, recanalization, calcification, cysts, and cholesterol crystals are common (32,34,43,50,65–68). A gliomatous reaction of the surrounding parenchyma is characteristic and may form a capsule around the lesion. Hemosiderin-laden macrophages are nearly always present in perilesional tissue and within the lesions themselves, and a robust infiltration of inflammatory cells has been recently characterized in CCM lesions (69). The preponderant B cells and plasma cells infiltrating lesions produce a monoclonal antibody, likely triggered by an antigen in the lesional milieu, unrelated to recent overt bleeding or lesion proliferation (70). Ultrastructural analysis of CCM lesions reveals a partially compromised blood-brain barrier at the site of CCMs, which facilitates erythrocyte diapedesis and the eventual deposition of hemosiderin in perilesional tissue (71,72).

The CCMs are dynamic lesions with demonstrated neuroimaging changes in lesion size and signal characteristics in up to 38% of patients as well as in the appearance of new lesions over time (33,36,42,49,50,53,73–77). In a recent study of familial CCMs, with an average follow-up of 2.2 years, 29% of the patients developed new lesions, with an average rate of 0.4 new lesions per patient per year (36). In a patient with multiple lesions, the excision of one previously active lesion does not deter the growth, dynamics, or development of symptoms of novel or previously quiescent lesions. These changes are thought to be attributable to intralesional hemorrhage, thrombosis, organization, calcification, cyst formation, and involution of the caverns (36,55,56,74,75). Less commonly, a lesion may expand after gross hemorrhage and then involute as the hematoma organizes and is resorbed. A review of the literature demonstrates several features, some intrinsic to the lesion like microhemorrhages that may promote hemorrhagic angiogenic proliferation and others to the patient, that seem to influence the dynamics of CCMs. Patients with familial CCMs have been shown to develop new lesions during prospective follow-up with serial MRI (36). Other new lesions consistent with de novo CCM genesis have been reported after radiation therapy (62) and along the path of a stereotactic biopsy (78). New CCMs have developed in association with pre-existing venous malformations (47). The possibility of evolution of the new CCMs from smaller lesions or other precursors not visible on earlier imaging studies, rather than total de novo lesion genesis, cannot be totally excluded. In particular, capillary telangiectases have been associated with CCMs (12,79), and it is possible that CCMs evolve from hemorrhagic coalescence of pre-existing telangiectases.

There is a marked difference in clinical presentation and neurological disability in patients with CCMs based on gender. Female patients are more likely to manifest gross hemorrhage, multiple lesions, and neurological deficits, whereas male patients are more likely to present with epilepsy (42,45,50,76,80–82). Furthermore, female patients with CCMs display a significantly greater degree of neurological disability compared with male patients (5,54). This trend is also demonstrable in pediatric patients (75). There is also a preponderance among female patients of mixed vascular malformations (75). Several preliminary studies have suggested that the reproductive cycle may have an impact on the rate of growth and the hemorrhagic risk of CCMs with documented aggressive clinical course during pregnancy (53,58,83).

Among patients with multiple lesions, the larger lesion is usually symptomatic (36,84). It has been observed that certain morphological criteria (the presence of dense calcifications, ossifications, a thick glial capsule, and a greater degree of intralesional organization) are associated with a less aggressive clinical course (44,50,85–87). Calcifications may be associated with greater epileptogenicity (50). The only correlation between the MRI characteristics and the clinical behavior of CCMs was the observation that as long as gross hemorrhage occurred within the hypodense perilesional hemosiderin ring, the patient would likely remain asymptomatic. However, if the bleed ruptured through this margin, the patient would be likely to manifest acute symptoms (88).

There is an increased risk of recurrent hemorrhage and progressive neurological decline after an initial bleed from a CM (54,56,57). It is not known whether hemorrhage per se causes the lesion to behave more aggressively or whether patient or extrinsic factors are responsible for repetitive hemorrhagic tendencies. A series examining certain pathological features at surgery and autopsy with a retrospective analysis of clinical and biological behavior of the lesion found that lesions with calcifications, evidence of chronic intralesional hemorrhage with thrombus organization, and thicker glial pseudocapsules were more likely to appear with seizures than with gross hemorrhage (87). It is possible that thrombus organization and the consequent glial reaction may protect patients from gross hemorrhage while predisposing them to seizures.

An evidence-based definition of significant hemorrhage in CCM has recently been proposed, to allow more consistent reporting in clinical series and therapeutic trials (2).

Pathogenesis of CCM lesions

There is growing evidence that the cellular pathology in CCM lies in dysregulation of vascular development and endothelial permeability. Familial form of CCM is associated with three separate genes: *CCM1/KRIT1*, *CCM2/MGC4607*, and *CCM3/PDCD10*. Each exhibits a Mendelian autosomal dominant inheritance due to a heterozygous loss-of-function mutation at one of three distinct loci. The respective encoded proteins appear to interact with cytoskeletal and interendothelial cell junction proteins. CCMs are caused by germline mutations in *CCM1*, which are involved in 40% of familial CCMs and nearly half of those patients will have neurological symptoms before 25 years of age. With familial CCM disease roughly 100 distinct mutations in this gene have been identified to date. *CCM1* is located on chromosome locus 7q11–q22 and produces Krev interaction trapped 1 or KRIT1 protein, a cytoplasmic ankyrin repeat containing protein that interacts with RAP-1A (Krev-1), a member of the RAS family of GTPases involved in interendothelial junction integrity, and integrin cytoplasmic domain-associated protein-1a (ICAP-1), a nuclear protein that shuttles between nucleus and cytoplasm and is involved in b1-integrin mediated signal transduction. KRIT1 is localized, in part, to interendothelial cell junctions and its loss results in disruption of junctional stability that leads to increased permeability in vitro and in vivo. Loss of endothelial cell junctions readily explains the leakage of blood in CCMs and their associated hemosiderosis, and can account for the observed inflammatory response in CCM lesions (89). *CCM2* mutations are involved in up to 40% of familial CCMs. Patients with *CCM2*-associated disease have a lower number of gradient-echo sequence lesions than those with *CCM1* or *CCM3* disease, and the number of lesions increases less rapidly with age than in patients with *CCM1* disease. *CCM2*, localized at chromosome 7p15–13, produces malcavernin protein, and shows similar temporal expression patterns as *KRIT1*. *CCM2* binds to *KRIT1* via a phosphotyrosine-binding domain, in a manner similar to ICAP-1, and is able to sequester *KRIT-1* in the cytoplasm. The *KRIT1-CCM2* interaction also stabilizes endothelial cell junctions by suppressing a protein called RhoA and its effector protein ROCK that are involved in actin stress fiber formation and endothelial monolayer permeability. Loss of either *KRIT1* or *CCM2* disinhibits RhoA and ROCK activity leading to interendothelial barrier instability and vascular leaking. Increased ROCK activity is noticed in the endothelial cells lining sporadic and familial CCM lesions. This suggests that a final common signaling aberration involving ROCK activation takes place in both sporadic and inherited lesions (90). Inhibition of ROCK activation has emerged as a potential therapeutic approach to prevent lesion genesis, or possibly to alter lesional permeability (91). The third and most recently discovered gene is *CCM3*, localized at 3q25.2–q27, which encodes programmed cell death protein 10 (PDCD10). *CCM3* mutation carriers are less common than *CCM1* or *CCM2* carriers, but they are more likely to present with hemorrhage and to have symptom onset before 15 years of age (92). The temporal expression of *CCM3* mRNA correlates with that of *CCM2* in meningeal and parenchymal cerebral vessels. Aberrant apoptosis, in the endothelium or neural cells, may play a role in the pathogenesis of CCMs. *CCM3* protein precipitates and co localizes with *CCM2*. Thus, all three CCM proteins interact to form a complex that then interacts with other proteins such as b1-integrin and ICAP-1 (91).

Diagnostic imaging

CCMs have very sluggish blood flow, or stasis and thrombus at different stages of organization within the caverns, thus they are not visible during conventional angiogram. The inability of angiography to adequately detect CCMs, capillary telangiectases, and thrombosed AVMs led to the grouping of these lesions as angiographically occult vascular malformations. A review of the literature shows that angiographic results are normal in the majority of patients with CCMs (26,34,43,50,64,77,93,94). Occasional abnormalities shown on angiography may include an avascular mass, minimal vascular abnormalities (including early, late, or widened draining veins), a capillary blush or stain, and evidence of neovascularity (27,42,44,50,53,56,68,81,93–96).

Plain computed tomographic (CT) scanning has a sensitivity of 70% to 100% for CCMs in published series (51,56,97). However, despite excellent sensitivity at detecting the presence of a lesion, the specificity of CT scanning for accurate diagnosis of a CM is quite poor in most series (34,51,68). Because of isodense appearance related to subacute hemorrhage or microcalcifications, CCMs are commonly missed or misdiagnosed on CT scans of the brain. The CT scan of a CCM typically exhibits a conspicuous, well-circumscribed, nodular lesion of uniform or variegated mixed density reflecting the juxtaposition of calcifications, hemorrhage, and cystic components that is known to comprise these lesions. In patients who have recently experienced hemorrhage, the homogeneous hyperdensity of a hematoma may overlie and obscure the lesion (27,50,52,56,73,93). The addition of contrast may elicit faint enhancement. The CT scan documents a hematoma or calcification but frequently does not delineate an underlying lesion or differentiate the lesion type.

MRI is the most sensitive and specific diagnostic tool for the evaluation of CCMs (98). The appearance of CCMs on MRI scans is sufficiently characteristic to allow confident preoperative evaluation of symptomatic lesions, identification, screening, and follow-up of incidental lesions, and depiction of lesion behavior including expansion, hemorrhage, and thrombosis (34,68,73,88,99). They are characterized by a mixed signal within the lesion itself on T1- and T2-weighted sequences, surrounded by a ring of T2 hypointensity from hemosiderin, reflecting blood leakage. Smaller CCM lesions may only be revealed by gradient-echo MR images, in which they can be identified because of the lesions' hemorrhagic signal. Lesions confirmed by pathological findings correlate with this MRI scan appearance in 80% to 100% of patients (68). The mixed signal intensities reflect the spectrum of lesion behavior of CCMs. Repeated subclinical intralesional and perilesional hemorrhages lead to ferritin deposition secondary to erythrocyte breakdown and account for the typical 'ring' of low T2 signal around CCMs. The reticulated low T2 signal within the lesions also reflects speckled intra-lesional calcification (27,42,68,73). Areas of hyperintensity correspond to acute and subacute hemorrhages and different stages of thrombus organization. Associated cysts most likely represent residua of previously expanded hemorrhagic caverns that have since involuted with thrombus organization and resolution (50,64,65,67,100–104). A classification system based on imaging and pathological features has been reported to stratify these heterogeneous lesions (15).

- Type I lesions are characterized by hyperintensity on both T1- and T2-weighted images (depending on the state of methemoglobin), which is consistent with subacute hemorrhage.
- Type II malformations, loculated regions of hemorrhage are surrounded by gliosis and hemosiderin-stained brain parenchyma. These CCMs exhibit a mixed-signal intensity core on both T1- and T2-weighted images, with a well-circumscribed hypointense rim on T2-weighted images; these lesions are the classic CCMs, with a 'popcorn' appearance and a predilection to produce recurrent symptoms.
- Type III lesions demonstrate a core that is iso- or hypointense on T1-weighted sequences and hypointense on T2-weighted sequences as well as a rim that is hypointense on T2-weighted sequences, compatible with chronic resolved hemorrhage or hemosiderin within and surrounding the lesion.
- Type IV malformations are minute lesions often seen as punctate hypointense foci on GRE MR images. Pathologically, Type 4 lesions may represent capillary telangiectasias or early-stage CCMs seen frequently in the familial form.

Susceptibility-weighted (SW) imaging provides a new mode that is particularly suited for imaging vascular malformations as it is very sensitive to deoxyhemoglobin and iron content. SW imaging increases the sensitivity of lesion detection in familial multifocal CCM lesions (14), but does not per se reveal lesion multiplicity that had not been already demonstrated by T2*GRE. The SW images are highly sensitive to delineation of associated venous anomalies, and possibly telangiectasias, without the need for contrast enhancement, and may be a more sensitive imaging biomarker of lesion burden in tracking disease progression in future therapeutic trials (15)

Clinical presentation

CCMs manifest a full clinical spectrum, from the asymptomatic lesion, discovered incidentally at autopsy or on neuroimaging, to the rare reported case of fatal intracranial hemorrhage. The clinical course is highly variable. Patients may present with acute or chronic neurological deficits, periods of remission and exacerbation, or progressive, insidious deterioration. Patients with asymptomatic lesions have traditionally included those presenting with mild headaches and nonspecific symptoms. Earlier autopsy series demonstrated asymptomatic lesions in up to 95% of patients (43,84). Solitary and multiple CMs of all sizes and locations may be clinically silent. Asymptomatic patients with MRI-documented lesions account for 11% to 44% of patients in clinical series (5,42,45,79). Headache may be the sole clinical manifestation in more than one-fourth of patients (26). In one study, 40% of patients with initially clinically silent lesions became symptomatic within an interval of 6 months to 2 years (5).

Because a majority of CCM lesions are supratentorial with a lobar predilection, it is not altogether surprising that in 38% to 100% of patients with CCM, seizure is the presenting symptom (Figs. 28.2 and 28.7) (26,43,50,52,53,56,93,94,105). All seizure types have been observed, including simple seizures in 27% to 31% of patients, complex partial seizures in 6% to 45%, and generalized seizures in 27% to 63% (27,44,50). In patients with intractable seizures, one series reported a predominance of complex partial seizures. CCMs are almost twice as likely to be associated with seizures when compared with other lesions, such as AVMs and tumors with similar volume distributions and in virtually identical locations. CCMs located in the temporal lobes are more commonly associated with medically refractory epilepsy. In one series, which included 27 vascular malformations associated with intractable epilepsy, 74.7% of the malformations were CCMs and only 14.8% were AVMs. The pathophysiology of seizures in CCMs is postulated to be related to irritation and compression secondary to mass effect and multiple local hemorrhages with the exposure of the surrounding brain to blood breakdown products, particularly iron, and the subsequent local gliomatous reaction (34,44,68,87,106). Adequately localizing the epileptogenic zone before ascribing a CCM as the cause of seizures is important, particularly in cases with multiple lesions. Unfortunately, in the majority of patients, it is not possible to localize or even lateralize the seizure focus by scalp electroencephalography because the results of the study may be normal or of indeterminate localizing value.

Another common clinical presentation of patients with CCMs is with acute or progressive focal neurological deficit. This is usually associated with intralesional or perilesional hemorrhage that can be documented by MRI. The frequency in clinical series ranges from 15.4% to 46.6% (4,5,26,27,34,36,42,45,50,51,53,54,56,57,76,81,82,88,107). The precise syndrome depends on the lesion location and size (Figs. 28.6, 28.8, and 28.9). The deficit may be transient, progressive, recurrent, or fixed. Recurrent hemorrhagic episodes result in cumulative disability, often with severe fixed impairments (4,5,26,34,42,52,54,56,57,76,107,108).

CCM and intracranial hemorrhage

A distinction must be made between apoplectic or gross hemorrhage and ongoing microhemorrhages and intralesional hemorrhagic expansion in CCMs. Al Shahi *et al.* (2) systematically reviewed the published literature and suggested evidence-based criteria for defining CCM-related hemorrhage as follows.

A clinical event involving both:

- Acute or subacute onset symptoms (any of headache, epileptic seizure, impaired consciousness, new/worsened focal neurological deficit referable to the anatomic location of the CM).
- Radiological, pathological, surgical, or rarely only cerebrospinal fluid evidence of recent extra- or intralesional hemorrhage.

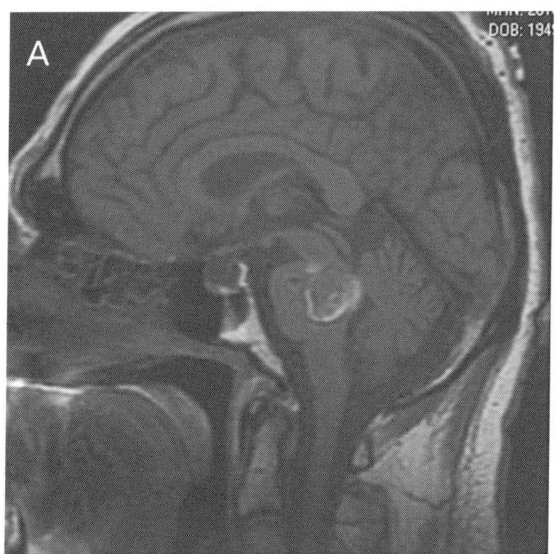

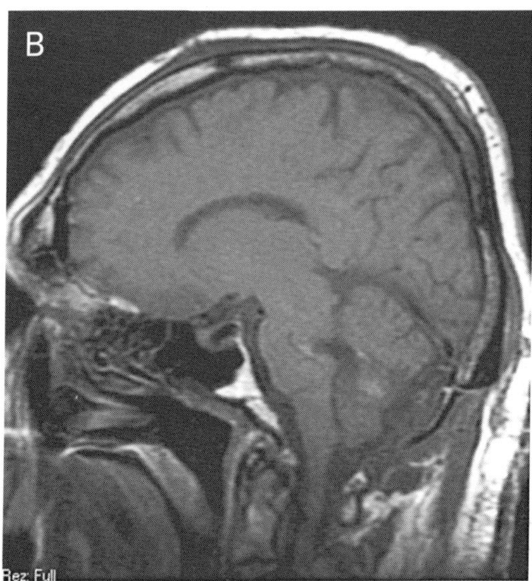

Fig. 28.6 (A) T1-weighted MRI of pontine lesion presenting with progressive symptoms. This was resected via a transvermian corridor through the floor of the fourth ventricle, with multimodality evoked potential and facial nerve monitoring. (B) Postoperative scan showing lesion excision and surgical corridor. The patient achieved excellent functional recovery, including independent gait and binocular vision.

The mere existence of a hemosiderin halo, or solely an increase in CM diameter without other evidence of recent hemorrhage, is not considered a clinically significant hemorrhage. Evidence of occult bleeding is a defining feature that is present in every lesion, regardless of clinical history. Overt hemorrhage, however, is a less common but clinically more significant event and has been reported in 8% to 37% of lesions in clinical studies (4,5,26,27,33,34,36,42,51–54,74,105,108). A higher association has been reported in children, with a range of 36% to 60% (43,48,49,109). The annual clinically significant hemorrhagic risk has been estimated at 0.7% to 1.1% per lesion per year (4,5,36). A majority of hemorrhages are intraparenchymal within the region of the CCM. Rarely they are subarachnoid (frequently seen with optic nerve or chiasmal CMs) or intraventricular (53,110,111). In mixed lesions comprising a CCM and a venous malformation, the hemorrhage is invariably secondary to the CCM (12). In contrast to a bleeding episode from an AVM, hemorrhage from a CCM is rarely life threatening. There are rare documented cases of patient death and few cases of rapid neurological deterioration from an acute apoplectic episode (50,81). More recent large series have also reported rare mortality attributable to a first hemorrhage from a CCM (5,50,110). The precise clinical presenting syndrome depends upon the location of the lesion. Typically, there is an acute onset of headache, which may be accompanied by a neurological deficit and a change in the level of consciousness (108). In the posterior fossa, hemorrhages cause neurological sequelae with greater frequency because of the concentration of vital tracts and nuclei and the possibility of obstruction of cerebrospinal fluid pathways. In the cerebellum, hemorrhages cause patients to present with headache, emesis, ataxia, vertigo, and nystagmus, whereas in the brain stem, typical signs of hemorrhage include diplopia, hemiparesis, sensory deficits, and change in mental status (5,82,97,107,112–116). In general, however, initial bleeds are self-limited and patients generally achieve a good or fair neurological recovery (5). In contrast, recurrent clinically overt hemorrhages are associated with progressive neurological decline and severe residual deficits. When hemorrhage occurs in the brain stem, periods of exacerbation and then

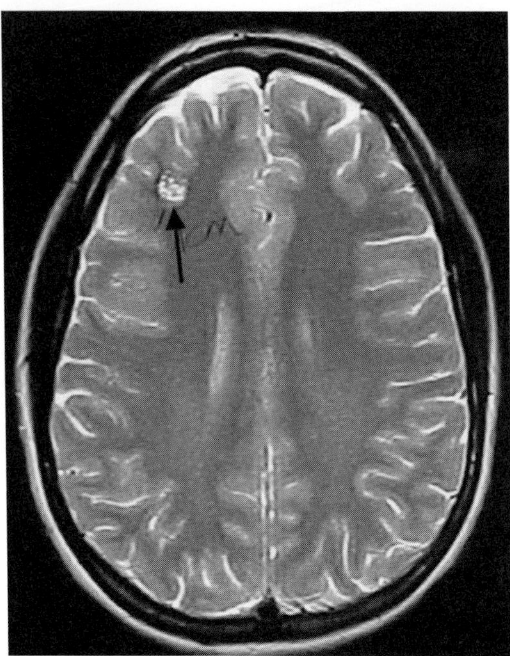

Fig. 28.7 Right frontal CCM presented with new onset seizures in a young patient. Lesion was resected with a generous margin including hemosiderin-stained brain ('lesionectomy plus'), achieving seizure-free state despite tapering off anticonvulsant medications. Mapping of perilesional tissue is performed in such cases, with option of resection of cortical tissue with epileptiform activity, in non-eloquent location.

remission may occur, mimicking demyelinating disease. Regardless of how patients present, data from several studies suggest that the risk of recurrent hemorrhage increases after an initial bleed (5,26,45,50,51,56–58,76,81,82,107,108). Several studies have suggested that female patients may have a higher risk of hemorrhage, particularly during pregnancy (5,42,54).

Management strategy

There are not sufficient firm scientific data to guide all relevant clinical decisions regarding the optimal management of CCMs. However, the existing information does provide a fundamental framework for rational clinical decisions. Patients with CCMs may be considered in clinical categories with distinct risk of hemorrhage and neurological disability. Patients may have only headache or nonspecific symptoms or may present with neurological deficits (either fixed, fluctuating, or progressive) or seizures. Each clinical scenario requires the proposal of a distinct management approach aimed at weighing the treatment risk against the best estimate of the cumulative natural risk.

Expectant management

Asymptomatic patients with single or multiple lesions and only vague complaints, such as headache or dizziness in the absence of focal neurological deficits, present a low annualized risk of a first debilitating hemorrhage. There are no current data to support an aggressive approach in this group or in patients with purely incidental lesions, in either sporadic or familial CCMs. Yet, surgical intervention for accessible solitary lesions carries a very small risk and virtually eliminates all subsequent serious risk from the lesions. Follow-up of these patients clinically and with sequential MRI seems reasonable. Alternatively, elective excision of readily accessible lesions may be considered in younger patients whose cumulative risk over time may not be negligible. Young patients with mild or non-disabling symptoms and solitary, accessible (usually supratentorial or cerebellar) lesions should be followed up closely, and lesion excision should be considered at the first manifestation of lesion growth or exacerbation of symptoms. We have more recently favored surgical excision of solitary, accessible lesions, even when minimally symptomatic, because follow-up of numerous such patients has shown that the psychological burden of living with the lesion, the costs, the stress and inconvenience of repeated imaging, and the outlook toward childbearing among young female patients has not been negligible. Patients with less accessible lesions and those associated with dominant venous anomalies require a correspondingly higher threshold for lesion excision (Fig. 28.5).

Medical management

The major role of medical management in CMs is to control epilepsy. The epileptogenicity may often be localized to a single lesion. The clinical spectrum

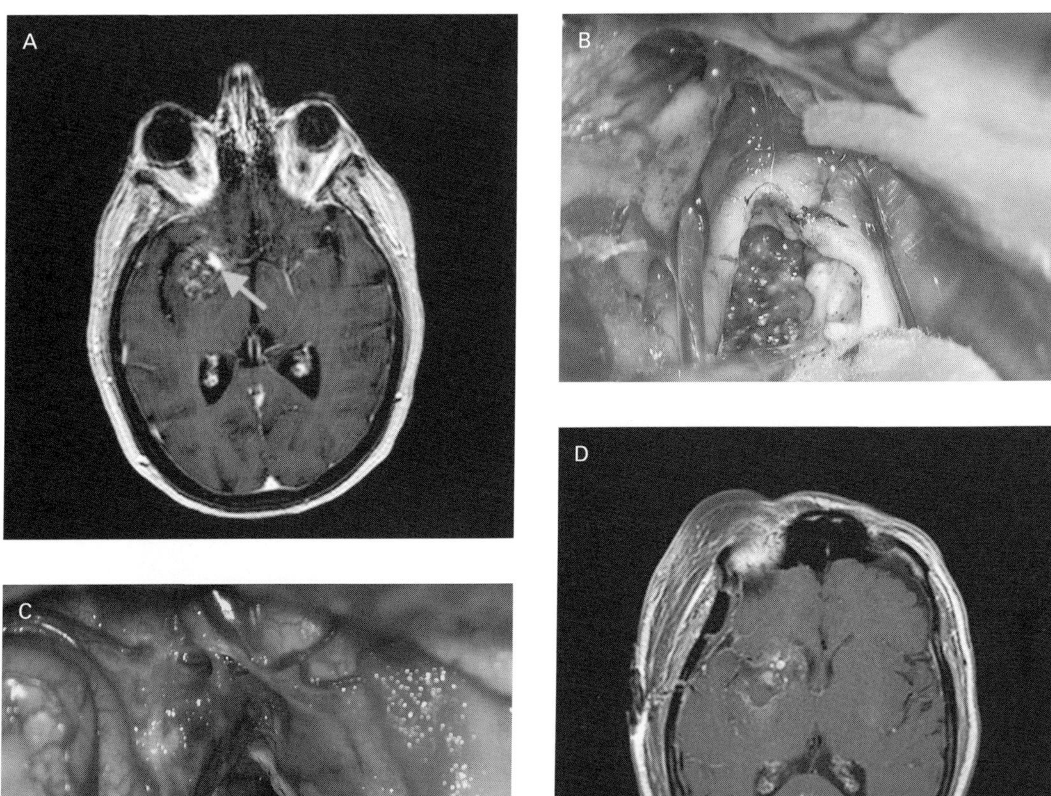

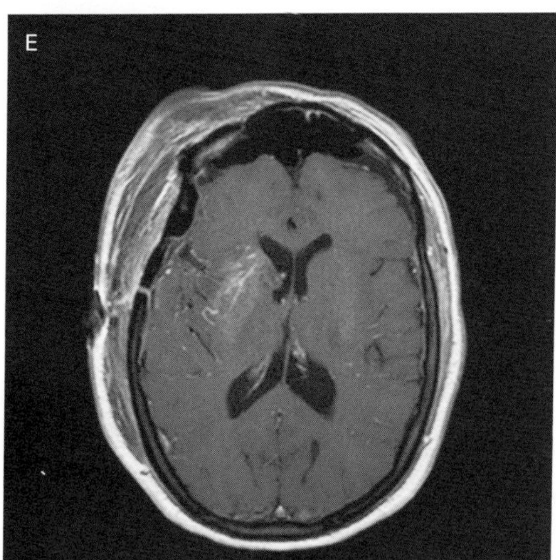

Fig. 28.8 (A) T1-weighted MRI scan of middle-aged female presenting with left hemiparesis and disabling left arm dystonia, reveals a large CCM lesion involving the lentiform nucleus and anterior limb of the internal capsule. Arrow reveals prominent venous anomaly at the medial aspect of the CCM. Other images (not shown) confirmed a large associated DVA. (B) Lesion was exposed via transylvian approach, with adjunct image guidance and evoked potential monitoring. (C) CCM lesion was resected with significant

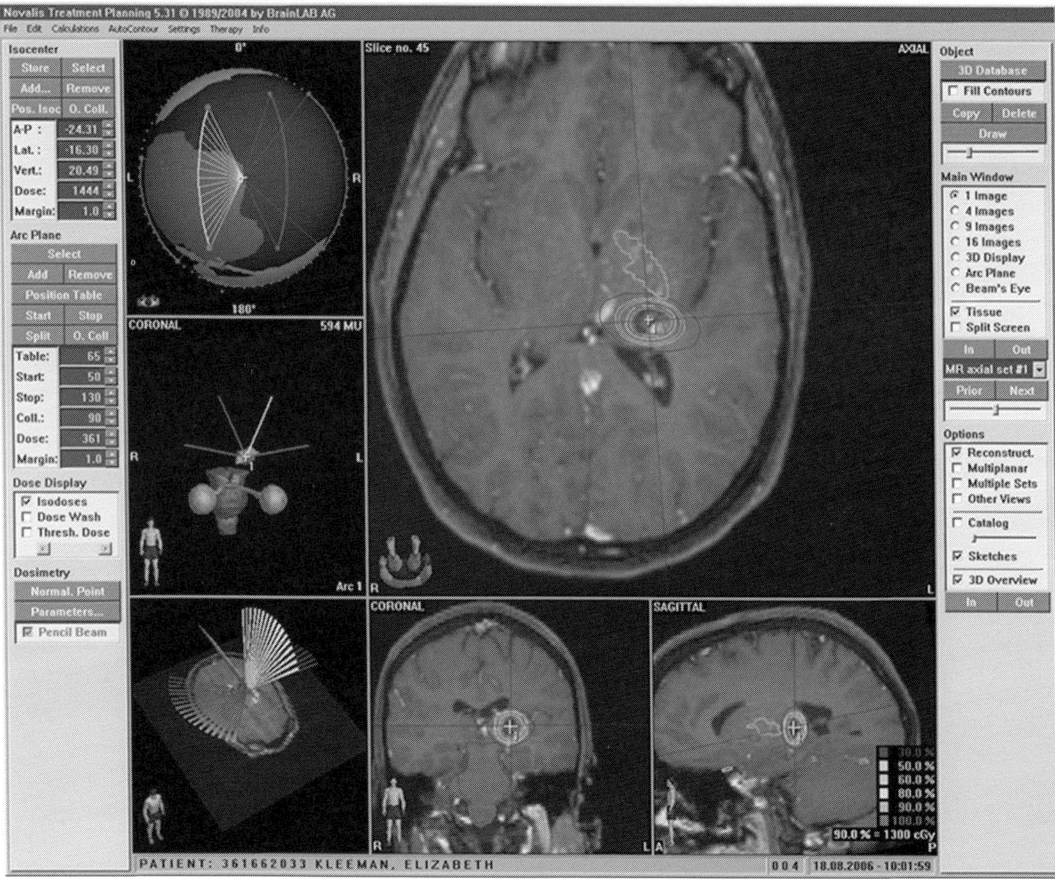

Fig. 28.9. Stereotactic radiosurgery using linear accelerator and micromultileaf collimator (13 Gy to 90% isodose line at lesion periphery) targeting posterior capsular CCM lesion. The patient had suffered from repeated symptomatic hemorrhages with partial hemisensory residual deficit during the 2 years preceding treatment. Patient had no further hemorrhagic episodes or symptom exacerbations in 4 years of follow up after radiosurgery. (See plate section for color version).

ranges from those patients who respond well to anticonvulsant medication to those patients with medically intractable and functionally debilitating seizures. Several studies have shown that the symptoms of patients with severe epilepsy who received anticonvulsant treatment persisted unabated with significant clinical and social disability from seizures (5,44). Other medical recommendations include the avoidance of blood thinners for questionable indications, and a higher threshold and closer monitoring if anticoagulation is otherwise recommended. No specific lifestyle restrictions are imposed except those

Fig. 28.8 (cont.)
effort at carefully preserving several lenticulostriate arteries coursing nearby, and also the large DVA. (D) Postresection MRI scan showing the resection cavity and surgical corridor. (E) MRI scan reveals the preserved venous anomaly with its caput medusae-like branches adjacent to the lesion resection. The patient experienced immediate relief of disabling dystonia. Her left hemiparesis, which worsened transiently postoperatively, resolved completely within 2 weeks of surgery.

related to epileptogenicity, and the avoidance of extreme strenuous activities beyond normal fitness.

Surgical resection

It is currently agreed that accessible symptomatic CMs should be considered for resection. The current firmly established indications for surgical management are overt hemorrhage, focal neurological symptoms, and/or medically intractable epilepsy. As previously noted, patients presenting with initial hemorrhage are at greater risk for recurrent hemorrhage. The resection of accessible symptomatic supratentorial lesions has been accompanied by a very low rate of morbidity (5,43,44,48–50,82,94,117). Deep supratentorial lesions require a higher threshold for surgical intervention, reserving surgery for lesions causing disabling or recurrent hemorrhages (Fig. 28.8) (118). Favorable results have also been reported in the resection of brain stem lesions that appear at a pial or ventricular surface (Fig. 28.6) (4,49,107,119). There is no consensus as to whether the excision of these lesions should be performed after a first bleed or should await symptom recurrence or progression (120). Lesion accessibility reflects on surgical risk (4,43,44,49,51,76,93,107,108,114,117,121). The mortality risk in surgery for brain stem CMs has ranged from 0% to 20%, with transient neurological worsening in 20% to 40% of patients and permanent worsening in <20% (76,82,114,119,121). In one series of patients with brain stem lesions who presented with neurological deficits and did not undergo surgery, 70% of patients had unremitting or fatal outcomes (50). In patients with multiple lesions, only the offending lesion should be resected, and the patients should receive expectant follow-up for the remaining lesions, as do patients with asymptomatic lesions. Recurrences have been reported with subtotal removal of lesions and are found more commonly in less accessible and infratentorial locations.

Special considerations in patients with CCM and epilepsy

Patients with CCMs in cortical locations, especially in temporal, frontal, and perilimbic locations, are subject to a prospective lifetime risk of new seizures. Lesionectomy with resection of adjacent hemosiderin-stained brain tissue in less-eloquent brain locations (Fig. 28.7) is associated with excellent postoperative seizure control in many patients. The likelihood of postoperative seizure control following simple lesion excision is greater, approximately 65–95%, in patients with less intractable preoperative epilepsy and also in patients with extratemporal lesions (122,123). Several studies have shown that complete lesion excision is necessary for seizure control in the majority of patients who harbor a CCM that has been shown to be responsible for their seizures (123). It is also well documented that lesion excision alone may not always be sufficient for seizure control, especially in patients with truly intractable epilepsy. Thus another strategy of epilepsy control involves resection of the lesion and a tailored resection of the epileptogenic cortex to avoid the eloquent cortex. In patients with temporal lobe lesions and intractable epilepsy, lesionectomy without resection of mesiotemporal lobe structures has documented relatively low seizure control rates, ranging from only 20% to 45% (122,124,125). However, some of these patients became seizure free after additional resection of epileptogenic brain tissue in the same region. When epileptogenic brain tissue is resected in addition to the lesion during a first operation, it may provide the patient with seizure control and avoid a second surgical intervention. But the potential functional impact of resection of additional brain tissue must be considered, especially when contemplating resection of mesial structures in the presence of high or normal material-specific memory function, or resection involving other eloquent areas (such as the dominant temporal neocortex). Intraoperative electrocorticography is sometimes performed to further delineate the extent of the cortical epileptogenic zone. This technique may provide prognostic information by indicating the areas of residual electric discharges after the resection of the vascular malformation or what was thought to be the seizure focus (126,127). It is important to remember, however, that residual spikes in adjacent brain areas do not reliably predict residual epileptogenicity, nor does their absence guarantee postoperative seizure control (126,127).

Often lesionectomy is performed as a first procedure, especially with CCM in more eloquent locations

(Fig. 28.2), and only those patients with persistent uncontrolled seizures are subjected to epilepsy surgery evaluation and a second respective procedure if this becomes necessary. Several studies (123,124,128,129) have compared lesionectomy with the combination of lesionectomy and cortisectomy with controversial results. A meta-analysis evaluating seizure outcome following either lesionectomy or the combination of lesionectomy and corticectomy concluded that at 2-year follow up, the prevalence of persistent seizures following lesionectomy ranged from 1.4 to 4 times the prevalence following the more extensive respective procedures. In contrast, patients with fewer seizures before presentation, shorter preoperative seizure histories, or seizures that responded to antiepileptic medications were more likely to be seizure free following lesionectomy alone (130–136).

Most patients in whom seizures are fully controlled postoperatively will still require long-term anticonvulsant therapy, although often with fewer agents and at lower dosages than they required preoperatively. When the decision is made to reduce or discontinue anticonvulsant therapy, it is important to taper the dosage cautiously to avoid precipitating new or recurrent seizures. Of patients who harbor a single CCM, undergo lesionectomy for treatment of recent-onset, localization-related seizures, and are seizure free postoperatively, up to half may be successfully tapered off all anticonvulsant medications (Fig. 28.2) (106,137–139). This promising outcome, and its associated positive impact on quality of life, may play a role in the decision to excise a solitary accessible cortical CCM, even when seizures are not truly intractable to medical therapy.

Surgical adjuncts in CCM resection

CCMs of eloquent locations pose a special challenge since in these cases benefits of improving the patient's clinical condition must be weighed against surgical risks of the procedure. With the advancement of image guidance technique and intraoperative monitoring now it is becoming possible to tackle these lesions with minimal untoward consequences (140). A study comparing clinical and surgical data of patients with cavernoma treated surgically with and without intraoperative navigation showed that use of neuronavigation was associated with a more effective and safer surgery of smaller and more deep-seated cavernomas (141). In an attempt to evaluate tools that can improve surgical precision and minimize surgical trauma for removal of cavernomas in the paracentral area Zhou *et al.* defined four key factors that influence successful excision of these lesions (142):

- First, the precise location of the lesion;
- Second, the precise evaluation of the functional area;
- Third, the choice of a minimally invasive surgical approach;
- Fourth, the entire removal of cavernoma and careful removal of hemosiderin-stained tissue.

In this study by Zhou *et al.* of 17 patients with paracentral cavernoma, by combining preoperative fMRI and intraoperative neurophysiological monitoring, including SEP, MEP, and cortical mapping, and with the aid of ultrasonography-assisted neuronavigation, the damage to the primary motor area was successfully avoided while achieving complete resection via trans-sulcal microsurgical approach without neurological deficits (142). Another retrospective study looking at the results of 26 patients operated for supratentorial deep-seated or near eloquent brain area cavernomas concluded that intraoperative visualization of eloquent cortex areas by integration of functional data for identification and exemption of eloquent brain areas combined with neuronavigation and intraoperative MR-guided resection allows safe and complete resection of supratentorial cavernomas in critical brain areas with low morbidity (143).

Surgical considerations in CCM associated with developmental venous anomalies

Surgery may be indicated for resection of symptomatic CCMs, even when associated with DVA (Fig. 28.8). In such cases, the surgical approach and strategy should aim to separate the CCM component of the lesion and excise it, while avoiding injury to associated DVA. While some reports have reported uneventful resection of small supratentorial DVA associated with CCM (23), many reports have described catastrophic complications of injury or resection of a DVA, resulting in serious and life threatening edema, hemorrhage and/or venous infarcts (144–146). Other cases of clustering of smaller CCMs with large predominant DVA should not ideally be treated surgically (Fig. 28.5).

Radiosurgical treatment of CCMs

Radiosurgery has been established as an effective alternative treatment option for small AVMs in eloquent and inaccessible areas (77,117,147,148). With standard doses as used for AVMs, CCMs exhibit a poor clinical response and a high rate of complications (26,149). In one series of 16 patients (13 with CCM alone and three with CCM associated with a venous malformation), there was no radiographic change in 80% but 37.4% eventually developed radiation-induced changes, one out of 16 (6.25%) experienced a second hemorrhage, and 12.5% had persistent neurological deficits (150). When lower margin doses are used, the results may be more promising (Fig. 28.9) (149,151,152). One such report used doses of 12–16 Gy for 39 deep-seated CMs, with an average follow-up of 23 months. The authors reported temporary neurological sequelae with MRI changes secondary to radiation in 10 patients (25.4%). There were four deaths, two reportedly unrelated to radiosurgery and two after 'delayed microneurosurgery'. After 15 months, there were no patients with delayed hemorrhage (149,151,152). These data correlate with published data on angiographically occult vascular malformations in general (149). The use of radiosurgery needs further investigation. In particular, issues of patient selection, follow-up, long-term risks, and safe dose levels must be addressed (153). End points of therapeutic success or failure have been difficult to establish in view of the variability of the natural behavior of the lesions. The results of the treatment of CCMs must be judged against the known natural history of the disease.

REFERENCES

1. Maraire JN, Awad IA. Intracranial cavernous malformations: lesion behavior and management strategies. *Neurosurgery.* 1995;**37**(4):591–605.
2. Al-Shahi Salman R, Berg MJ, Morrison L, Awad IA. Hemorrhage from cavernous malformations of the brain: definition and reporting standards. Angioma Alliance Scientific Advisory Board. *Stroke.* 2008;**39**(12):3222–30.
3. Beck L, Jr., D'Amore PA. Vascular development: cellular and molecular regulation. *FASEB J.* 1997;**11**(5):365–73.
4. Del Curling O, Jr., Kelly DL, Jr., Elster AD, Craven TE. An analysis of the natural history of cavernous angiomas. *J Neurosurg.* 1991;**75**(5):702–8.
5. Robinson JR, Awad IA, Little JR. Natural history of the cavernous angioma. *J Neurosurg.* 1991;**75**(5):709–14.
6. Dey M, Turner MS, Wollmann R, Awad IA. Fatal 'hypertensive' intracerebral hemorrhage associated with a cerebral cavernous angioma: case report. *Acta Neurochir* (Wien). **153**(2):421–3.
7. Chusid JG, Kopeloff LM. Epileptogenic effects of pure metals implanted in motor cortex of monkeys. *J Appl Physiol.* 1962;**17**:697–700.
8. Hoang TA, Hasso AN. Intracranial vascular malformations. *Neuroimaging Clin N Am.* 1994;**4**(4):823–47.
9. McCormick PW, Spetzler RF, Johnson PC, Drayer BP. Cerebellar hemorrhage associated with capillary telangiectasia and venous angioma: a case report. *Surg Neurol.* 1993;**39**(6):451–7.
10. Van Roost D, Kristof R, Wolf HK, Keller E. Intracerebral capillary telangiectasia and venous malformation: a rare association. *Surg Neurol.* 1997;**48**(2):175–83.
11. Wyburn-Mason R. *The vascular abnormalities and tumours of the spinal cord and its membranes.* London: Henry Kimpton;1943.
12. Awad IA, Robinson JR, Jr., Mohanty S, Estes ML. Mixed vascular malformations of the brain: clinical and pathogenetic considerations. *Neurosurgery.* 1993;**33**(2):179–88; discussion 188.
13. McDonald DA, Shenkar R, Shi C, *et al.* A novel mouse model of cerebral cavernous malformations based on the two-hit mutation hypothesis recapitulates the human disease. *Hum Mol Genet.* 2011;**20**(2):211–22.
14. de Champfleur NM, Langlois C, Ankenbrandt WJ, *et al.* MRI evaluation of cerebral cavernous malformations with susceptibility-weighted imaging. *Neurosurgery.* 2011;**68**(3):641–8.
15. Campbell PG, Jabbour P, Yadla S, Awad IA. Emerging clinical imaging techniques for cerebral cavernous malformations: a systematic review. *Neurosurg Focus.* 2010;**29**(3):E6.
16. Awad IA. On telangiectasia. *Am J Neurorad.* 1996;**17**:1799–800.
17. Abdulrauf SI, Kaynar MY, Awad IA. A comparison of the clinical profile of cavernous malformations with and

without associated venous malformations. *Neurosurgery.* 1999;**44**(1):41–6; discussion 46–7.
18. Awad IA, Robinson JR. Comparison of the clinical presentation of symptomatic arteriovenous malformations (angiographically visualized) and occult vascular malformations. *Neurosurgery.* 1993;**32**(5):876–8.
19. Mullan S, Mojtahedi S, Johnson DL, Macdonald RL. Cerebral venous malformation -arteriovenous malformation transition forms. *J Neurosurg.* 1996;**85**(1):9–13.
20. Petersen TA, Morrison LA, Schrader RM, Hart BL. Familial versus sporadic cavernous malformations: Differences in developmental venous anomaly association and lesion phenotype. *AJNR Am J Neuroradiol.* 2010;**31**(2):377–82.
21. Aksoy FG, Gomori JM, Tuchner Z. Association of intracerebral venous angioma and true arteriovenous malformation: a rare, distinct entity. *Neuroradiol.* 2000;**42**(6):455–7.
22. Chang SD, Steinberg GK, Rosario M, Crowley RS, Hevner RF. Mixed arteriovenous malformation and capillary telangiectasia: a rare subset of mixed vascular malformations. Case report. *J Neurosurg.* 1997;**86**(4):699–703.
23. Wurm G, Schnizer M, Fellner FA. Cerebral cavernous malformations associated with venous anomalies: surgical considerations. *Neurosurgery.* 2005;**57**(1 Suppl):42–58.
24. Yanaka K, Hyodo A, Nose T. Venous malformation serving as the draining vein of an adjoining arteriovenous malformation. Case report and review of the literature. *Surg Neurol.* 2001;**56**(3):170–4.
25. Labauge P, Enjolras O, Bonerandi JJ, *et al.* An association between autosomal dominant cerebral cavernomas and a distinctive hyperkeratotic cutaneous vascular malformation in four families. *Ann Neurol.* 1999;**45**(2):250–4.
26. Giombini S, Morello G. Cavernous angiomas of the brain. Account of fourteen personal cases and review of the literature. *Acta Neurochir* (Wien). 1978;**40**(1–2):61–82.
27. Lonjon M, Roche JL, George B, *et al.* Intracranial cavernoma. 30 cases. *Presse Med.* 1993;**22**(21):990–4.
28. Jabbour P, Gault J, Awad IA. What genes can teach us about human cerebrovascular malformations. *Clin Neurosurg.* 2004;**51**:140–52.
29. Gault J, Sarin H, Awadallah NA, Shenkar R, Awad IA. Pathobiology of human cerebrovascular malformations: basic mechanisms and clinical relevance. *Neurosurgery.* 2004;**55**(1):1–16; discussion 117.
30. Bicknell JM, Carlow TJ, Kornfeld M, Stovring J, Turner P. Familial cavernous angiomas. *Arch Neurol.* 1978;**35**(11):746–9.
31. Dobyns WB, Michels VV, Groover RV, *et al.* Familial cavernous malformations of the central nervous system and retina. *Ann Neurol.* 1987;**21**(6):578–83.
32. Duong H, del Carpio-O'Donovan R, Pike B, Ethier R. Multiple intracerebral cavernous angiomas. *Can Assoc Radiol J.* 1991;**42**(5):329–34.
33. Hayman LA, Evans RA, Ferrell RE, *et al.* Familial cavernous angiomas: natural history and genetic study over a 5-year period. *Am J Med Genet.* 1982;**11**(2):147–60.
34. Rigamonti D, Hadley MN, Drayer BP, *et al.* Cerebral cavernous malformations. Incidence and familial occurrence. *N Engl J Med.* 1988;**319**(6):343–7.
35. Steichen-Gersdorf E, Felber S, Fuchs W, Russeger L, Twerdy K. Familial cavernous angiomas of the brain: observations in a four generation family. *Eur J Pediatr.* 1992;**151**(11):861–3.
36. Zabramski JM, Wascher TM, Spetzler RF, *et al.* The natural history of familial cavernous malformations: results of an ongoing study. *J Neurosurg.* 1994;**80**(3):422–32.
37. Mason I, Aase JM, Orrison WW, *et al.* Familial cavernous angiomas of the brain in an Hispanic family. *Neurology.* 1988;**38**(2):324–6.
38. Gunel M, Awad IA, Finberg K, *et al.* A founder mutation as a cause of cerebral cavernous malformation in Hispanic Americans. *N Engl J Med.* 1996;**334**(15):946–51.
39. Gallione CJ SA, Awad IA, Weber JL, Marchuk DA. A founder mutation in the Ashkenazi Jewish population affecting mRNA splicing of the CCM2 gene is associated with cerebral cavernous malformations. *Genetics in Medicine.* 2011;**13** (7):662–6.
40. Clark JV. Familial occurrence of cavernous angiomata of the brain. *J Neurol Neurosurg Psychiatry.* 1970;**33**(6):871–6.
41. Kidd HA, Cumings JN. Cerebral angiomata in an Icelandic family. *Lancet.* 1947;**1**(6457):747.
42. Sage MR, Brophy BP, Sweeney C, *et al.* Cavernous haemangiomas (angiomas) of the brain: clinically significant lesions. *Australas Radiol.* 1993;**37**(2):147–55.
43. Voigt K, Yasargil MG. Cerebral cavernous haemangiomas or cavernomas. Incidence, pathology, localization, diagnosis, clinical features and treatment. Review of the literature and report of an unusual case. *Neurochirurgia* (Stuttg). 1976;**19**(2):59–68.
44. Weber JP, Silbergeld DL, Winn HR. Surgical resection of epileptogenic cortex associated with structural lesions. *Neurosurg Clin N Am.* 1993;**4**(2):327–36.
45. Requena I, Arias M, Lopez-Ibor L, *et al.* Cavernomas of the central nervous system: clinical and neuroimaging manifestations in 47 patients. *J Neurol Neurosurg Psychiatry.* 1991;**54**(7):590–4.
46. Bergeson PS, Rekate HL, Tack ED. Cerebral cavernous angiomas in the newborn. *Clin Pediatr* (Phila). 1992;**31** (7):435–7.

47. Ciricillo SF, Dillon WP, Fink ME, Edwards MS. Progression of multiple cryptic vascular malformations associated with anomalous venous drainage. Case report. *J Neurosurg.* 1994;**81**(3):477–81.
48. Mazza C, Scienza R, Dalla Bernardin B, *et al.* Cerebral cavernous malformations (cavernomas) in children. *Neurochirurgie.* 1989;**35**(2):106–8.
49. Scott RM, Barnes P, Kupsky W, Adelman LS. Cavernous angiomas of the central nervous system in children. *J Neurosurg.* 1992;**76**(1):38–46.
50. Simard JM, Garcia-Bengochea F, Ballinger WE, Jr., Mickle JP, Quisling RG. Cavernous angioma: a review of 126 collected and 12 new clinical cases. *Neurosurgery.* 1986;**18**(2):162–72.
51. Vaquero J, Leunda G, Martinez R, Bravo G. Cavernomas of the brain. *Neurosurgery.* 1983;**12**(2):208–10.
52. Vaquero J, Salazar J, Martinez R, Martinez P, Bravo G. Cavernomas of the central nervous system: clinical syndromes, CT scan diagnosis, and prognosis after surgical treatment in 25 cases. *Acta Neurochir* (Wien). 1987;**85**(1–2):29–33.
53. Yamasaki T, Handa H, Yamashita J, *et al.* Intracranial and orbital cavernous angiomas. A review of 30 cases. *J Neurosurg.* 1986;**64**(2):197–208.
54. Robinson JR, Jr., Awad IA, Magdinec M, Paranandi L. Factors predisposing to clinical disability in patients with cavernous malformations of the brain. *Neurosurgery.* 1993;**32**(5):730–5; discussion 735–6.
55. Lechevalier B. Neuropathologic study of cavernomas. *Neurochirurgie.* 1989;**35**(2):78–81.
56. Lobato RD, Perez C, Rivas JJ, Cordobes F. Clinical, radiological, and pathological spectrum of angiographically occult intracranial vascular malformations. Analysis of 21 cases and review of the literature. *J Neurosurg.* 1988;**68**(4):518–31.
57. Lobato RD, Rivas JJ, Gomez PA, *et al.* Comparison of the clinical presentation of symptomatic arteriovenous malformations (angiographically visualized) and occult vascular malformations. *Neurosurgery.* 1992;**31**(3):391–6; discussion 396–7.
58. Abe M, Kjellberg RN, Adams RD. Clinical presentations of vascular malformations of the brain stem: comparison of angiographically positive and negative types. *J Neurol Neurosurg Psychiatry.* 1989;**52**(2):167–75.
59. Robinson JR, Jr., Awad IA, Masaryk TJ, Estes ML. Pathological heterogeneity of angiographically occult vascular malformations of the brain. *Neurosurgery.* 1993;**33**(4):547–54; discussion 554–5.
60. Bourgouin PM, Tampieri D, Johnston W, *et al.* Multiple occult vascular malformations of the brain and spinal cord: MRI diagnosis. *Neuroradiology.* 1992;**34**(2):110–11.
61. Savoiardo M, Strada L, Passerini A. Intracranial cavernous hemangiomas: neuroradiologic review of 36 operated cases. *AJNR Am J Neuroradiol.* 1983;**4**(4):945–50.
62. Wilson CB. Cryptic vascular malformations. *Clin Neurosurg.* 1992;**38**:49–84.
63. Batra S, Lin D, Recinos PF, Zhang J, Rigamonti D. Cavernous malformations: natural history, diagnosis and treatment. *Nat Rev Neurol.* 2009;**5**(12):659–70.
64. Tomlinson FH, Houser OW, Scheithauer BW, *et al.* Angiographically occult vascular malformations: a correlative study of features on magnetic resonance imaging and histological examination. *Neurosurgery.* 1994;**34**(5):792–9; discussion 799–800.
65. Bellotti C, Medina M, Oliveri G, Barrale S, Ettorre F. Cystic cavernous angiomas of the posterior fossa. Report of three cases. *J Neurosurg.* 1985;**63**(5):797–9.
66. McCormick WF, Boulter TR. Vascular malformations ('angiomas') of the dura mater. *J Neurosurg.* 1966;**25**(3):309–11.
67. Ramina R, Ingunza W, Vonofakos D. Cystic cerebral cavernous angioma with dense calcification. Case report. *J Neurosurg.* 1980;**52**(2):259–62.
68. Rigamonti D, Drayer BP, Johnson PC, *et al.* The MRI appearance of cavernous malformations (angiomas). *J Neurosurg.* 1987;**67**(4):518–24.
69. Shenkar R, Shi C, Check IJ, Lipton HL, Awad IA. Concepts and hypotheses: inflammatory hypothesis in the pathogenesis of cerebral cavernous malformations. *Neurosurgery.* 2007;**61**(4):693-702; discussion 693.
70. Shi C, Shenkar R, Du H, *et al.* Immune response in human cerebral cavernous malformations. *Stroke.* 2009;**40**(5):1659–65.
71. Wong JH, Awad IA, Kim JH. Ultrastructural pathological features of cerebrovascular malformations: a preliminary report. *Neurosurgery.* 2000;**46**(6):1454–9.
72. Clatterbuck RE, Eberhart CG, Crain BJ, Rigamonti D. Ultrastructural and immunocytochemical evidence that an incompetent blood-brain barrier is related to the pathophysiology of cavernous malformations. *J Neurol Neurosurg Psychiatry.* 2001;**71**(2):188–92.
73. Biondi A, Scotti G, Scialfa G, Landoni L. Magnetic resonance imaging of cerebral cavernous angiomas. *Acta Radiol Suppl.* 1986;**369**:82–5.
74. Lechevalier B, Houtteville JP. Intracranial cavernous angioma. *Rev Neurol* (Paris). 1992;**148**(3):173–9.

75. Pozzati E, Giuliani G, Nuzzo G, Poppi M. The growth of cerebral cavernous angiomas. *Neurosurgery.* 1989;**25**(1):92–7.
76. Sakai N, Yamada H, Tanigawara T, *et al.* Surgical treatment of cavernous angioma involving the brainstem and review of the literature. *Acta Neurochir* (Wien). 1991;**113**(3–4):138–43.
77. Wilkins RH. Natural history of intracranial vascular malformations: a review. *Neurosurgery.* 1985;**16**(3):421–30.
78. Ogilvy CS, Moayeri N, Golden JA. Appearance of a cavernous hemangioma in the cerebral cortex after a biopsy of a deeper lesion. *Neurosurgery.* 1993;**33**(2):307–9; discussion 309.
79. Rigamonti D, Johnson PC, Spetzler RF, Hadley MN, Drayer BP. Cavernous malformations and capillary telangiectasia: a spectrum within a single pathological entity. *Neurosurgery.* 1991;**28**(1):60–4.
80. Farmer JP, Cosgrove GR, Villemure JG, *et al.* Intracerebral cavernous angiomas. *Neurology.* 1988;**38**(11):1699–704.
81. Tagle P, Huete I, Mendez J, del Villar S. Intracranial cavernous angioma: presentation and management. *J Neurosurg.* 1986;**64**(5):720–3.
82. Weil SM, Tew JM, Jr. Surgical management of brain stem vascular malformations. *Acta Neurochir* (Wien). 1990;**105**(1–2):14–23.
83. Zauberman H, Feinsod M. Orbital hemangioma growth during pregnancy. *Acta Ophthalmol* (Copenh). 1970;**48**(5):929–33.
84. Otten P, Pizzolato GP, Rilliet B, Berney J. 131 cases of cavernous angioma (cavernomas) of the CNS, discovered by retrospective analysis of 24,535 autopsies. *Neurochirurgie.* 1989;**35**(2):82–3, 128–31.
85. DiTullio MV, Jr., Stern WE. Hemangioma calcificans. Case report of an intraparenchymatous calcified vascular hematoma with epileptogenic potential. *J Neurosurg.* 1979;**50**(1):110–14.
86. Sanchis Fargueta J, Iranzo R, Garcia M, Jorda M. Hemangioma calcificans – a benign epileptogenic lesion. *Surg Neurol.* 1981;**15**(1):66–70.
87. Steiger HJ, Markwalder RV, Reulen HJ. Is there a relationship between the clinical manifestations and the pathologic image of cerebral cavernomas? *Neurochirurgie.* 1989;**35**(2):84–8.
88. Sigal R, Krief O, Houtteville JP, *et al.* Occult cerebrovascular malformations: follow-up with MR imaging. *Radiology.* 1990;**176**(3):815–19.
89. Leblanc GG, Golanov E, Awad IA, Young WL. Biology of vascular malformations of the brain. *Stroke.* 2009;**40**(12):e694–702.
90. Stockton RA, Shenkar R, Awad IA, Ginsberg MH. Cerebral cavernous malformation proteins inhibit Rho kinase to stabilize vascular integrity. *J Exp Med.* 2010;**207**(4):881–96.
91. Yadla S, Jabbour PM, Shenkar R, *et al.* Cerebral cavernous malformations as a disease of vascular permeability: from bench to bedside with caution. *Neurosurg Focus.* 2010;**29**(3):E4.
92. Denier C, Labauge P, Bergametti F, *et al.* Genotype-phenotype correlations in cerebral cavernous malformations patients. *Ann Neurol.* 2006;**60**(5):550–6.
93. Rapacki TF, Brantley MJ, Furlow TW, Jr., *et al.* Heterogeneity of cerebral cavernous hemangiomas diagnosed by MR imaging. *J Comput Assist Tomogr.* 1990;**14**(1):18–25.
94. Servo A, Porras M, Raininko R. Diagnosis of cavernous haemangiomas by computed tomography and angiography. *Acta Neurochir* (Wien). 1984;**71**(3–4):273–82.
95. Diamond C, Torvik A, Amundsen P. Angiographic diagnosis of teleangiectases with cavernous angioma of the posterior fossa. Report of two cases. *Acta Radiol Diagn* (Stockh). 1976;**17**(3):281–8.
96. Numaguchi Y, Fukui M, Miyake E, *et al.* Angiographic manifestations of intracerebral cavernous hemangioma. *Neuroradiology.* 1977;**14**(3):113–16.
97. Yamasaki T, Handa H, Moritake K. Cavernous angioma in the fourth ventricle. *Surg Neurol.* 1985;**23**(3):249–54.
98. de Souza JM, Domingues RC, Cruz LC, Jr., *et al.* Susceptibility-weighted imaging for the evaluation of patients with familial cerebral cavernous malformations: a comparison with t2-weighted fast spin-echo and gradient-echo sequences. *AJNR Am J Neuroradiol.* 2008;**29**(1):154–8.
99. Bien S, Friedburg H, Harders A, Schumacher M. Intracerebral cavernous angiomas in magnetic resonance imaging. *Acta Radiol Suppl.* 1986;**369**:79–81.
100. Hatashita S, Miyajima M, Koga N. Cystic cavernous angioma–case report. *Neurol Med Chir* (Tokyo). 1991;**31**(7):414–16.
101. Iplikcioglu AC, Benli K, Bertan V, Ruacan S. Cystic cavernous hemangioma of the cerebellopontine angle: case report. *Neurosurgery.* 1986;**19**(4):641–2.
102. Khosla VK, Banerjee AK, Mathuriya SN, Mehta S. Giant cystic cavernoma in a child. Case report. *J Neurosurg.* 1984;**60**(6):1297–9.
103. Nakasu S, Yoshida M, Nakajima M, Handa J. Cystic cavernous angioma in an infant: CT features. *J Comput Assist Tomogr.* 1991;**15**(1):163–5.
104. Vaquero J, Cabezudo JM, Leunda G. Cystic cavernous haemangiomas of the brain. *Acta Neurochir* (Wien). 1983;**67**(1–2):135–8.

105. Houtteville JP. Rare localizations. Review of the literature. *Neurochirurgie.* 1989;**35**(2):98:128–31.
106. Kraemer DL, Awad IA. Vascular malformations and epilepsy: clinical considerations and basic mechanisms. *Epilepsia.* 1994;**35** Suppl 6:S30–43.
107. Zimmerman RS, Spetzler RF, Lee KS, Zabramski JM, Hargraves RW. Cavernous malformations of the brain stem. *J Neurosurg.* 1991;**75**(1):32–9.
108. Wakai S, Ueda Y, Inoh S, Nagai M. Angiographically occult angiomas: a report of thirteen cases with analysis of the cases documented in the literature. *Neurosurgery.* 1985;**17**(4):549–56.
109. Hubert P, Choux M, Houtteville JP. Cerebral cavernomas in infants and children. *Neurochirurgie.* 1989;**35**(2):104–5.
110. Tung H, Giannotta SL, Chandrasoma PT, Zee CS. Recurrent intraparenchymal hemorrhages from angiographically occult vascular malformations. *J Neurosurg.* 1990;**73**(2):174–80.
111. Ueda S, Saito A, Inomori S, Kim I. Cavernous angioma of the cauda equina producing subarachnoid hemorrhage. Case report. *J Neurosurg.* 1987;**66**(1):134–6.
112. de Tribolet N, Kaech D, Perentes E. Cerebellar haematoma due to a cavernous angioma in a child. *Acta Neurochir* (Wien). 1982;**60**(1–2):37–43.
113. Stahl SM, Johnson KP, Malamud N. The clinical and pathological spectrum of brain-stem vascular malformations. Long-term course stimulates multiple sclerosis. *Arch Neurol.* 1980;**37**(1):25–9.
114. Symon L, Jackowski A, Bills D. Surgical treatment of pontomedullary cavernomas. *Br J Neurosurg.* 1991;**5**(4): 339–47.
115. Takahashi A, Kamiyama H, Abe H, *et al.* Cavernous angioma of the cerebellum and cerebellar atrophy – case report. *Neurol Med Chir* (Tokyo). 1992;**32**(10):762–4.
116. Yoshimoto T, Suzuki J. Radical surgery on cavernous angioma of the brainstem. *Surg Neurol.* 1986;**26**(1):72–8.
117. Ojemann RG, Crowell RM, Ogilvy CS. Management of cranial and spinal cavernous angiomas (honored guest lecture). *Clin Neurosurg.* 1993;**40**:98–123.
118. Gross BA, Batjer HH, Awad IA, Bendok BR. Cavernous malformations of the basal ganglia and thalamus. *Neurosurgery.* 2009;**65**(1):7–18; discussion 719.
119. Fahlbusch R, Strauss C, Huk W. Pontine-mesencephalic cavernomas: indications for surgery and operative results. *Acta Neurochir Suppl* (Wien). 1991;**53**:37–41.
120. Gross BA, Batjer HH, Awad IA, Bendok BR. Brainstem cavernous malformations. *Neurosurgery.* 2009;**64**(5): E805–18; discussion E18.
121. LeDoux MS, Aronin PA, Odrezin GT. Surgically treated cavernous angiomas of the brain stem: report of two cases and review of the literature. *Surg Neurol.* 1991;**35**(5): 395–9.
122. Cascino GD, Kelly PJ, Sharbrough FW, *et al.* Long-term follow-up of stereotactic lesionectomy in partial epilepsy: predictive factors and electroencephalographic results. *Epilepsia.* 1992;**33**(4):639–44.
123. Awad IA, Rosenfeld J, Ahl J, Hahn JF, Luders H. Intractable epilepsy and structural lesions of the brain: mapping, resection strategies, and seizure outcome. *Epilepsia.* 1991;**32**(2):179–86.
124. Jooma R, Yeh HS, Privitera MD, Gartner M. Lesionectomy versus electrophysiologically guided resection for temporal lobe tumors manifesting with complex partial seizures. *J Neurosurg.* 1995;**83**(2):231–6.
125. Moore JL, Jr. Open and closed heart massage. *J Med Assoc Ga.* 1962;**51**:239.
126. Bengzon AR, Rasmussen T, Gloor P, Dussault J, Stephens M. Prognostic factors in the surgical treatment of temporal lobe epileptics. *Neurology.* 1968;**18**(8):717–31.
127. Dodrill CB, Wilkus RJ, Ojemann GA, *et al.* Multidisciplinary prediction of seizure relief from cortical resection surgery. *Ann Neurol.* 1986;**20**(1):2–12.
128. Britton JW, Cascino GD, Sharbrough FW, Kelly PJ. Low-grade glial neoplasms and intractable partial epilepsy: efficacy of surgical treatment. *Epilepsia.* 1994;**35** (6):1130–5.
129. Spencer DD, Spencer SS, Mattson RH, Williamson PD. Intracerebral masses in patients with intractable partial epilepsy. *Neurology.* 1984;**34**(4):432–6.
130. Cappabianca P, Alfieri A, Maiuri F, *et al.* Supratentorial cavernous malformations and epilepsy: seizure outcome after lesionectomy on a series of 35 patients. *Clin Neurol Neurosurg.* 1997;**99**(3):179–83.
131. Cohen DS, Zubay GP, Goodman RR. Seizure outcome after lesionectomy for cavernous malformations. *J Neurosurg.* 1995;**83**(2):237–42.
132. Packer RJ, Sutton LN, Patel KM, *et al.* Seizure control following tumor surgery for childhood cortical low-grade gliomas. *J Neurosurg.* 1994;**80**(6):998–1003.
133. Rassi-Neto A, Ferraz FP, Campos CR, Braga FM. Patients with epileptic seizures and cerebral lesions who underwent lesionectomy restricted to or associated with the adjacent irritative area. *Epilepsia.* 1999;**40**(7):856–64.
134. Rossi GF, Pompucci A, Colicchio G, Scerrati M. Factors of surgical outcome in tumoural epilepsy. *Acta Neurochir* (Wien). 1999;**141**(8):819–24.

135. Yeh HS, Tew JM, Jr., Gartner M. Seizure control after surgery on cerebral arteriovenous malformations. *J Neurosurg.* 1993;**78**(1):12–18.
136. Zevgaridis D, van Velthoven V, Ebeling U, Reulen HJ. Seizure control following surgery in supratentorial cavernous malformations: a retrospective study in 77 patients. *Acta Neurochir* (Wien). 1996;**138**(6):672–7.
137. Dorsch NWC, McMahon JHA. Intracranial cavernous malformations-natural history and management. *Crit Rev Neurosurg.* 1998;**8**(3):154–68.
138. Siegel AM, Roberts DW, Harbaugh RE, Williamson PD. Pure lesionectomy versus tailored epilepsy surgery in treatment of cavernous malformations presenting with epilepsy. *Neurosurg Rev.* 2000;**23**(2):80–3.
139. Stefan H, Hammen T. Cavernous haemangiomas, epilepsy and treatment strategies. *Acta Neurol Scand.* 2004;**110**(6):393–7.
140. Gumprecht H, Ebel GK, Auer DP, Lumenta CB. Neuronavigation and functional MRI for surgery in patients with lesion in eloquent brain areas. *Minim Invasive Neurosurg.* 2002;**45**(3):151–3.
141. Winkler D, Lindner D, Strauss G, *et al.* Surgery of cavernous malformations with and without navigational support – a comparative study. *Minim Invasive Neurosurg.* 2006;**49**(1):15–19.
142. Zhou H, Miller D, Schulte DM, *et al.* Transsulcal approach supported by navigation-guided neurophysiological monitoring for resection of paracentral cavernomas. *Clin Neurol Neurosurg.* 2009;**111**(1):69–78.
143. Gralla J, Ganslandt O, Kober H, *et al.* Image-guided removal of supratentorial cavernomas in critical brain areas: application of neuronavigation and intraoperative magnetic resonance imaging. *Minim Invasive Neurosurg.* 2003;**46**(2):72–7.
144. Biller J, Toffol GJ, Shea JF, Fine M, Azar-Kia B. Cerebellar venous angiomas. A continuing controversy. *Arch Neurol.* 1985;**42**(4):367–70.
145. Porter RW, Detwiler PW, Spetzler RF, *et al.* Cavernous malformations of the brainstem: experience with 100 patients. *J Neurosurg.* 1999;**90**(1):50–8.
146. Rigamonti D, Spetzler RF. The association of venous and cavernous malformations. Report of four cases and discussion of the pathophysiological, diagnostic, and therapeutic implications. *Acta Neurochir* (Wien). 1988;**92**(1–4):100–5.
147. Alexander E, 3rd, Loeffler JS. Radiosurgery for intracranial vascular malformations: techniques, results, and complications. *Clin Neurosurg.* 1992;**39**:273–91.
148. Ogilvy CS, Heros RC, Ojemann RG, New PF. Angiographically occult arteriovenous malformations. *J Neurosurg.* 1988;**69**(3):350–5.
149. Coffey RJ, Lunsford LD, Bissonette D, Flickinger JC. Stereotactic gamma radiosurgery for intracranial vascular malformations and tumors: report of the initial North American experience in 331 patients. *Stereotact Funct Neurosurg.* 1990;**54–55**:535–40.
150. Steiner L LL, Forster D, Backlund E-O. *Radiosurgery: baseline and trends.* New York, Raven Press;1991.
151. Lunsford LD, Kondziolka D, Bissonette DJ, Maitz AH, Flickinger JC. Stereotactic radiosurgery of brain vascular malformations. *Neurosurg Clin N Am.* 1992;**3**(1): 79–98.
152. Lunsford LD, Kondziolka D, Flickinger JC. Stereotactic radiosurgery: current spectrum and results. *Clin Neurosurg.* 1992;**38**:405–44.
153. Pham M, Gross BA, Bendok BR, Awad IA, Batjer HH. Radiosurgery for angiographically occult vascular malformations. *Neurosurg Focus.* 2009;**26**(5):E16.

SECTION 6

Critical Care of Subarachnoid Hemorrhage

Medical interventions for subarachnoid hemorrhage

Joji B. Kuramatsu and Hagen B. Huttner

Medical management of SAH

Introduction

Subarachnoid hemorrhage (SAH) is a devastating neurovascular disease entity and accounts for 5% of all stroke sup-types, with case fatality rates as high as 50% including those 10–15% of patients that die before reaching the hospital, striking at a fairly young age and leaving those who survive in almost half of the cases severely disabled [1–3]. Therefore, a conjunct effort of a multidisciplinary team is needed to provide optimal care, preferably at high-volume centers. The team should consist of neuro-intensivists, neuro-interventionalists, neurosurgeons, and specialized nursing staff and health therapists, to anticipate, recognize, and promptly treat and manage the frequent neurological and systemic complications of SAH [3–5]. The general approach for the management of SAH seems intuitively simple: 'make the diagnosis, and occlude the aneurysm'. But still, one sees relatively high death rates even though there have been notable advances in treatment. The overall case fatality rate has decreased by 17% over the last three decades, coinciding with the implementation of improved management strategies [1,5,6].

Epidemiology

Epidemiological multinational studies documented a variation in age-adjusted annual incidence rates for different ethnic populations from 'Finland to China' ranging from 2 to 23 cases per 100 000, and these rates have not changed dramatically over the past decades [1,3,7,8]. Generally, all age groups are affected by SAH, but it most commonly affects patients between 40 and 60 years of age and occurs in women 1.6 times more frequently than in men [1,5,8–10]. Also temporal factors might contribute to SAH incidence, occurring more often in winter and spring, as well as more often early in the morning [1,8].

Pathogenesis

The major cause of SAH in 85% of all cases is a ruptured saccular aneurysm, versus other causes like non-aneurysmal peri-mesencephalic hemorrhage accounting for 10% of cases, and about 5% of other rare causes [9–12] (see Table 29.1). Most aneurysms are developing at branching sites of intracerebral arteries at the base of the brain, such as the circle of Willis and nearby locations. The most common aneurysm location with 40–45% is at the branching site of the anterior communicating artery, followed by 10–15% at the bifurcation of the medial cerebral artery, then internal carotid artery 10–15%, and with approximately 5% at the basilary artery [10,12,13]. The majority of aneurysms will never rupture, but risk of rupture increases with size. Interestingly, those which do rupture are small in diameter (Ø < 12 mm), probably due to the great proportion of small aneurysms in general [2,9,11]. The hemorrhage spreads through the subarachnoid space, along the

Critical Care of the Stroke Patient, ed. Stefan Schwab, Daniel Hanley, and A. David Mendelow. Published by Cambridge University Press.

Table 29.1 Rare causes of SAH

Congenital syndromes	Non-inflammatory lesions of intracerebral vessels
- Familial intracranial aneurysms	- Arterial dissection
- Ehlers-Danlos syndrome type IV	- Cerebral arteriovenous malformations
- Autosomal dominant polycystic kidney disease	- Fusiform aneurysms
- α1-antitrypsin deficiency	- Cerebral dural arteriovenous fistulae
- Infantile fibromuscular dysplasia	- Cerebral venous thrombosis
- Parry-Romberg disease	- Cerebral amyloid angiopathy
- Neurofibromatosis	- Moyamoya disease
- Marfan syndrome	- Vascular lesions in the spinal cord
	- Saccular aneurysm of spinal artery
Inflammatory lesions of cerebral arteries	- Spinal arteriovenous fistula or malformation
	- Cavernous angioma at spinal level
- Mycotic aneurysms	
- Borreliosis	**Tumors**
- Behçet's disease	
- Primary angiitis	- Cerebral metastases
- Polyarteritis nodosa	- Malignant glioma
- Churg-Strauss syndrome	- Acoustic neuroma
- Wegener's granulomatosis	- Angiolipoma
	- Schwannoma of cranial nerve
Hematologic diseases	- Cervical spinal cord hemangioblastoma
	Drugs
- Sickle cell disease	
- Coagulopathies	
- Myeloproliferative	- Cocaine abuse
- Leukemia	- Anticoagulant drugs
	- Phenylpropanolamine
Trauma	- Ethanol
	- Lead
- Traumatic brain injury	
- Strangulation	
- Barotraumas	
- Altitude sickness	

intracranial arteries and disperses often in a typical fashion within the basal cisterns, the sylvian fissures, and the interhemispheric fissure (Fig. 29.1). Blood itself can ascend retrograde or even break into the ventricular system, leading to an increased risk of developing an acute occlusive hydrocephalus, or it can lead to an intraparenchymal hematoma with a consecutive mass effect [11–14].

The pathophysiological mechanisms of aneurysm rupture are still not fully understood. Multivariate models have revealed hypertension, smoking, and alcohol abuse to be independent risk factors, all of which roughly double the risk of SAH [8,15,16]. Therefore, the formation of saccular aneurysms is supposed to develop during life, and is not primarily a congenital disorder as still described in some textbooks. The general idea of aneurysm development is a structural weakness or defect of the external muscular layer of arteries [8–10,15]. Especially, intracerebral arteries are lacking the adventitia which could further promote structural weakness. High flow rates and high arterial pressure might as well contribute to aneurysm formation and a sudden increase in transmural pressure might lead to rupture of the weakened aneurysmatic arterial walls. In up to 20% of SAH patients, strenuous physical activity is reported before the occurrence of rupture, which might support this theory [8,9,15].

Peri-mesencephalic SAH is a rather harmless type of SAH and it is not associated with aneurysm rupture, instead it is supposed to be a venous hemorrhage [3,10]. This condition is defined by its characteristic distribution of blood which is dispersed anterior to the midbrain or pons with a normal angiographic study. Its onset is more gradual and complications like re-bleeding and delayed cerebral infarction are seldom appreciated.

For the prevention of SAH only cessation of smoking is indirectly associated with a risk reduction [8,15,16]. The relationship of hypertension and SAH remains uncertain, but treatment of hypertension is generally recommended for stroke patients. The cost-effectiveness of screening for unruptured aneurysms

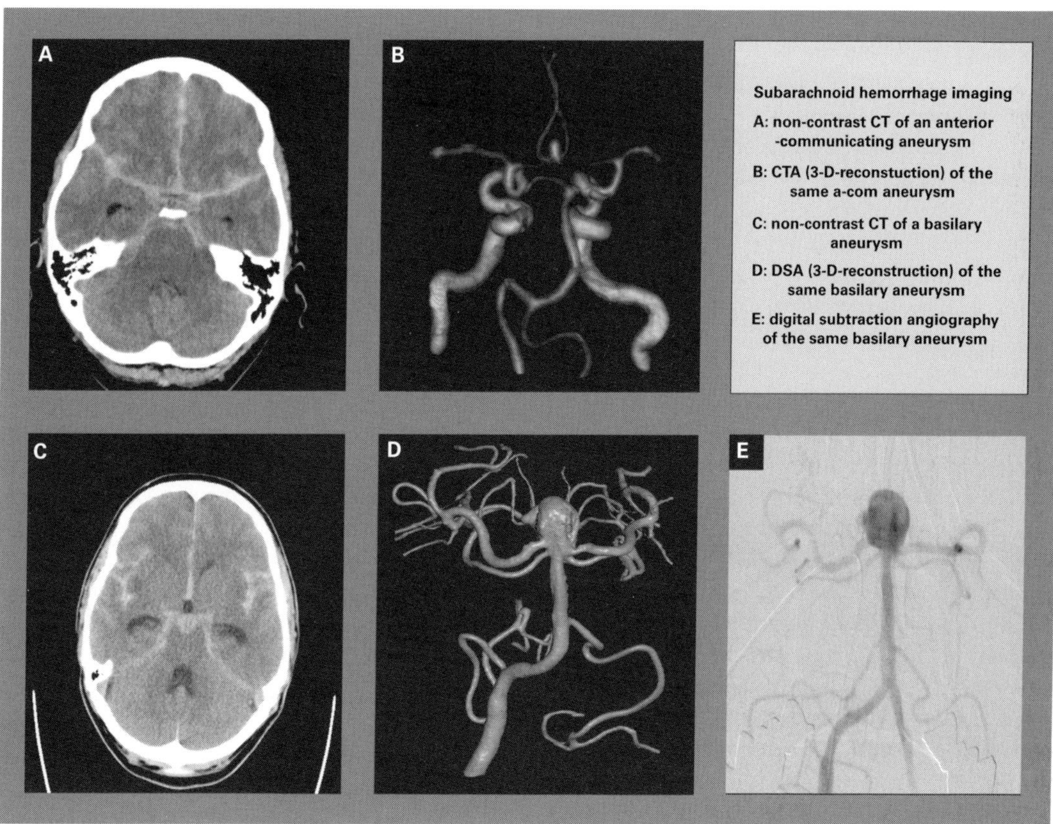

Fig. 29.1 CT/A and DSA imaging of two aneurysms. (See plate section for color version).

in certain high-risk populations still remains to be determined and should be made on an individual basis.

Prognosis

A historical population-based study estimated that of all SAH patients approximately 15% die before even reaching the hospital, and nearly half of all SAH patients die within 30 days, and of those who survive another half of the patients remains severely disabled; hence, only around one third of all SAH patients are able to resume previous daily activities or work [1–3,7,9]. Factors influencing outcome after SAH can be separated into (i) patient, (ii) aneurysm, and (iii) institutional factors. (i) Influential patient characteristics are: status on admission (grade), hemorrhage severity, age, sex, time to treatment, and general medical co-morbidities [7]. (ii) Aneurysm size, location (i.e. posterior circulation), and morphology are outcome-associated factors [17,18]. (iii) Institutional factors include the availability of endovascular services, the volume of SAH treated annually, and the type of facility where the patient is first evaluated [4,5]. The major outcome influencing parameter, however, is the effect of the hemorrhage itself [1,9,11].

In several systematic reviews and the largest randomized controlled trial (international subarachnoid aneurysm trial (ISAT)) there has been a reported decrease in mortality rates. The Cooperative Study on Intracranial Aneurysms in 1966 reported a 30-day mortality of 50%, in 1994 Broderick *et al.* reported in a population-based study a 30-day mortality of 45%, and recently Lovelock *et al.* reported a 50% decline in overall mortality rates, and the ISAT reported a 30-day mortality of only 12.9% [1,2,4,6,7,11]. Coinciding, rates of an unfavorable outcome are also declining, as reported by Langham *et al.* in 2009; still, 38.5% of patients at 6 months reach 5–8 points on the 8-point extended Glasgow outcome scale, documenting the severity of this disease [2,7]. In the future, with declining mortality rates we will have to take care of a growing burden of functionally dependent SAH survivors requiring specialized care [1,2,5].

Clinical presentation

In most cases of SAH the first patient encounter is out in the field by emergency services. It should be emphasized that if intracranial hemorrhage is suspected fast transportation, similarly to thrombolytic transport models, to high-volume centers is requisite [4,5]. Upon arrival in the emergency department rapid assessment of the patient is vital and has good prognostic power [5]. The two most commonly used grading scales are given in Table 29.2a.

Most SAH patients are asymptomatic before the 'classical' clinical presentation consisting of 'the worst headache in my life', a sudden onset of severe headache (74%), often accompanied by nausea and vomiting (77%), loss of consciousness (54%), and nuchal rigidity (35%) [12]. Therefore, on admission roughly two-thirds of SAH patients present with depressed consciousness and about half of those patients are comatose [5,9,12,19]. One out of five patients report retrospectively of having experienced sentinel headaches, which could be attributed to previous extravasation of blood, so called 'warning leaks' [3,9,19]. The timing of headache onset and brief loss of consciousness are important anamnestic features, because most patients seek medical advice only for the severity of the pain. The absence of neck stiffness cannot exclude the diagnosis of SAH, since it takes between 3 and 12 hours to develop and might not be appreciated in deeply comatose patients. Also possibly present are focal neurological deficits like cranial nerve palsies, especially the third cranial nerve being most commonly involved [12]. Extension of hemorrhage into the brain parenchyma or acute vasoconstriction after aneurysm rupture can also mimic ischemic stroke-like symptoms [10,11]. Further symptoms are seizures which are strong indicators for SAH when a patient with sudden 'thunderclap' headache presents to the ED [19,20].

Headache is a very common complaint in the ED, and 1% of all evaluated headaches accounts for SAH, therefore a high yield of suspicion should exist, which might be lifesaving [19]. Even with its classical presentation, SAH is still misdiagnosed commonly at a rate of 12%, because of individual patient characteristics, variable headache severity, and inconsistent findings such as focal neurological deficits [5,10,19]. Of those patients being misdiagnosed, there is a four-fold higher likelihood of death or disability at 1 year [10,19]. In the course of SAH management, fundoscopy should be performed, since one out of seven patients experiences intraocular hemorrhage, mostly subhyloid linear bleeds with extensions into the vitreous body, the so-called Terson's syndrome [21]. Moreover, features of systemic disease like hypertension, hypoxemia, and ECG abnormalities can be mistaken as acute myocardial infarction leading to an erroneous diagnostic work up.

Diagnosis

CT and CTA

The first and essential diagnostic tool for the evaluation of SAH is getting a non-contrast CT. Sensitivity and specificity are high and it can be rapidly done even in severely compromised patients without much effort and delay. The diagnostic sensitivity depends on the amount of blood, resolution of the scanner, skill of the radiologist, and importantly on timing of ictus versus scanning [3,18,22,23]. It is highest in the first 12 hours with 98–100%, and declines to 93% at 24 hours, and rapidly declines further after the following days, which warrants early imaging [22–24]. A typical pattern of blood dispersal often gives initial hints to the localization of the ruptured aneurysm, and the amount of blood is predictive for delayed infarctions [18,22]. Various grading systems exist, though the modified Fisher grading score is widely used and easily applied, which scores not only cisternal blood but also includes

Table 29.2a Clinical grading scales for patients presenting with SAH

Grade	Hunt and Hess	WFNS
I	asymptomatic, or mild headache	GCS of 15, absent motor deficit
II	moderate-severe headache, nuchal rigidity, no deficit other than cranial nerve palsy	GCS of 13–14, absent motor deficit
III	alteration in mental status (confusion, lethargy), mild focal neurological deficits	GCS of 13–14, present motor deficit
IV	stupor, severe focal neurological deficits (hemiparesis), vegetative disturbances	GCS of 7–12, present or absent motor deficit
V	comatose, decerebrate rigidity, moribund patient	GCS of 3–6, present or absent motor deficit

(WFNS = World Federation of Neurological Surgeons; GCS = Glasgow Coma Scale)

Table 29.2b Fisher grading score and modified Fisher grading score and proposed risk of DCI

Grade	Fisher grading score	Modified Fisher grading score	DCI risk
0		no SAH or IVH	minimal
1	no blood detected	minimum/thin SAH, no IVH in both lateral ventricles	low risk
2	diffuse, thin SAH, no clot > 1 mm in thickness	minimum/thin SAH, with IVH in both lateral ventricles	intermediate
3	localized thick layer of SAH, clot > 1 mm in thickness	thick SAH, no IVH in both ventricles	intermediate
4	predominant IVH or ICH with diffuse or no SAH	thick SAH, with IVH in both ventricles	high risk

(DCI = Delayed Cerebral Ischemia; IVH = Intraventricular Hemorrhage; ICH = Intracerebral Hemorrhage)

intraventricular extensions and has predictive power for delayed cerebral infarction (see Table 29.2b) [22,23].

CT angiography (CTA) is a steadily improving technique which is fast and readily available, and it is suitable for the critical patient for rapid diagnosis and treatment planning. Digital subtraction angiography (DSA) still remains the 'gold standard', but diagnostic sensitivity of CTA for aneurysms larger than 4 mm, in centers with neuroradiological expertise, equals that of DSA [18,23]. Recently a meta-analysis documented an overall sensitivity of only 93% for CT angiography, possibly due to inclusion of many early studies with limited CTA experience [18]. Further, it has been reported that in 74% of cases when DSA was performed after CTA, DSA did not provide any further information [3,6,23]. Due to quick and less expensive data assessment, with more complete anatomical detail, such as adjacent vessels, bony structures, atheromas, and neck-dome relationship, it becomes increasingly helpful in the assessment of treatment planning; 'coiling *versus* operation'. Therefore, when indicated, many neurosurgeons today operate solely by three-dimensional reconstruction images of SAH patients when a delay of surgery is not justified. CTA imaging techniques are evolving, its widespread availability and rapid imaging acquisition will increasingly supplement or maybe replace conventional angiography in the emergency setting, for decision making and for preoperative evaluation [6,18,23].

Regarding the development of vasospasm, CT angiography and perfusion studies are increasingly used with good correlations to conventional catheter studies. Initial baseline CTA in comparison with follow-up imaging provides useful information for the assessment of vessel diameter changes [17,22,23]. CT perfusion imaging evaluates actual brain perfusion, its measures can be quantified and it can detect ischemia without angiographic vasospasms. The mean transit time (MTT > 6.5 s) was reported to be a sensitive parameter with a negative predictive value of 98.7%, as well as another study which reported delayed time-to-peak measurements as most reliable for the diagnosis of vasospasms [17,23,25]. Disadvantages of CT imaging are radiation exposure and contrast nephropathy limiting its repeated use.

MRI and MRA

The use of MRI/MRA in the diagnosis of SAH is evolving, but often limited in the emergency setting, due to availability, logistics, patient compliance of the acutely ill, longer study time, and cost. MRI with proton density and *flair* imaging is comparably sensitive to CT scanning [26]. MRA can be a valuable diagnostic tool for the etiologic evaluation of the hemorrhage, and for the detection of delayed cerebral infarction with diffusion- and perfusion-weighted imaging, as well as in special situations such as pregnancy.

Lumbar puncture

For an accurate diagnostic work-up in the small minority of patients with a negative CT scan, lumbar puncture is essential [3,9,19,24]. When a decision for lumbar puncture is made, timing is detrimental since blood-tinged CSF obtained within 0–12 hours after ictus will be indistinguishable from a traumatic tap versus genuine subarachnoid hemorrhage [10,19,24,27]. Cerebrospinal fluid (CSF) samples need to be spun down immediately, to detect true xanthochromia, and should be stored in darkness to avoid UV-light breakdown of bilirubin. For the formal diagnosis of SAH by lumbar puncture wait at least 6 hours, but preferably 12 hours to detect bilirubin which can only be formed in vivo, and if the time interval is longer search for erythrophages which can be detected up to months after SAH [10,19,27]. To exclude other differential diagnosis if CSF is clear, measurement of opening pressure can be helpful to establish a diagnosis of central vein thrombosis, and CSF culture and antibody indexes are important if infections are in the differential diagnosis [10,19,27].

Digital subtraction angiography

Conventional angiography is still the 'gold standard' for the detection of ruptured aneurysms in SAH [3,5,9,18]. The reported sensitivity is currently around 95%, and three-dimensional reconstructions allow optimal depiction of neck-dome relationships, precise anatomical configurations, and the proximity of adjacent vessels for treatment planning of coiling vs. clipping [18,28]. Angiography is a rather complex and invasive procedure with associated complications like peri-procedural ischemia in 1.8%, and re-rupture of aneurysms in 1–2% of cases [18,28]. In approximately one out of five patients aneurysms will not be detected as the bleeding source, and repeat angiography will reveal the bleeding source in only 1–2% of cases. Therefore repeat angiography in aneurysm-negative patients is controversial; however, it should at least be performed in those 'initially non-aneurysmal SAH' patients who require an external ventricular drain because of occlusive hydrocephalus [3,18].

Complications

Clinical problems arising after SAH can be divided into acute and delayed complications. Various pathophysiological mechanisms have been postulated to cause acute and delayed brain injury. *Reduction in cerebral blood flow* (CBF), caused by the mass effect of the hemorrhage, is the major determinant when considering acute effects of SAH [9,11,13,29]. Reductions in CBF are caused by the global impact of the hematoma, by impaired cerebral autoregulation and by acute ischemia. Responsible for these processes are raised intracranial pressure (ICP) and consecutively decreased cerebral perfusion pressure (CPP) [3,11,13,29].

Recurrent hemorrhage is one of the most serious but treatable and avoidable complications with a reported case fatality rate of 70% [11]. Re-bleeding in general has been described to occur at a rate of 4% on the first day after SAH, and then ranges between 1% and 2% for each consecutive day [11]. Without treatment the risk of re-bleeding has been described to be between 20% and 30%, and stabilizes after a year at 3% per year [5]. Another study stated, after surviving this early 24 hours time window, the cumulative re-bleeding risk is around 40% over the next 4 weeks without intervention [3,5]. Most early re-bleedings occur within the first 24 hours, and 13.6% of re-bleedings peak at 2 hours after the initial ictus [3,5]. Other authors reported that all re-hemorrhages occurred within the first 12 hours, emphasizing the rapid temporal manner of SAH growth [3,23,30].

Further acute complications are *extensions of the hematoma into the ventricular system* possibly leading to an acute hydrocephalus, prompting immediate surgery with placement of an external ventricular drainage. One out of five of SAH patients will show a dilated ventricular system on initial imaging – and in respect to the level of consciousness – this should emphasize a primary operative approach of EVD placement and secondary decision making of how to occlude the aneurysm [23,28]. Moreover, involvement of brain parenchyma or subdural space may also require surgery with trepanation or craniectomy for decompression [9,11].

There are several different complications alongside the course of SAH. *Delayed cerebral infarction (DCI)* is one feared complication leading to a decrease in functional outcome [12,13,17,22]. Historically it was presumed that DCI was caused by vasospasms of proximal cerebral vessels that were occurring at day three through seven, which is coherent with the occurrence of ischemic lesions [13,22]. Although vasospasms are detectable in about 60% of SAH patients, only half of them become symptomatic [13,23]. Therefore, several other mechanisms have been postulated to influence and possibly cause DCI. Exposure of endothelial antigens with a consecutive inflammatory reaction caused by leukocyte–endothelial cell interactions after rupture may propagate mechanisms leading to microthrombosis and disturbances of perfusion and permeability of the microvasculature [31]. After lysis of erythrocytes, vasogenic substances are released that might contribute to an altered vascular reactivity, such as calcium, potassium, and magnesium as well as hemoglobin as NO-scavenger [31]. Recently a novel mechanism of delayed ischemic neurological deficits has been described, by the COSBID research group, who postulated that recurrent spreading depolarizations may be responsible for ischemic events in the brain [32]. A propagating wave of mass neuronal depolarization is presumed to be associated with dysfunctional ion channels inducing alterations in vessel resistance leading to hypoxia and ischemia, especially in metabolically disturbed neuronal tissue [32]. Currently, expert opinion considers DCI development to be a multifactorial process rather than solely caused by vasospasms [32].

In the course of SAH electrolyte disturbances are commonly appreciated, with *hyponatremia* and *hypomagnesemia* being the most frequent alterations, possibly promoting vasospasms and delayed cerebral ischemia [29,33,34]. Hyponatremia caused by either cerebral salt wasting syndrome or the syndrome of inappropriate secretion of antidiuretic hormone (SIADH) due to excessive natriuesis with subsequent volume contraction is potentially promoting vasospasms [29,33]. Magnesium is supposed to have vasodilator and neuroprotective properties which in turn might lead to DCI and poor outcome at 3 months in a state of hypomagnesemia [29,34].

Another delayed complication in more than 20% of SAH patients might be the development of a *communicating hydrocephalus* caused by inflammation of the Paccioni granulations with resulting impaired CSF absorption necessitating permanent ventriculo-peritoneal shunt placement [14].

Further systemic complications are the development of *neurogenic pulmonary edema, cardiac complications like arrhythmias, infarction and takostubo cardiomyopathy*, and more general issues like infections and fever and blood glucose control [5,10,29]. More long-term sequelae are the development of post-stroke epilepsia possibly caused by cortical involvement, *anosmia* more often appreciated after surgical clipping of a-com aneurysms, and cognitive and psychosocial dysfunction should not be underestimated [5,10,20].

Medical management

ED management

An overview of the proposed diagnostic and treatment pathway is given in Figure 29.2. First of all, stabilization of the patient in the ED is essential: check airway, breathing, and circulation. Most SAH patients initially do not present as severely compromised, but airway surveillance and continuous oxymetrie is paramount. If necessary, intubation should not be delayed and should be performed according to protocols, meticulously avoiding hypoperfusion. Continuous ECG monitoring and blood pressure (BP) monitoring at short

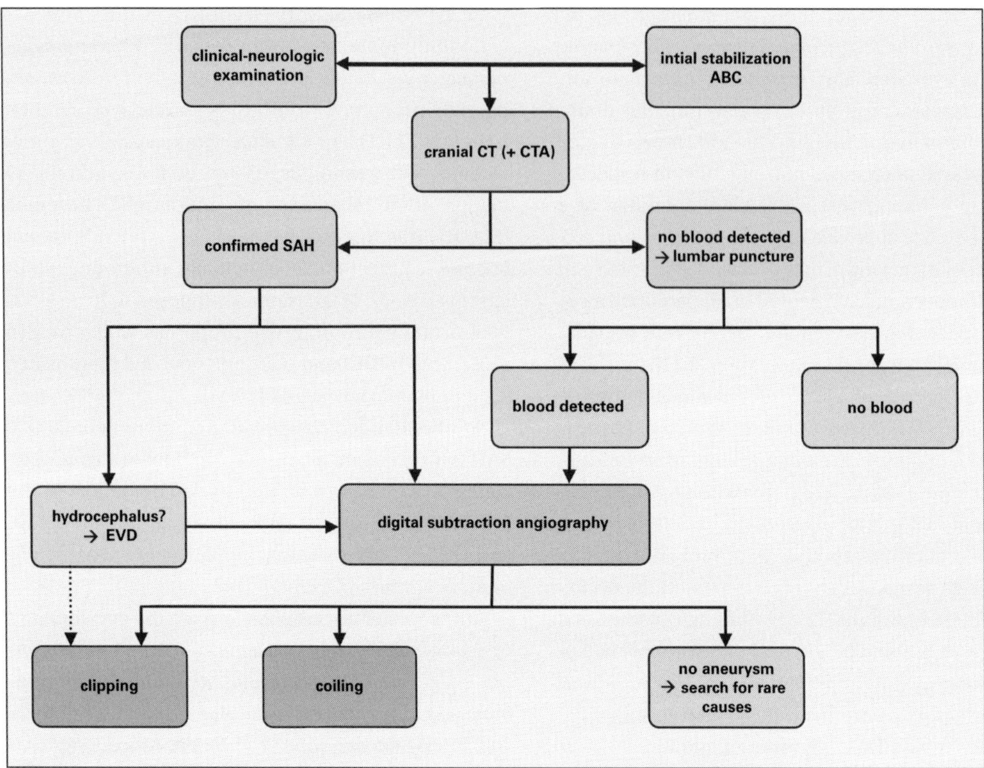

Fig. 29.2 Diagnostic and treatment pathway.

intervals for the surveillance of dysrhythmias and signs of neurogenic cardiopulmonary disturbances should be conducted, or if possible in a timely fashion an arterial blood pressure catheter should be placed [5,9].

After initial stabilization of the patient, a rapid diagnosis should be obtained for adequate and fast triage to surgeons, either for EVD placement or surgical clipping, or to interventionalists for coil-embolization [4,5,28]. The prevention of re-bleeding is crucial and obviously the most effective treatment is the elimination of the bleeding source. Before aneurysm occlusion, the only measure proposed so far, which impacts re-bleeding rates, is the avoidance of excessive blood pressure surges. Therefore, systolic blood pressure (BP) should be kept below 160 mmHg, which is a widely used cut-off point [3,28]. Up to now, there is no direct evidence suggesting a certain BP range, but retrospective studies yielded evidence suggesting an increased re-bleeding rate at a systolic BP greater than 150–160 mmHg [3]. Interpretation of these studies is limited, though rapid occlusion of the aneurysm is the best choice for re-bleeding prevention. Treatment should be initiated with short-acting continuous infusion intravenous agents with a favorable safety profile. Labetalol, Nicardipin and Esmolol seem to meet these criteria [3]. Vice versa, especially in patients with an elevated ICP, it is prudent to avoid sudden drops in BP to reduce time periods of decreased CBF [3]. Sodium nitroprusside should be avoided due to its tendency to increase ICP. Antifibrinolytics have been investigated, and re-bleeding rates were reduced, but treated patients were significantly more likely to develop cerebral infarction, which counterbalanced this positive effect on outcome. Therefore, antifibrinolytics are not recommended in the treatment of SAH [3,5,9].

More general recommendations should include strict bed rest, consecutively bladder catheterization, nasogastric tube placement for the avoidance of aspiration, laxatives to avoid strain, and intravenous catheters should be placed. Pain management to reduce sympathetic activation should be carried out [5,9]. If swallowing is not compromised, oral medications should be started at regular intervals, avoid aspirin, and if pain relief is not sufficient perfusion pumps should be added, preferably using medications with analgesic and anxiolytic properties, i.e. midazolam. Sedating agents should be avoided in the awake patient [5,9]. The last resort should be opiates, but adequate fluid intake and stool softeners are necessary in these situations. Continuous clinical surveillance from trained personnel is mandatory, because sudden deterioration is almost exclusively associated with rehemorrhage or hydrocephalus. Checking at regular intervals for new focal neurological deficits, temperature, blood glucose, pupillary responses, and changes in vigilance is obligatory. Treatment of fever and hyperglycemia from the start cannot be overemphasized, since these are well-known negative outcome predictors in stroke patients [4,5,29].

ICU management

The main management issue to consider in SAH patients after aneurysm treatment is the prevention of delayed complications [5,9,29]. Delayed cerebral infarction is a great threat to poor functional outcome [9,17]. Standard neuro-ICU care and neuro-monitoring should be applied (see Table 29.3), with special focus on the frequent complications occurring after SAH; electrolyte disturbances, arrhythmias, cardiomyopathy, neurogenic pulmonary edema, seizures, and post-hemorrhagic hydrocephalus [3,5,9,29].

Vasospasm

Vasospasms of proximal cerebral arteries are thought to be associated with delayed cerebral infarctions. These observations were concluded by angiographic evidence of vasospasm starting to occur 2–3 days after the ictus and prevailing between 5 and 20 days [13,23,25]. The

Table 29.3 Neuromonitoring in SAH patients

Methods	Importance	Risks and complications
Mandatory surveillance		
Clinical monitoring		
Pupils	+++	operation, optical tract lesion
Brainstem reflexes	+++	-
Reaction to stimuli	++	sedation
General ICU monitoring		
ECG	++	none
Invasive BP	++	thrombosis
CVP	+	infection, hemorrhage
$FetCO_2$	+	none
SpO_2	++	centralization
Temperature	++	measuring site
Clinical chemistry		
Blood gas analysis	++	none
Glucose	+	none
Sodium	+	none
Osmolarity	+	none
ICP monitoring		
Ventricular	+++	infection, hemorrhage
Intraparenchymal	++	infection, drift, cost
Lumbar	++	experimental
Facultative surveillance		
TCD	+++	interpretation, examiner skill
Central-venous oximetry	+	puncture, infection
$ptiO_2$-probes	++	dislocation, placement
Microdialysis	++	infection, cost
Thermo-sensor	+	little experience
EEG	++	not specific
SEP	++	artifacts
BaEP	++	artifacts
NIRS	+	little experience

(ECG = electrocardiography; BP = blood pressure; CVP = central venous pressure; $FetCO_2$ = end-tidal CO_2 fraction; SpO_2 = peripheral oxygen saturation; TCD = transcranial Doppler; $ptiO_2$ = brain tissue oxygen; EEG = electroencephalography; SEP = somatosensory evoked potential; BaEP = brainstem auditory evoked potential; NIRS = near infrared spectroscopy) onset of vasospasms is variable, from sudden to gradual, but there is an increased tendency to develop in poor grade patients, with thick arachnoid blood clots, intraventricular hemorrhage, and with a history of smoking [3,13,23,25,35]. The definition of a symptomatic vasospasm is the occurrence of a new focal neurological deficit with an according perfusion deficit. Studies on ultrasound flow velocities revealed increases in velocity that were coinciding with new neurological deficits, but the reported sensitivity and specificity range between 70 and 80%, and approximately only half of these patients actually develop DCI, which has led to some controversy regarding its use in SAH patients [36]. Beyond these aspects, ultrasonography is greatly operator dependent, and its use is often limited in older women with poor temporal ultrasonographic windows. The Lindegaard ratio has been shown to be helpful in the estimation of vasospasms, with ratios greater than 5–6 indicating severe spasms and greatest reliability for MCA vasospasms [37]. Even with its disadvantages, ultrasonography is a widely used and accepted method for screening and monitoring vasospasms, because its strengths are low cost, non-invasiveness, it can be done at bedside, and it has a good correlation with catheter angiography. Also, testing of vasomotor reactivity can be undertaken and most importantly it can be used daily to follow trends [36]. Catheter angiography is the most sensitive tool for vasospasm detection and its ability to directly undertake endovascular manoeuvres is a major advantage. It plays an important role in patients' refractory to medical treatment with good short-term clinical response rates [4]. The role of prophylactic balloon angioplasty still remains to be determined especially in poor grade patients. In a recent publication patients were randomly assigned to treatment, but there was no significant difference in vasospasm protection, outcome measures were equal in both arms and one important clinical aspect was the risk of vessel perforation, which was between 3 and 5% [4]. This risk seems too high to employ this strategy in good grade patients with a decreased risk of vasospasm development, but in poor grade patients this strategy might be beneficial, which has to be investigated. The evidence for intra-arterial application of vasodilators, such as papaverine, is inconclusive and cannot be recommended [9, 25].

Triple-H-therapy

Hemodynamic augmentation or historically called 'triple-H-therapy', since its introduction has been the mainstay of vasospasms treatment [3,5,38]. The objective was to improve cerebral perfusion by means of overcoming the increased vascular resistance induced by vessel narrowing, through induced hypervolemia, hypertension and hemodilution. However, evidence from randomized control trials is lacking, and more recently its components have been studied more rigorously, which has led to increased controversy. The only evidence for a net benefit exists for the induction of hypertension, which has been documented in several studies to increase cerebral blood flow and oxygenation [3,5,38]. The goal of this therapy is a systolic BP between 160 and 180 mmHg or an approximate mean arterial pressure of 110 mmHg and above [3,5]. Medications studied and recommended for this use are dopamine, dobutamine, milrinone, and norepinephrine. Vasopressin should be avoided, due to its potential of exacerbating hyponatremia.

Hemodilution with a target hematocrit of 30% is supposed to decrease viscosity, which is now less commonly used because of lacking evidence to actually improve oxygenation. This seems plausible with a reduction of the oxygen carrying capacity which consecutively compromises oxygen delivery to the brain, and therefore cannot be recommended for routine use any more [3–5,29]. In addition, more recently studies have revealed anemia to be a negative predictor for good outcome in patients with intracranial hemorrhage, but on the other hand aggressive transfusion strategies may contribute to a higher mortality rate, therefore should not be recommended [4,29,38].

Hyperdynamic therapy with induced hypertension and hypervolemia has led to positive results in some studies regarding an increased CBF [3,38]. The major issue when considering hypervolemic therapy is the initial volume status of the patient. There might be a true benefit of this therapy in euvolemic patients, but there is an increased risk of complications in volume expanded patients [9]. Encountered problems with fluid overload are the development of mostly pulmonary edema, brain edema, hemorrhagic diathesis due to relatively decreased clotting factors, and cardiac complications such as infarction and arrhythmias [38]. Aggressive treatment of cardiopulmonary complications with diuretics or vasodilators should be avoided, due to an increased risk of hypoperfusion with consecutive secondary brain injury [3,38].

Nimodipine

Originally introduced as a specific agent against vasospasms, the Ca-channel blocker nimodipine gained recognition as an outcome influencing parameter in prospective randomized studies, positively impacting functional outcome and morbidity [3,10]. Currently, nimodipine is considered a neuroprotective agent rather than a causal anti-vasospastic agent, though its precise mechanisms are unclear. Through available data the beneficial effects of oral nimodipine have been documented, and therefore are highly recommended in the routine of SAH therapy [3,9,39]. Advocated dosing is 60 mg six times a day taken orally for 20 days, data for intravenous administration are less conclusive with a reported decrease of vasospasm but without a reported outcome benefit [3,9,39]. Complications of this therapy are lowering of blood pressure, which should be strictly avoided and aggressively treated, and the development of pulmonary shunting with rapid decreases of arterial oxygen partial pressure, and further the occurrence of GI-tract complications such as subileus [3,39].

'Salt wasting' and hypertonic saline

The management of the volume status can be a challenging task after SAH, with electrolyte disturbances being commonly appreciated with increased natriuresis [29,33,38]. In the ICU setting adequate volume monitoring should be mandatory especially for poor grade patients, preferentially with central lines and continuous central venous pressure measurements, aiming at a CVP between 8 and 12 mmHg. Hyponatremia and volume contraction is a frequently encountered problem in SAH patients, occurring with a reported rate between 10 and 30%, most often asymptomatic, but being associated with vasospasms and delayed cerebral infarction as well as being associated with seizures, triggered by a rapid sodium decline. The mainstay of therapy is salt and fluid replacement, with hypertonic saline solutions (1.5% or 3%) solely or in combination with fludrocortisone being useful treatment options [3,33,38]. Hypernatremia is reported to be independently associated with a poor prognosis after SAH and therefore should be avoided [33].

General considerations

Fever management and blood glucose control are prerequisite in ICU patients. Body temperature should be measured at frequent intervals, and fever must be distinguished from infectious origins requiring adequate antibiotic treatment, versus central fever which is associated with a persistently increasing body temperature rather than spikes [4,9].

Infection prevention, especially hospital-acquired infections, has recently gained an increased focus in stroke patients. Selective digestive tract decontamination (SDD) and selective oropharyngeal decontamination (SOD) versus standard care has been investigated in a large randomized trial in critically ill patients [40]. Results were a significant reduction in mortality by both measures, indicating a transferable benefit to critically ill stroke patients. In respect of these special environments with a high prevalence of multi-drug-resistant colonization, SOD with the use of topical oral agents exclusively might be the better choice for the long-term prevention of resistant organisms, instead of intravenous antibiotics used in SDD [41].

Recently, a 6000 patient trial (NICE-SUGAR) documented a higher mortality with a strict glycemic control regimen of 80–110 mg/dl compared with a more liberal glucose target of below 180 mg/dl in ICU patients [42]. Further, a different study stated an association of sudden hypoglycemic drops with intensive insulin therapy, possibly causing brain energy metabolic crisis, which has been linked to poor outcome in brain-injured patients. Therefore, a more liberal glucose management regime of 120–180 mg/dl should be recommended [42].

Neurogenic pulmonary edema tends to develop early in the course after SAH, often in a rapid fashion. Although rare it is potentially life threatening and is more common in poor grade patients. It may be caused by a surge of catecholamines after cerebral injury leading to alterations of vascular permeability and hydrostatic changes with consequent pulmonary edema. On initial imaging edema might be massive but it responds well to high levels of positive end-expiratory pressures and diuretics. PiCCO-catheter monitoring can be very helpful in these situations [29].

Another general ICU problem is ventilator weaning in neurological patients. In a recent investigation prolonged mechanical ventilation was associated with diaphragmatic atrophy, which might contribute to weaning failure. Therefore, daily spontaneous breathing trials might prevent accelerated atrophy in these patients [43].

The frequency of seizures has been reported at a rate of 6–18% after SAH [3]. Risk factors for the development have been reported in retrospective studies, which are MCA aneurysms, intraparenchymal hematoma, and infarction. Data on prophylactic or long-term anti-epileptic treatment are inconclusive, demanding further investigations, and therefore treatment should be based on individual characteristics of the patients [20].

Finally, post-hemorrhagic hydrocephalus is reported to occur in 18–26% of surviving patients, and it is associated with older age, poor grade, intraventricular hemorrhage, early ventriculomegaly and female sex. Patients suffering from post-hemorrhagic hydrocephalus require permanent shunt placement, like ventriculo-atrial, ventriculo-peritoneal, and lumbo-peritoneal shunting, to improve clinical status [14].

Novel strategies

Endothelin antagonists: clazosentan

The system of endothelin-1 with its activation of the endothelin 1A receptor seems to play a major role in vasoconstriction of cerebral arteries, possibly through nuclear transduction pathways. Clazosentan, an endothelin-receptor antagonist, has been investigated in the double-blind CONCIOUS-trial (Clazosentan to Overcome Neurological Ischemia and Infarction Occuring After SAH). Clazosentan was able to reduce moderate to severe vasospasms in a dose-dependent manner, but was not able to influence outcome positively. Only post-hoc analysis revealed a trend towards a better outcome, therefore yielding inconclusive data. Thereafter, two phase III studies were initiated for clipped and coiled SAH patients (CONCIOUS 2 and 3). Overall, in both trials functional outcome was not significantly influenced by clazosentan treatment, even though for coiled SAH patients an influence on vasospasm-related morbidity and all-cause mortality was documented with the highest treatment dose [44,45].

Statins

Different mechanisms for statins have been postulated to lead to pleiotropic alterations, such as the attenuation of oxygen-radicals, up-regulation of NO-synthase and amelioration of glutamate mediated toxicity [46]. Various randomized studies have investigated its effects in SAH patients with divergent results. Positive influences have been reported on sonographically-detected vasospasms, duration of impaired autoregulation, delayed ischemic deficits, and outcome. But a recent meta-analysis has reported no net benefit for statins in SAH patients [47]. Currently, there are a few ongoing RCTs investigating statin therapy in subarachnoid hemorrhage [48].

Magnesium sulfate

Magnesium with its proposed vasodilator properties has been investigated in animal studies showing potential positive influence on vasospasms and delayed ischemic deficits. Almost half of all SAH patients develop hypomagnesemia during the course [5]. The MASH (Magnesium in Subarachnoid Hemorrhage) study group has initially reported a reduction of delayed infarctions and a better functional outcome, although confidence intervals of these results were too wide. Nevertheless, these promising findings have been counterbalanced by the recent results of the large MASH-II trial and further meta-analyses documenting no impact on outcome. Therefore, recommendations for the use of magnesium sulfate infusions cannot be made [49].

Albumin

Albumin has been used in SAH for hemodilution and volume expansion in triple-H-therapy. In one retrospective study albumin showed a trend towards a better 3-month functional outcome. A phase-II multi-center pilot trial has recently been completed and documented the safety of albumin treatment in SAH patients, but its influence on clinical end points will be determined in a randomized phase III trial; ALISAH (Treatment of SAH with Albumin) [50].

REFERENCES

1. Nieuwkamp, D. J., *et al.*, Changes in case fatality of aneurysmal subarachnoid haemorrhage over time, according to age, sex, and region: a meta-analysis. *Lancet Neurol*, 2009;**8**(7):635–42.
2. Lovelock, C. E., G. J. Rinkel, P. M. Rothwell, Time trends in outcome of subarachnoid hemorrhage: Population-based study and systematic review. *Neurology*, 2010;**74**(19):1494–501.
3. Connolly, E. S., Jr., *et al.*, Guidelines for the management of aneurysmal subarachnoid hemorrhage: a guideline for healthcare professionals from the American Heart Association/American Stroke Association. *Stroke*, 2012;**43**(6):1711–37.
4. Mayer, S. A., S. Schwab, Advances in critical care and emergency medicine. *Stroke*, 2010;**41**(2):e74–6.
5. Rabinstein, A. A., G. Lanzino, E. F. Wijdicks, Multidisciplinary management and emerging therapeutic strategies in aneurysmal subarachnoid haemorrhage. *Lancet Neurol*, 2010;**9**(5):504–19.
6. Molyneux, A., *et al.*, International Subarachnoid Aneurysm Trial (ISAT) of neurosurgical clipping versus endovascular coiling in 2143 patients with ruptured intracranial aneurysms: a randomised trial. *Lancet*, 2002;**360**(9342):1267–74.
7. Langham, J., *et al.*, Variation in outcome after subarachnoid hemorrhage: a study of neurosurgical units in UK and Ireland. *Stroke*, 2009;**40**(1):111–18.
8. Feigin, V. L., *et al.*, Risk factors for subarachnoid hemorrhage: an updated systematic review of epidemiological studies. *Stroke*, 2005;**36**(12):2773–80.
9. van Gijn, J., R. S. Kerr, G. J. Rinkel, Subarachnoid haemorrhage. *Lancet*, 2007;**369**(9558):306–18.
10. van Gijn, J., G. J. Rinkel, Subarachnoid haemorrhage: diagnosis, causes and management. *Brain*, 2001;**124**(Pt 2):249–78.
11. Broderick, J. P., *et al.*, Initial and recurrent bleeding are the major causes of death following subarachnoid hemorrhage. *Stroke*, 1994;**25**(7):1342–7.
12. Fontanarosa, P. B., Recognition of subarachnoid hemorrhage. *Ann Emerg Med*, 1989;**18**(11):1199–205.
13. Fisher, C. M., G. H. Roberson, R. G. Ojemann, Cerebral vasospasm with ruptured saccular aneurysm – the clinical manifestations. *Neurosurgery*, 1977;**1**(3):245–8.
14. Gruber, A., *et al.*, Chronic shunt-dependent hydrocephalus after early surgical and early endovascular treatment of ruptured intracranial aneurysms. *Neurosurgery*, 1999;**44**(3):503–9; discussion 509–12.
15. Qureshi, A. I., *et al.*, Risk factors for subarachnoid hemorrhage. *Neurosurgery*, 2001;**49**(3):607–12; discussion 612–13.
16. Longstreth, W. T., Jr., *et al.*, Cigarette smoking, alcohol use, and subarachnoid hemorrhage. *Stroke*, 1992;**23**(9):1242–9.
17. Pham, M., *et al.*, CT perfusion predicts secondary cerebral infarction after aneurysmal subarachnoid hemorrhage. *Neurology*, 2007;**69**(8):762–5.
18. Chappell, E. T., F. C. Moure, M. C. Good, Comparison of computed tomographic angiography with digital subtraction angiography in the diagnosis of cerebral aneurysms: a meta-analysis. *Neurosurgery*, 2003;**52**(3):624–31; discussion 630–1.
19. Edlow, J. A., Diagnosis of subarachnoid hemorrhage in the emergency department. *Emerg Med Clin North Am*, 2003;**21**(1):73–87.
20. Butzkueven, H., *et al.*, Onset seizures independently predict poor outcome after subarachnoid hemorrhage. *Neurology*, 2000;**55**(9):1315–20.
21. Stiebel-Kalish, H., L. S. Turtel, M. J. Kupersmith, The natural history of nontraumatic subarachnoid hemorrhage-related intraocular hemorrhages. *Retina*, 2004;**24**(1):36–40.
22. Fisher, C. M., J. P. Kistler, J. M. Davis, Relation of cerebral vasospasm to subarachnoid hemorrhage visualized by computerized tomographic scanning. *Neurosurgery*, 1980;**6**(1):1–9.
23. Dupont, S. A., *et al.*, Timing of computed tomography and prediction of vasospasm after aneurysmal subarachnoid hemorrhage. *Neurocrit Care*, 2009;**11**(1):71–5.
24. Boesiger, B. M., J. R Shiber, Subarachnoid hemorrhage diagnosis by computed tomography and lumbar puncture:

are fifth generation CT scanners better at identifying subarachnoid hemorrhage? *J Emerg Med,* 2005;**29**(1):23–7.

25. Rabinstein, A. A., *et al.*, Predictors of cerebral infarction in aneurysmal subarachnoid hemorrhage. *Stroke,* 2004;**35**(8):1862–6.
26. Fiebach, J. B., *et al.*, Stroke magnetic resonance imaging is accurate in hyperacute intracerebral hemorrhage: a multicenter study on the validity of stroke imaging. *Stroke,* 2004;**35**(2):502–6.
27. Absalom, S. R., Revised national guidelines for the analysis of cerebrospinal fluid for bilirubin in suspected subarachnoid haemorrhage. *Ann Clin Biochem,* 2009;**46**(Pt 2):177–8; author reply 178.
28. Molyneux, A. J., *et al.*, Risk of recurrent subarachnoid haemorrhage, death, or dependence and standardised mortality ratios after clipping or coiling of an intracranial aneurysm in the International Subarachnoid Aneurysm Trial (ISAT): long-term follow-up. *Lancet Neurol,* 2009;**8**(5):427–33.
29. Wartenberg, K. E., S. A. Mayer, Medical complications after subarachnoid hemorrhage. *Neurosurg Clin N Am,* 2010;**21**(2):325–38.
30. Laidlaw, J. D., K. H. Siu, Poor-grade aneurysmal subarachnoid hemorrhage: outcome after treatment with urgent surgery. *Neurosurgery,* 2003;**53**(6):1275–80; discussion 1280–2.
31. Chaichana, K. L., *et al.*, Role of inflammation (leukocyte-endothelial cell interactions) in vasospasm after subarachnoid hemorrhage. *Surg Neurol,* 2009;**73**(1):22–41.
32. Dreier, J. P., The role of spreading depression, spreading depolarization and spreading ischemia in neurological disease. *Nat Med,* 2011;**17**(4):439–47.
33. Qureshi, A. I., *et al.*, Prognostic significance of hypernatremia and hyponatremia among patients with aneurysmal subarachnoid hemorrhage. *Neurosurgery,* 2002;**50**(4):749–55; discussion 755–6.
34. van den Bergh, W. M., *et al.*, Hypomagnesemia after aneurysmal subarachnoid hemorrhage. *Neurosurgery,* 2003;**52**(2):276–81; discussion 281–2.
35. de Rooij, N. K., *et al.*, Delayed cerebral ischemia after subarachnoid hemorrhage: a systematic review of clinical, laboratory, and radiological predictors. *Stroke,* 2013;**44**(1):43–54.
36. Naval, N. S., C. E. Thomas, V. C. Urrutia, Relative changes in flow velocities in vasospasm after subarachnoid hemorrhage: a transcranial Doppler study. *Neurocrit Care,* 2005;**2**(2):133–40.
37. Lindegaard, K. F., *et al.*, Cerebral vasospasm diagnosis by means of angiography and blood velocity measurements. *Acta Neurochir (Wien),* 1989;**100**(1–2):12–24.
38. Dankbaar, J. W., *et al.*, Effect of different components of triple-H therapy on cerebral perfusion in patients with aneurysmal subarachnoid haemorrhage: a systematic review. *Crit Care,* 2010;**14**(1):R23.
39. Dorhout Mees, S. M., *et al.*, Calcium antagonists for aneurysmal subarachnoid haemorrhage. *Cochrane Database Syst Rev,* 2007(3):CD000277.
40. Berman, M. F., *et al.*, Impact of hospital-related factors on outcome after treatment of cerebral aneurysms. *Stroke,* 2003;**34**(9):2200–7.
41. de Smet, A. M., *et al.*, Decontamination of the digestive tract and oropharynx in ICU patients. *N Engl J Med,* 2009;**360**(1):20–31.
42. Finfer, S., *et al.*, Intensive versus conventional glucose control in critically ill patients. *N Engl J Med,* 2009;**360**(13):1283–97.
43. Ely, E. W., *et al.*, Effect on the duration of mechanical ventilation of identifying patients capable of breathing spontaneously. *N Engl J Med,* 1996;**335**(25):1864–9.
44. Macdonald, R. L., *et al.*, Clazosentan, an endothelin receptor antagonist, in patients with aneurysmal subarachnoid haemorrhage undergoing surgical clipping: a randomised, double-blind, placebo-controlled phase 3 trial (CONSCIOUS-2). *Lancet Neurol,* 2011;**10**(7):618–25.
45. Macdonald, R. L., *et al.*, Randomized trial of clazosentan in patients with aneurysmal subarachnoid hemorrhage undergoing endovascular coiling. *Stroke,* 2012;**43**(6):1463–9.
46. Lynch, J. R., *et al.*, Simvastatin reduces vasospasm after aneurysmal subarachnoid hemorrhage: results of a pilot randomized clinical trial. *Stroke,* 2005;**36**(9):2024–6.
47. Vergouwen, M. D., *et al.*, Effect of statin treatment on vasospasm, delayed cerebral ischemia, and functional outcome in patients with aneurysmal subarachnoid hemorrhage: a systematic review and meta-analysis update. *Stroke,* 2010;**41**(1):e47–52.
48. Wong, G. K., *et al.*, High-dose simvastatin for aneurysmal subarachnoid hemorrhage: a multicenter, randomized, controlled, double-blind clinical trial protocol. *Neurosurgery,* 2013;**72**(5):840–4.
49. Dorhout Mees, S. M., *et al.*, Magnesium for aneurysmal subarachnoid haemorrhage (MASH-2): a randomised placebo-controlled trial. *Lancet,* 2012;**380**(9836):44–9.
50. Suarez, J. I., *et al.*, The Albumin in Subarachnoid Hemorrhage (ALISAH) multicenter pilot clinical trial: safety and neurologic outcomes. *Stroke,* 2012;**43**(3):683–90.

Craniotomy for treatment of aneurysms

Patrick Mitchell

Indications

Prior to the early 1990s, the only means of securing cranial aneurysms was with surgery. Of the techniques of Huntarian ligation, wrapping, and clipping, clipping came to be the favored default option. The early 1990s saw the introduction of endovascular coil embolization, which spread rapidly in popularity because of its minimally invasive nature. This spread was accelerated by the results of the ISAT trial that became available in 2002 [1], showing that in the short term at least, endovascular treatment was the safer option. The argument about the long-term security of the treatment continued for several years. With more recent publication of long-term follow-up from the ISAT trial it has become clear that the increase in hemorrhage rates feared after coiling has not materialized, at least up to about 10 years after treatment [2–4]. This coupled with the natural history suggests that treatment of aneurysms should be primarily aimed at securing them in the short to medium term. In the longer term, beyond 5 years or so, it would appear that the re-hemorrhage rate from aneurysms is fairly similar, and very low, whether they are coiled, clipped, or probably even if they are untreated. Endovascular treatment has become the option of choice. Surgical craniotomy is therefore undertaken only in cases where endovascular treatment is either not available or deemed unsuitable.

In those areas of the world where endovascular treatment is available, it has had a significant impact on the nature of cases having surgery. Cases that are not coilable tend to be those that have wide necks or those where important arterial branches arise from the aneurysm sack directly. While these factors do not preclude surgical clipping, they do make it more difficult, and probably more dangerous. A further factor is that the current generation of surgeons has far less experience of clipping than their predecessors. Relatively inexperienced surgeons currently tackle difficult aneurysms. This should be borne in mind when considering the relative risks of coiling and clipping. The results of large series by surgeons with great experience extending back over many years probably do not reflect the reality in many current clinical settings. That said, the co-operative aneurysm study dates from a period when clipping was uncommon and did show that the results from surgical clipping were better than the results of Huntarian ligation or conservative treatment [5–7]. If coiling is not considered to be a favorable option for a dangerous aneurysm, then the argument for clipping is a strong one. The principal reasons why aneurysms come to surgery are discussed below.

Wide-necked aneurysms

In order to retain a coil basket without it prolapsing into the lumen of the parent vessel and any loops obstructing it, aneurysm needs to have a neck. The majority of aneurysms do have such a neck but there are some with a more sessile origin on the arterial wall where coiling

Critical Care of the Stroke Patient, ed. Stefan Schwab, Daniel Hanley, and A. David Mendelow. Published by Cambridge University Press.

would carry a substantial risk of occluding the parent vessel. There are various endovascular techniques that can get round this and it is ultimately a radiological judgment whether attempted coiling is advisable not.

Difficult endovascular access

Endovascular coiling requires the manipulation of fine catheters through a convoluted approach path from the groin to the neck, past the carotid bifurcation, around the carotid siphon, and beyond. In some cases this approach path is complicated by the atheromatous disease or excessive tortuosity. This technical consideration may make coil manipulation difficult or unfeasible.

Branches coming off the aneurysm sack

As a coil ball obstructs an aneurysm, it will also obstruct any branches arising from its dome or distal neck. If this risk is high and the threatened branches are important, coiling may be deemed inappropriate.

Failed attempted coiling

In cases where the feasibility of coiling is not clear, it is common to attempt to coil. If this attempt is found to involve excessive risk or proves unfeasible, then the coiling procedure can be abandoned and instead the aneurysm can be clipped.

Surgery necessary for another reason

The usual situation here is when an aneurysm has bled and caused a hematoma in the Sylvian fissure or temporal lobe and that this hematoma requires surgical removal. As the aneurysm is already exposed it is commonly clipped at the same time. The declining familiarity of non-vascular neurosurgeons with clipping has led to a trend to surgically remove the clot only and coil the aneurysm before or after clot removal [8].

Timing of surgery

There has been a long-running debate about the timing of surgery. Late surgery has better surgical outcomes but exposes patients to an increased risk of re-hemorrhage. Early surgery avoids this risk but is associated with more post-operative complications. There may be a high-risk period between days three and six after the hemorrhage [9]. The issue remains unresolved with high-class evidence but the fashion has moved towards a strategy of timing of surgery based on patient condition. Surgery is considered as soon as the patient's clinical condition has recovered to a certain point. This is often the point of communicative engagement with the surgeon such as 'when the patient looks you in the eye' or 'smiles at you' (personal communication, RP Sengupta, J. Sugita).

Preoperative preparation

Much preoperative preparation overlaps with the medical management of subarachnoid hemorrhage and its consequences. Measures of preoperative preparation specific to craniotomy and surgical clipping include the following.

Appropriate imaging

If craniotomy and clipping are considered, it is useful to have imaging of specific views of the aneurysm appropriate to the operative approach. These will generally not be available from diagnostic and endovascular imaging. A facility that has recently become more widely available is the three dimensional (3D) surface rendering of angiographic data. Current systems generally allow geometric rotation of virtual models of the aneurysm and its associate vessels on the angiographic workstation. What is exported from the workstation to image viewing technology used in theatre is not, however, the 3D model, but simply two-dimensional (2D) graphic representations of specific views. If this is the case it is useful to have specific views arranged which are from the same direction of view as the surgical approach, as well as from the opposite direction to facilitate surgical orientation in theatre and mental visualization of structures obscured by the aneurysm itself. Some branches that appear to be coming from the aneurysm sac on 2D angiogram images are actually coming from the parent vessel and are running adjacent to the sac. With 3D rendering this can often be better appreciated.

Site marking

Preoperative site marking is recommended as a security against operating on the wrong side.

Lumbar drain

Many surgical approaches to aneurysms are through relatively minimally invasive incisions with minimal access. In these cases, removal of sufficient CSF to allow space to operate is not as easy as in a wider craniotomy. Specifically in these cases it is suggested that the lumbar drain be inserted before the operation commences. The same measure can also be used for more conventional craniotomies but as CSF is generally easier to remove it is less critical.

Access to blood

Occasionally, an intraoperative aneurysm rupture can lead to substantial hemorrhage and the need for urgent blood transfusion. Local policies on blood availability will vary according to ease of access to the blood transfusion service. In general, where the neurosurgery operating theatres and blood transfusion service are in the same building, preoperative group and save is sufficient and on those rare occasions when urgent blood is needed, blood can be given. Full preoperative cross matching and issuing of blood from the blood bank are likely to be necessary in cases where access to blood would otherwise be unacceptably delayed. Also the risk of rapid blood loss is greater with some ophthalmic and basilar tip aneurysms that do not allow proximal control at surgery. If a cell saver is available it is advisable to have it deployed or on standby against an intraoperative rupture.

Positioning

Head positioning for aneurysm surgery is aimed at two objectives. The first of these is a position in which the surgeon can comfortably perform what could be several hours of microsurgery. The second is to position the head in such a way that when CSF is removed, gravity draws the brain away from the operative approach, thus minimizing the need for retraction. In general, the initial approach to aneurysms of the internal carotid and anterior cerebral arteries is along the sphenoid wing. The head is positioned to make this approximately downwards, so is tilted around 30° away from the side of the aneurysm. The approach path to the middle cerebral artery is from a more anterior point above the pterion or over the eye and along the anterior fossa floor. The head is tilted at 10–20° away from the side of the aneurysm. In both cases it is tilted slightly back so gravity pulls the brain off the skull base.

Operative technique

The basic strategy for aneurysm clipping is to make an extra cerebral approach. The intention is to expand the gap between the brain and skull base or frontal and temporal lobes, while allowing the brain to fall away on removal of CSF rather than be pushed away by retractors. In most cases it is not possible to get adequate access purely by gravity alone and retractors are necessary. They should be deployed slowly, allowing time for CSF removal.

Scalp flap

The intention when designing a scalp flap is to allow optimal surgical access, which is usually through a craniotomy flap that extends from the squamous temporal bone into the frontal bone above the lateral eyebrow, while keeping the incision hidden behind the hairline. This is generally done with an incision extending from just in front of the ear, above the zygomatic arch, to the anterior-most point of scalp that is covered by hair. The flap is then folded over its base and the middle of the base is stretched anteriorly with sutures of elastic to expose as much frontal bone as possible. This unilateral scalp flap is usually satisfactory but alternatives exist. If an approach that comes further medial onto the forehead is desired, a bi-coronal scalp flap is an option.

There has been recent interest in minimally invasive operations using an incision hidden in the eyebrow or eyelid [10–13]. A small 'eyebrow craniotomy' measuring about 3 cm × 1.5 cm is then fashioned. Several authors have reported the effectiveness and safety of these approaches. They have advantages and disadvantages. They are minimally invasive with smaller incisions than more conventional approaches. However, the incisions are moved from being hidden behind the hairline to the face, where any complications resulting in prominent scarring or alteration of bony contours are poorly tolerated. Another limitation is that operative access is restricted which means that the options for viewing the aneurysm from different directions during the operation are minimal. Endoscope-assisted open surgery is helpful in this situation but is itself demanding of equipment and skill. Careful selection and planning are therefore necessary.

Muscle dissection

After the scalp flap is turned, or together with the scalp flap, the temporalis muscle must be mobilized from the skull. This is a significant cosmetic issue because wasting of the temporalis muscle in the postoperative period leads to an unsightly cadaverous hollow behind the eye which is a common cause of concern. No reliable way of avoiding this wasting has been described, but avoidance of excessive diathermy and reattachment of the muscle in an anatomical position at the end of the operation have been advocated to minimize the risk.

Craniotomy

The intention is to approach the aneurysm underneath the brain so the craniotomy is positioned at the lower edge of the skull vault. The craniotomy need not extend more than 3 cm above this but a wide opening of 5–8 cm allows variable angles of view that make it easier to identify and protect arterial branches. The front of the craniotomy should be as far forward as possible for middle cerebral aneurysms unless they are peripheral and being approached directly rather than via the ICA/MCA. After turning the skull flap, the lower edge of the craniotomy is examined to see if it rises above the plane of the anterior fossa floor. Any part of this lower edge that does so will obstruct the view and is removed with a drill or hand tools.

Dural opening

Hemostasis is secured before the dura is open. The dural opening is restricted to the area necessary for the approach. Dura is often left intact over the upper part of the craniotomy to protect the brain from inadvertent injury. It is usual to open the dura as a flap with the base downwards. This flap is then secured with stay sutures that keep it under tension over the edge of the craniotomy. Any bleeding at this point is controlled and the fixed retraction systems deployed before proceeding to microdissection.

Microscopic approach

The first step in the microscopic approach is to open the space underneath the brain and move the microscope in order to look directly into the space, parallel with the skull base. This is done progressively. A protective layer is placed on the brain and a retractor passed a short way into the subdural space. This is done slowly and patiently, allowing time for CSF removal. As the brain yields to CSF removal, the space is widened and deepened. As this happens, the exact direction of the skull base will become more apparent and the microscope will be adjusted to look directly into the space.

Disorientation is a risk when looking down the microscope and for surgeons with limited experience it is suggested that the general direction of approach is checked every so often by macroscopic inspection to ensure that it is towards the desired structure, usually the optic nerve.

Once the optic nerve has been identified and adequate space to operate made around it, the sequence in which arteries are exposed depends on the aneurysm. As a general rule dissection starts away from the aneurysm and moves towards it along the artery. This minimizes the risk of an inadvertent rupture.

Posterior communicating artery aneurysms

The arachnoid membrane between the optic nerve and frontal lobe is incised at its anterior end. This opening is extended backwards around the lateral side of the optic nerve to reveal the anterior border of the carotid artery. The carotid artery is then dissected from the anterior side distally for a few millimeters. The aneurysm is located posterior to the carotid at this point.

Internal carotid and A1 aneurysms

The carotid artery is exposed as for posterior communicating artery aneurysms and the dissection followed along the carotid distally to its bifurcation. Bifurcation aneurysms will then be found at the bifurcation pointing laterally. A1 aneurysms are rare and difficult to clip because they frequently arise on the medial side of the carotid out of sight. Endoscope-assisted open surgery with a 30° or 70° side-viewing endoscope on a fixed holder is helpful for this but requires experience to do safely.

Middle cerebral artery aneurysms

Two alternative strategies may be adopted for middle cerebral artery aneurysms. The surest approach is to expose the carotid artery as with a posterior communicating artery aneurysm, then follow it to its bifurcations and follow the middle cerebral artery into the Sylvian fissure to the aneurysm. The anterior inferior surface of the terminal carotid and middle cerebral arteries can be readily dissected. The dissection should not be extended around to the posterior superior surface because of the numerous lenticulostriate arteries that arise from it.

This approach has the advantage of leading the surgeon reliably to the aneurysm without dissecting in the wrong direction. It has the disadvantage that with laterally placed aneurysms, operating time and Sylvian fissure dissection are increased. The alternative approach is to enter the Sylvian fissure at a point appropriate to the aneurysm's location, identify arterial vessels within the fissure, and follow them to the middle cerebral trunk and aneurysm. This approach is quick and minimizes dissection but in inexperienced hands carries a risk of getting lost in the wrong plane and also does not give such ready proximal control. This is the most commonly used approach used with minimal access craniotomies. Image guidance is a useful adjunct in this approach as it provides the orientation that is lacking from the anatomy.

Anterior communicating artery aneurysms

The anterior side of the optic nerve is avoided initially because of risk of causing a rupture. The arachnoid membrane at the back of the optic nerve and over the carotid is instead incised first. The carotid is then identified. The dissection follows the carotid into the proximal Sylvian fissure until its bifurcation. The anterior cerebral artery is then followed medially and anteriorly to the anterior communicating artery above the chiasm. The position of the A1, anterior communicating complex and A2 in relation to the gyrus rectus is variable. In many cases it is possible to visualize the arteries without resecting any gyrus but often they are tucked up between the hemispheres and a small part of the gyrus rectus may need to be removed to expose them. A primary approach through the gyrus rectus is an option and has the advantage that the aneurysm and arteries are on the far side of the gyrus' medial arachnoid membrane, affording some protection from inadvertent rupture before the dissection is complete.

Pericallosal artery aneurysms

Aneurysms of the pericallosal arteries are relatively uncommon but when they do arise, they frequently come to surgery. Their distal location makes the access pathway for endovascular treatment difficult and they are generally easy to clip. Unlike other anterior circulation aneurysms, the approach is interhemispheric with a parafalcine craniotomy located behind the hairline at a point that minimizes the distance between the craniotomy and aneurysm. The interhemispheric fissure is then dissected to identify the pericallosal or callosomarginal arteries. A difficulty then arises in knowing which way to follow them to find the aneurysm as this is not obvious from the anatomy. This is another area where image guidance can be very helpful.

Posterior fossa aneurysms

Basilar tip aneurysms

Basilar tip aneurysms are difficult to approach surgically. They are a long way back for a pterional or subfrontal operation and they are also between the upper cranial nerves. Proximal control in the event of an interoperative rupture is a problem. If the neck is low the feeding arteries will not be accessible to temporary clipping. An endovascular balloon can be deployed preoperatively in the basilar artery but this carries a risk of embolic complications. Furthermore it is difficult to visualize all the perforators from the basilar and posterior cerebral arteries that must be preserved. The endovascular approach path to basilar tip aneurysms is relatively straight and for these reasons, in most institutions, it is rare for basilar tip aneurysms to come to surgery.

Proximal control

Ophthalmic aneurysms

Proximal control means gaining access to the parent artery of the aneurysm proximal to it so that in the event of a rupture, blood loss can be contained by temporarily occluding the feeding vessel. In most cases this is achieved as part of the approach to the aneurysm. The issue is at its most critical in cases where the aneurysm is proximal on the carotid artery as they bleed most briskly. These are unfortunately also situations where proximal control is difficult to achieve because little of the proximal artery is accessible surgically. The problem is at its worst with carotid ophthalmic aneurysms where the aneurysm arises just as the carotid artery emerges from the skull base. The proximal carotid cannot be readily exposed via a craniotomy. One approach to this problem is to perform a neck dissection to expose and sling the internal carotid artery below the skull base before doing the craniotomy. This allows the artery to be occluded in the neck if proximal control is required but does involve the morbidity of the second operation. An alternative is to angiographically place a catheter in the internal carotid artery with a view to deploying a balloon if proximal control is necessary. This avoids the second operation but carries its own risk of embolic complications, and deployment of the balloon is likely to require on-table angiography to avoid arterial damage. Some surgeons do neither and rely on external compression of the carotid in the neck by an un-scrubbed team member if proximal control is needed. This has the limitation that occlusion is not likely to be as complete as with the other two methods.

Basilar tip aneurysms

Proximal control of basilar tip aneurysms is difficult because the terminal basilar artery is generally out of view during the operation. Preoperative catheter placement with a view to balloon occlusion is complicated by there being two vertebral arteries supplying the basilar, so occluding one is unlikely to achieve much control. Basilar tip aneurysms are usually operated on without proximal control. Extracorporal bypass with cooling and cardiac arrest has been tried but with high complication rates.

Anterior communicating artery aneurysms

Proximal control in anterior communicating artery aneurysm surgery is complicated by there being a bilateral supply to the aneurysm. Frequently there is asymmetry of the A1 arteries in which case approaching from the side of the dominant A1 makes it readily available for proximal control should it be necessary. Many surgeons have a preference for approaching the anterior communicating artery from the non-dominant right-hand side. If the left A1 is dominant it is still accessible during the approach by dissecting beyond the ipsilateral right A1 to locate the contralateral left A1 as it travels along the gyrus rectus towards the anterior communicating artery. In cases without a dominant A1, it is usual to approach from the right and both A1s will be accessible using this method.

Techniques for aneurysm repair

The objective of aneurysm clipping is to secure the aneurysm while preserving flow in arterial branches. The uncoilable aneurysms now reaching surgery present major challenges in this. It is recommended that a wide range of techniques and clips are available.

Simple clipping

With simple clipping the aneurysm is dissected, its branches exposed and identified, and a single clip applied to the aneurysm in a position and direction calculated to maintain flow in the parent vessel and its branches while minimizing the amount of pathological arterial wall that is proximal to the clip. This is the usual method adopted. It is complicated by the need to visualize branches that may be located behind the aneurysm sack and manipulations necessary to do this risk rupturing it.

Fenestrated clips

Fenestrated clips allow branches or the parent vessel to be located in the fenestration of the clip, the blades of which occlude the aneurysm. Location of the clip so that the fenestration does not allow persistent filling of the aneurysm can be difficult. A series of fenestrated clips can be lined up to encircle a vessel that is aneurysmal on the far side.

Another advantage fenestrated clips have over ordinary clips is occasionally relevant. With thick-walled aneurysms, the thickness of the wall proximal in the clip may splint the jaws open so that distally they do not close. This problem can be overcome by placing one conventional clip and a second fenestrated clip parallel and adjacent to it.

Wrapping

The idea of wrapping is to place around the aneurysm an irritant substance that induces intense fibrosis, reinforcing the aneurysm wall. It is a treatment without good evidence of effectiveness. It probably reduces aneurysm hemorrhage rates but is less effective than clipping [16]. It is only considered as a primary treatment where clipping is for some reason not feasible but is often used as an adjuvant to clipping to wrap areas of pathological aneurysm wall which must remain proximal to clips in order to allow flow in associated vessels. Cotton wool wisps or wisps from the absorbent middleware of dressings like eye pads are frequently used.

Slinging

With aneurysm slinging the intention is to produce a secure aneurysm repair that is not dependent on future fibrosis. A thin strip of non-absorbable flexible sheeting is cut and passed around the parent vessel and aneurysm. This strip is then pulled tight around the vessel and clipped to cover the aneurysm. It is used for small inaccessible aneurysms where there is a high risk of clipping important branches such as anterior choroidal aneurysms.

Temporary clipping

The use of temporary clips is a controversial issue with some surgeons advocating their frequent use and others avoiding whenever possible. Aneurysm clip manufacturers make two ranges of clips. Permanent clips with a high closing force and usually gold colored clips with lower closing force. These low-force clips are intended for temporary occlusion of vessels without excessive damage to the arterial wall. They are deployed proximal to an aneurysm before clipping to reduce the blood pressure in the aneurysm. Temporary clipping generally does not lead aneurysm collapse unless several arteries are occluded as backflow from branches usually provides some blood pressure, but it certainly makes them much softer and easier to manipulate with reduced risk of rupture. When temporary clips are used it is conventional to start a stopwatch when a clip is applied and record the time of application in the notes. The surgeon attempts to keep this time a short as possible in the hope of minimizing ischemic complications.

Adenosine cardiac standstill

Adenosine cardiac standstill is a useful technique that increases the safety of clipping many aneurysms. It requires close collaboration between surgical and anesthetic teams. The administration of a bolus of intravenous adenosine in a dose of 0.3 mg/kg (three to four times the starting dose used for cardioversion) leads to a period of asystole lasting 10 to 30 seconds. During this period, blood pressure falls to 0. Unlike temporary clipping, this allows the aneurysm to collapse completely. It is particularly useful in the situation where the conical neck of a large aneurysm makes clips slip proximally and occlude the parent vessel on closing. It is also useful for aneurysm slinging. The short duration of asystole means that the technique is of no use to control a bleeding aneurysm. When the technique is to be used the surgeon informs the anesthetist who draws up the drug and connects it, then waits for the indication to administer the bolus. The sound volume of the cardiac monitor is turned up so that the surgeon can hear the heartbeat. The surgeon prepares to apply the clip. Then, poised with clip applicator over the aneurysm, they request the dose. When the heart has stopped they close the clip on the aneurysm.

Management of intraoperative aneurysm rupture

Intraoperative aneurysm rupture is a stressful situation that is inevitably associated with an increased operative risk. When it occurs, the priority is to stop the bleeding. Continuing hemorrhage from an aneurysm not only carries risk of significant blood loss but also markedly compromises the perfusion pressure not only in the territory of the affected artery, but other areas of the brain via a steal phenomenon. Retaining perspective in a crisis is difficult and surgical teams can function poorly without specific measures. These in order of priority are listed below.

Communication

You are going to need all the help you can get. Explain to the surgical team that there has been an aneurysm rupture. All members' full attention is required. You will need a larger sucker on a cell saver if available, appropriate patties or cotton wool balls, temporary clips, and possible blood transfusion quickly. You will get what you need fastest and most accurately if the team senses you are in control, and making urgent but specific and courteous requests. Achieving this is not always easy!

It is impossible accurately to estimate the amount of blood loss occurring while looking down the microscope. For this reason it is helpful to ask somebody to 'call the hundreds' – to notify you of every hundred mls of blood that collects in the suction jar.

Visualization

Ideally you would visualize where the blood is coming from the aneurysm so that the hole can be covered with a patti or cotton wool. Failing that, you need to visualize the parent artery to apply a temporary clip. This will often require the use of a larger bore sucker on a high setting. Many surgeons clip aneurysms with a second, larger sucker on standby for this purpose.

Hemostasis

A small leak can be packed with oxidized cellulose, a patti or cotton wool which is pressed onto the aneurysm. In a couple of minutes the leak frequently clots so that the surgeon's hand can be freed from holding the pack in place. A more recalcitrant bleed can be controlled by holding a pack on with a micro fixed retractor. This allows dissection of the aneurysm to continue ready for clip application. If the bleeding cannot be controlled while allowing necessary dissection a temporary clip may be applied to the proximal parent artery. This slows but will not usually stop bleeding which continues via back flow from branches. Application of a temporary clip often brings a sense of urgency to repair the bleeding site. This should be resisted as a measured approach is likely to be faster and more effective than a panicked one.

Recovery

Recovery from the rupture involves stabilization of the patient's hemodynamics if necessary and continuing with dissection to apply the clip. This is likely to be hampered by the presence of either a temporary clip or a pack on the rupture site. A partial clipping of the aneurysm across its equator rather than its neck may allow the bleeding site to be isolated while dissection of its associated vessels proceeds.

Galvanic corrosion

Galvanic corrosion affects objects made of dissimilar metals that are connected together by direct metal to metal contact and by contact with an aqueous fluid in which both are immersed. One of the objects suffers anodic corrosion over years in which metal atoms in the surface are ionized and dissolve in the fluid. This can affect aneurysm clips which are made of different metals, in contact with each other, and immersed in CSF. For this reason all clips used on the same aneurysm must be of compatible metals. The practical consequence of this is that the aneurysm trays available in the neurosurgery theatres are quite likely not compatible with each other. Manufacturers produce differing designs of aneurysm clips and it is frequently necessary to have several types available to pick the ideal one but once a clip has been inserted, the choice of subsequent clips is restricted to those that are compatible with the first one.

Platinum has a positive electrode potential compared with metals found in clips which means that if coils and clips are involved in galvanic corrosion, the coils will act as the cathode and the clips suffer anodic corrosion. Though possible in theory, this has not become a practical issue to date.

Neuro-navigation aids

With most aneurysm surgery, dissection is done according to anatomical structures that lead directly to the aneurysm and neuro-navigation aids are of limited use. There are some exceptions to this rule. In the case of pericallosal aneurysms, neuro-navigation is of great assistance in minimizing the amount of the dissection necessary to localize the lesion. It is of similar use in the eyebrow approach to the middle cerebral artery where considerable dissection can be saved by using neuro-navigation to locate the medial to lateral position of the aneurysm in the Sylvian fissure. Ultrasound with color flow Doppler has also been used in this role, with some success, but the method is very operator dependent, and gives information that is difficult to interpret. It can be surprisingly difficult to tell the difference between an aneurysm and its parent vessel.

Craniotomy closure

The craniotomies used for aneurysms usually extended in front of the hairline to the pterional region and onto the forehead. In this area cosmetic considerations are important in reconstruction. The bone flap is replaced with a rigid fixation system, such as plates and screws or similar. If plates are required in the area in front of the hairline, they can be let into the bone by drilling small recesses to prevent them being visible or palpable through the skin. It is usual to move the craniotomy flap slightly forwards from its original position to close the gap left by the craniotome at the front, while allowing the gap to be wider where it is not visible behind the hairline. Rapid-setting hydroxyapatite plasters such as Hydroset® can be used to improve the bony contour once the bone flap has been fixed. Re-attachment of the superior margin of mobilized temporalis muscle with sutures passing through the bone flap may assist in reducing the incidence of postoperative temporalis wasting.

Conclusion

Craniotomy and clipping of cerebral aneurysms is a treatment that has undergone radical change in its application in recent years, as endovascular coil embolization has come to be the treatment of choice. Currently surgical clipping is more widely available around the world than coil embolization, but this situation is likely to change in favor of coiling. In response to these changes, aneurysm clipping has evolved from a general neurosurgical skill. Centers specializing in the treatment of aneurysms have been able to use subspecialization to concentrate surgical experience, skills, and team familiarity to optimize performance while developing endovascular services in parallel. At the time of writing it appears that the future role of aneurysm clipping is dependent more on technical developments in interventional radiology than in surgery. What is clear is that the treatment of aneurysms has become, and will remain, a multidisciplinary service, a development welcomed by all those involved.

REFERENCES

1. Molyneux, A., *et al.*, International Subarachnoid Aneurysm Trial (ISAT) of neurosurgical clipping versus endovascular coiling in 2143 patients with ruptured intracranial aneurysms: a randomised trial. *Lancet*, 2002;**360**(9342):1267–74.
2. Campi, A., *et al.*, Retreatment of ruptured cerebral aneurysms in patients randomized by coiling or clipping in the International Subarachnoid Aneurysm Trial (ISAT). *Stroke*, 2007;**38**(5):1538–44.
3. Molyneux, A. J., *et al.*, Risk of recurrent subarachnoid haemorrhage, death, or dependence and standardised mortality ratios after clipping or coiling of an intracranial aneurysm in the International Subarachnoid Aneurysm Trial (ISAT): long-term follow-up. *Lancet Neurol*, 2009;**8** (5):427–33.
4. Molyneux, A. J., *et al.*, International subarachnoid aneurysm trial (ISAT) of neurosurgical clipping versus endovascular coiling in 2143 patients with ruptured intracranial aneurysms: a randomised comparison of effects on survival, dependency, seizures, rebleeding, subgroups, and aneurysm occlusion. *Lancet*, 2005;**366**(9488):809–17.
5. Sahs, A. L. and D. W. Nibbelink, *Aneurysmal subarachnoid haemorrhage*. 1981: Urban & Schwarzenberg.
6. Graf, C. J. and D. W. Nibbelink, Cooperative study of intracranial aneurysms and subarachnoid hemorrhage. Report on a randomized treatment study. 3. Intracranial surgery. *Stroke*, 1974;**5**(4):557–601.
7. Nishioka, H., Report on the cooperative study of intracranial aneurysms and subarachnoid hemorrhage. Section VII. I. Evaluation of the conservative management of ruptured intracranial aneurysms. *J Neurosurg*, 1966;**25** (5):574–92.
8. Niemann, D. B., *et al.*, Treatment of intracerebral hematomas caused by aneurysm rupture: coil placement followed by clot evacuation. *J Neurosurg*, 2003;**99**(5):843–7.
9. Mahaney, K. B., M. M. Todd, J. C. Torner, Variation of patient characteristics, management, and outcome with timing of surgery for aneurysmal subarachnoid hemorrhage. *J Neurosurg*, 2011;**114**(4):1045–53.
10. Brydon, H. L., *et al.*, Supraorbital microcraniotomy for acute aneurysmal subarachnoid haemorrhage: results of first 50 cases. *Br J Neurosurg*, 2008;**22**(1):40–5.
11. Mori, K., *et al.*, Pterional keyhole approach to middle cerebral artery aneurysms through an outer canthal skin incision. *Minim Invasive Neurosurg*, 2007;**50**(4):195–201.
12. Reisch, R., A. Perneczky, Ten-year experience with the supraorbital subfrontal approach through an eyebrow skin incision. *Neurosurgery*, 2005;**57**(4 Suppl):242–55; discussion 242–55.
13. Mitchell, P., *et al.*, Supraorbital eyebrow minicraniotomy for anterior circulation aneurysms. *Surg Neurol*, 2005;**63** (1):47–51; discussion 51.

Endovascular interventions for subarachnoid hemorrhage

Arnd Dörfler

The primary treatment goal of cerebral aneurysms is prevention of rupture. Surgical clipping has been the treatment modality of choice for both ruptured and unruptured cerebral aneurysms for decades. Just over 20 years ago endovascular treatment was mainly restricted to those patients with aneurysms unsuitable or inaccessible for clipping due to size or location, or in whom surgical clipping was contraindicated because of the general medical condition. Nowadays, the increasing experience and development of appropriate devices has widened the indications, and endovascular therapy has become more than an alternative to surgical treatment.

Attempts to induce thrombosis of systemic aneurysms either by introducing foreign bodies or by application of electrical or thermic injury date back to the first half of the 19th century. Velpeau (1831) independently described a method of introducing arterial thrombosis by inserting a needle into the aneurysmal lumen and withdrawing it after thrombus had formed. In 1941 Werner *et al.* reported successful electrothermic thrombosis of an acute ruptured intracranial aneurysm through a transorbital approach. In 1963 Gallagher proposed a technique of inducing thrombosis of intracranial aneurysms by high-speed delivery of dog or horse hairs into the aneurysm using a pneumatic gun ('pilojection'). However, despite encouraging early results these methods did not gain acceptance.

Further improvements in endovascular devices, balloon techniques, and arterial catheterization rapidly led to the idea of endovascular navigation and occlusion of the aneurysmal sac. The first successful balloon embolization was performed by Serbinenko in 1974, establishing the way for modern endovascular treatment of cerebral aneurysms. However, several drawbacks of latex balloons, such as deflation, aneurysm rupture, protrusion into the parent vessel, distal embolization, and frequent rebleedings, prompted the search for better materials for aneurysm occlusion. Although balloon occlusion of parent vessels is still a therapeutic option for large, giant, or fusiform aneurysms, this technique has been mainly abandoned in favour of coil embolization.

In 1991, the Italian neurosurgeon Guido Guglielmi published his preliminary experience with electrolytically detachable platinum coils (Guglielmi Detachable Coils, GDC), opening a new era in aneurysm treatment. Since the introduction of controlled detachable coils for packing of aneurysms, endovascular embolization is increasingly used and the 'coiling' technique nowadays represents the current 'gold standard' in endovascular aneurysm therapy.

Endovascular techniques and devices

Owing to its excellent spatial resolution conventional cerebral angiography is still the gold standard for the detection of a cerebral aneurysm. Ideally, this is performed during the first available moment after presentation of the SAH patient at the hospital. The precise visualization of the aneurysm neck, the shape and the

Critical Care of the Stroke Patient, ed. Stefan Schwab, Daniel Hanley, and A. David Mendelow. Published by Cambridge University Press.

size of the aneurysm, and its relationship to parent vessels are important factors for clinical decision making, especially in favor of endovascular therapy. Rotational angiography in a 2D or 3D mode is available on most new generation neurointerventional angio suites and represents a valuable supplement to standard biplane DSA series. Using rotational angiography, multiple oblique views are obtained as a source for 3D reconstruction. Rotational angiography helps to define the aneurysm neck, find the appropriate working position, and perform accurate measurements. 3D angiography thereby improves planning of surgical and interventional procedures, especially in complex aneurysms.

There are mainly two strategies to treat cerebral aneurysms via the endovascular approach: first, occlusion of the aneurysmal sac with embolic material preserving the parent artery and second in otherwise untreatable aneurysms occlusion of the parent artery in order to exclude the aneurysm from the blood circulation.

Occlusion of the parent artery is a therapeutic alternative especially in patients with giant broad-based aneurysms of the internal carotid artery which are surgically inaccessible. The basic assumption for this treatment modality is that the patient will tolerate parent vessel occlusion without ischemic complications. Although there is no general consensus about the protocol to predict patient's tolerance to permanent vessel occlusion, some authors recommend blood flow studies to decide which patient will tolerate acute balloon occlusion and who will need an extracranial-intracranial (EC-IC) bypass to avoid ischemic complications. Complex scenarios include balloon test occlusion with SEP monitoring, SPECT imaging before, during and after test occlusion, and different degrees of hypotension during test occlusion. In our experience, a pretty simple test has a high predictive value: the compression test with injection into the contralateral ICA while the symptomatic ICA gets compressed. If the veins of the compressed side opacify not more than 1 s later than those of the injected site, anatomical preconditions for ICA occlusion are excellent. Also important is how to take care of the patient after the procedure. Blood pressure should be above the normal level in order to adapt to the different blood flow. After the third day the patient is allowed to sit on the bed, on day four the patient can walk with assistance. In case of any problems during the first walk around, the period of lying down should be prolonged. In experienced hands occlusion of the parent artery has proved to be safe, convenient, and effective. Vessel occlusion could be done either with a detachable balloon or detachable coils positioned proximal to the aneurysm. Some authors recommend lesion trapping in order to prevent retrograde filling of the aneurysm.

In order to reconstruct an aneurysm-bearing vessel there exist different techniques nowadays. In the past aneurysmal sac occlusion with a detachable balloon was performed but this is now clearly obsolete. Although it is technically feasible there is no detachable balloon with different configurations which could be navigated over a microwire in order to access the aneurysm lumen in an arbitrary manner. In addition, the relatively high risk of complications – mainly due to thromboembolic events as well as aneurysm rupture during or after the procedure – with a high procedure-related mortality (reported up to 18%), as well as the fact that the balloon would not keep its configuration over time, necessitated a more sophisticated endovascular technique for aneurysm embolization. Over the last 20 years, improvement in the development of flexible microcatheters which can navigate through cerebral vessels to lesions distally has allowed the treatment of an increasing range of intracranial aneurysms. The focus of modern endovascular therapy has shifted to the use of detachable platinum coils. Through a guiding catheter a microcathether is coaxially advanced into the cerebral vasculature and over a soft microwire it can be navigated into the aneurysm lumen, optimally placed in the aneurysm center in a stable position. Pioneering in the development was that these coils are retrievable until the operator is satisfied with placement and then could be detached (Fig. 31.1).

In the meantime there is a great variety of different neurointerventional devices currently available. Detachable platinum coils are most frequently used for endovascular aneurysm therapy. Usually the coils are attached to a stainless steel delivery wire. This allows repositioning and selective placement of the

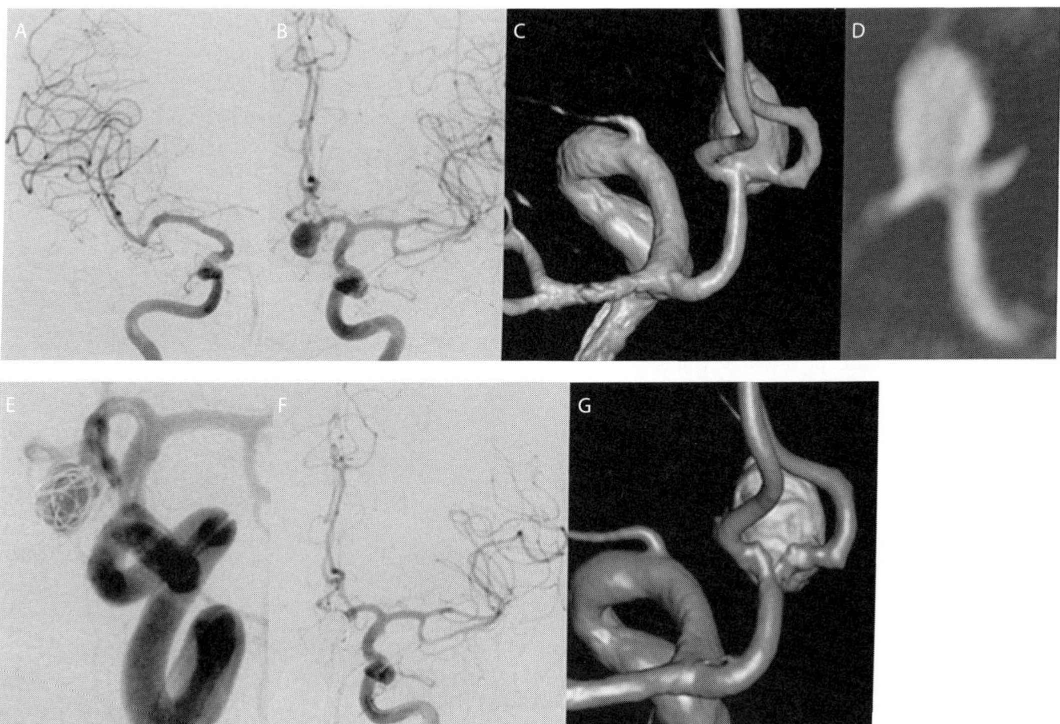

Fig. 31.1 Endovascular coil embolization of an acutely ruptured Acom aneurysm using detachable platinum coils. Note the superiority of 3D rotational angiography in displaying the angioarchitecture of the aneurysm neck (See plate section for color version).

coil within the aneurysm. This coil design combines the advantage of very soft, compliant platinum and retrievability resulting in markedly improved safety and efficacy. Over the last several years, many new designs in coil configuration, such as two- or three-dimensional shape have become available by numerous vendors and have significantly increased the versatility of this device for aneurysm therapy. Due to its spherical-shaped memory 3D coils spontaneously form a complex cage after deployment thereby serving as a basket for subsequent coils. Softer coils allow safer initial and last coil placement.

Recently, there has been growing interest in modifying platinum coils by coating the surface with extracellular matrix proteins, non-biodegradable polymers, fibroblasts, and vascular endothelial growth factors. Experimental studies indicate that these modifications might promote endothelialization, clot organization, and tissue integration of the coils, and thereby may lead to improved aneurysm occlusion and outcome. Hydrogel coils consist of a carrier platinum coil coupled to an expandable hydrogel material, which undergoes a tremendous increase in volume when placed into a physiological environment with a certain pH value, e.g. blood. Distinct from previous devices aimed at speeding the organization of thrombus, the new device has been designed to entirely fill the aneurysm cavity, with complete or near-complete exclusion of thrombus. Unlike thrombus, the hydrogel material is stable and unaffected by natural thrombolytic processes and thus may reduce observed rates of aneurysm recanalization. The HEAL study, which is a multicenter registry randomizing aneurysms to treatment with hydrogel versus treatment with bare coils, did show that when

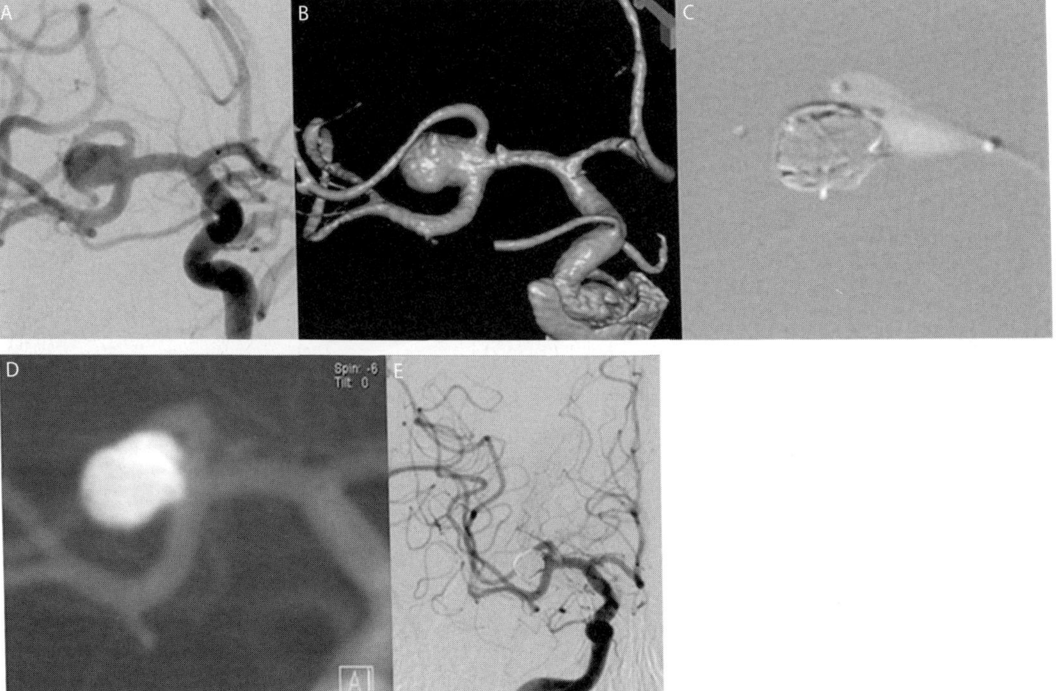

Fig. 31.2 Endovascular coil embolization of an acutely ruptured MCA aneurysm using the 'balloon-remodeling-technique' with an additional balloon placed in the superior branch of the MCA thus narrowing the broad aneurysm neck resulting in dense coil packing and complete aneurysm occlusion. (See plate section for color version).

used, 75% or more hydrogel coil length aneurysm recurrence rate at 3–6 month follow-up was 0%. But when less than 75% of hydrogel coil length was implanted recurrence was not lower than published rates.

Although there are several advantages of coil embolization over surgery, there is a disadvantage of endovascular treatment. Due to coil compaction and residual inflow in initially incompletely obliterated aneurysms a potential risk of recanalization with aneurysmal regrowth exists. In particular, the geometry of wide-necked aneurysms is less favorable for obtaining maximal coil packing. In cases of an unfavorable dome-to-neck ratio endovascular treatment can be feasible and sometimes more effective by simultaneous temporary balloon protection, widely known as the 'remodeling technique'. Hereby, a microcatheter-mounted nondetachable balloon provides a temporary barrier across the aneurysmal neck while introducing the coils into the aneurysmal sac. The use of simultaneous temporary balloon protection may allow denser intra-aneurysmal coil packing, especially at the neck, without parent artery compromise than did the use of coils alone. A potential risk might be induced by higher pressure inside the aneurysm during inflation of the balloon and inserting coils, facilitating aneurysm rupture. But in this case reinflation of the balloon and immediate further coiling is the consequence (Fig. 31.2 and Fig. 31.3).

Despite enormous advances in the development of flexible microcatheters, coil configurations, and embolic materials and use of remodeling technique, wide-necked aneurysms still remain a therapeutic challenge. With the recent development and refinement of endovascular stents, the significant potential for these devices in the treatment of wide-necked and fusiform

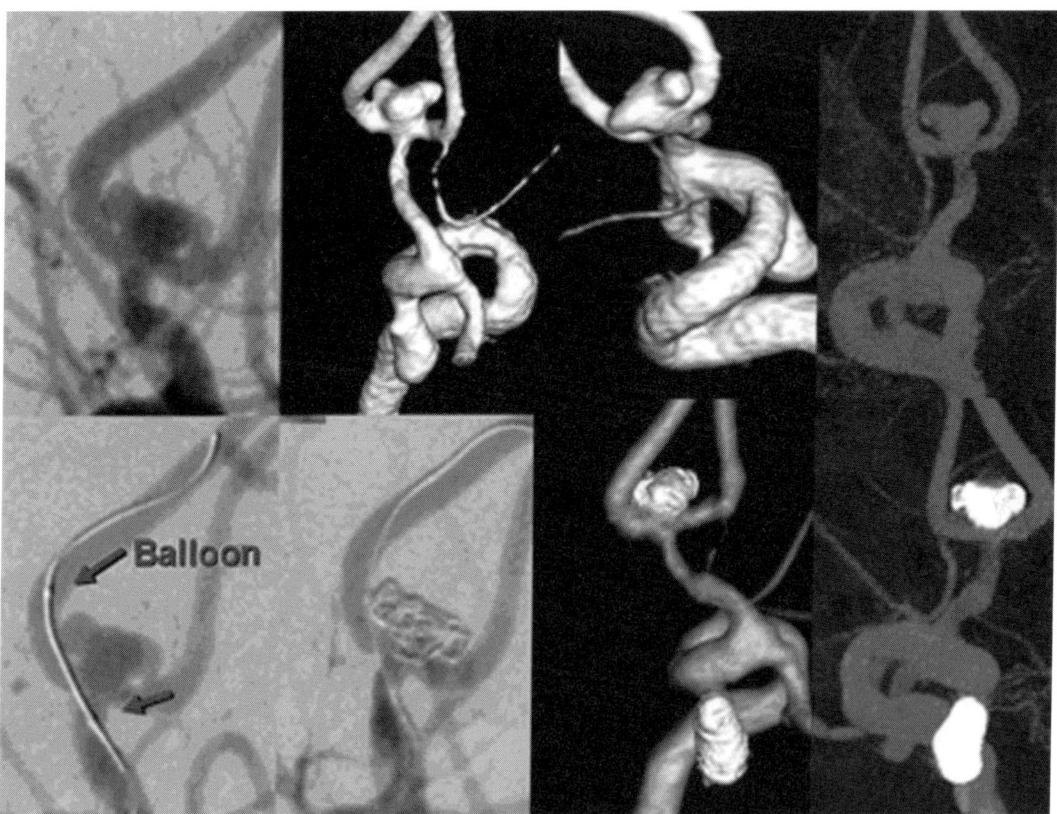

Fig. 31.3 Endovascular coil embolization in a patient presenting with SAH. Since the bleeding source was uncertain endovascular therapy of both an Acom aneurysm using the 'balloon-remodeling-technique' and of an additional aneurysm at the internal carotid artery was performed.

aneurysms has become apparent. Hereby, an intravascular stent is used to create a bridging scaffold followed by endovascular placement of coils through the interstices of the stent into a wide-necked or fusiform aneurysm. This is a treatment option in patients with a wide-necked aneurysm in which direct surgical clipping or conventional endovascular therapy would be difficult or impossible, and in whom parent artery occlusion is not a viable option. Stents are deployed either by balloon expansion or release of a self-expanding nitinol or steel stent from a constraining sheath. Balloon-expandable stents had been used for intracranial treatment, usually coronary stents (covering size ranges up to 4 mm), but these stents are very stiff and carry the risk of damaging a dysplastic aneurysm-bearing segment of the artery with eventual rupture of the vessel. The large profile and relative stiffness of these stent delivery systems limit the locations that are able to be accessed and increase the risk of vessel dissection. In summary, the balloon-expandable stents were not a real treatment option. Complication rates were too high and in the majority of patients it was impossible to obtain access to the intracranial target vessel. Nowadays, there are several self-expanding stents, Neuroform (Boston Scientific), Enterprise (Cordis), Solitaire (ev3), and Leo (Balt) specifically designed for intracranial use available. These stents are extremely flexible and access through tortuous vessels is facilitated. Even distal arteries can be reached easily. Since they are not

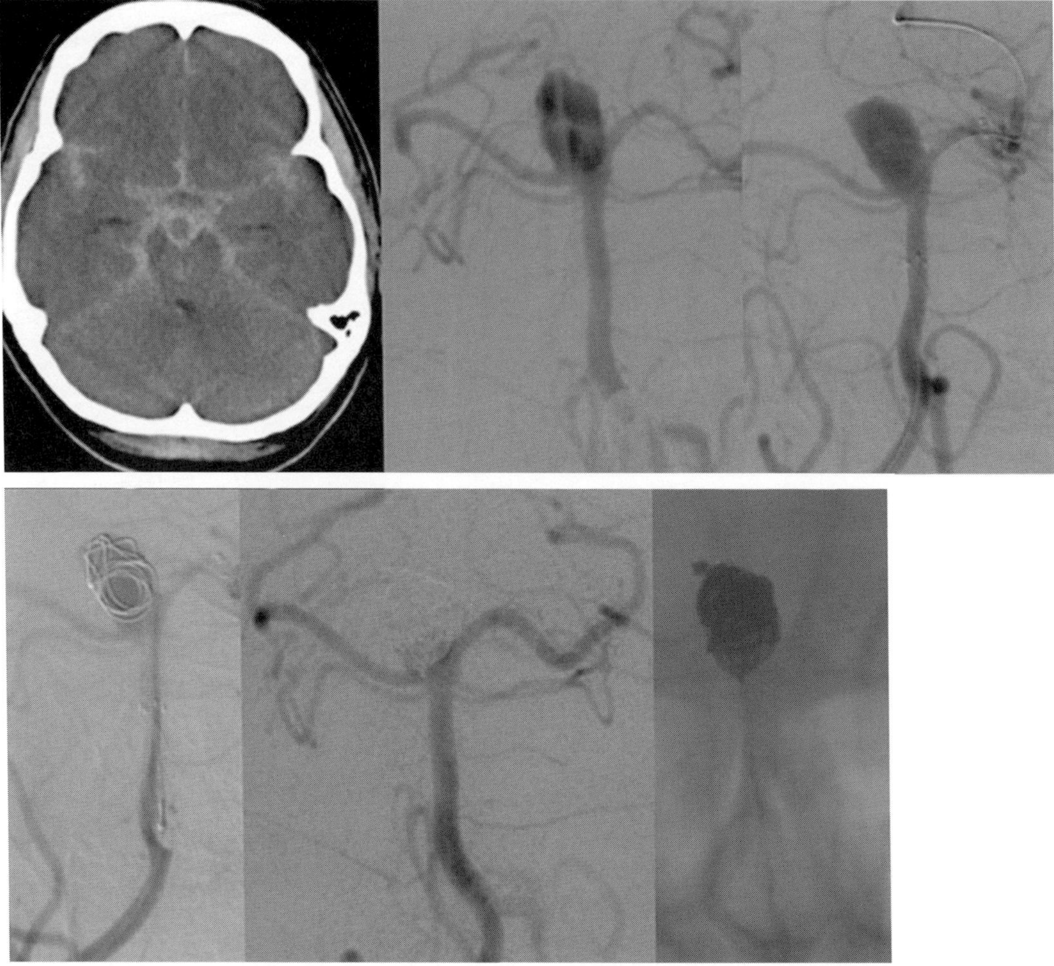

Fig. 31.4 SAH due to a broad-based aneurysm of the basilar tip. Complete endovascular coil embolization was performed after placement of a self-expandable stent (Neuroform) across the aneurysm neck.

balloon mounted the risk of damaging the artery is reduced. Another advantage is that these stents, beside the Neuroform, could be withdrawn even if more than 75% of the stent is already deployed.

Since anticoagulation therapy is mandatory in patients treated with an intravascular stent, patients with an acute SAH are not 'ideal stent candidates'. For patients presenting with an acutely ruptured broad-based aneurysm necessitating stent-assisted coil embolization, the risk of thromboembolic complications has always to be balanced with the increased risk of re-/hemorrhage. Our policy in these SAH patients is to start heparin and aspirin immediately prior to stent placement. At the same time we administer a loading dose of clopidogrel via a gastric tube (Fig. 31.4).

Future developments such as covered or coated or high-profile stents lining the neck of the aneurysm would effectively exclude the aneurysm from the circulation and might theoretically present a perfect cure for selected aneurysms. Depending on the stent design coiling might not be necessary any more since a dense stent mesh would promote aneurysm thrombosis. Covered stents would be extremely useful in large or giant aneurysms as long they are located along vessel segments without perforating arteries. They can exclude aneurysms located at the extracranial part of the ICA up to the paraophthalmic segment and at the vertebral artery. The advantage is that filling of the aneurysm with embolic material is not necessary, but the disadvantages are first the limited locations where deployment is suitable and second the stiffness of the system which makes access to the target vessel sometimes impossible.

Recently, a new therapeutic option, i.e. **flow diverting stents** is available. This novel type of vascular stent features a smaller wires diameter and a denser mesh compared to conventional stents. The concept of flow diversion is a strong modulation of intra-aneurysmal hemodynamics, guiding blood flow towards its physiological path and off the aneurysm, thereby facilitating thrombosis of the aneurysm. Yet, valid long-term data of the use of these new tools is still limited. Intravascular stents always act as a thrombogenic device, by stimulating platelet aggregation as soon as they are exposed to the patient's blood. Especially for patients scheduled for these highly thrombogenic flow diverters, it is mandatory that they receive prophylactic antiplatelet therapy with aspirin and clopidogrel (or an equivalent). Thus flow-diverting stents are usually not used in the acute phase of SAH for therapy of an acutely ruptured aneurysm. We used flow diverters in SAH patients only in very exceptional clinical situations, where this device was used as an individual 'ultima ratio' treatment attempt (Fig. 31.5).

Onyx is a nonadhesive liquid embolic agent composed of 20% ethylene vinyl alcohol (EVAL) copolymer dissolved in dimethyl sulfoxide and suspended micronized tantalum powder to provide a contrast for visualization under fluoroscopy. Onyx was first developed for the treatment of brain arteriovenous malformations and works by reducing the vascular supply of arteriovenous malformations and minimizing the potential bleeding during surgical resection. When onyx is placed in the target vessels, the dimethyl sulfoxide solvent dissipates into the blood, causing the EVAL copolymer to precipitate into a spongy, coherent embolus.

Onyx has been used to combine with the coils for the treatment of patients with aneurysms unsuitable for or previously failed coiling. The combination with the liquid embolic agent eliminates the interstices of coils that allow for regrowth and brings about a lower recanalization rate than that previously reported with coiling. Recently, the use of onyx itself for embolization of cerebral aneurysms has been reported in the literature. However, even with protective devices such as balloons or stents it is difficult to prevent the protrusion or migration of onyx into the parent vessel. Thus the onyx-technique does not represent a standard therapy for cerebral aneurysms.

Specific anatomical locations and clinical considerations

MCA aneurysms are often small and wide necked, and often incorporate neighboring arterial branches in the aneurysm base. Additionally, they are frequently associated with multiple intracranial aneurysms ('mirror aneurysms'). Due to the local anatomy and neck configuration, MCA aneurysms need particular consideration. For aneurysms with a very wide neck or difficult geometry surgery is still the therapy of choice. If a space-occupying hematoma is present, immediate evacuation of the hematoma is mandatory, in combination with clipping of the aneurysm. Major angioanatomic features that might hinder endovascular treatment in this location are an unfavorable dome-to-neck ratio of less than 1.5, and/or arterial branching from the aneurysm base. Compared to other aneurysm locations, the risk of thromboembolic complications or local compression of surrounding neighboring vessels seems to be increased. Therefore, for endovascular therapy of MCA aneurysms appropriate patient selection is mandatory. Careful evaluation of the angioarchitecture using rotational 3D angiography or 3D helical CT angiography might be helpful here in the precise visualization of the aneurysm neck, shape, and the size of the aneurysm, supporting further treatment decisions and planning. In selected cases the remodeling technique in broad-based MCA bifurcation aneurysms can be helpful.

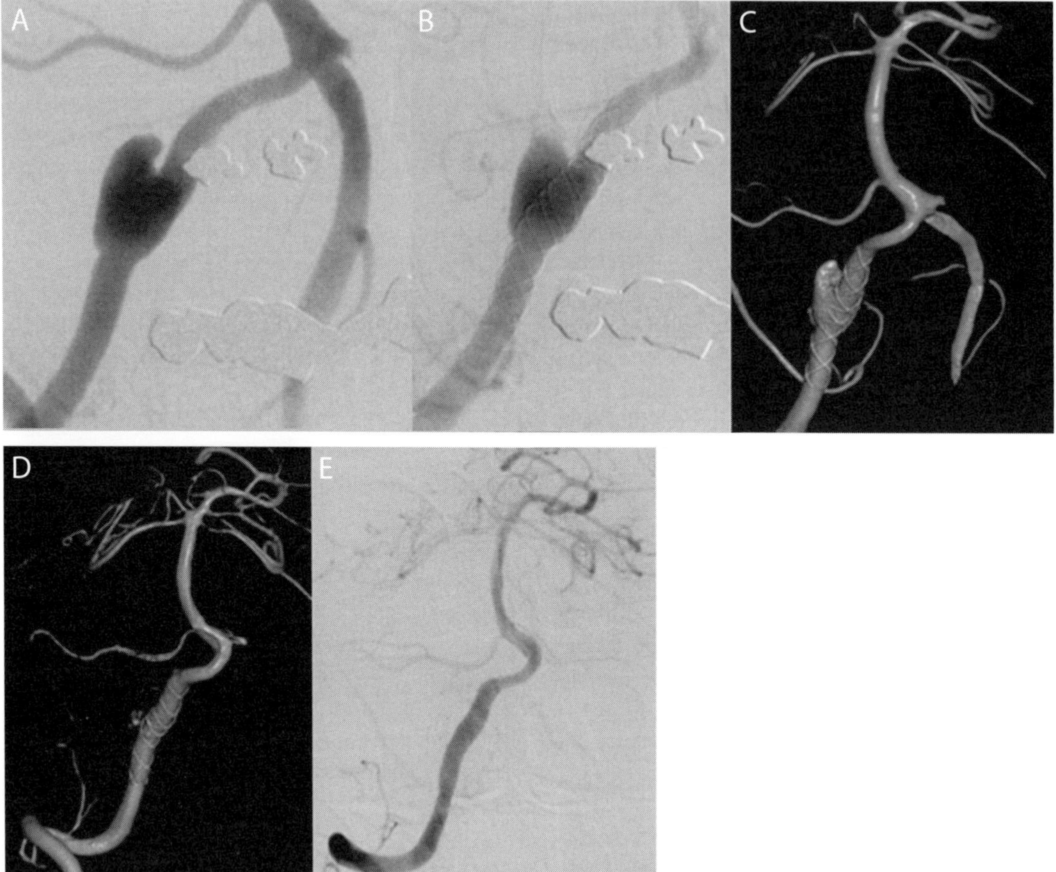

Fig. 31.5 Endovascular therapy of a dissecting fusiform aneurysm of the distal vertebral artery using a flow diverting stent (Silk) resulting in complete aneurysm obliteration at 6-month angiographic follow-up. (See plate section for color version).

Aneurysms of the posterior circulation account for about 15% of all intracranial aneurysms. Saccular aneurysms and those of the basilar tip are the most frequent, accounting for 5–8% of all intracranial aneurysms. Ruptured aneurysms in the posterior circulation have a worse prognosis than patients with a ruptured aneurysm in another location and early rerupture occurs more often in this location. Despite improvement in microsurgical therapy, clipping for posterior circulation aneurysms remains challenging. Furthermore, SAH and cerebral edema increase the difficulties of the surgical approach much more than in any other location. Nowadays, it is accepted worldwide that endovascular treatment should be done as the first treatment option since clinical outcome is much improved compared to clipping. The early recognition and acceptance that coiling is clearly better than clipping in posterior circulation aneurysms is the reason that these aneurysms are underrepresented in the ISAT study.

Aneurysms of the basilar tip remain an extreme surgical challenge, both in terms of technical difficulties associated with the access and the significant postoperative morbidity and mortality rates reported by experienced centers following direct clipping. In contrast, the endovascular approach is relatively easy (unless the patient has severe arteriosclerotic disease with increased vessel elongation and stenosis). However, the access to the basilar tip plays a minor role in most cases. The main technical challenge of the endovascular procedure depends on the shape of the aneurysm and not on its location. But since the introduction of flexible neurostents and the development of different coil designs most of the basilar tip aneurysms are now treatable with the endovascular approach.

Aneurysms of the vertebral artery leading to SAH are frequently located at the V4 segment. Dissecting aneurysms are more frequent in this location than non-dissecting berry aneurysms. Aneurysms are located proximal to the origin of the PICA, at the origin of the PICA (so-called PICA aneurysms) or slightly distal to the origin of the PICA. In patients with a dissecting aneurysm of the vertebral artery resulting in subarachnoid hemorrhage, either occlusion of the vertebral artery at the site of the aneurysm or trapping of the lesion is commonly advocated to prevent subsequent rupture. Fusiform aneurysms are usually considered due to atherosclerosis in adults. But, more common in the vertebrobasilar system, there is a subset of cerebral aneurysms with fusiform morphology, apparently unrelated to cerebral atherosclerosis or systemic connective tissue disease, thin-walled in part or whole, possibly containing thrombus. These aneurysms can rupture or cause cranial nerve or brain stem compression.

In contrast to vertebral aneurysms located at the origin of the PICA, real PICA aneurysms are located either proximally or distally at the PICA itself. Endovascular therapy with preservation of the parent artery was thought to be very difficult in this location. Like in basilar tip aneurysms and brain stem aneurysms the access to aneurysms at the PICA is easy to perform and this is in contrast to the surgical approach. Although PICA aneurysms tend to be fusiform or at least broad based, most of these aneurysms can be occluded sufficiently and often with preservation of the PICA via the endovascular route. If parent artery occlusion is necessary to exclude the aneurysm the PICA is a very resistant artery which is normally not easy to occlude. In proximal location the artery could be occluded with very little morbidity.

There is considerable uncertainty regarding the best treatment options for SAH patients grades IV and V on admission. Evidence from case series in the literature, local practice results, ethical issues, and cost should be taken into consideration. These patients have in general a poorer prognosis than patients in grades 0–III, but a subgroup appears to benefit from aggressive management (ICU care, ventricular drainage, angiography, and endovascular or surgical treatment of the aneurysm) at a cost-effective ratio.

Despite the lack of information of good quality (no randomized trials specifically designed for the elderly age group, very few elderly patients included in RCTs of SAH treatment, no matched or stratified case-control studies), the available evidence of case-series from centers in different world regions indicates that both surgical repair and endovascular treatment are feasible in this age group with acceptable rates of morbidity. Elderly patients more likely to benefit are those in good condition prior to the intervention.

SAH during pregnancy is an important cause of maternal death. Ruptured aneurysms during pregnancy should be treated, surgically or by coiling. If the gestational age allows, it is better to carry out the delivery by cesarean before aneurysmal treatment.

Periprocedural care

The role of anesthesia in interventional neuroradiology consists in providing patient comfort by analgesia and sedation, adequate monitoring, maintenance of vital functions, and (if required) management of systemic heparinization. The patient's underlying condition, duration and kind of intervention have to be considered to decide on the anesthetic management. Embolization of (ruptured) intracranial aneurysms is performed with the patient in general anesthesia. Although such an approach does not allow intraprocedural evaluation of the patient's neurological status and carries additional risks associated with general anesthesia and mechanical ventilation, we clearly prefer it during all (ruptured and unruptured) endovascular procedures occluding intracranial aneurysms. In order to minimize thromboembolic complications anticoagulation and/or antiplatelet therapy is useful. We recommend administration of i.v. aspirin, which we usually start also in ruptured aneurysms after insertion of the first coils. In unruptured aneurysms administration of aspirin is started optimally prior to the intervention. Usually, every patient receives aspirin (100 mg/d) for 3 months after the procedure. There are no evidenced-based data recommending a standard therapy against blood clotting, some groups heparinize all patients during the intervention. If thrombus formation occurs during treatment and does not resolve after elevation of the blood pressure and aspirin i.v. than glycoprotein receptor antagonists are recommended since they have a partial lytic effect. Clearly, local fibrinolysis with urokinase or rt-PA is not recommended in patients with ruptured aneurysms since fatal rebleeding is often observed. Mechanical lysis should be tried instead. If the patient was in good condition before the treatment or had an unruptured aneurysm he/she should be extubated in the angio suite. This is specifically important after treatment of MCA and basilar tip aneurysms, as these are associated with a higher risk of thrombotic complications resulting in morbidity. After the procedure the patient should be supervised on an intensive care unit and must be monitored by an experienced neurovascular team in order to detect symptomatic vasospasms before occurrence of infarction.

Complications of endovascular therapy

Endovascular treatment is potentially associated with procedural complications induced by the treatment itself. Mainly, there are two categories of complications: thromboembolic events and aneurysm rupture.

Ischemic complications are either due to a thrombosis of the aneurysm-bearing arterial segment or due to an embolus either into the aneurysm-bearing artery or into another artery. Thrombosis of the parent artery probably develops at the interface of the platinum coils due to aggregation of platelets. This complication is observed more often in broad-based aneurysms. Procedural morbidity of endovascular treatment ranges between 3.7% and about 10%, mortality between 0% and 2.1%. These numbers are well evaluated in patients with unruptured aneurysm to exclude complications due to the SAH itself. However, thromboembolic complications do not necessarily lead to neurologic deterioration of the patient. To reduce the risk of thromboembolic events, most of the neurointerventional centers anticoagulate the patient periprocedurally. Thereby, most of the groups at least double the ACT to 250–300 s. Although no evidence-based data exist about antiplatelet therapy and prevention of thromboembolic events during or after endovascular treatment, administration of aspirin might reduce symptomatic ischemic events.

Aneurysm rupture is another complication which can occur during the intervention. Aneurysm rupture has continued to be one of the most feared complications of endovascular aneurysm therapy. Any interventional neuroradiologist treating acutely ruptured aneurysms may be confronted with this complication. Some data regarding frequency, causes, management, and outcome of such ruptures during endovascular treatment are available and reveal that rupture does occur more often in previously ruptured aneurysms than in unruptured and if management is appropriate good clinical outcome is often achieved. Aneurysm rupture might be due to perforation with the guidewire or microcatheter, or might occur during coil placement. Clinical sequelae may be variable, ranging from slight leakage of contrast into the subarachnoid space to massive SAH or intraparenchymal hematoma with severe intracranial hypertension. Embolization of the aneurysm can be continued in most cases, and the majority of patients with treatment-related SAH survive without serious sequelae and with a better outcome than anticipated. It is very helpful in this situation to have the external CSF drainage in place before endovascular therapy starts. Some groups routinely use a microballoon in place to perform remodeling or, in case of intraprocedural aneurysm rupture, balloon inflation. Clearly, the use of a microballoon might be beneficial in aneurysms with a high risk of intraprocedural rupture: small Pcom aneurysms and, to a lesser extent, small para-ophthalmic aneurysms.

If aneurysm perforation occurs during an endovascular procedure, the patient usually has to be transported from the angiography suite to the CT scanner to determine the extent of hemorrhage. Flat-panel detector (FD) CT imaging combining angiography with rotational CT may overcome this temporal delay.

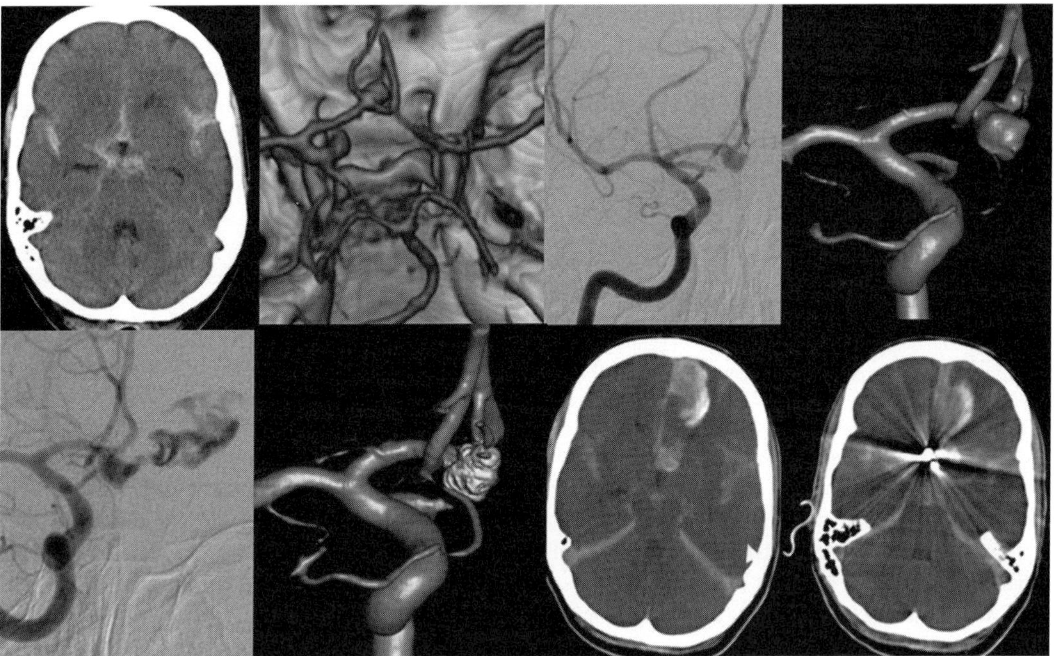

Fig. 31.6 Perforation of an acutely ruptured Acom aneurysm during diagnostic angiography prior to endovascular coil embolization. Immediate subsequent coil embolization resulted in complete aneurysm occlusion. Flat-panel-detector CT imaging (DYNA-CT) within the angio suite revealed the additional hemorrhage in the left frontal lobe. (See plate section for color version).

Although not of the same quality as conventional CT, current FD-CT image quality seems to be sufficient to assess the extent of intracranial hemorrhage and the width of the ventricles. FD imaging can be assessed within minutes, thus facilitating the management of rupture-related complications within the angio suite and overall resulting in an improved safety and outcome (Fig. 31.6).

Endovascular therapy of vasospasm

Vasospasms secondary to subarachnoid hemorrhage may be responsible for severe ischemic complications. Roughly 40% of patients with aneurysmal SAH develop angiographically visible vasospasm; about 20% have neurologic signs of vasospasm and 10% present with vasospasm-related infarction. If vasospasm is present at the time of patient administration and before treatment of the aneurysm, a combined approach might be necessary in order to occlude the aneurysm and to resolve vasospasm. After treatment of the ruptured aneurysm, approaches to treat aneurysmal vasospasm currently include medical treatment with Ca-antagonists, 'triple-H' therapy and endovascular methods.

There are two main endovascular treatment methods, i.e. balloon angioplasty and intra-arterial infusion of spasmolytic agents, respectively. If clinical deterioration is progressive despite intravenous medical therapy, endovascular methods to treat vasospasm should be discussed. Balloon angioplasty is superior to intra-arterial pharmacologic therapy for treatment of proximal vessel vasospasm and has a more sustained effect on the vessels. Although there is less data available of series documenting a significance of cerebral blood flow increase or improvement of delayed ischemic neurologic deficits induced by vasospasm compared to controls, our clinical experience and

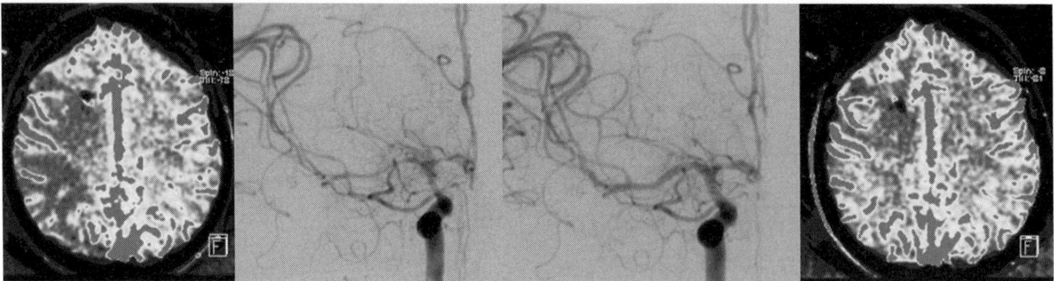

Fig. 31.7 Endovascular treatment of severe cerebral vasospasm in a patient with an acutely ruptured Acom aneurysm using intra-arterial nimodipine. Note perfusion CT imaging before and after administration of the vasoreactive drug resulting in a significantly improved brain perfusion. (See plate section for color version).

single case studies suggest that balloon angioplasty does reverse vasospasms and – if performed early enough – can improve the patient's condition. Papaverine or nimodipine can be useful as an adjunct to balloon angioplasty and also for the treatment of distal vessels that are not accessible for balloon angioplasty. However, this effect is short-lived and these drugs can cause severe hypotension and brain stem depression.

Although isolated series documenting clinical successes have prompted the increased use of papaverine or nimodipine as a treatment for vasospasm after SAH, some authors found, as it is currently being used, the drug does not provide added benefits, compared with medical treatment of vasospasm alone, but do not preclude the possibility that alterations in the timing of or indications for drug treatment might produce beneficial effects (Fig. 31.7).

Incompletely treated aneurysms/aneurysm remnants

Incomplete treatment of an aneurysm, either by clipping or coiling, may result in recurrent hemorrhage with serious or devastating consequences. Data on cerebral aneurysms treated by an endovascular approach also confirmed that a significant number of cases had either a residual or recurrent aneurysm. The incidence of aneurysm regrowing after incomplete treatment may have been underestimated. Even a small portion of aneurysm neck has the potential to enlarge over time. Although small aneurysm remnants measuring from 1 to 2 mm may not justify retreatment, the risk of progressive enlargement to a dangerous aneurysm should be considered. Long-term angiographic – preferentially done with MR – reassessment may be valuable not to miss aneurysm enlargement. There are some predisposing factors for postoperative aneurysm remnants such as aneurysm size and topographic peculiarities. Large or giant aneurysms are associated with a higher frequency of aneurysm remnants as well as neurosurgically difficult anatomic localizations such as the carotido-ophthalmic region, which requires removal of the clinoid process. Since nowadays endovascular aneurysm therapy is an important part in the management of SAH, comparison of surgical and endovascular methods regarding completeness of obliteration is of great importance. The reported results with coil embolization are very variable according to the series, techniques used, and aneurysmal size.

Since intra-operative techniques like checking exact clip location and absence of neighboring perforators under the microscope, and needle puncture of the aneurysm are standard parts of aneurysm surgery the need of postoperative angiography may be questioned. Although postoperative angiography is the method of choice for confirming the absence of any aneurysmal remnant, the widespread trend is not to perform postoperative angiography after microsurgical clipping. However, even opening of the aneurysm sac after clipping, a standard procedure in many neurosurgical institutions, does not exclude residual neck remnants proximal to the clip. Additionally, imperfect clip placement or delayed clip dislocation may remain unrecognized until postoperative angiography is performed. We think that postoperative angiography is at least justified in all 'difficult' and large aneurysms and in those in whom the surgeon is in doubt of leaving a remnant. There is another perspective that supports postoperative angiograms in all patients: incomplete clipped aneurysm can be managed very often via endovascular approach. A broad neck may be pretty small after incomplete clipping, a giant aneurysm may be turned into just a large one or the anatomy may have become clearer after inspection.

Recurrence of aneurysm after successful coiling might occur and impairs the long-term efficacy of endovascular treatment. The recurrence rates reported in the literature range from 4.7% to 50% for common aneurysms but up to 90% for giant aneurysms. There could be many causes for recurrence, including the recovery or displacement of coils, embolization during the acute bleeding period, large size or wide neck (more than 4 mm in diameter), and especially, incomplete embolization. A follow-up angiographic study demonstrated that among aneurysms that were considered to be 90% to 100% occluded in the initial examination, recurrence was rare. However, even in cases with complete occlusion as shown by angiographic imaging, only about 32% of the total volume of the aneurysm was filled by coils. If the opening of the rupture is properly occluded by coils, an occlusion of 50% to 90% of the total volume of aneurysm may alter the hemodynamics and prevent the recurrence of rupture.

Follow-up after endovascular therapy

The goal of intracranial aneurysm treatment is to achieve complete aneurysm occlusion in order to avoid rebleeding. One problem that might occur in endovascularly treated aneurysms is the relatively high number of suboptimal obliterated aneurysms with a tendency to recanalize. Therefore, no endovascular procedure should be performed without an appropriate follow-up imaging protocol. In our institution, every patient gets a MR scan (MRI and MRA: TOF and contrast enhanced technique) within 3 days after the procedure. In cases of satisfied occlusion rate (total or subtotal occlusion) the patient should be scheduled for a control MRA 6 months after the procedure followed by another control MRI 18 months after therapy. We try to get follow-up imaging for at least 3 years but try to continue follow-up as long as the patient collaborates (Fig. 31.8).

Clinical trial outcomes

Numerous observational studies have published complications rates, occlusion rates, and short-term follow-up results. These have been summarized in a systematic review of 48 eligible studies of 1383 patients with ruptured and unruptured aneurysms by Brilstra *et al.* (1999). Permanent procedural complications occurred in 3.7% of 1256 patients. More than 90% occlusion of the aneurysm was achieved in around 90% of patients.

Randomized trials in which coiling was compared with neurosurgical clipping have included 2272 patients, of which 2143 were from the International Subarachnoid Aneurysm Trial (ISAT). Most patients were in good clinical condition and had a small (<1 cm) aneurysm on the anterior circulation. The study was prematurely stopped after the results of a planned interim analysis were available: at 1 year, 23.7% of the patients allocated to endovascular treatment were dependent or dead, as compared with 30.6% of patients in the surgical group. Later on, the study group reported the revised outcome results with an even greater absolute risk reduction of 8.7% and a relative risk reduction of 26.8% for patients after coiling compared to patients after clipping. In addition, patients after coiling experienced significantly fewer seizures and needed to a significantly lesser extent CSF drainage. Patients older than 70 years were under-represented in this comparison – in view of the perceived advantage of coiling in elderly people – as were patients with aneurysms of the middle cerebral artery,

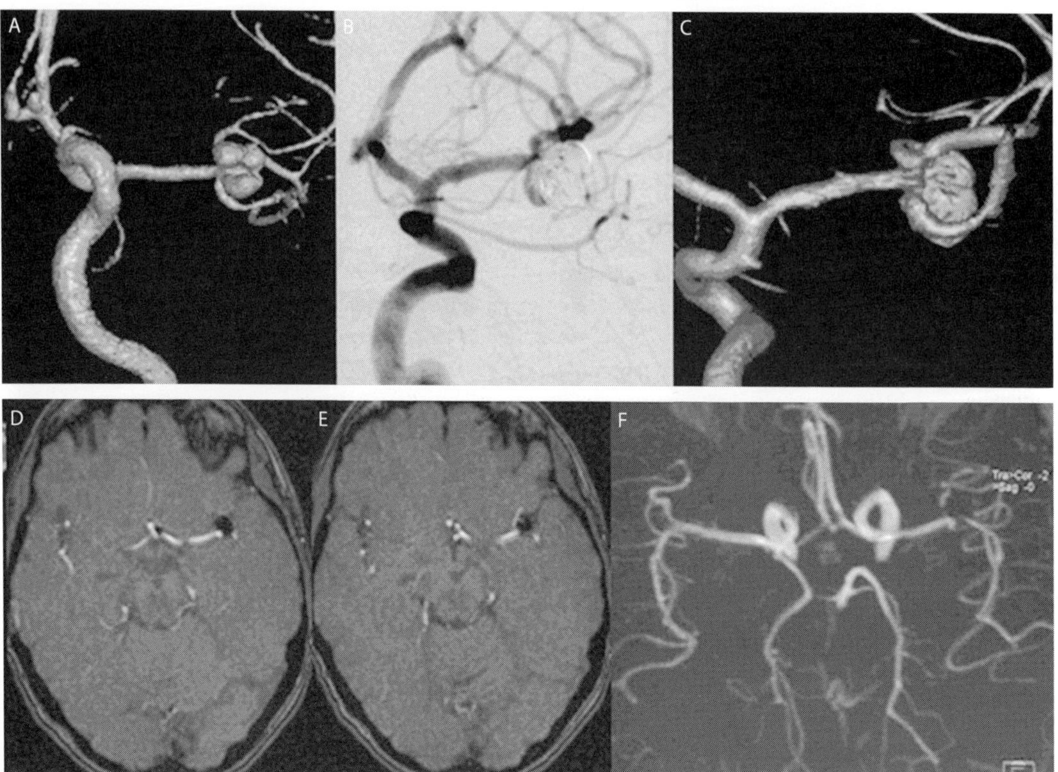

Fig. 31.8 Noninvasive follow-up of a completely embolized MCA aneurysm using TOF-MR angiography 6 months after therapy. Note the additional small aneurysm at the Acom also treated by coil embolization. (See plate section for color version).

because the anatomical configuration is often unfavorable for coiling, with branches arising near the neck of the aneurysm. Ideally, after coiling, the remaining lumen becomes occluded by a process of reactive thrombosis, but early or late rebleeding can occur after technically correct procedures. Nevertheless, in ISAT, the 7% absolute advantage over surgical treatment in the rate of death or dependence was maintained after 1 year, and the early survival advantage was maintained for up to 7 years. Uncertainty exists about the length of time that patients need to be followed up after coiling, about the most suitable radiological technique, and about the need for a second procedure for aneurysm necks that have recanalized by impaction of the coils, through recoiling or surgical occlusion.

The results of the ISAT study were not readily accepted, particularly not in the neurosurgical community. Some important features of the ISAT trial should be considered when transposing its results into practice. It followed the incertitude principle and therefore many patients were treated surgically or by endovascular techniques outside the trial; it only included aneurysms of the anterior circulation; the majority of treated aneurysms were < 10 mm in size; patients were treated very shortly (mean 2 days) after the diagnosis, so the results cannot be generalized to centers where the endovascular procedures cannot be performed on an emergency basis. Finally, to transpose ISAT results into practice it is crucial to know the local figures for morbidity and mortality after coiling and clipping. The selection of the best treatment depends also on the morphology and location of the aneurysm (e.g. posterior circulation aneurysms are best treated by endovascular techniques)

Another major issue is the durability of aneurysm occlusion after coiling. It is true that long-term durability of endovascular therapy remains to be determined. The present data, however, suggest that it is very unlikely that late aneurysm rebleeding after coiling will occur at a rate that would significantly affect the difference in outcome between surgery and coiling. The ISAT data indicate a risk of rebleeding after 1 year to be 2 per 1276 (0.16%) patient-years of follow-up. Thus it would take more than 40 years to overcome the benefit seen at 1 year with endovascular treatment. A recently published evidence-based review provides an objective comparison on clipping and coiling in ruptured and unruptured aneurysms analyzing single-center studies, multicenter studies with and without independent outcome ascertainment, and randomized clinical trials. The authors found that outcome at discharge, at 2 to 6 months, and at 1 year, and later survival, were all better after endovascular treatment than after surgery. Their results suggest that the higher rates of incomplete obliteration and the need of retreatment in patients after endovascular treatment do not affect patient's clinical outcome. Observational studies confirmed better discharge outcome and lower costs for patients treated for an unruptured aneurysm, no difference concerning outcome and rebleeding rate was revealed after 1 year in this patient group but only a few data were available for the latter comparison.

The clear benefit of the endovascular-treated patients did definitely change treatment strategies for patients with intracranial aneurysms in a lot of centers. The endovascular approach has become the first line treatment option, whenever this option is available. Since ISAT it is mandatory that all patients should be seen by a neurointerventionalist to decide whether the aneurysm is suitable for coiling or not. If one treatment is recommended over another, the reasons for this decision should be documented as in accordance with the usual standards for informed consent. Furthermore, the ISAT data add support for the treatment of patients with aneurysmal SAH in high-volume centers that offer both surgery and endovascular therapy.

The decision to treat an aneurysm endovascularly or surgically is best made in a multidisciplinary discussion. This collaboration requires both the neurosurgeon and the interventionalist to be honest about what they think they can achieve with each approach. Neurosurgery and interventional neuroradiology are not competitive facilities, but the complementary nature of techniques offers the best chance for reducing treatment morbidity and improving long-term outcome in difficult aneurysms.

Promoted by scientific data and by the institutional experience, currently more and more aneurysms are treated via the endovascular approach and in complete contrast to the situation of two decades ago – surgery is increasingly indicated in difficult endovascularly inaccessible aneurysms. Due to this circumstance the question of how to maintain the neurosurgeon's expertise is becoming increasingly important.

Regarding timing, in recent years, the strategy of overall management has changed, focussing on early referral and immediate therapeutic intervention to minimize the risk of rebleeding and enhance the possibilities of aggressive neurointensive care to prevent vasospasm and secondary ischemic complications. One benefit of the endovascular arm in ISAT was the earlier treatment compared to the surgical group.

Conclusion

Aneurysm therapy has changed in recent years. At some centers already before ISAT and in many since ISAT, endovascular therapy is the method of choice for those aneurysms that are suitable for this technique. In specialized centers, the majority of aneurysms could be treated via the endovascular approach. In addition, for selected patients stents and flow diverters have further expanded the endovascular therapeutic options especially for unruptured aneurysms. The remaining aneurysms are difficult and it will be a major challenge to maintain neurosurgical expertise for exactly these 'non-coilable' aneurysms. However, despite all the technical improvements, occlusion of a ruptured aneurysm is often not the most difficult part of the therapy. The disease is the subarachnoid hemorrhage and that determines patient outcome. Instead of fighting about 'who should do what', all disciplines should now focus on the remaining problems of the disease.

READING LIST

Asgari S, Doerfler A, Wanke I, *et al.* Complementary management of partially occluded aneurysms by using surgical or endovascular therapy. *J Neurosurg* 2002; **97**: 843–50.

Bavinzski G, Killer M, Gruber A, *et al.* Treatment of basilar artery bifurcation aneurysms by using Guglielmi detachable coils: a 6-year experience. *J Neurosurg* 1999; **90**: 843–52.

Brilstra EH, Rinkel GJ, van der Graaf Y, *et al.* Treatment of intracranial aneurysms by embolization with coils: a systematic review. *Stroke* 1999; **30**: 470–6.

Byrne JV, Beltechi R, Yarnold JA, *et al.* Early experience in the treatment of intra-cranial aneurysms by endovascular flow diversion: a multicentre prospective study. *PLoS One* 2010; **5**: e12492.

Cognard C, Pierot L, Boulin A, *et al.* Intracranial aneurysms: endovascular treatment with mechanical detachable spirals in 60 aneurysms. *Radiology* 1999; **202**: 783–92.

Cognard C, Weill A, Spelle L, *et al.* Long-term angiographic follow-up of 169 intracranial berry aneurysms occluded with detachable coils. *Radiology* 1999; **212**: 348–56.

Diringer MN. Management of aneurysmal subarachnoid hemorrhage. *Crit Care Med* 2009; **37**: 432–40.

Doerfler A, Wanke I, Egelhof T, *et al.* Aneurysmal rupture during embolization with Guglielmi detachable coils: causes, management, and outcome. *AJNR Am J Neuroradiol* 2001; **22**: 1825-32

Ferro JM, Canhão P, Peralta R. Update on subarachnoid haemorrhage. *J Neurol* 2008; **255**: 465–79.

Gallagher JP. Obliteration of intracranial aneurysms bypilojection. *JAMA* 1963; **183**: 231–6.

Guglielmi G, Vinuela F, Sepetka I, *et al.* Electrothrombosis of saccular aneurysms via endovascular approach, part 1. Electrochemical basis, technique, and experimental results. *J Neurosurg* 1991a; **75**: 1–7.

Guglielmi G, Vinuela F, Dion J, *et al.* Electrothrombosis of saccular aneurysms via endovascular approach, part 2. Preliminary clinical experience. *J Neurosurg* 1991b; **75**: 8–14.

Guglielmi G, Vinuela F, Duckwiler G, *et al.* Endovascular treatment of posterior circulation aneurysms by electrothrombosis using electrically detachable coils. *J Neurosurg* 1992; **77**: 515–24.

Hieshima GB, Grinnell VS, Mehringer CM. A detachable balloon for therapeutic transcatheter occlusions. *Radiology* 1981; **138**: 227–8.

Johnston SC, Dudley RA, Gress DR, *et al.* Surgical and endovascular treatment of unruptured cerebral aneurysms at university hospitals. *Neurology* 1999a; **52**: 1799–1805.

Johnston SC, Wilson CB, Halbach VV, *et al.* Endovascular and surgical treatment of unruptured cerebral aneurysms: comparison of risks. *Ann Neurol* 2000; **48**: 11–19.

Kassell NF, Torner JC, Haley EC Jr, *et al.* The International Cooperative Study on the Timing of Aneurysm Surgery, part 1. Overall management results. *J Neurosurg* 1990a; **73**: 18–36.

Kassell NF, Torner JC, Jane JA, *et al.* The International Cooperative Study on the Timing of Aneurysm Surgery, part 2. Surgical results. *J Neurosurg* 1990b; **73**: 37–47.

Koivisto T, Vanninen R, Hurskainen H, *et al.* Outcomes of early endovascular versus surgical treatment of ruptured cerebral aneurysms. A prospective randomized study. *Stroke* 2000; **31**: 2369–77.

Kulcsár Z, Wetzel SG, Augsburger L, *et al.* Effect of flow diversion treatment on very small ruptured aneurysms. *Neurosurgery* 2010; **67**: 789–93.

Kulcsár Z, Ernemann U, Wetzel SG, *et al.* High-profile flow diverter (silk) implantation in the basilar artery: efficacy in the treatment of aneurysms and the role of the perforators. *Stroke* 2010; **41**: 1690–6.

Lin T, Fox AJ, Drake CG. Regrowth of aneurysm sacs from residual neck following aneurysm clipping. *J Neurosurg* 1989; **70**: 556–60.

McGuinness B, Gandhi D. Endovascular management of cerebral vasospasm. *Neurosurg Clin N Am* 2010; **21**: 281–90.

Molyneux A, Kerr R, Stratton I, *et al.* International Subarachnoid Aneurysm Trial (ISAT) of neurosurgical clipping versus endovascular coiling in 2143 patients with ruptured intracranial aneurysms: a randomised trial. *Lancet* 2002; **360**: 1267–74.

Moret J, Cognard C, Weill A, *et al.* Reconstruction technique in the treatment of wide-neck intracranial aneurysms. Long-term angiographic and clinical results. Apropos of 56 cases. *J Neuroradiol* 1997; **24**: 30–44.

Murayama Y, Vinuela F, Tateshima S, *et al.* Endovascular treatment of experimental aneurysms by use of a combination of liquid embolic agents and protective devices. *AJNR Am J Neuroradiol* 2000; **21**: 1726–35.

Murayama Y, Vinuela F, Tateshima S, *et al.* Bioabsorbable polymeric material coils for embolization of intracranial aneurysms: a preliminary experimental study. *J Neurosurg* 2001; **94**: 454–63.

Natarajan SK, Sekhar LN, Ghodke B, *et al.* Outcomes of ruptured intracranial aneurysms treated by microsurgical clipping and endovascular coiling in a high-volume center. *AJNR Am J Neuroradiol* 2008; **29**: 753–9.

Nelson PK. Neurointerventional management of intracranial aneurysms. *Neurosurg Clin North Am* 1998; **9**: 879–95.

Newell DW, Elliott JP, Eskridge JM, *et al.* Endovascular therapy for aneurysmal vasospasm. *Crit Care Clin* 1999; **15**: 685–99.

Qureshi Al, Mohammad Y, Yahia AM, *et al.* Ischemic events associated with unruptured intracranial aneurysms: multicenter clinical study and review of the literature. *Neurosurgery* 2000a; **46**: 282–9; discussion 289–90.

Qureshi Al, Luft AR, Sharma M, *et al.* Prevention and treatment of thromboembolic and ischemic complications associated with endovascular procedures, part II. Clinical aspects and recommendations. *Neurosurgery* 2000b; **46**: 1360–75; discussion 1375.

Raaymakers T, Rinkel G, Limburg M, *et al.* Mortality and morbidity of surgery for unruptured intracranial aneurysms. *Stroke* 1998a; **29**: 1531–8.

Raymond J, Roy D. Safety and efficacy of endovascular treatment of acutely ruptured aneurysms. *Neurosurgery* 1997; **41**: 1235–45; discussion 1245.

Rinkel GJ, Prins NE, Algra A. Outcome of aneurysmal subarachnoid hemorrhage in patients on anticoagulant treatment. *Stroke* 1997; **28**: 6–9.

Schievink WI, Wijdicks EF, Piepgras DG, *et al.* The poor prognosis of ruptured intracranial aneurysms of the posterior circulation. *J Neurosurg* 1995; **82**: 791–5.

Scott RB, Eccles F, Molyneux AJ, *et al.* Improved cognitive outcomes with endovascular coiling of ruptured intracranial aneurysms: neuropsychological outcomes from the International Subarachnoid Aneurysm Trial (ISAT). *Stroke* 2010; **41**: 1743–7.

Serbinenko FA. Balloon occlusion of saccular aneurysms of the cerebral arteries. *Vopr Neirokhir.* 1974a; Jul–Aug; (4): 8–15.

Serbinenko FA. Balloon catheterization and occlusion of major cerebral vessels. *J Neurosurg* 1974b; **41**: 125–45.

Song JK, Elliott JP, Eskridge JM. Neuroradiologic diagnosis and treatment of vasospasm. *Neuroimaging Clin North Am* 1997; **7**: 819–35.

Van Rooij WJ, Sluzewski M, Metz NH, *et al.* Carotid balloon occlusion for large and giant aneurysms: evaluation of a new test occlusion protocol. *Neurosurgery* 2000; **47**: 116–21; discussion 122.

Velpean A. Memoir sur la piqûre ou l'acupuncture des artères dans le traitement des anéurismes. *Gaz Méd De Par.* 1831; **2**: 1.

Vinuela F, Duckwiler G, Mawad M. Guglielmi detachable coil embolization of acute intracranial aneurysm: perioperative anatomical and clinical outcome in 403 patients. *J Neurosurg* 1997; **86**: 475–82.

Wanke I, Doerfler A, Dietrich U, *et al.* Combined endovascular therapy of ruptured aneurysms and cerebral vasospasm. *Neuroradiology* 2000; **42**:926–9.

Wanke I, Doerfler A, Dietrich U, *et al.* Endovascular treatment of unruptured intracranial aneurysms. *AJNR Am J Neuroradiol* 2002; **23**: 756–61.

Wanke I, Doerfler A, Schoch B, *et al.* Treatment of wide-necked intracranial aneurysms with a self-expanding stent system: initial clinical experience. *AJNR Am J Neuroradiol* 2003; **24**: 1192–9.

Werner SC, Blakemore AH, King BG. Aneurysm of the internal carotid artery within the skull: wiring and electrothermic coagulation. *JAMA* 1941; **116**: 578–82.

32

Management of vasospasm in subarachnoid hemorrhage

Rajat Dhar and Michael C. Diringer

Introduction

Delayed cerebral ischemia and the vasospasm: concepts and history

The early brain injury from aneurysmal rupture is associated with substantial morbidity and mortality, including the risks of rebleeding, elevations in intracranial pressure, and development of hydrocephalus. However, even those surviving this initial period after subarachnoid hemorrhage (SAH) in good clinical condition may subsequently deteriorate, developing neurological deficits and/or cerebral infarction. This process is termed *delayed cerebral ischemia* (DCI) and is the major contributor to secondary brain injury and residual neurological disability in survivors of SAH (1).

Pathologic narrowing of proximal intracranial arteries was first noted after SAH with the advent of cerebral angiography in the 1950s (2). This phenomenon, termed cerebral vasospasm, has been associated with neurological deterioration (3), reductions in cerebral blood flow (CBF) (4), and ischemic brain lesions (5). Angiographic vasospasm develops in as many as two-thirds of patients after SAH, with peak onset 4–10 days post-bleeding and usually regresses by the third week (6). The association of vasospasm with neurological deficits and DCI has fostered the interchangeable but misleading use of these terms. Vasospasm should be reserved to only describe the vascular/radiographic abnormality (7).

Development of vasospasm is strongly linked to the volume of cisternal and ventricular blood in SAH (8,9). Clinically useful predictive scales for vasospasm grade degree of SAH and intraventricular hemorrhage (IVH) on initial head CT (see Table 32.1) (10). Extravasated red blood cells release vasoactive and inflammatory mediators as they break down within the subarachnoid space (12). Oxy-hemoglobin, for example, is a potent stimulant of the inflammatory cascade, leading to ingress of activated neutrophils to the CSF (13). This process leads to an imbalance between the endogenous vasodilator, nitric oxide, which is scavenged by erythrocytes, and the powerful vasoconstrictor, endothelin-1 (14), resulting in vasoconstriction as well as inflammatory changes in the vessel wall. Reduction in arterial caliber, when severe, may reduce distal perfusion and regional CBF sufficiently to impair neuronal function, resulting in deficits and eventually irreversible ischemic injury.

However, the link between vasospasm and DCI is increasingly being questioned, and is at least not as straightforward or linear as first presumed (15). Firstly, the majority of patients with angiographic vasospasm do not develop ischemic deficits or infarction. Capacity for distal vasodilation, adequacy of collateral circulation, blood pressure, and volume status all modulate tissue perfusion in addition to severity of arterial narrowing. There are also patients with delayed neurological deterioration after SAH who do not have any angiographic vasospasm, and a similar proportion (33% in one study)

Critical Care of the Stroke Patient, ed. Stefan Schwab, Daniel Hanley, and A. David Mendelow. Published by Cambridge University Press.

Table 32.1 Modified Fisher Scale

Grade	Cisternal blood	Intraventricular hemorrhage	Risk of DCI
0	None	Absent	Negligible
1	Thin	Absent	12–24%
2	Thin	Present	21–33%
3	Thick	Absent	19–33%
4	Thick	Present	40%

Thick SAH considered present if at least one cistern is filled; IVH considered present if blood is seen layering in at least both lateral ventricles. Data from (10,11).

of those with infarction on brain imaging who do not exhibit abnormality in the corresponding vascular supply (16,17). Finally, a poor concordance has been found between treatments that are able to reduce vasospasm and a reduction in cerebral infarction or poor outcomes (18). Focusing on reducing vasospasm alone may not adequately combat the complex interplay of processes leading to ischemic brain injury. Investigators are now looking beyond the basic vascular theory of ischemia at other factors contributing to delayed ischemic brain injury (19).

Cerebral ischemia results from reductions in CBF such that oxygen delivery is inadequate to meet metabolic demands (see Chapter 2). Almost all patients exhibit some reduction in CBF after SAH, even prior to or in the absence of vasospasm, although this reduction appears matched to a reduction in cerebral metabolism (4). Those developing vasospasm have lower CBF than those without it, along with elevated oxygen extraction fraction (resulting in oligemia) (20), with deficits developing when oxygen extraction cannot meet cellular demands. However, reductions in regional CBF do not correlate well with territories affected by vasospasm (21,22). Hypoperfusion and oligemia can be seen in vascular territories (and patients) without angiographic vasospasm. It may be that vasospasm is an imperfect marker of the complex vascular-inflammatory process underlying DCI that is occurring primarily at a microcirculatory/tissue level, with the large-vessel changes an epiphenomenon.

In the setting of autoregulatory dysfunction, as may occur after SAH, cerebral perfusion becomes pressure-dependent, meaning that reductions in systemic blood pressure can worsen CBF and precipitate ischemia. This may be further worsened by hypovolemia, a clear risk-factor for infarction, as is anemia (23,24). Ischemic deficits are often nonspecific (e.g. alterations in cognition and level of consciousness) and tend to fluctuate, a consequence of the multifocal non-occlusive ischemia common after SAH. Less often, focal neurological deficits develop, when ischemia occurs in eloquent (motor/language) brain regions. Ischemia may also be clinically silent (or difficult to detect) if localized to relatively silent brain regions or in patients remaining in poor clinical condition or requiring sedation. It may only be appreciated when infarction develops, at which point irreversible injury has already occurred (although subtle radiographic hypodensity is not always irreversible in the setting of acute DCI). As the strongest predictor of poor neurological recovery after SAH, therapeutic and research focus should be on minimizing cerebral infarction, rather than just reducing or reversing vasospasm (7,25,26).

Prevention of vasospasm and delayed cerebral ischemia

The time interval between aneurysmal rupture and onset of cerebral ischemia after SAH affords the opportunity to prevent infarction. A number of experimental and clinical studies aimed at the prevention of both vasospasm and ischemia after SAH have been performed. However, despite this unique window for neuroprotective therapies, such studies have largely been disappointing (27). In fact, the only intervention supported by good-quality evidence is the L-type calcium-channel blocker, nimodipine (28). Given enterally (or often intravenously in Europe), nimodipine improved outcomes and reduced ischemia in patients with SAH, but did not seem to reduce angiographic vasospasm, again highlighting the lack of correlation between these two measures. Its beneficial effect may not be mediated by its vasodilatory properties but via a neuroprotective mechanism. All patients with SAH should receive nimodipine (60 mg every 4 hours) for 21 days after bleeding; if significant drops in blood pressure occur, more frequent lower-dose administration (e.g. 30 mg every 4 hours, or lowering the infusion rate) can be attempted (29). Another calcium-channel antagonist, nicardipine, has been tested in SAH patients and reduced vasospasm without improving outcomes (30).

Clazosentan is an endothelin receptor antagonist; preliminary studies confirmed the dose-dependent ability of intravenous clazosentan to significantly reduce angiographic vasospasm (31). However, phase III studies were unable to demonstrate any associated improvement in neurological outcomes with clazosentan administration (32). This disappointing lack of benefit may be explained by the complexity of the association between vasospasm and ischemic brain injury after SAH, our improved ability to manage vasospasm and prevent infarction/disability, as well as potential adverse effects occurring from drug treatment, including a higher incidence of pulmonary edema and hypotension.

Magnesium is another vasodilator with neuroprotective properties that has been tested in SAH with conflicting results (33). A meta-analysis of six trials through 2011 found a reduction in cerebral infarction (OR 0.6, 95% CI 0.40–0.88) that did not persist when excluding a study of lower methodological quality, and no overall improvement in functional outcome with treatment (34). More recently, a phase three randomized multicenter study with 1204 patients found no difference in outcomes (35). Although magnesium infusion cannot be recommended at this time, targeting normal magnesium levels seems a reasonable goal for all SAH patients.

Circulating blood volume is often reduced after SAH as a result of natriuresis and cerebral salt wasting (36). The importance of preserving volume status was highlighted by the observation that SAH patients who were fluid restricted in response to hyponatremia demonstrated a much higher incidence of cerebral infarction than those allowed adequate fluid intake (23). Avoiding hypovolemia is of paramount importance after SAH; this necessitates strict monitoring of fluid intakes and outputs (although fluid balance correlates poorly with actual measurement of circulating blood volume) and continued intravenous fluid administration, with isotonic crystalloid solutions most often recommended, titrated to balance output. There is a general consensus that central venous pressure (CVP) or pulmonary artery pressures alone should not be used to guide volume resuscitation after SAH (29); newer noninvasive hemodynamic metrics such as stroke volume or pulse pressure variation may be useful for such monitoring, but require further study.

Given the importance of volume status to cerebral perfusion, studies have tested whether prophylactic hypervolemia can prevent ischemia better than maintaining euvolemia. One randomized study used boluses of 5% albumin to keep CVP above either 5 or 8 mmHg, but did not find that higher filling pressures were able to either improve CBF or prevent ischemia (37). The optimal fluid regimen for prevention of DCI after SAH appears to be the assiduous targeting of euvolemia. Clinical assessment of volume status and balancing intake and output may be the simplest (albeit suboptimal) means of achieving this goal. Hypervolemia incurs additional risks, including pulmonary edema, without any clear benefit. The mineralocorticoid fludrocortisone may prevent the natriuresis seen after SAH and minimize volume contraction, and is an option in cases where maintaining euvolemia and blood pressure is threatened by excessive natriuresis with negative fluid balance (38). While permissive hypertension (i.e. discontinuation of anti-hypertensive agents) is recommended to facilitate adequate perfusion after SAH (once the ruptured aneurysm has been definitely secured), prophylactic induced hypertension does not seem to confer any additional benefit (39).

Given the strong association between volume of cisternal blood after SAH with vasospasm (8), and the implication of blood breakdown in the pathophysiology of DCI, attempts to promote removal of subarachnoid blood have been evaluated. A lumbar drain may be one relatively simple and effective means of removing cisternal blood. A recent single-center study randomized good-grade SAH patients to insertion of lumbar drain or standard therapy (40). Of 105 patients in each arm, incidence of delayed ischemic neurological deficits was reduced from 35% to 21% in the lumbar drainage group

Table 32.2 Studies testing anti-inflammatory therapies for the prevention of delayed cerebral ischemia

Agent	Mechanism	Study	Vasospasm/DCI	Outcome
Corticosteroids (42)	Inhibit cyclo-oxygenase and lipid peroxidation	RCT n = 95	No change	Trend to better 1-year outcome
Tirilazad (43)	Inhibits lipid peroxidation Free radical scavenger	Meta-analysis n = 3821	OR 0.81 (95% CI 0.69–0.93) for delayed ischemic deficits/infarction	No change in death or poor outcome
Edaravone (44)	Free radical scavenger	RCT n = 91	Ischemic deficits 10% vs. 21% (p = 0.12) Cerebral infarction 4% vs. 21% (p = 0.01)	Trend to better outcome (92% vs. 83% favorable, p = 0.12)
Acetylsalicylic acid (45)	Anti-inflammatory Anti-platelet	RCT n = 161	Increased with ASA	No change in outcome
'Statins' (46)	Restore eNOS (increase NO) Block neutrophils Improve endothelial function, prevent apoptosis, etc.	Meta-analysis of four RCTs n = 190	No reduction in TCD-defined vasospasm. Trend to fewer ischemic deficits (OR 0.57, 95% CI 0.29–1.13)	No change in poor outcome but trend to lower mortality (OR 0.37, 95% CI 0.13–1.10)

DCI = delayed cerebral ischemia; TCD = transcranial Doppler; NO = nitric oxide; eNOS = endothelial NO synthase.

(p = 0.02). However, 6-month disability was not improved despite an improvement in acute neurological status.

A number of studies have linked inflammatory markers and evidence of inflammatory activation after SAH to development of vasospasm and outcome (41). This has led to considerable interest in therapies that block these inflammatory pathways as a means of reducing the burden of ischemia. Trials evaluating a number of these potential therapies, including statins, are summarized in Table 32.2. At this time, no agent has sufficient evidence to justify its routine use in SAH (29). However, for patients already on statins prior to SAH, these should be continued.

The observation that intracranial angioplasty durably reversed narrowing in vasospastic segments prompted a multi-center study of prophylactic angioplasty in high-risk SAH patients (47). Eighty-five patients with high Fisher grade SAH underwent angioplasty of most proximal intracranial arteries within 96 hours of SAH, once their ruptured aneurysm was secured. Three patients died as a result of complications from this procedure. The incidence of transcranial Doppler (TCD)-defined vasospasm and delayed ischemic deficits was not significantly reduced by pre-treatment. Fewer patients required therapeutic angioplasty for refractory vasospasm in the prophylactically-treated group (12% vs. 26%, p = 0.03) but there was no difference in neurological outcome. Prophylactic angioplasty cannot be recommended even for high-risk SAH patients.

Detection of vasospasm

Catheter angiography is the gold standard for evaluation of cerebral vasospasm, although newer and less invasive imaging modalities are increasingly being utilized, especially for screening and in asymptomatic patients. CT angiography may offer reliable visualization of proximal vasospasm, with sensitivity of 80% and specificity of 93% compared to catheter angiography (48). Limitations include contrast and radiation exposure (limiting repeat studies), overestimation of proximal vasospasm in some cases, and insensitivity for more distal vasospasm. The most noninvasive (albeit indirect) assessment of vessel diameter can be obtained by TCD measurement of proximal arterial blood flow velocities, allowing serial measurements (49). However, TCD is operator-dependent, not all patients have bone windows to allow adequate insonation, and correlation of elevated TCD velocities with both vasospasm and cerebral perfusion is limited (21). TCD evaluation has moderate sensitivity (67%) but high specificity (99%) for middle cerebral artery vasospasm (50). A trend of rapidly rising velocities and an increase in MCA velocity relative to the extracranial internal carotid artery (the Lindegaard ratio) are both additional specific markers of developing vasospasm. The accuracy of TCD for predicting vasospasm in other intracranial arteries is suboptimal, limiting the ability of TCD to reliably exclude vasospasm throughout the intracranial circulation.

Detection of delayed cerebral ischemia

An operational definition of clinical deterioration related to delayed cerebral ischemia has recently been outlined (7). It encompasses focal neurological deficits (e.g. hemiparesis, aphasia) or reduction in Glasgow Coma Scale (by at least two points), lasting for at least 1 hour. Onset is typically more than 3 days after SAH. Confounders must first be excluded, including fever, infection, metabolic abnormalities (such as hyponatremia, hypoglycemia or hypoxia), seizures (including non-convulsive seizures, or the post-ictal state), hydrocephalus, rebleeding, cerebral edema, and deficits that were present immediately after (and attributed to) aneurysm-securing procedures. Close clinical monitoring in a specialized neurological/neurosurgical intensive care unit (with trained bedside nurses) is optimal for early detection of such often subtle changes in neurological status. For this reason, and many others relating to the complexity of managing patients with SAH, an emphasis has been placed on caring for such patients in centers with adequate experience with SAH, including an organized neurointensive care unit (29). Detection of DCI is even more challenging in those in poor neurological condition as a result of SAH or those requiring sedative medications, in whom ischemia may be missed, leading to 'silent' cerebral infarction, a marker of poor outcome (51,52). Such clinically inaccessible patients may benefit from increased neuromonitoring, whether with TCD and/or CT angiography to evaluate for vasospasm, accompanied by measures of cerebral perfusion or tissue metabolism.

Intracranial probes are now available that continuously measure both local CBF and brain tissue tension of oxygen (P_bO_2). P_bO_2 appears to reflect a balance of oxygen delivery and extraction/utilization, but has not been adequately evaluated for detection of ischemia after SAH. A study of CBF monitoring in SAH found that a reduction in focal perfusion was associated with vasospasm more strongly than were changes in TCD velocities (53). Cerebral microdialysis (allowing measurement of lactate/pyruvate as markers of tissue ischemia) has shown some promise in small series, but it is unclear whether changes in metabolites can reliably be detected early enough to provide a useful marker of imminent ischemia (54). The fundamental limitation of all such focal measures of brain perfusion/metabolism lies in their inability to detect changes outside a very small radius around the probe. With vasospasm and DCI being multifocal processes, a single regional measurement may miss significant abnormalities elsewhere. Greater investigation of the role of such neuro-monitoring devices is required before they can be widely adopted in SAH.

Perfusion imaging offers an alternative physiological assessment of ischemia and may be able to detect reductions in CBF in asymptomatic patients at high risk for deterioration or in those without accessible neurological examination. CT perfusion may be performed concurrently with CT angiography and offers complementary information and assessment of multiple brain regions (55). Hypoperfusion may best be estimated by increased mean transit time (MTT). A study assessing CT perfusion in those with clinical deterioration after SAH found CTP to have better positive predictive value for DCI (at 88%) than both non-contrast CT and CT angiography (56). A follow-up study found that a MTT threshold of 5.9 seconds provided optimal sensitivity and specificity (57). MR perfusion is less widely available and less feasible in unstable critically ill patients, but can similarly be used to estimate perfusion delay; it offers the advantage of better visualizing cerebral infarcts than CT (58).

Perfusion imaging may be especially useful in patients with (TCD or angiographic) vasospasm but who are either asymptomatic (i.e. remain in good clinical condition) or whose exam is moribund and the implications of vasospasm (on perfusion and risk of ischemia) are therefore unclear.

Triggers and targets for aggressive interventions

Early detection of DCI allows prompt interventions to prevent permanent neurological deficits and infarction. High-risk patients may be identified by the modified Fisher scale (Table 32.1) and severity of clinical presentation, but positive predictive value of these remains poor (10). Aggressive interventions such as prophylactic hypertension or hypervolemia are not recommended even in high-risk subgroups. The development of new clinical deterioration due to ischemia (after exclusion of confounders) is a definite indication for aggressive intervention. It may also warrant angiographic evaluation for vasospasm, not only to corroborate the impression of vasospasm-associated DCI, but to allow endovascular interventions if vasospasm is severe. Softer triggers for intervening include asymptomatic elevation in TCD velocities or vasospasm on screening angiography. Specific thresholds to initiate therapy based on TCD or angiography are not clear (but should likely be limited to only severe vasospasm and/or if accompanied by symptoms or perfusion abnormality). Similarly, finding of a new vascular hypodensity on brain imaging may prompt interventions aimed at avoiding further ischemia, although aggressive hemodynamic augmentation in the face of a large infarct may risk exacerbating edema or inducing hemorrhagic transformation (59). A reduction in perfusion (e.g. using CT or MR perfusion techniques or intracranial monitoring) may serve as a useful marker that a patient is at high risk for imminent ischemic damage and warrants hemodynamic interventions and/or evaluation for vasospasm.

Hemodynamic interventions

The primary goal of interventions for DCI is restoration of adequate CBF and oxygen delivery. This may be assessed (depending on the trigger for treatment) based on reversal of neurological deficits, improvement in measures of perfusion, or reversal of severe angiographic vasospasm (if endovascular treatments are being employed). Notably, improvement (i.e. a reduction) in TCD velocities cannot be used as a marker of either improved perfusion or reduction in vasospasm when hemodynamic therapies are used (60).

The ability of increases in systemic blood pressure to augment CBF was first proposed by Denny-Brown in 1951 (61). The combination of induced hypertension, hypervolemia, and an element of hemodilution was systematically applied to patients with SAH in the 1970s and 1980s under the rubric 'triple-H therapy' (62,63), facilitated by a shift to early aneurysm treatment. Although no controlled studies have been performed to confirm the efficacy of this therapeutic approach, a number of series have documented high rates of neurological improvement (generally exceeding 70%) with such hemodynamic interventions (63,64).

It appears that induced hypertension is the central component responsible for the clinical and physiologic benefits provided by triple-H therapy (65). Increasing cerebral perfusion pressure (CPP) is the only intervention that clearly improves CBF after SAH (66). Induction of hypervolemia (e.g. with a fluid bolus) has minimal impact on CBF, although it provided benefit to regions with low CBF in a small study of symptomatic patients (67). Hemodilution may induce a small rise in CBF but this occurs at the expense of lower net oxygen delivery, as arterial oxygen content is reduced at lower hemoglobin levels (68). In fact, the addition of hypervolemic hemodilution abrogated the physiologic benefit of induced hypertension, likely by counteracting any rise in CBF with a reduction of oxygen delivery at lower hemoglobin (65).

Selection of fluids and vasopressors is largely empiric, with some recommending colloids such as albumin to maintain volume status and/or induce hypervolemia. No studies have demonstrated superiority of this approach over the cheaper (and potentially safer) use of crystalloids such as isotonic saline. A clinical trial of 25% albumin (albeit as a neuroprotectant not as a volume expander) is currently being conducted in SAH, based on dose-finding pilot data suggesting

studies of transfusion have included few if any patients with SAH and insufficient numbers of subjects with brain injury, in general (97). Further, there are conflicting data about an association between transfusion and worse outcomes after SAH, tempering any enthusiasm for excessive utilization of this limited resource (98).

RBC transfusion has been shown to improve cerebral oxygen delivery when given to anemic patients after SAH, at least up to hemoglobin of 10 g/dl (99). In fact, the rise in regional oxygen delivery after transfusion of one unit of RBCs appeared comparable to that seen with induced hypertension and likely superior to that seen after a fluid bolus (100). Nonetheless, it remains unclear whether this rise in oxygen delivery translates into improved oxygen utilization or a reduction in cerebral ischemia. No adequate controlled clinical studies have been performed testing transfusion in SAH, and so the optimal hemoglobin for patients at risk for delayed cerebral ischemia remains unclear. In the meantime, significant practice variability and uncertainty persist in this realm of SAH management (96). On balance, many argue that a target of 9–10 g/dl may provide the optimal balance between restriction of unnecessary transfusion and optimization of oxygen delivery, at least for patients with or at high risk for DCI.

Assessing response to therapy

It is critical to evaluate the patient's clinical response to each stage of intervention. This is easiest in patients with neurological deficits such as hemiparesis, but more challenging in those with fluctuating and/or non-focal alterations in cognition or mental status. This may not be feasible in those in whom therapy is initiated for radiographic findings of vasospasm, in whom targets must be empiric, especially when clinical examination is either normal or inaccessible; neuromonitoring or repeat perfusion studies may be useful in such cases. If deficits are reversed with therapy, then the level of hemodynamic augmentation (and specific targets) should be maintained for at least 24–72 hours before weaning is attempted. If response is incomplete, then further titration/escalation of hemodynamic therapy should be considered (e.g. initiation of vasopressors after failure of fluid bolus, see Fig. 32.1).

Endovascular therapies for vasospasm

Angiography provides the opportunity not only to confirm the presence of vasospasm but also allows therapeutic interventions to reverse arterial narrowing that may underlie some reductions in CBF and ischemic deficits. Such interventions should be considered in cases refractory to initial medical interventions, and may be more effective when initiated early after onset of deficits (101). Percutaneous transluminal angioplasty involves inflation of a balloon via a microcatheter placed across the segment of arterial narrowing. This results in a reliable and usually durable increase in luminal diameter. The procedure is limited by accessibility to smaller/distal vessel segments often including the proximal ACA and PCA as well as MCA beyond M_1. Rare complications include vessel perforation, dissection, or bleeding from a nearby aneurysm (especially if unsecured) (47). Reversal of vasospasm by angioplasty is usually sustained, with most segments not requiring retreatment. Treatment can be associated with prompt improvement in clinical deficits and an improvement in CBF.

For more distal vasospasm, intra-arterial infusion of vasodilators may reverse vessel narrowing. Use of papaverine has largely been abandoned with the advent of safer options and recognition of various complications, including raised intracranial pressure and seizures. Alternative intra-arterial vasodilators include nicardipine, nimodipine, verapamil, magnesium, and milrinone. The dilatory response to these agents is usually more transient than seen with angioplasty, and many segments require retreatment for recurrent vasospasm.

Endovascular treatment of vasospasm may also be preferred in patients with contraindications to or complications from hemodynamic therapy (e.g. cardiac instability and/or pulmonary edema), or in those who continue to experience deficits despite maximal medical therapy (especially if attributable to a focal stenosis amenable to angioplasty). In the case of focal, asymmetric vasospasm (e.g. unilateral ICA and/or MCA) with hemispheric deficits, endovascular treatment may be preferable to raising systemic pressure to reverse regional ischemia. The contralateral unaffected (and so 'unprotected') hemisphere is exposed to very high perfusion pressures from induced hypertension, with cases of

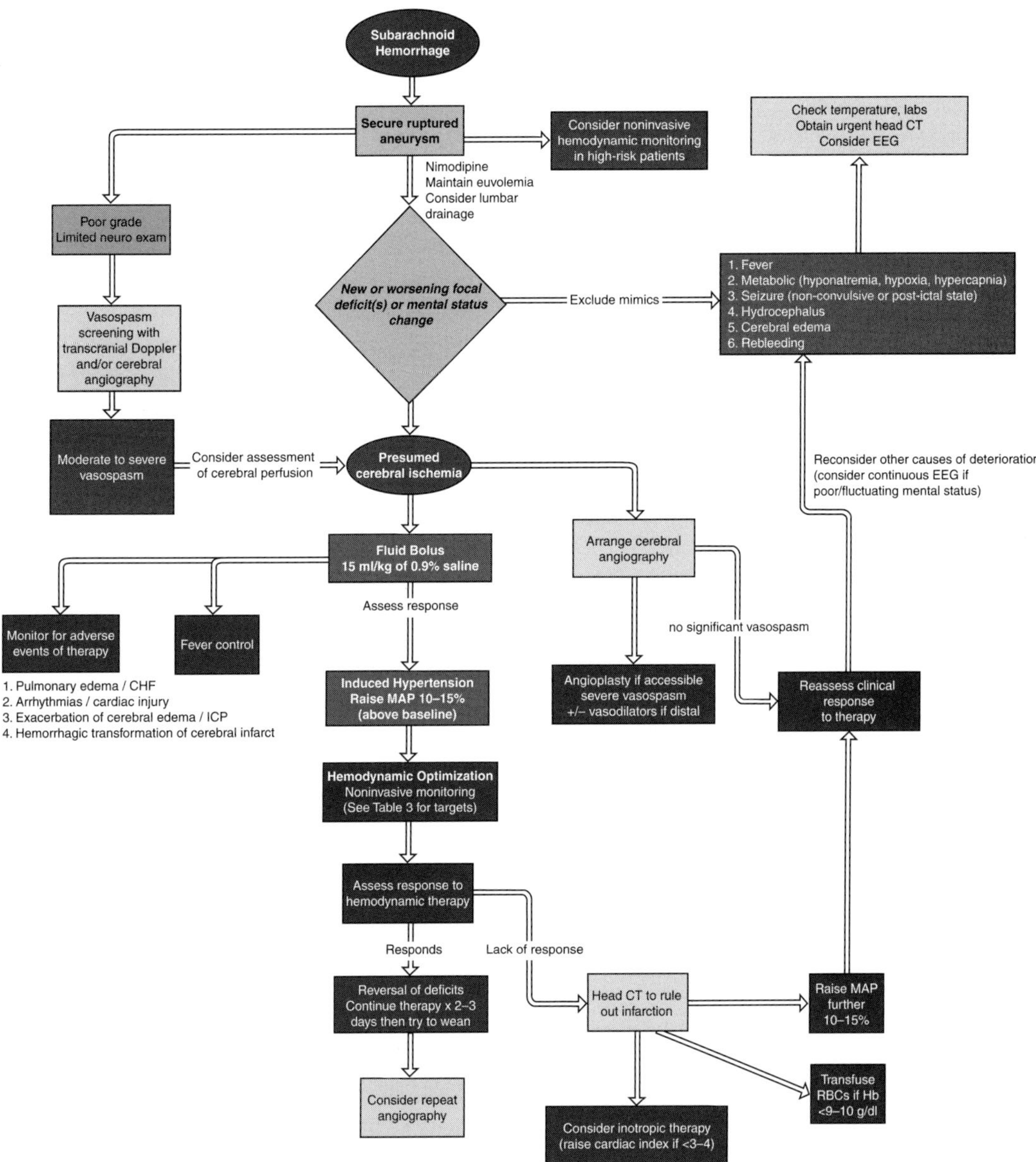

Fig. 32.1 Algorithm for management of vasospasm.

hypertensive encephalopathy ('PRES'; posterior reversible encephalopathy syndrome) being reported (102).

Complications of treatment

The benefits of preventing ischemic brain injury with hemodynamic interventions must be balanced against the risks of such aggressive physiologic manipulations. The most common adverse events with triple-H therapy are cardiopulmonary, with high rates of pulmonary edema in some series, mainly related to induction of hypervolemia with large volumes of fluids (39,63). Arrhythmias and even cardiac injury or stunning can be seen with high-dose vasopressors. Careful monitoring, whether invasively (e.g. PA catheters) or increasingly, utilizing noninvasive monitoring devices (64,79,86), may minimize these risks and allow more targeted titration of fluids and vasoactive medications. In rare cases, hemodynamic augmentation has been associated with worsening of cerebral edema and ICP (59); this was usually seen in cases with pre-existing brain injury (e.g. postoperative edema) or in cases with already developing cerebral infarction (in which hemorrhagic transformation was also seen). Caution should be exercised with hemodynamic augmentation when edema or infarction is already present (although subtle hypodensity should not serve as a contraindication). Hypertensive encephalopathy (i.e. PRES) has been reported with elevations in blood pressure and is important to distinguish from persistent/worsening ischemia, as this misattribution may lead to further efforts to raise blood pressure with the risk of worsening hydrostatic cerebral edema. Induced hypertension should also be avoided in the presence of an unprotected ruptured aneurysm, now not a common issue with near-universal early treatment of aneurysms after SAH. Rebleeding from unruptured aneurysms (even if unprotected) has not been described, and should not constitute a contraindication to hypertensive therapy if ischemia develops (103).

Adjunctive therapies for ischemia

The overarching goal of managing a patient with delayed cerebral ischemia is to minimize irreversible neuronal injury. While the focus of this approach is on restoring perfusion, and oxygen delivery, it is important to avoid exacerbating factors that increase metabolic demand and could worsen ischemic injury. For this reason, aggressive control of fever (almost ubiquitous after SAH and associated with worse outcome) in patients with or at high risk for ischemia has been advocated, but clinical benefit remains to be demonstrated. Induction of mild hypothermia for those with refractory ischemia has also been proposed as a salvage therapy, as has sedation with barbiturates (104). However, these therapies entail significant potential for adverse events and should not be used as first-line therapies. Reduction of ICP by CSF drainage in patients with ventriculostomy or lumbar catheters in place may be attempted as another approach to optimizing cerebral perfusion, especially in cases of intracranial hypertension. Hypertonic saline also reduces ICP while augmenting CBF in poor-grade SAH patients (70), and may be an ideal agent in patients with cerebral edema and vasospasm (while mannitol, with a tendency to induce diuresis and hypovolemia, should be avoided if ischemia is a concern).

Conclusions

Delayed ischemic deficits and cerebral infarction contribute significantly to poor outcome for survivors of SAH. Angiographic vasospasm does not account for the full extent of hypoperfusion underlying such delayed cerebral ischemia. Agents that combat the complex inflammatory and metabolic pathways underlying DCI are being evaluated in SAH. DCI is best detected by serial bedside evaluation, but, in patients without accessible neurological examination, monitoring with TCD, perfusion imaging and invasive neuro-monitoring devices can be considered. DCI is best treated with hemodynamic augmentation, primarily involving induced hypertension, titrated not only to hemodynamic targets, but clinical response. Noninvasive hemodynamic monitoring may aid in titrating vasoactive medications and fluids while minimizing complications such as pulmonary edema. Endovascular interventions including angioplasty should be considered if response to hemodynamic interventions is incomplete. Recommendations for critical care management of all aspects of SAH have recently been provided through in-depth recommendations from a multidisciplinary consensus conference (29).

REFERENCES

1. Heros RC, Zervas NT, Varsos V. Cerebral vasospasm after subarachnoid hemorrhage: an update. *Ann Neurol.* 1983;**14** (6):599–608.
2. Ecker A, Riemenschneider P. Arteriographic demonstration of spasm of the intracranial arteries, with special reference to saccular arterial aneurysms. *J Neurosurg.* 1951;**8**(6):660–7.

3. Fisher CM, Roberson GH, Ojemann RG. Cerebral vasospasm with ruptured saccular aneurysm – the clinical manifestations. *Neurosurgery*. 1977;**1**(3):245–8.
4. Grubb Jr RL, Raichle MEME, Eichling JOO, Gado MHH, Grubb RL. Effects of subarachnoid hemorrhage on cerebral blood volume, blood flow, and oxygen utilization in humans. *J Neurosurg*. 1977;**46**(4):446–53.
5. Allcock J, Drake C. Ruptured intracranial aneurysms – the role of arterial spasm. *J Neurosurg*. 1965;**22**:21–9.
6. Weir B, Grace M, Hansen J, Rothberg C. Time course of vasospasm in man. *J Neurosurg*. 1978;**48**(2):173–8.
7. Vergouwen MDI, Vermeulen M, Van Gijn J, *et al.* Definition of delayed cerebral ischemia after aneurysmal subarachnoid hemorrhage as an outcome event in clinical trials and observational studies: proposal of a multidisciplinary research group. *Stroke*. 2010;**41**(10):2391–5.
8. Fisher CM, Kistler JP, Davis JM. Relation of cerebral vasospasm to subarachnoid hemorrhage visualized by computerized tomographic scanning. *Neurosurgery*. 1980;**6**(1):1–9.
9. Harrod CG, Bendok BR, Batjer HH. Prediction of cerebral vasospasm in patients presenting with aneurysmal subarachnoid hemorrhage: A review. *Neurosurgery*. 2005;**56**(4):633–54.
10. Claassen J, Bernardini GL, Kreiter K, *et al.* Effect of cisternal and ventricular blood on risk of delayed cerebral ischemia after subarachnoid hemorrhage: the Fisher scale revisited. *Stroke*. 2001;**32**(9):2012–20.
11. Frontera J, Claassen J, Schmidt JM, *et al.* Prediction of symptomatic vasospasm after subarachnoid hemorrhage: the modified Fisher scale. *Neurosurgery*. 2006;**59**(1):21–7.
12. Macdonald RL, Weir BK. A review of hemoglobin and the pathogenesis of cerebral vasospasm. *Stroke*. 1991;**22**(8):971–82.
13. Chaichana KL, Pradilla G, Huang J, Tamargo RJ. Role of inflammation (leukocyte-endothelial cell interactions) in vasospasm after subarachnoid hemorrhage. *World Neurosurg*. 2010;**73**(1):22–41.
14. Seifert V, Löffler BM, Zimmermann M, Roux S, Stolke D. Endothelin concentrations in patients with aneurysmal subarachnoid hemorrhage. Correlation with cerebral vasospasm, delayed ischemic neurological deficits, and volume of hematoma. *J Neurosurg*. 1995;**82**(1):55–62.
15. Vergouwen MDI, Ilodigwe D, Macdonald RL. Cerebral infarction after subarachnoid hemorrhage contributes to poor outcome by vasospasm-dependent and -independent effects. *Stroke*. 2011;**42**(4):924–9.
16. Rabinstein A, Friedman J, Weigand SD, *et al.* Predictors of cerebral infarction in aneurysmal subarachnoid hemorrhage. *Stroke*. 2004;**35**(8):1862–6.
17. Brown RJ, Kumar A, Dhar R, Sampson TR, Diringer MN. The relationship between delayed infarcts and angiographic vasospasm after aneurysmal subarachnoid hemorrhage. *Neurosurgery*. 2013;**72**(5):702–8.
18. Etminan N, Vergouwen MDI, Ilodigwe D, Macdonald RL. Effect of pharmaceutical treatment on vasospasm, delayed cerebral ischemia, and clinical outcome in patients with aneurysmal subarachnoid hemorrhage? A systematic review and meta-analysis. *J Cerebral Blood Flow Metab*. 2011;**31**(6):1443–51.
19. Pluta RM, Hansen-Schwartz J, Dreier J, *et al.* Cerebral vasospasm following subarachnoid hemorrhage: time for a new world of thought. *Neurol Res*. 2009;**31**(2):151–8.
20. Carpenter DA, Grubb RL, Tempel LW, Powers WJ. Cerebral oxygen metabolism after aneurysmal subarachnoid hemorrhage. *J Cerebral Blood Flow Metab*. 1991;**11**(5):837–44.
21. Minhas PS, Menon DK, Smielewski P, *et al.* Positron emission tomographic cerebral perfusion disturbances and transcranial Doppler findings among patients with neurological deterioration after subarachnoid hemorrhage. *Neurosurgery*. 2003;**52**(5):1017–24.
22. Dhar R, Scalfani MT, Blackburn S, *et al.* Relationship between angiographic vasospasm and regional hypoperfusion in aneurysmal subarachnoid hemorrhage. *Stroke*. 2012;**43**(7):1788–94.
23. Wijdicks EF, Vermeulen M, Hijdra A, Van Gijn J. Hyponatremia and cerebral infarction in patients with ruptured intracranial aneurysms: is fluid restriction harmful? *Ann Neurol*. 1985;**17**(2):137–40.
24. Naidech AM, Drescher J, Ault ML, *et al.* Higher hemoglobin is associated with less cerebral infarction, poor outcome, and death after subarachnoid hemorrhage. *Neurosurgery*. 2006;**59**(4):775–9.
25. Rosengart AJ, Schultheiss KE, Tolentino J, Macdonald RL. Prognostic factors for outcome in patients with aneurysmal subarachnoid hemorrhage. *Stroke*. 2007;**38**(8):2315–21.
26. Vergouwen MDI, Etminan N, Ilodigwe D, Macdonald RL. Lower incidence of cerebral infarction correlates with improved functional outcome after aneurysmal subarachnoid hemorrhage. *J Cerebral Blood Flow Metab*. 2011;**31**(7):1545–53.
27. Laskowitz DT, Kolls BJ. Neuroprotection in subarachnoid hemorrhage. *Stroke*. 2010;**41**(10 Suppl):S79–84.
28. Dorhout Mees SM, Rinkel GJE, Feigin VL, *et al.* Calcium antagonists for aneurysmal subarachnoid haemorrhage. *Cochrane Database Syst Rev*. 2007;(3):CD000277.
29. Diringer MN, Bleck TP, Claude Hemphill J, *et al.* Critical care management of patients following aneurysmal

subarachnoid hemorrhage: Recommendations from the Neurocritical Care Society's Multidisciplinary Consensus Conference. *Neurocrit Care.* 2011;**15**(2):211–40.

30. Haley EC, Kassell NF, Torner JC. A randomized controlled trial of high-dose intravenous nicardipine in aneurysmal subarachnoid hemorrhage: A report of the Cooperative Aneurysm Study. *J Neurosurg.* 1993;**78**(4):537–47.
31. Macdonald RL, Kassell NF, Mayer S, *et al.* Clazosentan to overcome neurological ischemia and infarction occurring after subarachnoid hemorrhage (CONSCIOUS-1): randomized, double-blind, placebo-controlled phase 2 dose-finding trial. *Stroke.* 2008;**39**(11):3015–21.
32. Macdonald RL, Higashida RT, Keller E, *et al.* Clazosentan, an endothelin receptor antagonist, in patients with aneurysmal subarachnoid haemorrhage undergoing surgical clipping: a randomised, double-blind, placebo-controlled phase 3 trial (CONSCIOUS-2). *Lancet Neurol.* 2011;**10** (7):618–25.
33. Suarez JI. Magnesium sulfate administration in subarachnoid hemorrhage. *Neurocrit Care.* 2011;**15**(2):302–7.
34. Wong GK, Boet R, Poon WS, *et al.* Intravenous magnesium sulphate for aneurysmal subarachnoid hemorrhage: an updated systemic review and meta-analysis. *Crit Care.* 2011;**15**(1):R52.
35. Mees SMD, Algra A, Vandertop WP, *et al.* Magnesium for aneurysmal subarachnoid haemorrhage (MASH-2): a randomised placebo-controlled trial. *Lancet.* 2012;**380**:44–9.
36. Hoff RG, Van Dijk GW, Algra A, Kalkman CJ, Rinkel GJE. Fluid balance and blood volume measurement after aneurysmal subarachnoid hemorrhage. *Neurocrit Care.* 2008;**8**(3):391–7.
37. Lennihan L, Mayer S, Fink ME, *et al.* Effect of hypervolemic therapy on cerebral blood flow after subarachnoid hemorrhage: a randomized controlled trial. *Stroke.* 2000;**31** (2):383–91.
38. Moro N, Katayama Y, Kojima J, Mori T, Kawamata T. Prophylactic management of excessive natriuresis with hydrocortisone for efficient hypervolemic therapy after subarachnoid hemorrhage. *Stroke.* 2003;**34**(12):2807–11.
39. Egge A, Waterloo K, Sjøholm H, *et al.* Prophylactic hyperdynamic postoperative fluid therapy after aneurysmal subarachnoid hemorrhage: a clinical, prospective, randomized, controlled study. *Neurosurgery.* 2001;**49**(3):593–605.
40. Al-Tamimi YZ, Bhargava D, Feltbower RG, *et al.* Lumbar drainage of cerebrospinal fluid after aneurysmal subarachnoid hemorrhage: A prospective, randomized, controlled trial (LUMAS). *Stroke.* 2012;**43**(3):677–82.
41. Dhar R, Diringer MN. The burden of the systemic inflammatory response predicts vasospasm and outcome after subarachnoid hemorrhage. *Neurocrit Care.* 2008;**8**(3):404–12.
42. Gomis P, Graftieaux JP, Sercombe R, *et al.* Randomized, double-blind, placebo-controlled, pilot trial of high-dose methylprednisolone in aneurysmal subarachnoid hemorrhage. *J Neurosurg.* 2010;**112**(3):681–8.
43. Zhang S, Wang L, Liu M, Wu B. Tirilazad for aneurysmal subarachnoid haemorrhage. *Cochrane Database Syst Rev.* 2010;(**2**):CD006778.
44. Munakata A, Ohkuma H, Nakano T, *et al.* Effect of a free radical scavenger, edaravone, in the treatment of patients with aneurysmal subarachnoid hemorrhage. *Neurosurgery.* 2009;**64**(3):423–8.
45. Van den Bergh WM, Algra A, Dorhout Mees SM, *et al.* Randomized controlled trial of acetylsalicylic acid in aneurysmal subarachnoid hemorrhage: the MASH Study. *Stroke.* 2006;**37**(9):2326–30.
46. Vergouwen MDI, De Haan RJ, Vermeulen M, Roos YBWEM. Effect of statin treatment on vasospasm, delayed cerebral ischemia, and functional outcome in patients with aneurysmal subarachnoid hemorrhage: a systematic review and meta-analysis update. *Stroke.* 2010;**41**(1):47–52.
47. Zwienenberg-Lee M, Hartman J, Rudisill N, *et al.* Effect of prophylactic transluminal balloon angioplasty on cerebral vasospasm and outcome in patients with Fisher grade III subarachnoid hemorrhage: results of a phase II multicenter, randomized, clinical trial. *Stroke.* 2008;**39**(6):1759–65.
48. Greenberg ED, Gold R, Reichman M, *et al.* Diagnostic accuracy of CT angiography and CT perfusion for cerebral vasospasm: a meta-analysis. *Am J Neuroradiol.* 2010;**31** (10):1853–60.
49. Saqqur M, Zygun D, Demchuk A. Role of transcranial Doppler in neurocritical care. *Crit Care Med.* 2007;**35**(5 Suppl):S216–23.
50. Lysakowski C, Walder B, Costanza MC, Tramèr MR. Transcranial Doppler versus angiography in patients with vasospasm due to a ruptured cerebral aneurysm: A systematic review. *Stroke.* 2001;**32**(10):2292–8.
51. Rabinstein AA, Weigand S, Atkinson JLD, Wijdicks EF. Patterns of cerebral infarction in aneurysmal subarachnoid hemorrhage. *Stroke.* 2005;**36**(5):992–7.
52. Schmidt JM, Wartenberg KE, Fernandez A, *et al.* Frequency and clinical impact of asymptomatic cerebral infarction due to vasospasm after subarachnoid hemorrhage. *J Neurosurg.* 2008;**109**(6):1052–9.
53. Vajkoczy P, Horn P, Thome C, Munch E, Schmiedek P. Regional cerebral blood flow monitoring in the diagnosis

of delayed ischemia following aneurysmal subarachnoid hemorrhage. *J Neurosurg.* 2003;**98**(6):1227–34.
54. Sandsmark DK, Kumar MA, Park S, Levine JM. Multimodal monitoring in subarachnoid hemorrhage. *Stroke.* 2012;**43**:1440–45.
55. Binaghi S, Colleoni ML, Maeder P, *et al.* CT angiography and perfusion CT in cerebral vasospasm after subarachnoid hemorrhage. *Am J Neuroradiol.* 2007;**28**(4):750–8.
56. Dankbaar JW, De Rooij NK, Velthuis BK, *et al.* Diagnosing delayed cerebral ischemia with different CT modalities in patients with subarachnoid hemorrhage with clinical deterioration. *Stroke.* 2009;**40**(11):3493–8.
57. Dankbaar JW, De Rooij NK, Rijsdijk M, *et al.* Diagnostic threshold values of cerebral perfusion measured with computed tomography for delayed cerebral ischemia after aneurysmal subarachnoid hemorrhage. *Stroke.* 2010;**41**(9):1927–32.
58. Weidauer S, Lanfermann H, Raabe A, *et al.* Impairment of cerebral perfusion and infarct patterns attributable to vasospasm after aneurysmal subarachnoid hemorrhage: a prospective MRI and DSA study. *Stroke.* 2007;**38**(6):1831–6.
59. Shimoda M, Oda S, Tsugane R, Sato O. Intracranial complications of hypervolemic therapy in patients with a delayed ischemic deficit attributed to vasospasm. *J Neurosurg.* 1993;**78**(3):423–9.
60. Manno EM, Gress DR, Schwamm LH, Diringer MN, Ogilvy CS. Effects of induced hypertension on transcranial Doppler ultrasound velocities in patients after subarachnoid hemorrhage. *Stroke.* 1998;**29**(2):422–8.
61. Denny-Brown D. The treatment of recurrent cerebrovascular symptoms and the question of 'vasospasm'. *Med Clin North Am.* 1951;**35**:1470–4.
62. Kosnik EJ, Hunt WE. Postoperative hypertension in the management of patients with intracranial arterial aneurysms. *J Neurosurg.* 1976;**45**(2):148–54.
63. Kassell NF, Peerless SJ, Durward QJ, *et al.* Treatment of ischemic deficits from vasospasm with intravascular volume expansion and induced arterial hypertension. *Neurosurgery.* 1982;**11**(3):337–43.
64. Miller JA, Dacey RG, Diringer MN. Safety of hypertensive hypervolemic therapy with phenylephrine in the treatment of delayed ischemic deficits after subarachnoid hemorrhage. *Stroke.* 1995;**26**(12):2260–6.
65. Muench E, Horn P, Bauhuf C, *et al.* Effects of hypervolemia and hypertension on regional cerebral blood flow, intracranial pressure, and brain tissue oxygenation after subarachnoid hemorrhage. *Crit Care Med.* 2007;**35**(8):1844–51.
66. Dankbaar JW, Slooter AJ, Rinkel GJ, Schaaf IC Van Der. Effect of different components of triple-H therapy on cerebral perfusion in patients with aneurysmal subarachnoid haemorrhage: a systematic review. *Crit Care.* 2010;**14**(1):R23.
67. Jost SC, Diringer MN, Zazulia AR, *et al.* Effect of normal saline bolus on cerebral blood flow in regions with low baseline flow in patients with vasospasm following subarachnoid hemorrhage. *J Neurosurg.* 2005;**103**(1):25–30.
68. Ekelund A, Reinstrup P, Ryding E, *et al.* Effects of iso- and hypervolemic hemodilution on regional cerebral blood flow and oxygen delivery for patients with vasospasm after aneurysmal subarachnoid hemorrhage. *Acta Neurochir* (Wien). 2002;**144**(7):703–12.
69. Suarez JI, Martin RH, Calvillo E, *et al.* The Albumin in Subarachnoid Hemorrhage (ALISAH) multicenter pilot clinical trial: Safety and neurologic outcomes. *Stroke.* 2012;**43**(3):683–90.
70. Al-Rawi PG, Tseng M-Y, Richards HK, *et al.* Hypertonic saline in patients with poor-grade subarachnoid hemorrhage improves cerebral blood flow, brain tissue oxygen, and pH. *Stroke.* 2010;**41**(1):122–8.
71. Meyer R, Deem S, Yanez ND, *et al.* Current practices of triple-H prophylaxis and therapy in patients with subarachnoid hemorrhage. *Neurocrit Care.* 2011;**14**(1):24–36.
72. Muehlschlegel S, Dunser MW, Gabrielli A, Wenzel V, Layon AJ. Arginine vasopressin as a supplementary vasopressor in refractory hypertensive, hypervolemic, hemodilutional therapy in subarachnoid hemorrhage. *Neurocrit Care.* 2007;**6**:3–10.
73. Kim DH, Joseph M, Ziadi S, *et al.* Increases in cardiac output can reverse flow deficits from vasospasm independent of blood pressure: A study using xenon computed tomographic measurement of cerebral blood flow. *Neurosurgery.* 2003;**53**(5):1044–52.
74. Levy ML, Rabb CH, Zelman V, Giannotta SL. Cardiac performance enhancement from dobutamine in patients refractory to hypervolemic therapy for cerebral vasospasm. *J Neurosurg.* 1993;**79**(4):494–9.
75. Fraticelli AT, Cholley BP, Losser M-R, Saint Maurice J-P, Payen D. Milrinone for the treatment of cerebral vasospasm after aneurysmal subarachnoid hemorrhage. *Stroke.* 2008;**39**(3):893–8.
76. Romero CM, Morales D, Reccius A, *et al.* Milrinone as a rescue therapy for symptomatic refractory cerebral vasospasm in aneurysmal subarachnoid hemorrhage. *Neurocrit Care.* 2009;**11**(2):165–71.
77. Lannes M, Teitelbaum J, Corte P, Angle M. Milrinone and homeostasis to treat cerebral vasospasm associated

with subarachnoid hemorrhage: The Montreal Neurological Hospital Protocol. *Neurocrit Care.* 2012;**16**:354–62.

78. Lazaridis C, Pradilla G, Nyquist PA, Tamargo RJ. Intra-aortic balloon pump counterpulsation in the setting of subarachnoid hemorrhage, cerebral vasospasm, and neurogenic stress cardiomyopathy. Case report and review of the literature. *Neurocrit Care.* 2010;**13**(1):101–8.
79. Pritz MB, Giannotta SL, Kindt GW, McGillicuddy JE, Prager RL. Treatment of patients with neurological deficits associated with cerebral vasospasm by intravascular volume expansion. *Neurosurgery.* 1978;**3**(3):364–8.
80. Kim DH, Haney CL, Van Ginhoven G. Reduction of pulmonary edema after SAH with a pulmonary artery catheter-guided hemodynamic management protocol. *Neurocrit Care.* 2005;**3**(1):11–15.
81. Shah MR, Hasselblad V, Stevenson LW, *et al.* Impact of the pulmonary artery catheter in critically ill patients: meta-analysis of randomized clinical trials. *JAMA.* 2005;**294**(13):1664–70.
82. Rosenwasser RH, Jallo JI, Getch CC, Liebman KE. Complications of Swan-Ganz catheterization for hemodynamic monitoring in patients with subarachnoid hemorrhage. *Neurosurgery.* 1995;**37**(5):872–5.
83. Kumar A, Anel R, Bunnell E, *et al.* Pulmonary artery occlusion pressure and central venous pressure fail to predict ventricular filling volume, cardiac performance, or the response to volume infusion in normal subjects. *Crit Care Med.* 2004;**32**(3):691–9.
84. Berkenstadt H, Margalit N, Hadani M, *et al.* Stroke volume variation as a predictor of fluid responsiveness in patients undergoing brain surgery. *Anesth Analg.* 2001;**92**(4):984–9.
85. Thiel SW, Kollef MH, Isakow W. Non-invasive stroke volume measurement and passive leg raising predict volume responsiveness in medical ICU patients: an observational cohort study. *Critical Care.* 2009;**13**(4):R111.
86. Mutoh T, Kazumata K, Ajiki M, Ushikoshi S, Terasaka S. Goal-directed fluid management by bedside transpulmonary hemodynamic monitoring after subarachnoid hemorrhage. *Stroke.* 2007;**38**(12):3218–24.
87. Mutoh T, Kazumata K, Ishikawa T, Terasaka S. Performance of bedside transpulmonary thermodilution monitoring for goal-directed hemodynamic management after subarachnoid hemorrhage. *Stroke.* 2009;**40**(7):2368–74.
88. Mutoh T, Kazumata K, Kobayashi S, Terasaka S, Ishikawa T. Serial measurement of extravascular lung water and blood volume during the course of neurogenic pulmonary edema after subarachnoid hemorrhage: initial experience with 3 cases. *J Neurosurg Anesthesiol.* 2012;**24**:203–8.
89. Kramer AH, Zygun D, Bleck TP, *et al.* Relationship between hemoglobin concentrations and outcomes across subgroups of patients with aneurysmal subarachnoid hemorrhage. *Neurocrit Care.* 2009;**10**(2):157–65.
90. Sampson TR, Dhar R, Diringer MN. Factors associated with the development of anemia after subarachnoid hemorrhage. *Neurocrit Care.* 2010;**12**(1):4–9.
91. Awad IA, Carter LP, Spetzler RF, Medina M, Williams FC. Clinical vasospasm after subarachnoid hemorrhage: response to hypervolemic hemodilution and arterial hypertension. *Stroke.* **18**(2):365–72.
92. Mori K, Arai H, Nakajima K, Tajima A, Maeda M. Hemorheological and hemodynamic analysis of hypervolemic hemodilution therapy for cerebral vasospasm after aneurysmal subarachnoid hemorrhage. *Stroke.* 1995;**26**(9):1620–6.
93. Marik PE, Corwin HL. Efficacy of red blood cell transfusion in the critically ill: a systematic review of the literature. *Crit Care Med.* 2008;**36**(9):2667–74.
94. Hèbert PC, Wells G, Blajchman M, *et al.* A multicenter, randomized, controlled clinical trial of transfusion requirements in critical care. Transfusion Requirements in Critical Care Investigators, Canadian Critical Care Trials Group. *N Engl J Med.* 1999;**340**(6):409–17.
95. Napolitano LM, Kurek S, Luchette FA, *et al.* Clinical practice guideline: red blood cell transfusion in adult trauma and critical care. *Crit Care Med.* 2009;**37**(12):3124–57.
96. Kramer AH, Diringer MN, Suarez JI, *et al.* Red blood cell transfusion in patients with subarachnoid hemorrhage: a multidisciplinary North American survey. *Crit Care.* 2011;**15**(1):R30.
97. Mcintyre LA, Fergusson DA, Hutchison JS, *et al.* Effect of a liberal versus restrictive transfusion strategy on mortality in patients with moderate to severe head injury. *Neurocrit Care.* 2006;**5**(1):4–9.
98. Kramer AH, Gurka MJ, Nathan B, *et al.* Complications associated with anemia and blood transfusion in patients with aneurysmal subarachnoid hemorrhage. *Crit Care Med.* 2008;**36**(7):2070–5.
99. Dhar R, Zazulia AR, Videen TO, *et al.* Red blood cell transfusion increases cerebral oxygen delivery in anemic patients with subarachnoid hemorrhage. *Stroke.* 2009;**40**(9):3039–44.
100. Dhar R, Scalfani MT, Zazulia AR, *et al.* Comparison of induced hypertension, fluid bolus, and blood transfusion to augment cerebral oxygen delivery after subarachnoid hemorrhage. *J Neurosurg.* 2012;**116**(3):648–56.

101. Rosenwasser RH, Armonda RA, Thomas JE, *et al.* Therapeutic modalities for the management of cerebral vasospasm: timing of endovascular options. *Neurosurgery.* 1999;**44**(5):975–9.
102. Dhar R, Dacey R, Human T, Zipfel GJ. Unilateral posterior reversible encephalopathy syndrome with hypertensive therapy of contralateral vasospasm: case report. *Neurosurgery.* 2011;**69**(5):E1176–81.
103. Hoh BL, Carter BS, Ogilvy CS. Risk of hemorrhage from unsecured, unruptured aneurysms during and after hypertensive hypervolemic therapy. *Neurosurgery.* 2002;**50** (6):1207–11.
104. Seule MA, Muroi C, Mink S, Yonekawa Y, Keller E. Therapeutic hypothermia in patients with aneurysmal subarachnoid hemorrhage, refractory intracranial hypertension, or cerebral vasospasm. *Neurosurgery.* 2009;**64**(1):86–92.

33

Management of metabolic derangements in subarachnoid hemorrhage

Kara L. Krajewski and Oliver W. Sakowitz

Introduction

Approximately 10–15% of all patients with aneurysmal subarachnoid hemorrhage (SAH) die before reaching a hospital. Nowadays increasing numbers of patients can be salvaged with professional emergency medical services, early resuscitation, and diagnosis in the emergency room. Availability of means for immediate aneurysm securement by microsurgical and endovascular methods has improved. But even then, those who survive oftentimes remain critically ill for a sustained period of time, so that neurocritical care management is vital. Secondary injuries may arise from pathophysiological cascades originating from the primary injury site itself or from a distant (systemic) failure. The Multicenter Cooperative Aneurysm study was designed to test the efficacy of the calcium antagonist nicardipine on the development of cerebral vasospasm. Observational data from the placebo limb revealed that mortality from medical complications was 23%, which was tantamount to the rate associated with deaths after the initial hemorrhage (19%), rebleeding (22%), and vasospasm after aneurysmal rupture (23%) (1). These findings emphasize the complexity involved with SAH as well as the value of a differentiated neurointensive care setting.

Pathophysiology

The parenchyma surrounding the core primary insult is subject to a high degree of ischemic vulnerability and its fate largely determines the extent of the secondary injury and, ultimately, the patient's outcome.

Ischemia as the result of the primary injury can cause brain swelling, which leads to a rise in intracranial pressure. Any secondary insult that promotes hypotension and/or hypoxia may promote a concomitant decrease in cerebral perfusion pressure, spreading ischemia to areas of the brain that were initially intact.

A further and more important source of ischemia is vasospasm (VSP). Although the pathophysiology of VSP is ultimately unclear, the occurrence of a localized blood clot in a perivascular distribution seems to be a triggering factor (2). It is hypothesized that spasmogenic factors released from the clot disturb the equilibrium of vasodilatory and vasoconstricting mediators. Both calcium-dependent and calcium-independent pathways, triggered through G-protein-coupled receptors and receptor tyrosine kinases, have been suggested.

In addition to the well-described macroscopic vasospasm of the basal cerebral vasculature, microcirculatory changes have gained substantial interest in recent years (Fig. 33.1). Today, various pathophysiological cascades from protein kinase activation, nitric oxide scavenging by (de)oxyhemoglobin, increased endothelin activity, and changes in contractile receptor subtypes to altered intracellular calcium signaling and/or accompanying structural changes of the vasospastic arterial wall (e.g. inflammation, proliferation, apoptosis) have been revealed (for review, cf. (3,4)). Outcome studies have found a clear correlation with VSP and a poor outcome and, at present, the only risk factor that

Critical Care of the Stroke Patient, ed. Stefan Schwab, Daniel Hanley, and A. David Mendelow. Published by Cambridge University Press.

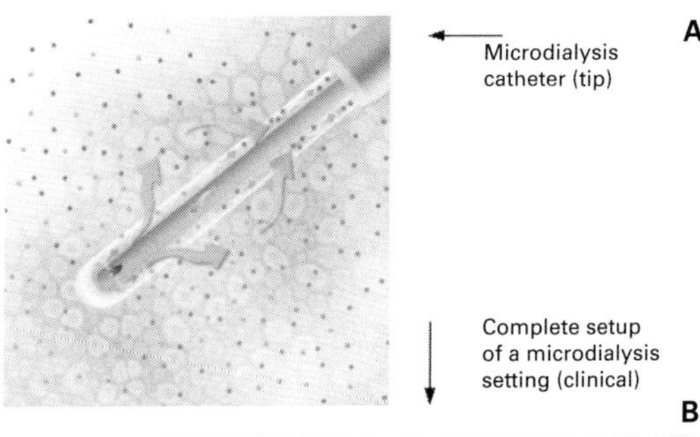

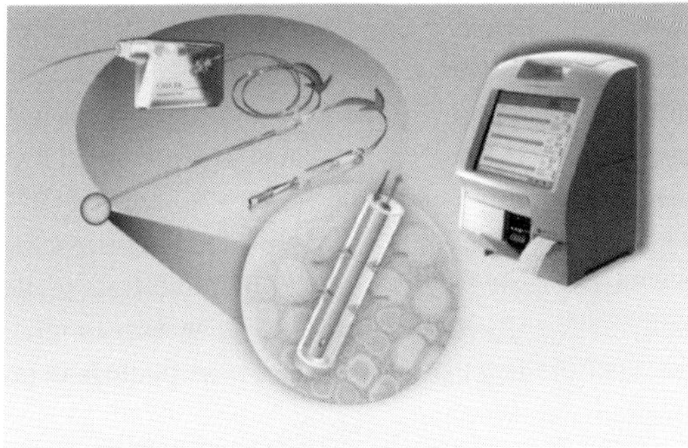

Fig. 33.1 A) Schematic drawing of the microdialysis (MD) principle: The MD inlet (inner tube) containing the dialysate and the outer probe (outer tube) are shielded by a semipermeable membrane at the tip. After this dialysate has reached an equilibrium with the extracellular fluid (ECF), the catheter fluid contains a 'mirror image' of the ECF, which can be analyzed and vital information about cell hypoxia and/or ischemia can thus be obtained. B) Complete microdialysis setup with a perfusion pump, microdialysis catheter, and bedside analysis system (left to right). Slightly modified graph of the supplier; artists' rights are with CMA Microdialysis AB (Solna, Sweden).

has been consistently associated with the occurrence of VSP is a large blood burden. Opinions differ on whether VSP inevitably implies ischemia and the best method of detection (5). The focus in neurocritical care, however, lies on detecting and preventing symptomatic vasospasm resulting from a perfusion-relevant decrease in vessel diameter resulting in delayed cerebral ischemia (DCI), which ultimately leads to ischemic stroke with permanent damage (6)

In addition, these cerebral dysfunctions cause systemic derangements. Obviously a high degree of primary cerebral injury renders the organism susceptible to a higher burden of systemic dysfunction as well. Neurotransmitter- and hormone-mediated changes lead to cardiopulmonary insufficiency, glycemic imbalance, and thermal regulation dysfunction. These changes are independently associated with poorer outcome and cause further breakdown in cerebral metabolism, a vicious circle (7).

Metabolic derangements

Systemic metabolic derangements

Systemic metabolic dysfunctions associated with subarachnoid hemorrhage are a combination of the end products of cerebral neuroendocrine and neurotransmitter dysfunction as well as common medical complications and general reactions related to the stress response. The most frequent medical complications in the SAH setting are fever, anemia, systemic hyperglycemia, hypertension, hypernatremia, pneumonia, hypotension, pulmonary edema, and hyponatremia. Those found to be statistically associated with poor outcome are fever, anemia, and systemic hyperglycemia, and have been found to occur in one-third to one-half of patients (6).

Medical complications

Fever is common in patients on intensive care units and can be associated with a wide variety of pathologies from infections to pharmacological side effects. Fever is also common in neurointensive care patients and can not only cause seizures and dehydration, but it has also been found to be associated with vasospasm and a worsening of ischemia as well as cerebral edema and increased ICP. (6)

Anemia is especially common in SAH patients and is often related to surgery and hemodilution associated with 'triple-H' therapy. Studies have shown a clear relationship between anemia and poor outcome in SAH (7). It is unknown whether the pathomechanism is related to reduced cerebral oxygen delivery, a general poor state of health, or a mixture of both. At the same time, red blood cell transfusions in SAH patients were found to be significantly associated with major medical complications, infections such as pneumonia as well as meningitis and septicemia (8).

Electrolyte disorders

In SAH patients, electrolyte disorders are common. In the study by Solenski and coworkers the combined frequency of electrolyte disorders was 33% (1). These findings included hypokalemia in 16%, hyponatremia in 9%, hypernatremia in 6%, and hyperkalemia in only 2%. There was no overall correlation with the use of corticosteroids, saline, or potassium chloride administration. However, hypokalemia was significantly associated with diuretic use. Especially hyponatremia (<130 mEq/l) may be deleterious to the injured brain. It can be simply the side effect of hypervolemic hemodilution, or it can be associated either with the syndrome of inappropriate antidiuretic hormone secretion (SIADH), which is characterized by hypotonic hyperhydration, hypophosphatemia, hypokalemia, metabolic alkalosis, as well as low albumin, creatinine and blood urea nitrogen levels (8). Less commonly it is the result of the cerebral salt wasting syndrome (CSW), which presents similarly but can be distinguished from SIADH via hypovolemia (9,10). Both syndromes are associated with a significantly longer length of stay in comparison to patients with normal sodium levels. Mortality and length of stay were found to be similar for both syndromes (8). Severe hyponatremia (<120 mEq/l) is associated with the development of neuromuscular hyperexcitability and the cerebral edema (11). As a rule of thumb, hypotonic fluids should be avoided in SAH patients. Fludrocortisone (0.1–0.3 mg/d) can be used to reduce natriuresis and maintain fluid balance. Correction of hyponatremia by hypertonic saline solutions should be performed slowly to avoid the development of central pontine myelinolysis; the rate of correction should not exceed 0.5 mEq/l/h and no more than 10 mEq/l over the first 24 hours (9, 10).

Glucose

Cerebral functional and structural integrity is ultimately based on systemic fuel supply, i.e. constant perfusion and euglycemia. With systemic derangements in neurologically impaired, critically-ill patients this is put at risk. Hyperglycemia is common in the intensive care setting as stress hormones stimulate hepatic gluconeogenesis and antagonize the effects of insulin. Systemic hyperglycemia has been repeatedly shown to be associated with poorer outcome, not only in stroke patients, but in all ICU patients (12). Mean blood glucose values on admission and inpatient serum glucose levels were found to be significantly higher in patients with vasospasm (13). Hyperglycemia was also found to be associated with longer stays on the ICU (13). Glucose burden, an alternative parameter to serum glucose levels, was also found to be associated with increased ICU stay, cardiopulmonary complications as well as brainstem compression from herniation, and after adjusting for SAH-specific factors such as Hunt and Hess grade and aneurysm size, this glucose burden was an independent predictor of death (14). These findings demonstrate that avoiding egregiously high serum glucose levels alone is not enough.

So-called intensive insulin therapy (IIT) has become *en vogue* over the past few years on surgical and non-surgical ICUs alike as a method to pre-emptively combat hyperglycemia-associated complications. Van den Berghe and colleagues compared IIT with conventional insulin therapy and found IIT to significantly decrease overall in-hospital mortality, infections, renal failure, anemia requiring blood transfusions, and critical illness polyneuropathy (15,16). A follow-up study a few years later addressed safety concerns concerning hypoglycemia: IIT was found to 'cause no harm'. Additionally, benefits were shown to be limited to non-diabetics and long-term ICU patients (17). On the other hand, the 'NICE-SUGAR' trial also compared IIT to conventional insulin therapy and found IIT to increase mortality (18). IIT has remained the subject of much controversy. It should be noted that a meta-analysis including the NICE-SUGAR data showed IIT to increase the risk of hypoglycemia and could not demonstrate decreases in mortality; however, surgical ICU patients were shown to have a slight benefit (19). The central question for neurosurgical patients is to what extent these systemic parameters correlate to local cerebral metabolism.

Cerebral metabolic derangements

In SAH local cerebral metabolism is challenged by secondary ischemia and tissue hypoxia due to the aforementioned systemic derangements, brain edema, seizures, and, last but not least, cerebral vasospasm. Thorough knowledge about changes in cerebral blood flow and metabolism may prove key to avoid secondary ischemia (i.e. DCI).

Global measurements

Several radiological imaging techniques provide valuable measurements of global cerebral perfusion and/or cerebral metabolism. While these techniques remain the most powerful in terms of spatial resolution, they are uniformly limited in their availability, can be performed only discontinuously and (with few exceptions) require patient transport to the imaging suite. This may in itself affect measurements and may pose a threat to patient safety unless carried out in highly experienced centers (20,21). In regards to SAH patients, it has been shown that there is a trend to a global transient reduction in cerebral blood flow, metabolism, and blood volume with normal oxygen extraction even without radiographically defined VSP. This may be due to a generalized reaction of the brain to toxic blood products, but may also suggest metabolic depression with decreased demand (22). Because in patients with DCI cerebral blood flow and oxygen metabolism decrease further, these complementary techniques are useful when coupled to continuous bedside monitoring techniques (i.e. to verify uncertain results that may represent VSP) (4).

Regional measurements

Microdialysis (MD) is a relatively young invasive monitoring tool (Fig. 33.2). Following intraparenchymal placement of an MD catheter (e.g. through a burr-hole craniotomy, or in addition to craniotomy and microsurgical aneurysm clipping) it allows neurocritical care specialists to analyze extracellular substances such as products of glucose metabolism, neurotransmitters and other amino acids at the bedside. These substances diffuse across the semipermeable dialysis membrane along the concentration gradient introduced by the constant dialysate flow within the catheter (23). Up to now MD has allowed for many insights on brain metabolism within the realm of tumor surgery to epilepsy and subarachnoid hemorrhage. For in-depth coverage of the technique the interested reader is referred to the following reviews (24,25).

Clinical studies comparing this technique with transcranial Doppler sonography have identified a similar sensitivity, but higher specificity in the detection of secondary ischemia in SAH patients with angiographical and symptomatic VSP (26,27). The order of metabolic changes thereby preceded clinical

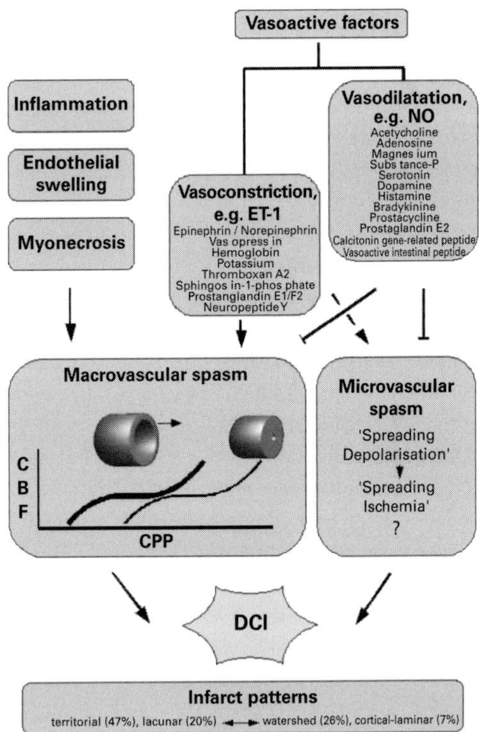

Fig. 33.2 Overview of pathomechanisms involved in the development of delayed cerebral ischemia (DCI) following subarachnoid hemorrhage. CBF: cerebral blood flow; CPP: cerebral perfusion pressure; DCI: delayed cerebral ischemia.

deterioration in 83% of cases, leaving the opportunity to initiate therapeutic measures earlier than the anticipated neurological worsening (28).

Clinical grades of SAH patients are reflected by deranged metabolic parameters such as increased tissue lactate and lactate/pyruvate (L/P) ratios. Similarly, clinical outcomes were significantly worse, independent of clinical grading or patient age (29,30).

The technical drawbacks of MD are mostly related to the restriction to a small volume of tissue parenchyma. Careful choices of the location are necessary to yield the low false-negative rates of 10–15% observed (26). Initial investment costs and maintenance intensity are high.

Glucose

Cerebral glucose concentrations are complex to interpret. Kett-White *et al.* found a slightly lower level of brain glucose in patients with a poor outcome and Sarrafzadeh *et al.* found a slight correlation, though not nearly as strong as glutamate and L/P as indicators of ischemia (29,30). Vespa and colleagues found reduced extracellular glucose concentrations to occur with seizures (per EEG), nonischemic reductions in CPP and jugular venous oxygen concentration as well as with terminal herniation (31). It has already been long-established that systemic hyperglycemia should be avoided in the brain-injured patient and studies on systemic hyperglycemia and vasospasm such as by Badjatia and colleagues have found a positive correlation between the two (13).

Although hypoglycemia in patients on regular intensive care units has been well documented as associated with poorer outcome (32), a review of the literature reveals that the dangers of hyperglycemia in the brain-injured patient have been much more appreciated during the past decade. Hypoglycemia – whether relative or absolute – has been shown to have deleterious effects in the neurointensive care setting. Decreases in systemic glucose concentrations were found to be associated with brain energy metabolic crisis, which has been defined by L/P ratios greater than or equal to 40 as detected by cerebral microdialysis. Important is the fact that acute reductions greater than or equal to 25%, even within normoglycemic limits, were shown to demonstrate this dysfunction in cerebral metabolism (33). Schlenk and colleagues found low cerebral glucose concentrations in normoglycemic SAH patients after insulin treatment that was not related to ischemia (34). Vespa and colleagues determined that glycemic control by IIT leads to lower cerebral glucose concentrations, but that L/P ratios and e.c. glutamate concentrations are increased at the same time (35). This was confirmed by Oddo and colleagues, who found that low systemic glucose concentrations were directly related to brain energy crisis, as defined by low cerebral glucose levels coupled with an elevated L/P ratio (defined here as >40), as well as lower cerebral glucose levels in nonsurvivors compared to survivors (36). In a nutshell, it is possible that a tight glycemic control by IIT, at least in patients with severe brain injury, is a 'double-edged sword'.

A recent study from our group focused on the cause and outcome analysis of transient microdialysis events (unpublished data). The initial (primary) injury was found to be associated with persistently low e.c. brain concentrations (<1 mM) of glucose in 53% of all detected episodes. In the remaining events, vasospasm accounted for 46%, while the other half of the cases (54%) were the result of variable other pathomechanisms. Seizures were found to account for less than 1% of cases. Vasoconstriction as a result of hypocapnia accounted for 3% of episodes. Further parameters found responsible for episodes of cerebral hypoglycemia include hyperthermia and systemic hypoglycemia.

Cerebral hyperglycemia, in contrast, was unexplainable in only 9% of the episodes and was found to be overwhelmingly caused by systemic hyperglycemia (91%). In contrast, systemic hypoglycemia only accounted for less than 4% of low cerebral glucose events.

Outcome as measured by the SF-36 physical score was found to correlate negatively with both systemic hypoglycemia and hyperglycemia in the first correlation and then only with severe systemic hyperglycemia after correcting for age, clinical SAH grade, and anisocoria.

Lactate and pyruvate

Based on experimental results the so-called astrocyte-neuron lactate shuttle hypothesis has been formulated. It may explain functional metabolic coupling between glutamatergic neurons and astrocytes through lactate as metabolic substrate for the activated neurons. It is suggested that glutamate, released by neurons, stimulates astrocytic glycolysis, thus producing lactate, which is then exported to neurons to be converted back to pyruvate and enter the neuronal tricyclic acid cycle (37).

In the clinical setting, however, increased e.c. lactate brain concentrations have been identified as a marker of anaerobic metabolism due to impending ischemia and as such as a useful marker of vasospasm after SAH (26,38,39).

We found an increased L/P ratio to be the result of the primary injury most of the time (74%). Of the factors found to cause transient episodes, vasospasm and systemic acidosis were the conditions accounting for the majority of instances, whereas intracranial hypertension accounted for less than 1% of instances and low CPP was not at all related to the L/P ratio.

Glutamate

Glutamate is the most abundant excitatory neurotransmitter in the central nervous system. Physiologically, the injurious potential of glutamate is limited by active transport into glia and neurons through high-affinity glutamate transporters. Excessive release of intracellular glutamate stores is thought to trigger cell death in the vicinity via at least two mechanisms, involving mitochondrial injury by excessive amounts of intracellular calcium and pro-apoptotic signaling cascades. Secondary brain injury subsequent to glutamatergic excitotoxicity may be involved in various neurological disorders such as traumatic brain injury, stroke, epilepsy, and neurodegeneration (40–42).

In SAH, several microdialysis studies have demonstrated that 'extracellular' glutamate accumulation is correlated with secondary ischemia and poor outcome (26,43–45).

In contrast to e.c. cerebral concentrations of glucose, lactate and pyruvate, no satisfactory 'cut-off' value for glutamate exists. Nilsson and colleagues found large variations in glutamate concentrations, both among patients and intra-individually, when they studied the use of microdialysis in detecting ischemia after SAH; thus, only a general increase in glutamate could be found to correlate with impending ischemia, whereas 'low and stable' levels were found to follow an uneventful clinical course (45). Sarrafzadeh and colleagues also investigated the relationship between glutamate and ischemia in several studies and found that although increased cerebral glutamate levels correlated with high ICP and although it was even the best of the MD parameters with respect to detecting low CBF, interpatient and intra-individual differences in glutamate concentrations were astoundingly high (32,46).

Oxygenation and pH

Brain tissue oxygen pressure ($p_{ti}O_2$) monitoring is a method to detect tissue hypoxia, which is theoretically more 'direct' than measuring end products of metabolism. One study on SAH patients showed that $p_{ti}O_2$ remained normal during the occurrence of vasospasm, while carbon dioxide pressure increased significantly and pH levels decreased significantly. Acidosis was thought to be directly related to decreases in cerebral blood flow and acidosis was found in the early stages of vasospasm, which may represent a future method for faster vasospasm detection (47). Of note, one study found that $p_{ti}O_2$ as well as ICP and CPP monitoring was not able to provide early detection of non-survival in SAH; pathological values in these parameters were not able to be detected until the last day prior to exitus (48).

Treatment

General guidelines

A comprehensive overview of target values for ICU parameters and suggested therapies is beyond the scope of this chapter: Table 33.1 summarizes the key systemic and cerebral metabolically relevant derangements and treatment recommendations.

Table 33.1 Overview of common systemic and cerebral metabolic derangements in SAH patients. Thresholds to indicate pathological values and treatment recommendations are given.

Systemic	Pathological values	Treatment recommendations
Fever	>38.5 °C	Rule out/treat infectious disease, drug-related fever, etc. Treat pharmacologically (e.g. acetaminophen) or by cooling blanket
Anemia	Hb <10 g/dl	In patients free of serious cardiac disease => restrictive transfusion policy; maintain Hb >8 g/dl, otherwise check for clinical transfusion triggers (cerebral metabolic derangements/neuromonitoring?, DCI?)
Hyponatremia (SIADH, CSW, iatrogenic)	<130 mEq/l	Avoid hypotonic fluids, consider fludrocortisone 0.1–0.3 mg/d to reduce natriuresis and maintain fluid balance; With SIADH first restrict fluids, otherwise replace with hypertonic saline at 0.5 mEq/l/h, not to exceed 10 mEq/l over the first 24 hours
Systemic hyperglycemia	>7.8 mM	Avoid glucocorticosteroids; use sliding scale insulin
Systemic hypoglycemia	<4.5 mM	Loosen glycemic control (IIT?); if <3 mM: 50 ml dextrose, 50% i.v. bolus
Cerebral		
Cerebral hyperglycemia	>3 mM	Normalize systemic glucose concentrations
Cerebral hypoglycemia	<1 mM	Normalize systemic glucose concentrations
Acidosis	pH <7.35	Check for systemic acidosis, treat causes (e.g. hypoventilation, sepsis, ischemia)
Increased cerebral glutamate levels, elevated L/P ratio, decreased partial pressure of oxygen in brain tissue ($ptiO_2$)	? >25 < 10 mmHg	1a) Rule out hydrocephalus, seizures, inadvertent hyperventilation, hypotension, hypoxia, anemia, and pyrexia; otherwise treat 1b) Consider angiography, perfusion imaging to confirm VSP /DCI 2) Perfusion augmentation ('HHH': CPP >90–120 mmHg, normovolemia to moderate hypervolemia as necessary to achieve pressure goal) 3) If therapy refractory: consider interventional perfusion augmentation (e.g. angioplasty)

SIADH: syndrome of inappropriate antidiuretic hormone secretion; CSW: cerebral salt wasting syndrome; CPP: cerebral perfusion pressure; HHH: hypervolemia, hypertension, hemodilution; DCI: delayed cerebral ischemia; VSP: (angiographic) vasospasm.

The main branches of SAH treatment can broadly be separated into stabilization and prevention. Raabe *et al.* identify the following four areas as the main targets in the reduction of secondary insults: 1) hypoxia and hypercapnia; 2) arterial hypotension and hypertension; 3) increased intracranial pressure as the result of expansive intracerebral/subdural bleeds and/or hydrocephalus; and 4) rebleeding from primary hemorrhagic foci, such as the aneurysm in the case of SAH (49).

Nimodipine

Prophylactic treatment with calcium antagonists, e.g. nimodipine, was implemented in the early 1980s, and is still the only substance proven to be beneficial following SAH. The oral dosing regimen is recommended over the intravenous application, which is currently not FDA-approved, but available outside the US (50). The neuroprotective effect of systemically applied nimodipine remains enigmatic. It neither affects angiographic vasospasm, nor has a significant affect on cerebral blood flow or oxygenation which is observable (51). Next to the angiographic (macrovascular) vasospasm, microvascular ischemia due to microthrombosis, inflammation, etc. has been declared a 'culprit' in the development of DCI (52) (cf. Fig. 33.1). The electrophysiological phenomenon of 'spreading depolarization' (aka cortical spreading depression), which is suppressed by calcium-channel blockers and NMDA-antagonists, has recently been linked to DCI following SAH (53).

Triple-H therapy

Traditionally, postoperative treatment for aneurysmal SAH to alleviate cerebral vasospasm includes triple-H (HHH) therapy (hypertension, hypervolemia, hemodilution) (54). Triple-H therapy is not recommended in every patient due to its aggressive nature and potentially severe cardiovascular complications. Indeed, in a prospective, randomized, controlled study, Egge and colleagues showed that *prophylactic* triple-H therapy had no effect on outcome, vasospasm or cerebral blood flow in comparison to the normovolemic control therapy (55). Although the individual value of each triple-H component is under debate, every attempt to increase CBF in patients with confirmed vasospasm and/or neurological deficits resulting from progressive ischemia is usually indicated (49,56). Surrogate parameters of tissue oxygenation and microdialysis glutamate, respectively, indicate a favorable effect of therapeutic triple-H therapy (28,57).

Summary

From the primary injury at the time of aneurysmal rupture, via peri-procedural perils to the delayed phase of cerebral vasospasm, the treatment of SAH patients remains a constant challenge for the neurocritical care specialist. In contrast to acute ischemic stroke, DCI from SAH is seen in a remarkable percentage of patients, who are already hospitalized at the peak time of occurrence. Therefore, the detection and treatment of ischemia following SAH, as well as understanding its underlying causes and pathophysiological cascades, are 'in reach' for the involved clinician, clinical researcher and basic scientist. A more profound knowledge of the intra- and extracerebral metabolic derangements associated with DCI by means of (invasive) neuromonitoring may be instrumental in future developments to avoid or treat secondary brain injuries in SAH patients.

REFERENCES

1. Solenski NJ, Haley EC, Kassell NF, *et al.* Medical complications of aneurysmal subarachnoid hemorrhage: a report of the multicenter, cooperative aneurysm study. Participants of the Multicenter Cooperative Aneurysm Study. *Crit. Care Med.* 1995;**23**:1007–17.
2. Fisher CM, Kistler JP, Davis JM. Relation of cerebral vasospasm to subarachnoid hemorrhage visualized by computerized tomographic scanning. *Neurosurgery.* 1980;**6**:1–9.
3. Dietrich HH, Dacey RG. Molecular keys to the problems of cerebral vasospasm. *Neurosurgery.* 2000;**46**:517–30.
4. Sakowitz OW, Unterberg AW. Detecting and treating microvascular ischemia after subarachnoid hemorrhage. *Curr. Opin. Crit. Care.* 2006;**12**(2):103–111.
5. Frontera JA, Fernandez A, Schmidt JM, *et al.* Defining vasospasm after subarachnoid hemorrhage: what is the most clinically relevant definition? *Stroke.* 2009;**40**(6):1963–8.
6. Vergouwen M, Vermeulen M, van Gijn J, *et al.* Definition of delayed cerebral ischemia after aneurysmal subarachnoid hemorrhage as an outcome event in clinical trials and observational studies: proposal of a multidisciplinary research group. *Stroke.* 2010;**41**(10):2391–5.
7. Barth M, Piepgras A, Thome C. Subarachnoidalblutung / Hirnarterienaneurysma. In: Piek J, Unterberg A, editors. *Grundlagen neurochirurgischer Intensivmedizin.* Zuckschwerdt; 2006: 331–47.
8. Kao L, Al-Lawati Z, Vavao J, Steinberg GK, Katznelson L. Prevalence and clinical demographics of cerebral salt wasting in patients with aneurysmal subarachnoid hemorrhage. *Pituitary.* 2009;**12**(4):347–51.

9. Harrigan MR. Cerebral salt wasting syndrome: a review. *Neurosurgery.* 1996;**38**:152–60.
10. Rahman M, Friedman WA. Hyponatremia in neurosurgical patients: clinical guidelines development. *Neurosurgery.* 2009;**65**(5):925–35; discussion 935–6.
11. Sterns RH, Silver SM. Brain volume regulation in response to hypo-osmolality and its correction. *Am. J. Med.* 2006;**119**(7 Suppl 1):S12–16.
12. Wartenberg KE, Schmidt JM, Claassen J, *et al.* Impact of medical complications on outcome after subarachnoid hemorrhage. *Crit. Care Med.* 2006;**34**:617–23.
13. Badjatia N, Topcuoglu MA, Buonanno FS, *et al.* Relationship between hyperglycemia and symptomatic vasospasm after subarachnoid hemorrhage. *Crit. Care Med.* 2005;**33**(7):1603–9.
14. Frontera JA, Fernandez A, Claassen J, *et al.* Hyperglycemia after SAH: predictors, associated complications, and impact on outcome. *Stroke.* 2006;**37**:199–203.
15. Van den Berghe G, Wilmer A, Hermans G, *et al.* Intensive insulin therapy in the medical ICU. *N. Engl. J. Med.* 2006;**354**(5):449–61.
16. Van den Berghe G, Wouters P, Weekers F, *et al.* Intensive insulin therapy in the critically ill patients. *N. Engl. J. Med.* 2001;**345**(19):1359–67.
17. Van den Berghe G, Wilmer A, Milants I, *et al.* Intensive insulin therapy in mixed medical/surgical intensive care units: benefit versus harm. *Diabetes.* 2006;**55**(11):3151–9.
18. Finfer S, Chittock DR, Su SY, *et al.* Intensive versus conventional glucose control in critically ill patients. *N. Engl. J. Med.* 2009;**360**(13):1283–97.
19. Griesdale DEG, de Souza RJ, van Dam RM, *et al.* Intensive insulin therapy and mortality among critically ill patients: a meta-analysis including NICE-SUGAR study data. *CMAJ.* 2009;**180**(8):821–7.
20. Coles JP. Imaging of cerebral blood flow and metabolism. *Curr. Opin. Anaesthesiol.* 2006;**19**(5):473–80.
21. Wintermark M, Sesay M, Barbier E, *et al.* Comparative overview of brain perfusion imaging techniques. *Stroke.* 2005;**36**(9):e83–99.
22. Carlson AP, Yonas H. Radiographic assessment of vasospasm after aneurysmal subarachnoid hemorrhage: the physiological perspective. *Neurol. Res.* 2009;**31**(6):593–604.
23. Ungerstedt U. Microdialysis – principles and applications for studies in animals and man. *J. Intern. Med.* 1991;**230**(4):365–73.
24. Goodman JC, Robertson CS. Microdialysis: is it ready for prime time? *Curr. Opin. Crit. Care.* 2009;**15**(2):110–17.
25. Hillered L, Vespa PM, Hovda DA. Translational neurochemical research in acute human brain injury: the current status and potential future for cerebral microdialysis. *J. Neurotrauma.* 2005;**22**(1):3–41.
26. Unterberg AW, Sakowitz OW, Sarrafzadeh AS, Benndorf G, Lanksch WR. Role of bedside microdialysis in the diagnosis of cerebral vasospasm following aneurysmal subarachnoid hemorrhage. *J. Neurosurg.* 2001;**94**:740–9.
27. Skjoth-Rasmussen J, Schulz M, Kristensen SR, Bjerre P. Delayed neurological deficits detected by an ischemic pattern in the extracellular cerebral metabolites in patients with aneurysmal subarachnoid hemorrhage. *J. Neurosurg.* 2004;**100**:8–15.
28. Sarrafzadeh AS, Sakowitz OW, Kiening KL, *et al.* Bedside microdialysis: a tool to monitor cerebral metabolism in subarachnoid hemorrhage patients? *Crit. Care Med.* 2002;**30**(5):1062–70.
29. Kett-White R, Hutchinson PJ, Al-Rawi PG, *et al.* Adverse cerebral events detected after subarachnoid hemorrhage using brain oxygen and microdialysis probes. *Neurosurgery.* 2002;**50**:1213–21.
30. Sarrafzadeh A, Haux D, Kuchler I, Lanksch WR, Unterberg AW. Poor-grade aneurysmal subarachnoid hemorrhage: relationship of cerebral metabolism to outcome. *J. Neurosurg.* 2004;**100**:400–6.
31. Vespa PM, McArthur D, O'Phelan K, *et al.* Persistently low extracellular glucose correlates with poor outcome 6 months after human traumatic brain injury despite a lack of increased lactate: a microdialysis study. *J. Cereb. Blood Flow Metab.* 2003;**23**(7):865–77.
32. Mechanick JI, Handelsman Y, Bloomgarden ZT. Hypoglycemia in the intensive care unit. *Curr. Opin. Clin. Nutr. Metab. Care.* 2007;**10**(2):193–6.
33. Helbok R, Schmidt JM, Kurtz P, *et al.* Systemic glucose and brain energy metabolism after subarachnoid hemorrhage. *Neurocrit. Care.* 2010;**12**(3):317–23.
34. Schlenk F, Graetz D, Nagel A, Schmidt M, Sarrafzadeh AS. Insulin-related decrease in cerebral glucose despite normoglycemia in aneurysmal subarachnoid hemorrhage. *Crit. Care.* 2008;**12**(1):R9.
35. Vespa P, Boonyaputthikul R, McArthur DL, *et al.* Intensive insulin therapy reduces microdialysis glucose values without altering glucose utilization or improving the lactate/pyruvate ratio after traumatic brain injury. *Crit. Care Med.* 2006;**34**(3):850–6.
36. Oddo M, Schmidt JM, Carrera E, *et al.* Impact of tight glycemic control on cerebral glucose metabolism after severe brain injury: a microdialysis study. *Crit. Care Med.* 2008;**36**(12):3233–8.

37. Pellerin L, Magistretti PJ. Glutamate uptake into astrocytes stimulates aerobic glycolysis: a mechanism coupling neuronal activity to glucose utilization. *Proc. Natl Acad. Sci. U S A.* 1994;**91**:106–259.
38. Sarrafzadeh A, Haux D, Plotkin M, *et al.* Bedside microdialysis reflects dysfunction of cerebral energy metabolism in patients with aneurysmal subarachnoid hemorrhage as confirmed by 15 O-H2 O-PET and 18 F-FDG-PET. *J. Neuroradiol.* 2005;**32**(5):348–51.
39. Nilsson OG, Brandt L, Ungerstedt U, Saveland H. Bedside detection of brain ischemia using intracerebral microdialysis: subarachnoid hemorrhage and delayed ischemic deterioration. *Neurosurgery.* 1999;**45**:1176–84.
40. Olney JW. Brain lesions, obesity, and other disturbances in mice treated with monosodium glutamate. *Science.* 1969;**164**:719–21.
41. Choi DW. Glutamate neurotoxicity in cortical cell culture is calcium dependent. *Neurosci. Lett.* 1985;**58**(3):293–7.
42. Faden AI, Demediuk P, Panter SS. The role of excitatory amino acids and NMDA receptors in traumatic brain injury. *Science.* 1989;**244**:798–800.
43. Enblad P, Valtysson J, Andersson J, *et al.* Simultaneous intracerebral microdialysis and positron emission tomography in the detection of ischemia in patients with subarachnoid hemorrhage. *J. Cereb. Blood Flow Metab.* 1996;**16**:637–44.
44. Persson L, Valtysson J, Enblad P, *et al.* Neurochemical monitoring using intracerebral microdialysis in patients with subarachnoid hemorrhage. *J. Neurosurg.* 1996;**84**:606–16.
45. Nilsson OG, Brandt L, Ungerstedt U, Saveland H. Bedside detection of brain ischemia using intracerebral microdialysis: subarachnoid hemorrhage and delayed ischemic deterioration. *Neurosurgery.* 1999;**45**:1176–84.
46. Sarrafzadeh AS, Thomale UW, Haux D, Unterberg AW. Cerebral metabolism and intracranial hypertension in high grade aneurysmal subarachnoid haemorrhage patients. *Acta Neurochir.* Suppl. 2005;**95**:89–92.
47. Charbel FT, Du X, Hoffman WE, Ausman JI. Brain tissue PO2, PCO2, and pH during cerebral vasospasm. *Surg. Neurol.* 2000;**54**:432–7; discussion 438.
48. Meixensberger J, Vath A, Jaeger M, Kunze E, Dings J, Roosen K. Monitoring of brain tissue oxygenation following severe subarachnoid hemorrhage. *Neurol. Res.* 2003;**25**: 445–50.
49. Raabe A, Beck J, Berkefeld J, *et al.* Recommendations for the management of patients with aneurysmal subarachnoid hemorrhage. *Zentralbl. Neurochir.* 2005;**66**:79–91.
50. Dorhout Mees SM, Rinkel GJE, Feigin VL, *et al.* Calcium antagonists for aneurysmal subarachnoid haemorrhage. *Cochrane Database Syst. Rev.* 2007;(3):CD000277.
51. Stiefel MF, Heuer GG, Abrahams JM, *et al.* The effect of nimodipine on cerebral oxygenation in patients with poor-grade subarachnoid hemorrhage. *J. Neurosurg.* 2004;**101** (4):594–9.
52. Macdonald RL, Pluta RM, Zhang JH. Cerebral vasospasm after subarachnoid hemorrhage: the emerging revolution. *Nat. Clin. Pract. Neurol.* 2007;**3**:256–63.
53. Leng LZ, Fink ME, Iadecola C. Spreading depolarization: A possible new culprit in the delayed cerebral ischemia of subarachnoid hemorrhage. *Arch. Neurol.* [Internet]. 2010 Sep 13 [cited 2011 Jan 9]; Available from: http://www.ncbi.nlm.nih.gov/pubmed/20837823
54. Kosnik EJ, Hunt WE. Postoperative hypertension in the management of patients with intracranial arterial aneurysms. *J. Neurosurg.* 1976;**45**(2):148–54.
55. Egge A, Waterloo K, Sjoholm H, *et al.* Prophylactic hyperdynamic postoperative fluid therapy after aneurysmal subarachnoid hemorrhage: a clinical, prospective, randomized, controlled study. *Neurosurgery.* 2001;**49**:593–605; discussion 605–6.
56. Dankbaar JW, Slooter AJ, Rinkel GJ, Schaaf ICVD. Effect of different components of triple-H therapy on cerebral perfusion in patients with aneurysmal subarachnoid haemorrhage: a systematic review. *Crit. Care.* 2010; **14**(1):R23.
57. Raabe A, Beck J, Keller M, *et al.* Relative importance of hypertension compared with hypervolemia for increasing cerebral oxygenation in patients with cerebral vasospasm after subarachnoid hemorrhage. *J. Neurosurg.* 2005;**103**: 974–81.

34

Management of cardiopulmonary dysfunction in subarachnoid hemorrhage

Jan-Oliver Neumann and Oliver W. Sakowitz

Introduction

Medical complications significantly add to morbidity and mortality after aneurysmal subarachnoid hemorrhage (SAH). It has been estimated that the risk of at least one life-threatening medical complication during the acute course of SAH is about 40% (1). The proportion of deaths from these complications (about 20–25%) is comparable to the rate of deaths attributable to cerebral vasospasm or re-bleeding (1).

Cardiopulmonary dysfunctions such as pulmonary edema or cardiac arrhythmia constitute very common problems after subarachnoid hemorrhage with an incidence of about 20% and 35%, respectively (1,2).

The etiology of these phenomena can be classified as either of primary neurologic origin or as secondary due to complications or side effects of SAH treatment.

Interconnections between the central nervous system (CNS) and the cardiopulmonary system, as well as the potentially detrimental effect of acute CNS pathology on the latter, were first described at the beginning of the 20th century (3–6). Following a series of experimental and clinical studies in the 1950s to 1970s, it became clear that acute dysregulation of the autonomous nervous system (ANS) plays an important role in these events. Because this has been shown particularly for the sympathetic leg of the ANS, the term 'sympathetic storm' has been coined.

Although our understanding of the underlying (patho-)physiology has improved profoundly since these times, the mechanisms, prognostic implications, and possible treatments of CNS-mediated cardiopulmonary dysfunction remain to be elucidated completely.

Pathophysiology

In animal experiments, a sudden rise in intracranial pressure as well as di- or mesencephalic electrical stimulation is able to produce distinct patterns of ECG changes and cardiac or pulmonary injury (7–12). Interruption of signal transduction in the ANS by measures such as spinal chord transsection, stellate gangliotomy, adrenalectomy or the treatment with sympatho- or vagolytic drugs are able to reduce or even abolish the development of these lesions. The suppression of the sympathetic ANS was found to have a much larger protective effect than the parasympathetic leg of the ANS. Consequently, it was hypothesized that sympathetic activation plays an important role in neurogenic cardiopulmonary injury.

Autonomic control of the cardiovascular system

A complex network of cortical and subcortical neurons usually performs the nervous system control of the cardiopulmonary system. Supraspinal regulation and feedback mechanisms of the cardiovascular system as well as the respiratory center are located in the lower

Critical Care of the Stroke Patient, ed. Stefan Schwab, Daniel Hanley, and A. David Mendelow. Published by Cambridge University Press.

medulla oblongata. These centers are controlled by descending tracts from the hypothalamus, which performs primary integration of behavioral, vegetative, humoral, and motor activity to sustain homeostasis of the body.

Sympathetic spinal nuclei located in the intermediate zone of the thoracolumbar spine are directly connected to the hypothalamic and medullar centers via neuronal tracts (13–15). These spinal centers conduct signals via cholinergic fibers to the para- or prevertebral ganglions. Synaptic nicotinergic receptors in the ganglion subsequently switch the signals to postganglionic fibers that ultimately reach the effector organs.

The adrenal medulla is a specialized sympathetic ganglion (paraganglion) although it lacks distinct synapses. It releases norepinephrine (NE) and epinephrine (EPI) directly into the circulation.

Sympathetic nervous activation acts on the cardiovascular system via four pathways (16): 1) NE released at the sinus and atrioventricular nodes causing positive chrono- and dromotropic effects as well as positive left ventricular inotropy by sympathetic noradrenergic plexus located subepicardially; 2) EPI and NE released by the adrenal medulla affecting both the myocardium and peripheral vessels via the humoral route; 3) local release of NE and EPI by paravascular nerve fibers reaching the entire vascular bed except the capillaries; 4) NE plasma spillover from activated sympathetic nerve fibers.

The main effect of sympathetic activation in vessels is vasoconstriction, but the individual response of each vessel system depends on the distinct distribution of various catecholamine receptor subtypes (α_1, α_2, $\beta_{1\text{-}3}$) in the postsynaptic membrane.

Parasympathetic control of the cardiopulmonary system originates from nuclei in the medulla oblongata that send cholinergic fibers via the vagal nerve to ganglions that are located in the proximity of the heart and lungs. Nicotinergic receptors of the short second neuron then switch the signal to the final muscarinergic postgangliotic receptors. The parasympathetic fibers run subendocardially and are mainly present in the atrial myocardium where they cause negative dromotropic, bathmotropic, and chronotropic effects.

Signal divergence, i.e. the ratio between post- and preganglionic fibers, in the parasympathetic leg of the ANS is about four times lower than in the sympathetic system, making massive discharges of the entire parasympathetic system less likely than in the sympathetic system.

Catecholamine surge

A remarkable similarity between cardiopulmonary distress after SAH and in pheochromocytoma crises does exist. Both diseases share the same clinical features, echocardiographic, and histological patterns. Other than in pheochromocytoma, direct paravascular and intracardial release of NE and EPI seems to play the dominant role in the pathophysiology of neurogenic cardiac dysfunction and NPE. This is supported by the fact that adrenalectomy in experimental SAH does not abolish cardiorespiratory sequelae and, ultrastructurally, the pathological changes in the myocardium decrease with growing distance from an intracardial nerve (17).

The existence of a catecholamine surge finds further proof by increased concentrations of plasmatic catecholamines and their urinary metabolites in patients with acute SAH (18). An evidence for sympathetic overactivity in SAH was given by Naredi *et al.* (19) by using an isotope dilution technique: compared with two different control groups, patients with subarachnoid hemorrhage exhibited a three-fold increase in total-body NE spillover from synapses into the plasma within 48 hours after the insult.

Cellular mechanisms

Histological analysis of the underlying ultrastructural changes is limited to autopsy series of fatal cases of SAH and animal models. A distinct histopathological pattern described as 'focal myocytolysis', 'myofibrillar degeneration' or 'contraction-band necrosis' has been identified in patients who died from SAH (20,21) and pheochromocytoma (22). This pattern is characterized by dense eosinophilic bands replacing the striated appearance of the cytoplasm and it differs substantially from the histological changes seen in ischemic infarction.

The exact cellular mechanisms that induce contraction-band necrosis are still not known today, but a sudden influx of calcium is a possible pathway by which irreversible contractures may occur. NE released locally is known to stimulate synthesis of cyclic adenosine monophosphate (cAMP), which in turn opens calcium channels and causes an influx of calcium and an efflux of potassium. Continuously high levels of NE may thus result in a failure of the calcium channel to close and may lead to a continuum of pathological changes from brief cardiac dysfunction to widespread myocardial necrosis.

In the lungs, an increase in transmural pulmonary vascular pressures by a combination of α- and β-adrenoreceptor activation is believed to cause hydrostatic transsudation of edema fluid. Further increase in capillary pressures may then cause disruption of the basal membrane causing fluid and protein exudation. This is supported by animal studies, in which intense pulmonary vasoconstriction caused by endothelin administration caused the aforementioned pattern.

Clinical features and diagnosis

Signal conduction and rhythm disturbances

Morphological electrocardiographic (ECG) changes were the first cardiac symptoms to be directly demonstrated in the setting of acute SAH (4). Since then, many studies and case reports have shown ECG abnormalities after SAH. Sakr *et al.* (23) systematically reviewed the literature and found the incidence of ECG abnormalities ranging from 49% to 100%. T-wave changes were most common (36%) followed by ST-segment changes (28%), the presence of U-waves (24%), QT-prolongation (23%), pathological Q-waves (3%), and other ECG changes (10%).

In a prospective study of 406 patients with SAH, Rudehill *et al.* (24) found ECG alterations in 82% of the patients regardless of underlying heart disease, electrolyte disturbances and medical treatments. Patients with at least one of these non-CNS conditions, however, showed a significantly greater incidence of ECG alterations, which underlines the possibility of an overestimation of the influence of SAH to these ECG changes. Nonetheless, in a prospective study on SAH patients without underlying heart disease, Brouwers *et al.* (25) reported ECG changes in all 61 patients. In a large, randomized, controlled trial of cerebral vasospasm protection with the calcium antagonist nicardipine, half of the patients in the placebo limb (n = 457) showed an abnormal admission ECG with approximately 25% having either ST-segment or T-wave changes (26).

As reviewed by Sakr *et al.* (23), the most commonly reported arrhythmias in the setting of SAH are sinus bradycardia (15%), sinus tachycardia (13%), and premature ventricular beats (13%). Atrial fibrillation and ventricular tachycardia were reported in 2% of cases, atrio-ventricular block in 1.5%, and asystole in 1% of cases.

Impaired ventricular function

Unexpected ventricular hypokinesis and stunned myocardium in the absence of coronary heart disease and ischemia have been described in the medical literature for a variety of pathophysiological triggers. Due to the similarity of the typical echocardiographical picture ('apical ballooning') to a traditional mug-shaped Japanese squid trap with short neck, the term of 'Takotsubo myopathy' was born.

Typical features of this acute and transient cardiomyopathy are 1) hypocontractility of the left ventricle (especially the apex) not corresponding to the vascular territory of a coronary artery, 2) exclusion of underlying coronary heart disease, 3) ECG abnormalities, and 4) temporal relation to a form of physiological stress.

Cardiac dysfunction and secondary failure, either as regional wall-motion abnormality (RWMA) or globally impaired myocardial contractility, have also often been reported in the setting of SAH. There is a wide range of the reported incidences in the literature from 8% to 100% (23). With technical improvements and the growing availability of echocardiography, the number of reported cases and prospective series is increasing.

In 1995, Mayer *et al.* (27) found RWMA in five (9%) of 57 patients with SAH and without a previous history of cardiac disease. Five years later, Parekh *et al.* (28)

reported that nine (15%) of 39 patients with SAH showed echocardiographic signs of RWMA with five (13%) individuals also having clinical or radiological evidence of myocardial dysfunction.

To test the hypothesis that regional wall motion patterns in SAH patients do not match the typical patterns observed in coronary artery disease, a segmental wall motion analysis was performed in 30 SAH patients with left ventricular dysfunction by Zaroff *et al.* (29). In contrast to the typical presentation of Takotsubo myopathy, a preservation of apical function in 17 (57%) cases was found. The authors stressed the fact that these 'wall motion patterns were atypical of coronary artery disease but correlated with the distribution of the myocardial sympathetic nerve terminals'. In recent times, more and more cases of this 'Inverted Takotsubo' syndrome in the setting of pheochromocytoma or acute cerebral injury were reported (30–34).

The largest and most profound study on left ventricular dysfunction in SAH was performed by Banki *et al.* (35). To assess prevalence, distribution, and rate of recovery of left ventricular dysfunction, echocardiography was performed three times over a 7-day period in 173 patients with acute SAH. An ejection fraction of less than 50% was found in 15% of the patients and 13% of patients showed RWMA with a normal ejection fraction. In two-thirds of the patients a recovery of left ventricular function over time was noted. Most affected segments of the left ventricle were the basal and middle ventricular portions of the anteroseptal and anterior walls. The apex was rarely affected.

In summary, patients with acute SAH may often present with global or regional left ventricular dysfunction in the absence of coronary heart disease. The echocardiographic pattern is atypical of coronary heart disease and often follows the likes of 'Inverted Takotsubo' myopathy. Most patients experience a partial or complete improvement of left ventricular function during the course of SAH recovery.

Enzymatic markers of myocardial injury

Myocardial damage and cell disintegration can be demonstrated by detecting the transfer of specific structural proteins from the heart muscle into the serum. Cardiac troponin I (cTnI) is the current standard method of serologic detection of myocardial infarction. Due to its high sensitivity and specificity, it is able to detect myocardial cell damage that is undetectable by conventional enzyme methods (36).

Consecutively, an elevation of cTnI levels in patients with SAH could be demonstrated in several studies and was often associated with a higher incidence of myocardial dysfunction (28, 37).

A recent study on 103 consecutive cases of SAH even demonstrated a positive association of highly positive cTnI levels with neurological severity, systolic and diastolic cardiac dysfunction, pulmonary congestion, and length of ICU stay (38).

While it seems clear that acute myocardial damage does occur during SAH and is reflected by cTnI elevation, clinical recovery with normalization of ECG and ventricular function occurs frequently (see above).

Neurogenic pulmonary edema

Neurogenic pulmonary edema (NPE) is defined as acute pulmonary edema following neurologic injury in the absence of any pre-existing cardiovascular or pulmonary pathology severe enough to explain the edema. The first cases of this phenomenon were reported in patients with epilepsy (6) or a gunshot wound to the head (5). Since then, NPE has been reported in numerous and various acute pathologies of the central nervous system.

The overall incidence of pulmonary complications in large cohorts of SAH patients has been reported to be in the range of 20–25% (1, 39). Due to confounding pulmonary co-morbidities influenced directly or indirectly by SAH such as pneumonia, congestive heart failure or water/electrolyte imbalances, the incidence of *true* NPE in SAH is still not established today. As an estimate, Friedman *et al.* have reported neurogenic pulmonary edema in five (2%) of 305 consecutive cases of SAH (39).

NPE shares its clinical presentation with other forms of acute pulmonary edema (tachypnea, tachycardia, basal pulmonary crackles, respiratory failure) and lacks the signs of left ventricular failure in its pure form. It usually starts in conjunction with the initial neurologic injury, but it can also occur in the time following, especially during secondary neurological deterioration due to cerebral vasospasm. Chest x-ray demonstrates bilateral pulmonary infiltrates while hemodynamic parameters are normal. The transient increase in pulmonary artery occlusion pressure (PAOP) described classically (40, 41) can often not be demonstrated in clinical practice due the early occurrence and short duration of this phenomenon.

Differential diagnosis of NPE versus aspiration or ventilator-associated pneumonia can be challenging. It is facilitated by appreciating the time-course of edema development and by seeking confirmation of bacterial infection. The onset of NPE usually begins within hours after the neurologic incident and evolves during the following days. Pneumonia usually develops within days and advances more slowly. In the absence of positive tracheal cultures, the serum concentration of pro-calcitonin is an important sign of underlying bacterial infection as the etiology of the pulmonary edema (42).

Treatment

Treatment of the underlying disease remains the most important therapeutic goal in SAH. Occlusion of the ruptured aneurysm, salvation of acute hydrocephalus and, if necessary, evacuation of an intracerebral hematoma take precedence over further diagnostic procedures to evaluate the etiology of acute cardiopulmonary dysfunction.

Nevertheless, the prevention of secondary brain damage by maintaining adequate perfusion and oxygenation of the brain is of highest importance. Consequently, measures that are necessary to perform proper resuscitation of the hemodynamically instable patient have to be taken immediately.

Following the initial neurosurgical and/or interventional treatment, more sophisticated medical diagnostics and treatment should be undertaken to achieve further stabilization of the patient.

It has to be kept in mind that a neurogenic origin of cardiopulmonary compromise should only be assumed if other possibly treatable reasons have been ruled out.

Monitoring

As in any other life-threatening disease, adequate monitoring is the key for any rational goal-directed therapy. The minimal diagnostic setup comprises ECG, pulse oximetry, and preferably invasive blood pressure monitoring as well as chest x-ray and lab parameters.

Especially in seriously hemodynamically compromised patients, advanced monitoring of cardiac function and volume status is indicated.

While catheterization of the pulmonary artery provides monitoring of cardiac output and filling pressures, its application is invasive and requires considerable experience with this method. Less invasive alternatives such as thermal indicator transpulmonary dilution and continuous pulse-contour cardiac output (PiCCO) monitoring are currently available and have been shown to be of considerable clinical value (43).

Echocardiography is an excellent, non-invasive tool to assess cardiac function and volume status. The spatial distribution of RWMAs can give valuable hints regarding the etiology of cardiac dysfunction. Patterns that are inconsistent with the distribution of coronary arteries (Takotsubo or inverted Takotsubo myopathy) are commonly associated with a neurogenic origin of the myopathy. Vice-versa, hypocontractibility matching the vascular territory of a coronary artery will often warrant coronary catheterization to rule out ongoing ischemia.

Continuous, transesophageal echocardiography provides the most extensive cardiac monitoring. Whether this invasive method is truly superior to discontinuous bed-side echocardiography remains to be elucidated.

Because cTnI levels are often raised moderately in SAH patients (see above), serial assessment of cTnI concentrations is usually only performed if hemodynamic deterioration occurs and concurrent ischemic heart disease has to be ruled out.

Fluid management

It is well known today that patients after SAH have a risk of hypovolemia and that hypovolemia is associated with delayed cerebral ischemia and poor outcome.

The avoidance of hypovolemia by ample fluid intake and, in some cases, the induction of hypervolemia, have been a mainstay of treatment after SAH. Systematic review of the literature has raised serious doubts about the effectiveness and safety of this treatment regime (44).

Especially cardiopulmonary-compromised patients are at risk of developing complications due to fluid overloading, and the careful use of fluids is necessary. Any prophylactic induction of hypervolemia in order to prevent cerebral vasospasm is contraindicated.

To achieve the goal of normovolemia, knowledge about the current volume status and cardiac output is necessary. This may often require additional hemodynamic monitoring (see above) as neither net fluid balance nor central venous filling pressures are good parameters of volume status.

Catecholamines and inotropes

The conventional pharmacologic management of heart failure following SAH is based on the use of norepinephrine, epinephrine, and dobutamine. Although it may seem counterintuitive to treat catecholamine-induced heart failure by the administration of catecholamines, positive inotropic support with dobutamine has been shown to be effective (45, 46) while vasopressors like norepinephrine may help to maintain cerebral perfusion pressure in an acceptable range.

It has been speculated that the endogenous catecholamine surge and subsequent intracellular calcium overload causes myocytes to become relatively insensitive to physiological inotropic stimuli. Consequently, supraphysiological inotropic stimulation may temporarily compensate this deficiency to some extent.

In cases in which the effects of catecholamines are not sufficient, additive use of alternative inotropic substances may help to improve cardiac pump function. Inhibitors of phosphodiesterase III (PDE-3) (e.g. milrinone) slow the breakdown of intracellular cAMP and cause a further rise of intracellular calcium levels while circumventing the adrenoreceptor pathway.

Novel substances that sensitize contractile filaments of the myocardium to calcium may pose a promising therapeutic alternative in the future. The idea of resensitizing the heart muscle to physiological inotropic stimuli following a catecholamine surge appears to be more pathophysiologically correct than the further pharmacological raise of catecholamine levels. Busani *et al.* recently reported successful application of such a drug, levosimendan, in a case of refractory ventricular dysfunction following SAH (47). Future studies are necessary to validate the value of this drug in cardiac failure after SAH.

Adrenoreceptor blockade

Although pharmacological or surgical blockade of autonomous signal transduction following SAH has been shown to be effective in animals, there are few data on adrenoreceptor blockade to reduce myocardial injury after SAH in humans. In a randomized study on 90 SAH patients without a history of cardiac disease and presenting within 48 hours of SAH, administration of propranolol and phentolamine caused no difference in mortality between the placebo and treatment group (48). In fatal cases, signs of typical contraction-band necrosis were only found in the placebo group indicating a potential protective effect.

Considering a potential upregulation of adrenoreceptors in patients already on α- or ß-blockers, it may be wise to continue this medication following SAH.

Cardiac assist devices

In cases of cardiac failure refractory to maximum medical therapy with concomitant cerebral vasospasm, sporadic reports of the successful application of intra-aortic balloon pump (IABP) counterpulsation do exist (49,50). The impact of IABP counterpulsation on cerebral hemodynamics has not been studied extensively. In a series of 23 non-SAH patients with IABP, Schachtrupp *et al.* (51) reported significantly changed blood-flow patterns in basal cerebral arteries and a transient reversal of intracranial blood flow counterbalanaced by a slight increase in mean antegrade flow. Where available, IABP counterpulsation may be considered as an *ultima ratio* in severe cardiac failure after SAH.

Ventilation

A rational ventilation strategy should be guided by oxygenation needs as well as current cerebral hemodynamic constraints and should try to avoid any additional lung injury due to mechanical ventilation. The selection between invasive or non-invasive ventilation should be guided by the severity of the cardiopulmonary compromise and the patient's level of consciousness. Some individuals with only moderate problems may be handled using non-invasive ventilation, but patients with serious conditions must be sedated, intubated, and properly ventilated.

Ventilator settings should be consistent with the guidelines for lung-protective ventilation with a tidal volume of 6–8 ml/kg and the application of positive end-expiratory pressure (PEEP).

It has to be stressed that PEEP values below 15 cm H_2O have been shown to be safe in neurosurgical patients and that they *do not* compromise cerebral perfusion pressures (52–54).

Permissive hypercapnia is not advisable as it may increase intracerebral pressure due to cerebral vasodilation. Equally, hyperventilation should be avoided due to its compromising effect on cerebral perfusion. Arterial partial CO_2 pressure should be measured frequently and maintained in a normoventilation range (35–40 mmHg). To prevent accidental hyperventilation, end-tidal CO_2 monitoring can also be applied.

If hyperventilation is inevitable, it should only be allowed if ICP monitoring and preferably brain perfusion (rCBF) or tissue oxygenation ($pTiO_2$) monitoring is available. Similar limitations should be observed for prone positioning of patients with acute SAH and raised ICP (55–57).

Summary

Cardiopulmonary dysfunction is a common and potentially reversible complication after acute subarachnoid hemorrhage. It is caused by a sudden overactivation of the sympathetic nervous system which causes a surge of catecholamines to reach the heart and central vasculature. Subsequent cardiac signal conduction or pump failure and neurologic pulmonary edema are life-threatening sequelae of SAH and should be taken as seriously as neurological complications. While the exact pathophysiological mechanisms of catecholamine-induced compromise are still not known today, the management is centered around sustaining and augmenting cardiopulmonary function within the constraints given by the neurological situation until natural recovery occurs.

REFERENCES

1. Solenski NJ, Haley EC, Jr., Kassell NF, *et al.* Medical complications of aneurysmal subarachnoid hemorrhage: a report of the multicenter, cooperative aneurysm study. Participants of the Multicenter Cooperative Aneurysm Study. *Crit Care Med.* 1995;**23**(6):1007–17.
2. Crago EA, Kerr ME, Kong Y, *et al.* The impact of cardiac complications on outcome in the SAH population. *Acta Neurol Scand.* 2004;**110**(4):248–53.
3. Cushing H. The blood pressure reaction of acute cerebral compression illustrated by cases of intracranial hemorrhage. *Am J Med Sc.* 1903;**125**:1017–44.
4. Byer E, Ashman R, Toth LA. Electrocardiograms with large, upright T waves and QT intervals. *Am Heart J.* 1947;**33**:796–806.
5. Moutier F. Hypertension et mort par oedème pulmonaire aigu, chez les blesses cranio-encephaliques. *Press Med.* 1918;**26**:108–9.
6. Shanahan W. Pulmonary edema in epilepsy. *NY Med J.* 1908;**87**:54–6.
7. Attar HJ, Gutierrez MT, Bellet S, *et al.* Effects of stimulation of hypothalamic and reticular activating systems on production of cardiac arrhythmias. *Circ Res.* 1963;**12**:14–21.
8. Hunt D, Gore I. Myocardial ultrastructural and hemodynamic reactions during experimental subarachnoid hemorrhage. *J Mol Cell Cardiol.* 1972;**4**:287–98.
9. Hawkins WE, Clover BR. Myocardial damage after head trauma and simulated intracranial hemorrhage in mice: the role of the autonomic nervous system. *Cardiovasc Res.* 1971;**5**:524–9.
10. Yanwowitz F, Preston JB, Abildskov JA. Functional distribution of right and left stellate innervation of the ventricles: Production of neurogenic electrocardiographic changes by unilateral alteration of sympathetic tone. *Circ Res.* 1966;**18**:416–28.

11. Weinberg SJ, Fuster JM. Electrocardiographic changes produced by hypothalamic stimulation. *Ann Intern Med.* 1960;**53**:332–8.
12. Manning JW, De Vacotter M. Mechanisms of cardiac arrhythmias induced by diencephalic stimulation. *Am J Physiol.* 1962;**203**:1120–4.
13. Beattie J, Brow GR, Long CN. Physiological and anatomical evidence for the existence of nerves connecting the hypothalamus with spinal sympathetic centers. *Proc R Soc Lond* (Biol). 1930;**106**:253–75.
14. Saper CB, Loewy AD, Swanson LW, Cowan WM. Direct hypothalamo-autonomic connections. *Brain Res.* 1976;**117**(2):305–12.
15. Magouin HW. Descending connection from the hypothalami and central levels of autonomic function. Procedures associated for research in nervous and mental disease. *Baltimore: Williams & Wilkins*; 1941: 270–85.
16. Triposkiadis F, Karayannis G, Giamouzis G, *et al.* The sympathetic nervous system in heart failure physiology, pathophysiology, and clinical implications. *J Am Coll Cardiol.* 2009;**54**(19):1747–62.
17. Jacob WA, Van Bogaert A, DeGroot-Lassed MHA. Myocardial ultrastructural and haemodynamic reactions during experimental subarachnoid hemorrhage. *J Mol Cell Cardiol.* 1972;**4**:287–98.
18. Kawahara E, Ikeda S, Miyahara Y, Kohno S. Role of autonomic nervous dysfunction in electrocardio-graphic abnormalities and cardiac injury in patients with acute subarachnoid hemorrhage. *Circ J.* 2003;**67**(9):753–6.
19. Naredi S, Lambert G, Eden E, *et al.* Increased sympathetic nervous activity in patients with nontraumatic subarachnoid hemorrhage. *Stroke.* 2000;**31**(4):901–6.
20. Connor RC. Myocardial damage secondary to brain lesions. *Am Heart J.* 1969;**78**:145–8.
21. Greenhoot JH, Reichenbach DD. Cardiac injury and subarachnoid hemorrhage. A clinical, pathological, and physiological correlation. *J Neurosurg.* 1969;**30**:521–31.
22. Kline IK. Myocardial alterations associated with phaeochromocytomas. *Am J Pathol.* 1961;**38**:539–51.
23. Sakr YL, Ghosn I, Vincent JL. Cardiac manifestations after subarachnoid hemorrhage: a systematic review of the literature. *Prog Cardiovasc Dis.* 2002;**45**(1):67–80.
24. Rudehill A, Olsson GL, Sundqvist K, Gordon E. ECG abnormalities in patients with subarachnoid haemorrhage and intracranial tumours. *J Neurol Neurosurg Psychiatry.* 1987;**50**(10):1375–81.
25. Brouwers PJ, Wijdicks EF, Hasan D, *et al.* Serial electrocardiographic recording in aneurysmal subarachnoid hemorrhage. *Stroke.* 1989;**20**(9):1162–7.
26. Haley EC, Jr., Kassell NF, Torner JC. A randomized controlled trial of high-dose intravenous nicardipine in aneurysmal subarachnoid hemorrhage. A report of the Cooperative Aneurysm Study. *J Neurosurg.* 1993;**78**(4): 537–47.
27. Mayer SA, LiMandri G, Sherman D, *et al.* Electrocardiographic markers of abnormal left ventricular wall motion in acute subarachnoid hemorrhage. *J Neurosurg.* 1995;**83**(5):889–96.
28. Parekh N, Venkatesh B, Cross D, *et al.* Cardiac troponin I predicts myocardial dysfunction in aneurysmal subarachnoid hemorrhage. *J Am Coll Cardiol.* 2000;**36**(4):1328–35.
29. Zaroff JG, Rordorf GA, Ogilvy CS, Picard MH. Regional patterns of left ventricular systolic dysfunction after subarachnoid hemorrhage: evidence for neurally mediated cardiac injury. *J Am Soc Echocardiogr.* 2000;**13**(8):774–9.
30. Di Palma G, Daniele GP, Antonini-Canterin F, Piazza R, Nicolosi GL. Cardiogenic shock with basal transient left ventricular ballooning (Takotsubo-like cardiomyopathy) as first presentation of pheochromocytoma. *J Cardiovasc Med* (Hagerstown). 2010;**11**(7):507–10.
31. Gervais MK, Gagnon A, Henri M, Bendavid Y. Pheochromocytoma presenting as inverted Takotsubo cardiomyopathy: a case report and review of the literature. *J Cardiovasc Med* (Hagerstown). 2010; Feb 11.
32. Riera M, Llompart-Pou JA, Carrillo A, Blanco C. Head injury and inverted Takotsubo cardiomyopathy. *J Trauma.* 2010;**68**(1):E13–15.
33. Marechaux S, Goldstein P, Girardie P, Ennezat PV. Contractile pattern of inverted Takotsubo cardiomyopathy: illustration by two-dimensional strain. *Eur J Echocardiogr.* 2009;**10**(2):332–3.
34. Marechaux S, Fornes P, Petit S, *et al.* Pathology of inverted Takotsubo cardiomyopathy. *Cardiovasc Pathol.* 2008;**17** (4):241–3.
35. Banki N, Kopelnik A, Tung P, *et al.* Prospective analysis of prevalence, distribution, and rate of recovery of left ventricular systolic dysfunction in patients with subarachnoid hemorrhage. *J Neurosurg.* 2006;**105**(1):15–20.
36. Adams JE, 3rd, Bodor GS, Davila-Roman VG, *et al.* Cardiac troponin I. A marker with high specificity for cardiac injury. *Circulation.* 1993;**88**(1):101–6.
37. Naidech AM, Kreiter KT, Janjua N, *et al.* Cardiac troponin elevation, cardiovascular morbidity, and outcome after subarachnoid hemorrhage. *Circulation.* 2005;**112** (18):2851–6.
38. Tanabe M, Crago EA, Suffoletto MS, *et al.* Relation of elevation in cardiac troponin I to clinical severity, cardiac dysfunction, and pulmonary congestion in patients with

subarachnoid hemorrhage. *Am J Cardiol.* 2008;**102**(11):1545–50.

39. Friedman JA, Pichelmann MA, Piepgras DG, *et al.* Pulmonary complications of aneurysmal subarachnoid hemorrhage. *Neurosurgery.* 2003;**52**(5):1025–31; discussion 1031–2.
40. Mertes PM, el Abassi K, Jaboin Y, *et al.* Changes in hemodynamic and metabolic parameters following induced brain death in the pig. *Transplantation.* 1994;**58**(4):414–18.
41. Novitzky D, Wicomb WN, Rose AG, Cooper DK, Reichart B. Pathophysiology of pulmonary edema following experimental brain death in chacma baboon. *Ann Thorac Surg.* 1987;**43**:288–94.
42. Pusch F, Wildling E, Freitag H, Weinstabl C. Procalcitonin as a diagnostic marker in patients with aspiration after closed head injury. *Wien Klin Wochenschr.* 2001;**113**(17–18):676–80.
43. Mutoh T, Kazumata K, Ajiki M, Ushikoshi S, Terasaka S. Goal-directed fluid management by bedside transpulmonary hemodynamic monitoring after subarachnoid hemorrhage. *Stroke.* 2007;**38**(12):3218–24.
44. Rinkel GJ, Feigin VL, Algra A, van Gijn J. Circulatory volume expansion therapy for aneurysmal subarachnoid haemorrhage. *Cochrane Database Syst Rev.* 2004(**4**):CD000483.
45. Deehan SC, Grant IS. Haemodynamic changes in neurogenic pulmonary oedema: effect of dobutamine. *Intensive Care Med.* 1996;**22**(7):672–6.
46. Parr MJ, Finfer SR, Morgan MK. Reversible cardiogenic shock complicating subarachnoid haemorrhage. *BMJ.* 1996;**313**(7058):681–3.
47. Busani S, Rinaldi L, Severino C, *et al.* Levosimendan in cardiac failure after subarachnoid hemorrhage. *J Trauma.* 2010;**68**(5):E108–10.
48. Neil-Dwyer G, Walter P, Cruickshank JM, Doshi B, O'Gorman P. Effect of propanolol and phentolamine on myocardial necrosis after subarachnoid hemorrhage. *BMJ.* 1978: 990–2.
49. Taccone FS, Lubicz B, Piagnerelli M, *et al.* Cardiogenic shock with stunned myocardium during triple-H therapy treated with intra-aortic balloon pump counterpulsation. *Neurocrit Care.* 2009;**10**(1):76–82.
50. Apostolides PJ, Greene KA, Zabramski JM, Fitzgerald JW, Spetzler RF. Intra-aortic balloon pump counterpulsation in the management of concomitant cerebral vasospasm and cardiac failure after subarachnoid hemorrhage: technical case report. *Neurosurgery.* 1996;**38**(5):1056–9; discussion 1059–60.
51. Schachtrupp A, Wrigge H, Busch T, Buhre W, Weyland A. Influence of intra-aortic balloon pumping on cerebral blood flow pattern in patients after cardiac surgery. *Eur J Anaesthesiol.* 2005;**22**(3):165–70.
52. McGuire G, Crossley D, Richards J, Wong D. Effects of varying levels of positive end-expiratory pressure on intracranial pressure and cerebral perfusion pressure. *Crit Care Med.* 1997;**25**(6):1059–62.
53. Huynh T, Messer M, Sing RF, *et al.* Positive end-expiratory pressure alters intracranial and cerebral perfusion pressure in severe traumatic brain injury. *J Trauma.* 2002;**53**(3):488–92; discussion 492–3.
54. Videtta W, Villarejo F, Cohen M, *et al.* Effects of positive end-expiratory pressure on intracranial pressure and cerebral perfusion pressure. *Acta Neurochir Suppl.* 2002;**81**:93–7.
55. Nekludov M, Bellander BM, Mure M. Oxygenation and cerebral perfusion pressure improved in the prone position. *Acta Anaesthesiol Scand.* 2006;**50**(8):932–6.
56. Thelandersson A, Cider A, Nellgard B. Prone position in mechanically ventilated patients with reduced intracranial compliance. *Acta Anaesthesiol Scand.* 2006;**50**(8):937–41.
57. Fletcher SJ, Atkinson JD. Use of prone ventilation in neurogenic pulmonary oedema. *Br J Anaesth.* 2003;**90**(2):238–40.

SECTION 7

Critical Care of Cerebral Venous Thrombosis

Identification, differential diagnosis, and therapy for cerebral venous thrombosis

José M. Ferro and Patrícia Canhão

Epidemiology

Thrombosis of the dural sinus and of the cerebral veins (CVT) is less common (0.5–1% of all strokes) than other types of stroke [1–3]. There are no population-based studies on the incidence of CVT. From hospital-based series incidence varies from 0.22/100 000/year (IC 95% = 0–47) in Portugal [4] to 1.23/100 000/year in Isfahan, Iran [5]. The incidence is higher in pregnant and puerperal females (11.6/100 000 deliveries in US) and in children (0.64/100 000 in infants and children <18 years in Canada) [6]. Among adults CVT predominates in females (3:1) and in younger adults, as less than 10% CVT patients are older than 65.

Clinical features

CVT can have an acute, subacute or less often chronic presentation. The most frequent symptoms are headaches, seizures, motor, sensory or language deficits, altered mental status, decreased consciousness, diplopia, and visual loss. Symptoms and signs can be grouped in three major presentation syndromes: isolated intracranial hypertension (headache, vomiting, papilloedema, and visual symptoms), focal syndrome (focal deficits, seizures or both), and encephalopathy (multifocal signs, mental status changes, stupor/coma) [3]. Less common syndromes include thunderclap headache, mimicking subarachnoid hemorrhage, cavernous sinus syndrome (cavernous sinus thrombosis), pulsating tinnitus, and multiple lower cranial nerve palsies (lateral sinus thrombosis).

The clinical presentation is influenced by the site and number of occluded sinus and veins, the presence and type of parenchymal lesions, the age [6,7] and gender [8] of the patient and the interval from onset to presentation [9]. Headaches and isolated intracranial hypertension syndromes are less frequent among elderly patients while altered mental status is more frequent [7]. Headache is more frequent in women than in men [8]. Not surprisingly, patients with more severe clinical presentation are admitted and diagnosed earlier, while those with isolated headache or intracranial hypertension syndrome are diagnosed later, allowing time for papilloedema to develop [9]. About two-thirds of CVT patients have parenchymal lesions on their admission computed tomography (CT) or magnetic resonance imaging (MR). These patients have a more severe clinical picture and more often thrombosis of the sagittal sinus and of the cerebral deep venous system. In contrast, isolated intracranial hypertension syndrome and isolated thrombosis of the lateral sinus are rare in patients with parenchymal lesions. There is a gradient of increasing clinical severity when patients with no parenchymal lesions, patients with venous 'infarcts', and with intracerebral hemorrhages are compared [10,11].

Of special interest for intensivists are the CVT patients who are admitted in coma. In the International Study on Cerebral Vein Thrombosis (ISCVT) [12] 5.2% of the

Critical Care of the Stroke Patient, ed. Stefan Schwab, Daniel Hanley, and A. David Mendelow. Published by Cambridge University Press.

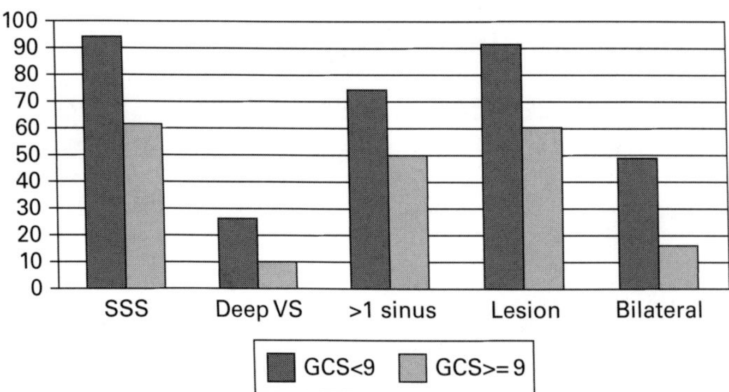

Fig. 35.1 Site and extension of sinus/vein thrombosis and parenchymal lesions in comatose and non-comatose CVT patients.

patients had admission Glasgow Coma Scale score < 9. Comatose patients had more often an acute onset, seizures and motor deficits, occlusion of the superior sagittal sinus and of the deep venous system, multiple sinus occlusions and parenchymal lesions, in particular bilateral brain lesions (Fig. 35.1)

Identification of CVT

Neuroimaging

The confirmation of the diagnosis of CVT requires the demonstration of an occluded sinus/vein and of the thrombus by neuroimaging. In emergency settings, CT is usually the first investigation to be performed in a patient with an 'unusual' headache, an inaugural seizure, hemiparesis or disturbed mental status or coma, which are the most common presenting symptoms of CVT. CT has a low sensitivity, as it may be normal in up to 30% of the patients. The specificity of direct and indirect signs of CVT disclosed by CT is moderate. Direct signs of CVT that can be depicted by CT include: 1) the cord sign due to the hyperdensity of a thrombosed cortical vein and/or dural sinus, and 2) the dense triangle sign. Indirect signs of CVT comprise: 1) dilated transcerebral veins, 2) small ventricles, and 3) parenchymal lesions. Parenchymal lesions may occur in 60–80% of cases and consist of A) hemorrhagic lesions: 1) intracerebral hematomas, 2) hemorrhagic infarct (Fig. 35.2), 3) subarachnoid hemorrhage (<1%) usually limited to the convexity, or B) non-hemorrhagic lesions, appearing as areas of hypodensity due to 1) focal edema or 2) venous infarction, usually not respecting the arterial boundaries, and 3) diffuse brain edema. After contrast injection the occluded superior sagittal sinus appears as the 1) empty delta sign and there may be 2) intense contrast enhancement of falx and tentorium or 3) areas of gyral enhancement. In serial CT the parenchymal lesions may disappear ('vanishing infarcts') or new lesions may appear. If CVT is suspected, plain or contrast CT should be supplemented by CT venography (CTV), which has a good visualization of major venous dural sinuses and can show the non-opacity of the occluded sinus or veins [13]. CTV is more available than MR, can be performed quickly and be used in unstable or agitated patients and in patients with contraindication to MR. The overall accuracy of CT/CTV is 90–100%, depending on the occlusion site. CTV may miss a cortical vein occlusion or a partial deep venous system occlusion. CT/CTV is at least equivalent to MR venography in the diagnosis of CVT [13] and has a 95% sensitivity and a 91% specificity compared to digital subtraction intra-arterial angiography [14]. Drawbacks to CTV include radiation exposure, contrast allergy, and the possibility of aggravating poor renal function. As for all angiography modalities, CTV alone cannot distinguish between non-opacity related to hypoplasia/aplasia and occlusion due to thrombosis. This is a frequent diagnostic dilemma in left lateral sinus occlusion. CTV also cannot

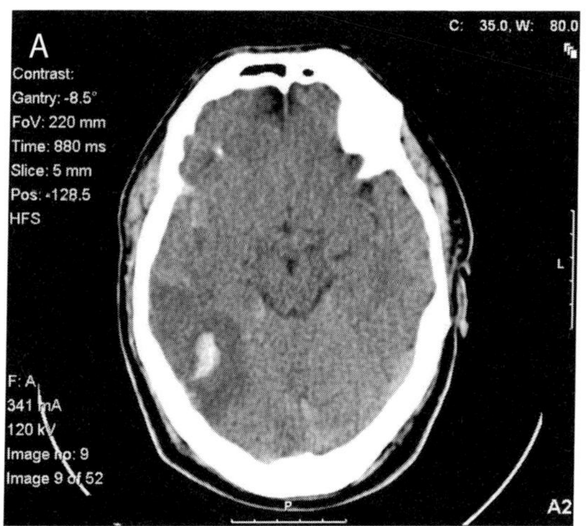

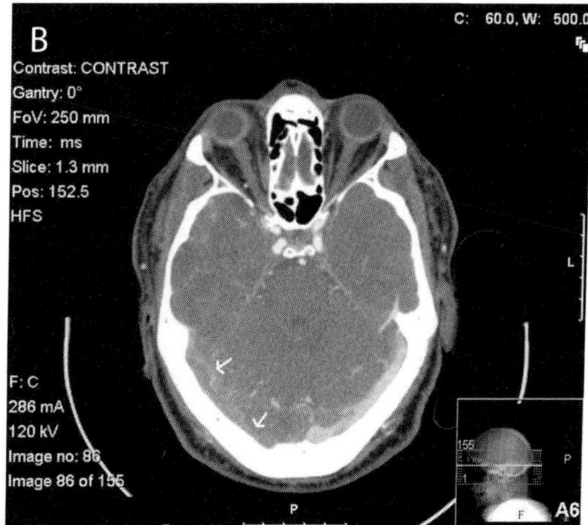

Fig. 35.2 (A) Right temporal hemorrhagic infarct in a patient with right lateral sinus thrombosis. (B) Contrast CT scan shows filling defects in the right lateral sinus (white arrows).

differentiate whether a non-visualized cortical vein is just an anatomical variation or is missing because it is thrombosed.

MR imaging combined with MR venography (MRV) is the most sensitive examination technique for the diagnosis of CVT [15]. The combination of an abnormal signal in a sinus and a corresponding absence of flow on MRV support the diagnosis of CVT (Fig. 35.3). MR images of the occluded sinus change with the age of the thrombus: in the first 5 days the thrombus is isointense on T1-weighted images and hypointense on T2-weighted images due to increased deoxyhemoglobin. After the fifth day there is increased signal on both T1- and T2-weighted images due to methemoglobin. After the first month there is a variable pattern of signal, which may become isointense. A chronically thrombosed sinus may still demonstrate low signal on gradient echo (GRE) and susceptibility-weighted image (SWI). Non-thrombosed hypoplastic sinus will not have abnormal low signal in the sinus on GRE and/or SWI. Gradient echo T_2*-weighted images improve the diagnosis of CVT, in particular of isolated cortical venous thrombosis, which is shown as an hypointense tubular or rounded image [16,17]. After contrast (gadolinium) injection the thrombus appears as a central isointense lesion in a venous sinus with surrounding enhancement. MR is less available and more time consuming than CT/CTV. MRV has several limitations including limited spatial resolution and saturation of flow signal. Turbulent, slow sinus flow and flow gaps are commonly seen on TOF MR venographic images, and may be misdiagnosed as thrombosis.

MRI is also useful to demonstrate non-hemorrhagic parenchymal lesions secondary to venous occlusion and differentiating its type. In contrast with arterial infarct, in venous infarct the area of increased T2 signal is larger than that on DWI. Venous infarcts have increased signal on T2 and DWI and corresponding decreased signal on ADC. T2 hyperintense lesions due to vasogenic edema can have increased signal on DWI but with normal or increased ADC. Non-hemorrhagic lesions in CVT are usually heterogeneous in DWI/ADC, because of the combination of areas of cytotoxic and vasogenic edema.

Intra-arterial venography has a spatial resolution superior to CT or MR venography but is nowadays rarely performed. Intra-arterial venography is reserved to cases with inconclusive or contradictory findings in the other imaging modalities or when intervention is planned.

Independently of the modality (CT, MR or IA), venography has limitations related to anatomical venous variations, such as hypoplasia of the anterior

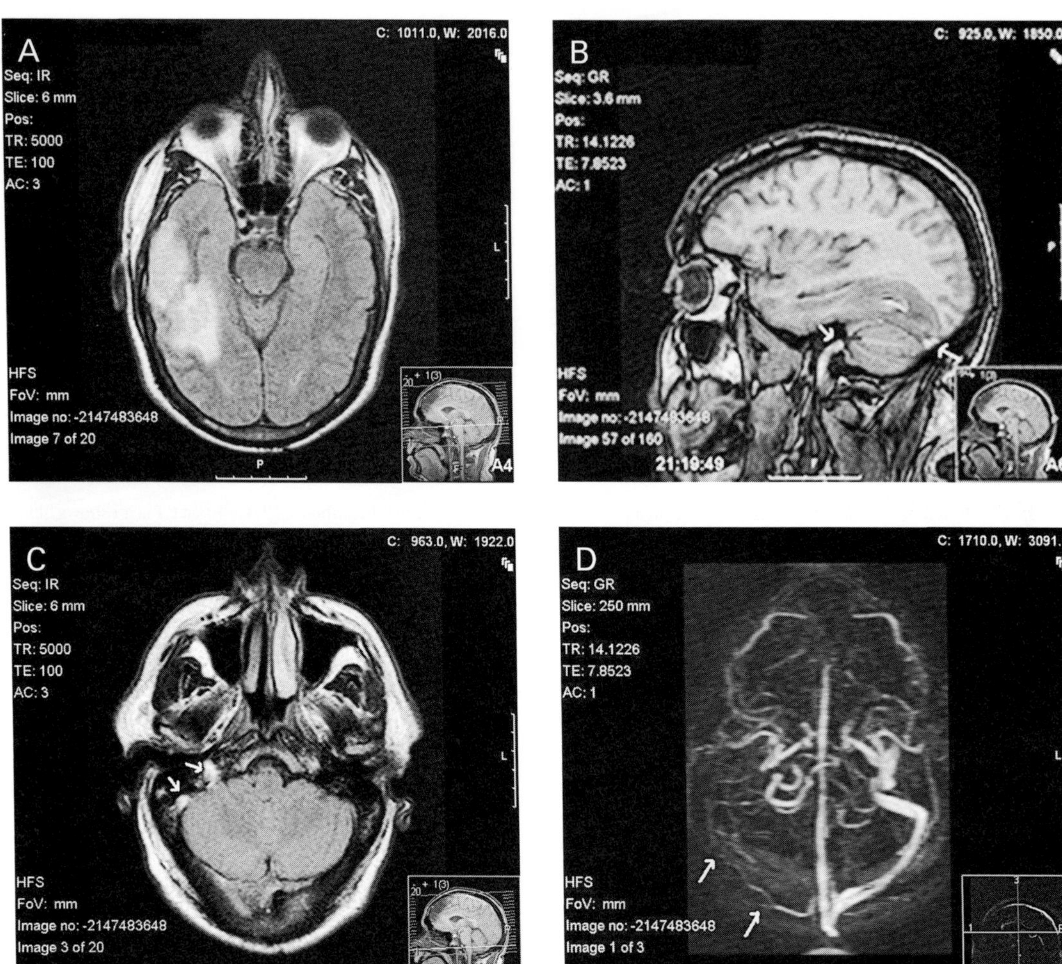

Fig. 35.3 (A) T2-weighted flair images of a temporal hemorrhagic infarct. T1-weighted MRI discloses a hyperintense signal in the right lateral sinus and jugular vein (arrows) corresponding to a thrombus ((B), sagittal; (C), axial); magnetic resonance venography confirms the absence of flow (D) consistent with the occlusion of the lateral sinus.

part of the superior sagittal sinus, duplication of the superior sagittal sinus, intrasinus septa, giant arachnoid granulations, and hypo- or aplasia of the transverse sinuses, which may be misdiagnosed as thrombosis.

The interobserver agreement on CVT diagnosis is not perfect. The proportion of agreement is 62% for angiography and 94% for MR plus angiography [18]. Agreement is lower in cortical vein thrombosis and left transverse sinus occlusion [19].

MR or CT venography is also useful to assess recanalization of the thrombosed sinus. Recanalization occurs in 40–90% of the patients. This percent varies with the site of occlusion, being lower for the lateral sinus. Recanalization happens mainly during the first 4 months post-CVT. Recanalization has no influence on long-term outcome and is apparently not influenced by oral anticoagulant treatment given after the acute phase. The presence of hyperintensities in the veins or sinus in DW MR predicts low recanalization rate [20]. Nevertheless, it is useful to obtain a follow-up venography, in order to have a post-acute study to compare if there is a suspicion of CVT recurrence.

Screening tests: D-dimers

A screening laboratorial test with a high sensitivity for CVT would be of evident clinical importance in emergency and other settings where MR is not readily available to confidently rule out CVT. Unfortunately such a test does not yet exist. Measurement of D-dimers, a product of fibrin degradation, is used in the diagnosis of deep venous thrombosis of the limbs and of pulmonary embolism. A systematic review of all studies using D-dimers in CVT showed that D-dimers have a sensitivity range from 83 to 100, specificity 90–95, positive predictive value 56–83, and negative predictive value 95–100. D-dimers may be helpful to identify patients with a low probability of CVT, who will have a level < 500 μg/l or equivalent using sensitive immunoassay or ELISA [21]. However, false negatives can occur, in particular in CVT patients presenting with isolated headache. D-dimers may also be normal in CVT patients with subacute or chronic presentations and in those with not very extensive sinus/vein thrombosis. In summary, D-dimers cannot be used to rule out CVT.

Differential diagnosis

Given the non-specificity of the symptoms, signs, and presenting syndromes of CVT, the key issue for a prompt diagnosis is a high suspicion rate in patients having appropriate etiologic context: women taking oral contraceptives, pregnant or puerperal females, patients with ear or sinus infection, known acquired or genetic prothrombotic condition, malignancies or other systemic diseases with prothrombotic potential.

Headaches are the most common symptom of CVT. Usually headaches are of the increased intracranial pressure type, worsening when the patient is recumbent or with Valsalva's maneuvers, often accompanied by nausea and vomiting or episodes of brief transient bilateral visual loss (visual obscurations). However, in other patients headaches have non-specific characteristics and may even mimic primary headaches including migraine with aura. In patients with new onset acute severe headache with or without vomiting or a syndrome of intracranial hypertension and meningismus, the differential diagnosis includes meningitis, subarachnoid hemorrhage, and thunderclap headache. CT and CSF examination will establish the diagnosis of the former two entities, meanwhile for the latter diagnosis will depend on history intake of vasoconstrictors or of medical conditions associated with increase in blood pressure and listed among the causes of the reversible cerebral vasoconstriction syndrome. For patients with headache with a subacute onset the differential diagnosis also includes brain tumors, subdural hematoma, and idiopathic intracranial hypertension (IIH). Patients with CVT and isolated headache presenting later usually have papilloedema and normal/nonspecific changes in brain CT. Lumbar puncture will show a normal CSF with high pressure in both CVT and IIH, whose differentiation relies on venography and MR that demonstrate the occluded sinus/vein and the thrombus.

In young or middle-age adults with an inaugural seizure the diagnoses to keep in mind include neoplasms and other brain tumors, AVMs, and cavernomas. CVT involving the superior sagittal sinus or the cortical veins can also present as seizures. Isolated cortical vein thrombosis can be missed unless the GRE T2* sequence is performed.

CVTs presenting as a combination of a focal deficit, such as aphasia or hemiparesis and seizure, also suggests a brain tumor or even encephalitis. The combination of focal deficits and seizures is much more frequent in venous than in arterial stroke.

Cavernous sinus thrombosis must be distinguished from other causes of complete or incomplete cavernous sinus syndrome including intracavernous carotid aneurysm and fistulae, cellulitis or pseudotumor of the orbit.

In patients with headaches, seizures, focal signs or mental changes that are imaged by CT/MR, two-thirds of CVT patients are expected to have parenchymal lesions, which in one-third of cases will be multiple. The differential diagnosis of multiple brain lesions includes brain embolism, secondary or multicentric neoplasms, some infectious diseases, in particular in the context of HIV infection, and less often granulomas and vasculitis. Some imaging patterns are suggestive of CVT, such as: infarct-like lesion not matching an arterial territory, multiple infarcts, infarcts combined with hemorrhagic lesions and hemorrhagic infarcts, early and disproportionate vasogenic edema, and larger lesion in T2 than in DWI. Some lesion locations are also suggestive of CVT, such as frontal or parietal paramedian lesions, in instances of superior sagittal sinus thrombosis, posterior temporal intracerebral hematomas in cases of lateral sinus thrombosis, or bilateral thalamic lesions in cases of deep venous system thrombosis. In a repeated scan, new lesions may appear, some may undergo hemorrhagic transformation, and some may vanish or disappear. Hemorrhagic transformation usually starts centrally and has a finger-like appearance on CT.

Diagnosis of the cause of CVT

Case reports, case-series reports, and less often case-control studies [22] have described the association of several predisposing conditions and precipitating risk factors for CVT (Table 35.1). In about 15% of the patients no underlying cause can be found despite extensive investigation (cryptogenic CVT) [12].

Table 35.1 Risk factors for CVT

Transient risk factors
Pregnancy and puerperium (or post-abortion)
Oral contraceptives
Post menopausal hormonal therapy
Other drugs with prothrombotic effect
Intracranial infection
Meningitis
Others
Infection of neighboring structure
Sinusitis, mastoiditis, otitis
Other (infections of the eye, tooth, skin of face, scalp)
Other infections
Mechanical causes
Head trauma
Lumbar puncture
Jugular catheter
Neurosurgery
Severe dehydration
Severe anemia
Permanent risk factors
Genetic thrombophilia
Severe: Protein C, protein S, and anti-thrombin deficiencies
Mild: Factor V Leiden and prothrombin G20210A mutations
Antiphospholipid syndrome
Nephrotic syndrome
Malignancies
Hematological diseases
Polycythemia
Thrombocythemia
Connective tissue diseases
Systemic lupus erythematous
Others
Behçet's disease
Other vasculitis
Other inflammatory systemic diseases
Inflammatory bowel diseases
Intracranial causes
Meningeoma
Cerebral vascular malformations

Treatment of intracranial hypertension

The more frequent risk factors are prothrombotic conditions, either genetic or acquired, oral contraceptives, puerperium or pregnancy, malignancy, and infection [12]. Infections are nowadays less frequent as a cause of CVT. ENT consultation may be required if otitis or sinusitis is suspected or detected and cerebrospinal fluid examination through a lumbar puncture is indicated if there is a clinical suspicion of meningitis.

Multiple risk factors may be found in about half of patients, including a prothrombotic condition which can be identified in one-third of patients, being genetically determined in one-quarter of patients and acquired in the remainder, mainly antiphospholipid syndrome (APL) [12]. The genetic background probably determines the inherent individual risk for CVT. In the presence of genetic prothrombotic conditions (e.g. antithrombin, protein C or protein S deficiency, factor

V Leiden; prothrombin gene mutation), patients are at increased risk of developing a CVT when exposed to transient risk factors such as oral contraceptives, pregnancy/puerperium, infections, head trauma, lumbar puncture, surgery or prothrombotic drugs. Therefore testing for APL and for genetic prothrombotic conditions is recommended in all CVT patients, even when another associated condition is already identified. The diagnosis of APL requires abnormal high titers of lupus anticoagulant, anticardiolipin IgG or anti-β2-glycoprotein IgG antibodies) on two or more occasions at least 12 weeks apart. Testing for deficiencies of protein C, S, and antithrombin must be performed at least 6 weeks after a thrombotic event, and should be confirmed with repeat testing and family studies. Heparin reduces antithrombin levels and protein C and S levels are lowered by oral anticoagulants. High levels of Factor VIII were also found in some CVT series, but high Factor VIII levels may be secondary to the acute CVT or to a systemic disease underlying CVT. Hyperhomocysteinemia also increase the risk of CVT. High levels of factors IX, XI, TAFI, and MTHFR mutation [23] are not established risk factors for CVT.

In elderly CVT patients the proportion of cases with malignancies and hematological disorders such as polycythemia is higher [7]. Therefore in the elderly patient and in cryptogenic CVT search for an occult neoplasm is recommended. In almost 15% of adult CVT patients extensive search is unable to reveal an underlying cause. Sometimes, the cause (e.g. vasculitis, antiphospholipid syndrome, malignancy, polycytemia, thrombocytemia) is discovered only weeks or months after the acute phase or after repeated testing.

Outcome and prognosis

Only a few cohort studies analyzed the prognostic factors for the short-term and the long-term outcome of CVT patients. In the largest cohort study (ISCVT) [12], complete recovery at last follow-up (median 16 months) was observed in 79% of the patients, overall death rate was 8.3% and there was a 5.1% dependency rate (mRS $\geq$3) at the end of follow-up. In a systematic review including both retrospective and prospective studies, overall mortality was 9.4% and the proportion of dependency (mRS $\geq$3 or GOS $\geq$3) was 9.7% [24]. Considering only cohort studies, the overall death and dependency rate is 15% (95% CI 13–18) [12].

Around one-quarter of CVT patients can have neurological deterioration after admission, even several days after diagnosis and starting treatment. Neurologic worsening can feature depressed consciousness, mental status disturbance, new seizure, worsening of or a new focal deficit, increase in headache intensity, or visual loss. About one-third of patients with neurologic deterioration will have new parenchymal lesions if neuroimaging is repeated [25]. Four to 15% of patients die in the acute phase of CVT. The main cause of acute death with CVT is transtentorial herniation secondary to a large hemorrhagic lesion [26] followed by herniation due to multiple lesions or to diffuse brain edema. Status epilepticus, medical complications, and pulmonary embolism are among other causes of early death. Deaths after the acute phase are mainly due to the underlying conditions, in particular malignancies [12]. Brain herniation leading to early death is more frequent in young patients, whereas late deaths due to malignancies are more frequent in elderly patients.

In the ISCVT cohort, among 31 patients with GCS score < 9 at admission, 16 (52%) worsened after diagnosis (new seizure in seven patients, worsening of or a new focal deficit in five patients each). Eight new intracerebral hemorrhages and six new venous infarcts were detected in the 25 patients who had repeated CT/MR. Concerning outcome nine of these comatose patients died in the acute phase (29%) and two others during follow up (total mortality: 35%). Among the survivors the outcome was in general good: 13 patients had mRS 0–1, six patientst mRS 2, and only one patient mRS 3. None was left severely disabled (mRS 4 or 5) (Fig. 35.4).

Risk factors for poor long-term prognosis in the ISCVT cohort were central nervous system infection, any malignancy, thrombosis of the deep venous system, intracranial hemorrhage on the admission CT/MR, Glasgow coma scale score (GCS) <9, mental status disturbance, age >37 years, and male gender [12]. Among comatose patients, those without thrombosis of the deep venous system had a better prognosis.

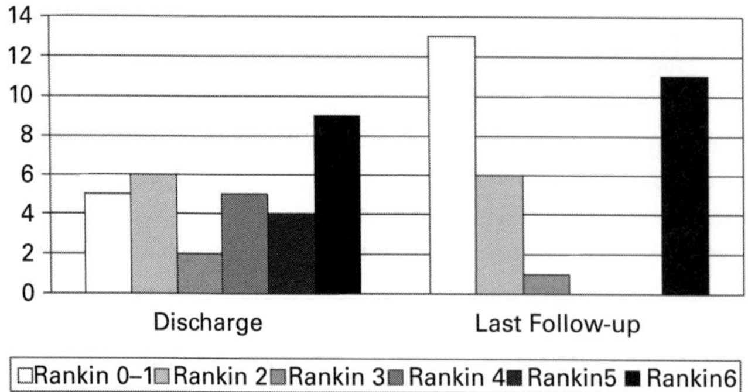

Fig. 35.4 Outcome at discharge from acute hospital and last follow-up of comatose CVT patients.

Table 35.2 CVT risk socre

Prognostic variable	HR (95% CI)	Risk points
Malignancy	4.53 (2.52–8.15)	2
Coma	4.19 (2.20–6.28)	2
Thrombosis of the deep venous system	3.03 (1.76–5.23)	2
Mental status disturbance	2.18 (1.37–3.46)	1
Male gender	1.60 (1.01–5.23)	1
Intracranial hemorrhage	1.42 (0.88–2.27)	1

The risk score model range from 0 (lowest risk) to 9 (highest risk) with a cut-off of ≥ 3 points indicating a higher risk of death or dependency at 6 months.

Risk stratification scores might improve the ability to inform CVT patients on their individual prognosis and to select those who might benefit most from intensive monitoring and invasive treatments [27–29] The ISCVT study group developed a risk score for poor outcome (mRS Scale > 2) (Table 35.2) which was tested in two validation samples of CVT patients. Using the risk score (range from 0 to 9) with a cut-off of ≥3 points, overall efficiency was 85.4%, 84.4% and 90.1% in the derivation and validation samples, respectively. Sensitivity and specificity in the three samples combined was 96.1% and 13.6%.

Long-term complications of CVT include seizures, headaches, visual loss, dural arteriovenous fistulae, and recurrent venous thrombosis of the brain, limbs, abdomen or pelvis [12,30].

Treatment

Besides the treatment of the associated condition/risk factors, treatment of CVT includes: 1) antithrombotic treatment, 2) symptomatic treatment, and 3) prevention/treatment of complications.

Treatment of the risk factors

Although the treatment of the multiple possible risk factors/associated conditions is outside the scope of this chapter, we would stress the importance of appropriate antibiotic treatment, whenever there is meningitis or other intracranial infection or an infection of a neighboring structure (e.g. otitis, mastoiditis). Sometimes these ENT infections need local surgery.

Anti-thrombotic treatment

Heparins

The use of heparins in acute CVT is supported by four clinical trials and a meta-analysis of two of these trials [31], which showed a non-significant relative risk of 0.33 (95% CI 0.08–1.21) for death and 0.46 (95% CI 0.16–1.31) of death or dependency after anticoagulant therapy as compared to placebo. Two trials performed in India were excluded from the meta-analysis, because one was performed only in puerperal CVT and in the other the diagnosis of CVT was based only on CT.

If these trials are included, the relative risk of death will be again 0.33 but significant (95% CI 0.14–0.78) (Ia/A).

Concerning safety of use of heparin in CVT with intracranial hemorrhagic lesions, several observational series showed that heparin is safe and can be used in acute CVT patients with intracranial hemorrhagic lesions. If lumbar puncture or other intervention are planned to be performed, heparin should be stopped to have a normalized APTT and then restarted.

LMWHs have longer half-life, more predictable clinical response and are less likely to decrease platelet counts compared with standard heparin. A non-matched case control study of cases treated with IV heparin and LMWH in ISCVT showed that death or dependency was more frequent in IV heparin treated patients (16% vs. 9%, $p = 0.05$). Inclusion of patients who received both IV and LMWH ($n = 96$), based on the therapy they received first, yielded similar results, although the difference in poor outcome was no longer statistically significant (15% vs. 9%, $p = 0.1$; OR 1.7, $p = 0.2$). These results suggest that LMWH is at least equally effective to IV heparin for the treatment of CVT [32].

Endovascular thrombolysis

Direct endovascular thrombolysis aiming to dissolve the venous clot and reopen the occluded sinus or vein is used as an alternative to heparin in severe cases or in patients who fail to improve or deteriorate despite anticoagulation or if there is an elevation in intracranial pressure that increases despite conventional treatment. Catheterization of the sigmoid, transverse, and superior sagittal sinuses via the femoral venous or jugular approach is followed by local injection of rtPA or urokinase. Mechanical thrombolysis by disruption, removal or suction may be additionally performed or utilized alone.

No randomized trials of endovascular treatment for sinus thrombosis have been performed. The published literature consists of case reports or uncontrolled case series. A systematic review including 169 patients with CVT treated with local thrombolysis, suggested a possible benefit for severe CVT cases, indicating that thrombolytics may reduce case fatality in critically ill patients. Intracranial hemorrhage after thrombolysis was reported in 17% of cases, and was associated with clinical worsening in 5% [33]. Several other series with encouraging results were published after the systematic review. However, the possibility of publication bias must be kept in mind. In a recent Dutch series of 20 patients treated with IV local thrombolysis, 12 patients recovered to independent living while six died [34]. Local thrombolysis was not useful in patients with large infarcts and impending herniation. A randomized trial (TO-ACT) to compare endovascular treatment vs. heparin in acute CVT is in the final preparation stages and will randomize patients with severe forms of CVT, as defined by the presence of one or more of intracranial hemorrhage, mental status disturbance, coma or thrombosis of the deep cerebral venous system, for endovascular or standard (any heparin) treatment. Patients with isolated intracranial hypertension or large hemispheric lesions with eminent herniation will be excluded. Pending the results of this trial, endovascular thrombolysis should be considered a treatment option for CVT patients who worsen despite anticoagulant therapy, in particular those with thrombosis of the cerebral deep venous system and without large hemispheric lesions with mass effect.

Oral anticoagulation

Prolonged oral anticoagulation with warfarin is used after the acute phase of CVT to prevent further venous thrombotic events, including the recurrence of CVT.

Four recent studies analyzed the risk and risk factors for the recurrence of venous thrombotic events in CVT patients. In the Rochester Mayo Clinic series, the likelihood of recurrent venous thrombosis was the same after CVT and lower extremity deep venous thrombosis. Recurrence of CVT was not influenced by warfarin therapy [35]. In children, age at CVT onset (after 2 years), persistent venous occlusion, the G20210A mutation, and non-administration of anticoagulation predict recurrent CVT or systemic venous thrombosis [36]. In the ISCVT the risk of all venous thrombotic events after the initial CVT was 4.1 per 100 person-years [37] and the rate of recurrence of CVT was 1.5 per 100 person-years.

Recurrence of venous thrombosis (all territories) after CVT was more frequent among men and in patients with polycythaemia/thrombocythemia. In the Martinelli *et al.* series [38], the risk of recurrent CVT was 0.5 per 100 persons/year and the risk of other venous thrombosis 2.0. Males and patients with severe thrombophilia (or combined defects) had an increased risk of further venous thrombotic events. Such risk was not increased in mild thrombophilia.

Optimal duration of anticoagulation has not yet been addressed in randomized controlled trials, although such a study is in the planning phase. Oral anticoagulation aims at an international normalized ratio (INR) of two to three. The EFNS Guidelines recommend that if CVT is related to transient risk factor, anticoagulants should be given for 3 months. In patients with cryptogenic CVT or in those with mild thrombophilia, the period of anticoagulation must be extended for 6 to 12 months. In patients with 'severe' thrombophilia or recurrent venous thrombosis, anticoagulants should be given for life (Table 35.1) [39].

In patients presenting a syndrome of isolated increased intracranial pressure, featuring severe headache and papilloedema, intracranial hypertension can be reduced and symptoms relieved through a therapeutic lumbar puncture, performed after CT or MR excludes large parenchymal lesions or hydrocephalus.

Corticosteroids do not improve outcome in the acute phase of CVT, as shown by a large case-control study [40]. Acetazolamide is used in some centers, despite a lack of supporting evidence. Other measures to control acutely increased ICP include elevating the head of the bed, osmotic diuretics such as mannitol, intensive care unit admission with sedation, hyperventilation to a target $PaCO_2$ of 30 to 35 mmHg with ICP monitoring.

Decompressive surgery

Herniation due to unilateral mass effect is the major cause of death in CVT [26]. Decompressive surgery can be life saving in these patients (Fig. 35.5). Recent case series, a case control study, a retrospective registry [41], and a systematic review of 68 cases of CVT [42] who were treated by decompressive surgery (hemicraniectomy or

A

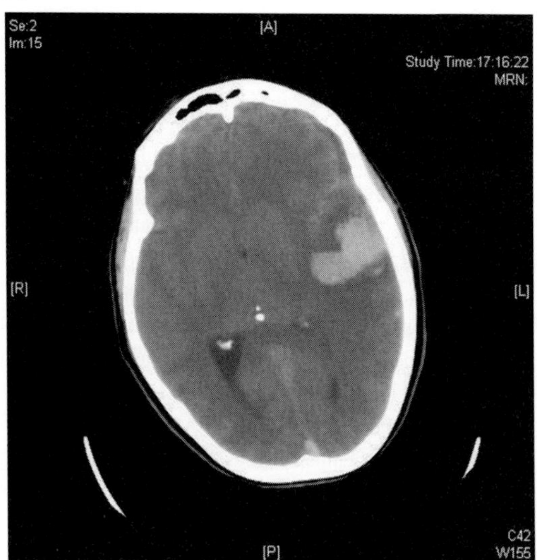

B

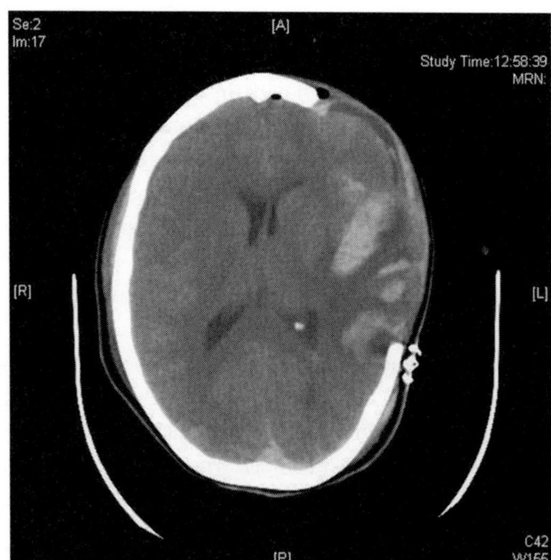

Fig. 35.5 Large temporal hemorrhage lesions with mass effect secondary to thrombosis of the left lateral and superior saggital sinus. CT before (A) and after (B) decompressive hemicraniectomy

hematoma drainage) showed that in CVT patients with large parenchymal lesions causing herniation, decompressive surgery was life saving, and often resulted in good functional outcome, irrespective of age, coma, aphasia, bilateral lesions or bilateral fixed pupils. In the systematic review, at last follow-up (median 13 months), 26 (38%) patients had mRS 0–1, 29 (43%) mRs$\geq$3, and only four (6%) were alive with mRS>3. Eleven (16%) patients died. A prospective registry is under way to confirm these encouraging results.

Shunting

Except in the rare occurrence of hydrocephalus, which can complicate CVT of the posterior fossa, ventriculostomy or ventriculo-peritoneal shunts are not indicated in acute CVT.

In patients presenting a syndrome of isolated increased intracranial pressure, lumbo-peritoneal shunt may be indicated if severe headaches and /or visual loss (decreased visual acuity or increasing visual field defects in serial perimetry) develop or do not improve with repeated lumbar punctures and with other measures to reduce intracranial pressure.

Headache

Headache is a common complaint during the follow-up of CVT patients. Severe headaches requiring bed rest or hospital admission were reported in 14% of patients in the ISCVT [12] and 11% in the VENOPORT [30]. In general, headaches are primary and not related to CVT. In patients with persistent or severe headaches, MR with MRV should be performed to rule out recurrent CVT. These MR results should be compared to a 'baseline' follow-up MR obtained 3 months following CVT diagnosis, looking for CVT at a new site or increase in size of a previous thrombus. Occasionally, MRV may show stenosis of a previously occluded sinus, but the clinical significance of this is unclear. If headache persists and MR is normal, lumbar puncture may be needed to exclude or confirm elevated intracranial pressure.

Visual Loss

Severe visual loss due to CVT rarely occurs (2–4%) nowadays [12,30,43]. Patients with papilledema or visual complaints should have a complete neuro-ophthalmological study, including visual acuity and visual field testing. Rapid diagnosis of CVT [9] and treatment of intracranial hypertension are the main measures to prevent visual loss. Surgical fenestration of the optic nerve may be performed in specialized centers, but is rarely required.

Treatment and prevention of seizures

Focal or generalized post-CVT seizures can be divided into early or remote (occurring more than 2 weeks after diagnosis) [44–46]. In general routine prescription of anti-epileptic drugs is not indicated to prevent seizures and should be reserved for high-risk patients. Concerning early seizures, a case control study showed that seizures prior to or at admission and supratentorial lesion are the risk factors for subsequent early seizures. Fifty-one percent of the patients with both risk factors who were not prescribed anti-epileptic drugs suffered a new seizure, contrasting with 0.7% of those who received antiepileptic medication [44]. This evidence indicates that patients with both supratentorial lesions and presenting seizures should be prescribed anti-epileptic drugs in the acute phase [39]. This may also be considered in patients with single seizure in the absence of parenchymal lesions.

Remote seizures affect 5% to 32% of patients. Most of these seizures occur in the first year of follow-up [45,46]. Risk factors for remote seizures are hemorrhagic lesion on admission CT/MR (HR = 2.6), early seizure (HR = 2.4), and paresis (HR = 2.2). Five percent of patients have post-CVT epilepsy (more than one remote seizure). Post-CVT epilepsy is also associated with hemorrhagic lesion on admission CT/MR (HR = 6.8), early seizure (HR = 4.0), and paresis (HR = 2.8) [46]. Prophylactic antiepileptics for a defined duration (usually 1 year) should be prescribed in patients with early seizure and parenchymal lesions and in those with post-CVT epilepsy [39]. It may also be considered in patients with single seizure in the absence of parenchymal lesions.

Contraception and pregnancy

Oral contraception and hormonal replacement therapy should be stopped. Emergency contraception is also contraindicated. Contraceptive methods other than oral or parental contraceptives should be used.

CVT and pregnancy or puerperium-related CVT are not a contraindication for future pregnancy. A comprehensive search for associated conditions and for prothrombotic genetic conditions and APL syndrome should be pursued. Although pregnancy and the puerperium are risk factors for CVT, the risk of complications during subsequent pregnancy among women who have a history of CVT is low. There is information in the literature on 114 women who became pregnant after a CVT, resulting in 145 pregnancies: 83% terminated in normal births. There were only three cases of deep venous thrombosis and none of recurrent CVT. However, a high proportion of spontaneous abortion was noticed [12,38,47–49].

CVT occurring during pregnancy should be preferentially treated with LMWH and this treatment should be continued for at least 6 weeks post-partum. Warfarin is teratogenic and should not be given in the first trimester of pregnancy. Oral anticoagulants may also induce fetal or placental hemorrhage, mainly in the last trimester of pregnancy and at delivery, because they cross the placenta.

REFERENCES

1. Bousser MG, Ferro JM. Cerebral venous thrombosis: an update. *Lancet Neurol* 2007;**6**:162–70.
2. Stam J. Thrombosis of the cerebral veins and sinuses. *N Engl J Med* 2005;**352**:1791–8.
3. Bousser MG, Russell RR. Cerebral venous thrombosis. In: Warlow CP, Van Gijn J, eds. *Major Problems in Neurology*. London, WB Saunders, 1997, Vol **33**.
4. Ferro JM, Correia M, Pontes C, *et al.* Cerebral Venous Thrombosis Portuguese Collaborative Study Group (Venoport). *Cerebrovasc Dis* 2001;**11**:177–82.
5. Janghorbani M, Zare M, Saadatnia M, *et al.* Cerebral vein and dural sinus thrombosis in adults in Isfahan, Iran: frequency and seasonal variation. *Acta Neurol Scand.* 2008;**117**:117–21.
6. deVeber G, Andrew M, Adams C, *et al.* and the Canadian Pediatric Ischemic Stroke Study Group. Cerebral sinovenous thrombosis in children. *N Engl J Med* 2001;**345**:417–423.
7. Ferro JM, Canhão P, Bousser MG, Stam J, Barinagarrementeria F. ISCVT Investigators. Cerebral vein and dural sinus thrombosis in elderly patients. *Stroke* 2005;**36**:1927–32.
8. Coutinho JM, Ferro JM, Canhão P, *et al.* Cerebral venous and sinus thrombosis in women. *Stroke* 2009;**40**:2356–61.
9. Ferro JM, Canhão P, Stam J, *et al.* ISCVT Investigators. Delay in the diagnosis of cerebral vein and dural sinus thrombosis: influence on outcome. *Stroke* 2009;**40**:3133–8.
10. Girot M, Ferro JM, Canhão P, *et al.* ISCVT Investigators. Predictors of outcome in patients with cerebral venous thrombosis and intracerebral hemorrhage. *Stroke* 2007;**38**:337–42.
11. Ferro JM, Canhão P, Bousser MG, *et al.* ISCVT Investigators. Cerebral venous thrombosis with nonhemorrhagic lesions: clinical correlates and prognosis. *Cerebrovasc Dis* 2010;**29**:440–5.
12. Ferro JM, Canhão P, Stam J, *et al.* ISCVT Investigators: Prognosis of cerebral vein and dural sinus thrombosis: results of the International Study on Cerebral Vein and Dural Sinus Thrombosis (ISCVT). *Stroke* 2004;**35**:664–70.
13. Linn J, Erti-Wagner B, Seelos KC, *et al.* Diagnostic value of multidetector-row CT angiography in the evaluation of thrombosis in the cerebral venous sinuses. *AJNR Am J Neuroradiol* 2007;**28**:946–52.
14. Wetzel SG, Kirsch E, Stock KW. Cerebral veins: comparative study of CT venography with intra-arterial digital subtraction angiography. *AJNR Am J Neuroradiol* 1999; **20**:249–55.
15. Lafitte F, Boukobza M, Guichard JP, *et al.* MRI and MRA for diagnosis and follow-up of cerebral venous thrombosis (CVT). *Clin Radiol* 1997;**52**:672–9.
16. Selim M, Fink J, Linfante I, *et al.* Diagnosis of cerebral venous thrombosis with echo-planar T2*-weighted magnetic resonance imaging. *Arch Neurol* 2002;**59**:1021–6.
17. Idbaih A, Boukobza M, Crassard I, *et al.* MRI of clot in cerebral venous thrombosis: high diagnostic value of susceptibility-weighted images. *Stroke* 2006;**37**:991–5.
18. de Bruijn SF, Majoie CB, Koster PA, *et al.* Interobserver agreement for MR-imaging and conventional angiography in the diagnosis of cerebral venous thrombosis. In: de Bruijn SF, ed. *Cerebral venous sinus thrombosis. Clinical and epidemiological studies.* Amsterdam, Thesis Publishers, 1998: 23–33.

19. Ferro JM, Morgado C, Sousa R, Canhão P. Interobserver agreement in the magnetic resonance location of cerebral vein and dural sinus thrombosis. *Eur J Neurol* 2007;**14**:353–6.
20. Favrole P, Guichard JP, Crassard I, *et al.* Diffusion-weighted imaging of intravascular clots in cerebral venous thrombosis. *Stroke* 2004;**35**:99–103.
21. Haapaniemi E, Tatlisumak T. Is D-dimer helpful in evaluating stroke patients? A systematic review. *Acta Neurol Scand* 2009;**119**:141–50.
22. Saadatnia M, Fatehi F, Basiri K, *et al.* Cerebral venous thrombosis risk factors. *Int J Stroke* 2009;**4**:111–23.
23. Gouveia LO, Canhão P. MTHFR and the risk for cerebral venous thrombosis meta-analysis. *Thromb Res* 2010;**125**: e153–8.
24. Dentali F, Gianni M, Crowther MA, Ageno W. Natural history of cerebral vein thrombosis: a systematic review. *Blood* 2006;**108**:1129–34.
25. Crassard I, Canhão P, Ferro JM, *et al.* Neurological worsening in the acute phase of cerebral venous thrombosis in ISCVT (International Study on Cerebral Venous Thrombosis). *Cerebrovasc Dis* 2003;**16**(suppl 4):60.
26. Canhão P, Ferro JM, Lindgren AG, *et al.* ISCVT Investigators. Causes and predictors of death in cerebral venous thrombosis. *Stroke* 2005;**36**:1720–5.
27. Barrinagarrementeria F, Cantú C, Arredondo H. Aseptic cerebral venous thrombosis: proposed prognostic scale. *J Stroke Cerebrovasc Dis* 1992;**2**:34–9.
28. Ferro JM, Bacelar-Nicolau H, Rodrigues T, *et al.* ISCVT and VENOPORT investigators. Risk score to predict the outcome of patients with cerebral vein and dural sinus thrombosis. *Cerebrovasc Dis* 2009;**28**:39–44.
29. Koopman K, Uyttenboogaart M, Vroomen PC, *et al.* Development and validation of a predictive outcome score of cerebral venous thrombosis. *J Neurol Sci* 2009;**276**:66–8.
30. Ferro JM, Lopes MG, Rosas MJ, *et al.* Cerebral Venous Thrombosis Portugese Collaborative Study Group (VENOPORT). Long-term prognosis of cerebral vein and dural sinus thrombosis: results of the VENOPORT Study. *Cerebrovasc Dis* 2002;**13**:272–8.
31. Stam J, de Bruijn SF, deVeber G. Anticoagulation for cerebral sinus thrombosis. *Cochrane Database Syst Rev* 2002;**4**:CD002005.
32. Coutinho J, Ferro JM, Bousser M-G, *et al.* Unfractioned or low-molecular weight heparin for the treatment of cerebral venous thrombosis: analysis of the ISCVT data. *Cerebrovasc Dis* 2010;**29**(suppl 2).
33. Canhão P, Falcão F, Ferro JM. Thrombolytics for cerebral sinus thrombosis: a systematic review. *Cerebrovasc Dis* 2003;**15**:159–66.
34. Stam J, Majoie BLM, van Delden OM, *et al.* Endovascular thrombectomy and thrombolysis for severe cerebral sinus thrombosis: a prospective study. *Stroke* 2008;**39**:1487–90.
35. Gosk-Bierska I, Wysokinski W, Brown RD Jr, *et al.* Cerebral venous sinus thrombosis: Incidence of venous thrombosis recurrence and survival. *Neurology* 2006;**67**:814–19.
36. Kenet G, Kirkham F, Niederstadt T, European Thromboses Study Group. Risk factors for recurrent venous thromboembolism in the European collaborative paediatric database on cerebral venous thrombosis: a multicentre cohort study. *Lancet Neurol* 2007;**6**:595–603.
37. Miranda B, Ferro JM, Canhão P, *et al.* and the ISCVT Investigators. Venous thromboembolic events after cerebral vein thromboembolic events after cerebral vein thrombosis. *Stroke* 2010, Jul 15 [Epub ahead of print].
38. Martinelli I, Bucciarelli P, Passamonti SM, *et al.* Long-Term evaluation of the risk of recurrence after cerebral sinus-venous thrombosis. *Circulation* 2010;**121**:2740–6.
39. Einhäupl K, Stam J, Bousser MG, *et al.* EFNS guideline on the treatment of cerebral venous and sinus thrombosis in adult patients. *Eur J Neurol* 2010 Apr 7 [Epub ahead of print].
40. Canhão P, Cortesão A, Cabral M, *et al.*, for the ISCVT investigators. Are steroids useful to treat cerebral venous thrombosis? *Stroke* 2008;**39**:105–10.
41. Ferro JM, Bousser M-G, Stam J, *et al.* Decompressive surgery in cerebrovenous thrombosis (CVT). A retrospective multicentre registry (ISCVT 2). *Cerebrovasc Dis* 2010;**29** (suppl 2).
42. Crassard I, Bousser M-G, Canhão P, *et al.* Decompressive surgery in cerebrovenous thrombosis (CVT). A systematic review of individual patient data. *Cerebrovasc Dis* 2010;**29** (suppl 2).
43. Biousse V, Ameri A, Bousser MG. Isolated intracranial hypertension as the only sign of cerebral venous thrombosis. *Neurology* 1999;**53**:1537–1542.
44. Ferro JM, Canhão P, Bousser MG, *et al.* ISCVT Investigators. Early seizures in cerebral vein and dural sinus thrombosis. Risk factors, and role of antiepileptics. *Stroke* 2008;**39**:1152–1158.
45. Ferro JM, Correia M, Rosas MJ, *et al.* Cerebral Venous Thrombosis Portuguese Collaborative Study Group [Venoport]. Seizures in cerebral vein and dural sinus thrombosis. *Cerebrovasc Dis* 2003;**15**:78–83.

46. Ferro JM, Vasconcelos J, Canhão P, *et al.* ISCVT Investigators. Remote seizures in acute cerebral vein and sinus thrombosis (CVT). Incidence and associated conditions. *Cerebrovasc Dis* 2007;**23** (suppl 2):48.
47. Srinivasan K. Cerebral venous and arterial thrombosis in pregnancy and puerperium. A study of 135 patients. *Angiology* 1983;**34**:731–746.
48. Lamy C, Hamon JB, Coste J, Mas JL. Ischemic stroke in young women: risk of recurrence during subsequent pregnancies. French Study Group on Stroke in Pregnancy. *Neurology* 2000;**55**:269–74.
49. Merhraein S, Ortwein H, Busch M, *et al.* Risk of recurrence of cerebral venous and sinus thrombosis during subsequent pregnancy and puerperium. *J Neurol Neurosurg Psychiatry* 2003;**74**:814–16.

SECTION 8

Vascular Disease Syndromes Associated With Traumatic Brain Injury

Ischemic brain damage in traumatic brain injury (TBI): extradural, subdural, and intracerebral hematomas and cerebral contusions

A. David Mendelow

The management of patients with severe traumatic brain injury (TBI) is very similar to that of patients with ischemic brain damage from stroke. Ever since Graham *et al.* showed that the incidence of ischemic brain damage in head-injured patients who died was consistently near 90% (1,2), it has been known that the prevention and treatment of ischemia should be an important component of the management of severe TBI. These patients are cared for in the same critical care environment as patients with ischemic stroke, often in intensive care units (ITUs) and in high-dependency units (HDUs) run by neuro-intensivists and neurosurgeons. Similar arguments can be made for including a description of the care of patients with subarachnoid and intracerebral hemorrhage in a book of this nature. In all these four conditions brain ischemia is one of the main underlying causes of neuronal damage (3–6). This fact has been one of the main reasons for undertaking experimental and clinical trials of neuroprotective agents in these four conditions.

Epidemiology of head-injured patients

Head injury affects ten times more people than stroke. Although the vast majority of these injuries are minor or mild, any one of them can later give rise to an extradural hematoma and it is impossible to predict with any certainty, in advance, which patient with a mild head injury will deteriorate. Many of the mild injuries do not even attend hospital, so data can only be based on attendees at emergency departments. Only 0.3% of all head-injured patients that present to emergency departments will have an extradural or a subdural hematoma, so that there is a real problem in recognizing those few who need immediate treatment. That is why the UK NICE Guidelines for the triage of head injury are so important. Their scientific foundation is based on the Canadian CT head rule (7) which was re-evaluated in a second set of patients (8) and found to have very high sensitivity and specificity for diagnosing clots that required neurosurgical evacuation. When compared with other diagnostic rules, the Canadian CT head rule produced the greatest reduction in the number of CT scans without missing a single surgical case (Fig. 36.1 (9)). Data that have been collected about head-injured populations depend very much on the population base from which they are gathered. If from neurosurgery units, the data only represent 1% or 2% of the entire head injury population. Attempts to compare head-injured populations depend upon the causes, definitions, denominators, and severity of the injury. Classifications are numerous and data suggest that the incidence per 100 000 population is somewhere between 56 and 430 (10). Comparing head-injured patients around the world, (11) describe the variations and mortality rates in different continents (Fig. 36.2). The important concept is to realise that neurosurgery operative treatment is needed in less than 1 in 200 patients while rapid triage and excellent critical care is needed in all. However, those few that do need surgery need it quickly.

Critical Care of the Stroke Patient, ed. Stefan Schwab, Daniel Hanley, and A. David Mendelow. Published by Cambridge University Press.

	Relevant CT Scan						
Authors & Year	% Sensitivity†	% Specificity†	% PPV†	% NPV†	% Accuracy†	% CT Scan Reduction	No. of Patients Lost‡
Stein, 1996	89.2 (82.5–95.8)	47.2 (44.2–50.3)	12.1 (9.5–14.7)	98.2 (97.0–99.4)	50.4 (47.5–53.4)	44.5	9 (3)
Tomei, et al., 1996	92.8 (87.2–98.3)	35.9 (32.9–38.8)	10.5 (8.3–12.8)	98.4 (97.1–99.7)	40.1 (37.2–43.0)	33.7	6 (0)
Arienta, et al., 1997	88.0 (80.9–95.0)	54.2 (51.2–57.2)	13.5 (10.7–16.4)	98.2 (97.1–99.3)	56.8 (53.8–59.7)	51.0	10 (2)
Lapierre, 1998	92.8 (87.2–98.3)	24.5 (21.8–27.1)	9.1 (7.2–11.0)	97.6 (95.8–99.5)	29.6 (26.9–32.3)	23.2	6 (0)
Murshid, 1998	60.2 (49.7–70.8)	81.1 (78.7–83.5)	20.7 (15.6–25.8)	96.2 (94.9–97.4)	79.6 (77.2–81.9)	78.0	33 (3)
Haydel, et al., 2000	95.2 (90.6–99.8)	18.7 (16.3–21.1)	8.7 (6.9–10.5)	97.9 (95.9–99.9)	24.4 (21.9–27.0)	17.6	4 (0)
Ingebrigtsen, et al., 2000	84.3 (76.5–92.2)	59.8 (56.8–62.8)	14.6 (11.5–17.8)	97.9 (96.8–99.0)	61.7 (58.8–64.5)	56.5	13 (2)
SIGN, 2000	65.1 (54.8–75.3)	74.5 (71.8–77.1)	17.2 (13.0–21.4)	96.3 (95.0–97.6)	73.8 (71.2–76.4)	71.5	29 (4)
Servadei, et al., 2001	97.6 (94.3–100)	13.9 (11.7–16.0)	8.5 (6.7–10.2)	98.6 (96.7–100)	20.2 (17.8–22.5)	13.0	2 (0)
Stiell, et al., 2001	85.5 (78.0–98.0)	50.4 (47.3–53.4)	12.3 (9.6–15.0)	97.7 (96.4–99.0)	53.0 (50.1–56.0)	47.7	12 (0)
Vos, et al., 2002	96.4 (92.4–100)	27.7 (25.0–30.5)	9.8 (7.8–11.8)	98.9 (97.8–100)	32.9 (30.1–35.7)	25.9	3 (0)

* NPV = negative predictive value; PPV = positive predictive value; SIGN = Scottish Intercollegiate Guidelines Network.
† The 95% CIs appear in parentheses.
‡ Values without parentheses represent absolute data; those within parentheses represent the number of surgical cases lost.

Fig. 36.1 CT reduction and diagnostic accuracy. From reference (9). Please see reference for further information on these studies.

	Place				
Parameter	Europe[1]	U.S.[2]	Australia[3]	Asia[4]	India[5]
Incidence rate[6,7]	235	103	226	344	160
Prevalence rate[6]	NR	1893	NR	709	97
Mortality rate[6]	15.4	18.1	NR	38	20
Severity (% Mi/Mo/Sev)	79/12/9	80/10/10	76/12/11	78/9/13	71/15/13
Case fatality rate[8]	2.7[a]	6.2	2.4	11	6
External cause (% Fall/MVC/Vio)	37/40/7	21/25/6	49/25/9	23/65/7	59/25/14
Outcomes[9] (% GOS unfavor)	50[b]	64[c]	NR	27	9

[1] Source: this report, [2] source: aggregate data from references 24, 23, 47,
[3] source: aggregate data from references 42, 16, 5, [4] source: Chiu, [8],
[5] source: Gururaj, [14], [6] per 100,000 population,
[7] includes hospitalized & deaths, [8] rate per 100 hospitalized,
[9] unfavorable includes deaths, PVS, and severe disability.
[a] Excludes outlier rates of 46.5, 30, and 52/100 from Table 2.
[b] Source: EBIC [29] includes moderate/severe TBI
[c] Source: U.S. Traumatic Coma Data Bank [47] severe cases.
NR not reported.

Fig. 36.2 Epidemiology of head injury (11). For further details and source references, please see reference (11).

The original findings of Graham *et al.* (1) were confirmed a decade later in more post-mortem studies (2). The demonstration of ischemia in living patients following TBI was more difficult but has now been confirmed with various monitoring techniques and with imaging. The monitoring techniques that demonstrate ischemia include the measurement of cerebral blood flow with heat clearance techniques (12), using

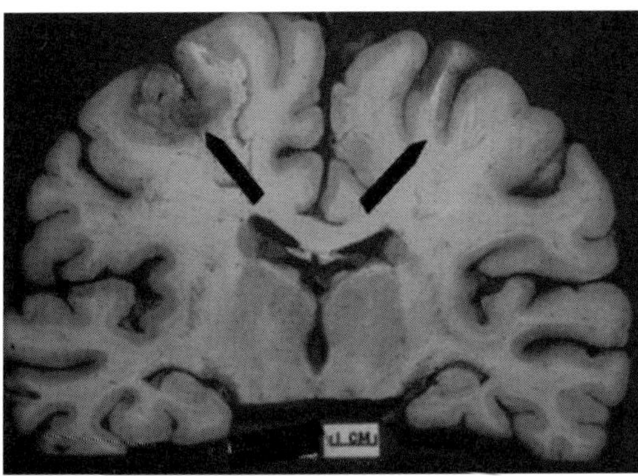

Fig. 36.3 Post-mortem slice showing infarcts in the arterial boundary zones.

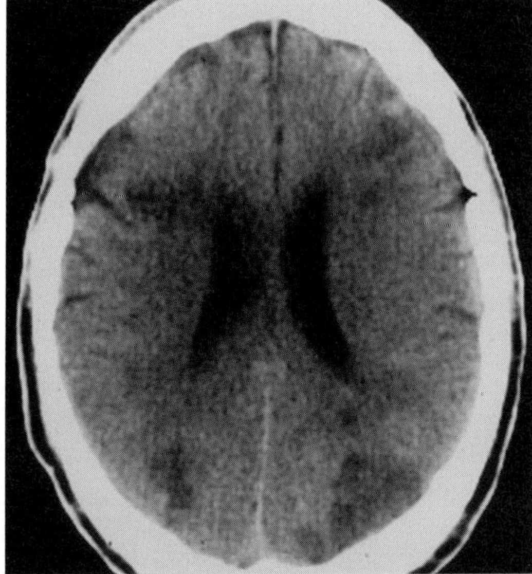

Fig. 36.4 CT scan a week after injury showing hypoxic brain damage characterized by boundary zone infarcts.

brain tissue oxygen (13–15) and with micro-dialysis (16–18). With the last form of monitoring, high levels of glutamate have been demonstrated in the brains of patients following TBI (16). The imaging techniques that have demonstrated ischemia include SPECT and PET (Fig. 36.3) scanning (19–21). Ischemic neuronal damage can also occur following trauma due to large vessel occlusion, dissection or compression. These focal lesions represent infarction that is identical to that seen with occlusive stroke because they are caused by occlusion of large cerebral arteries. Dissection of carotid and vertebral arteries within bony canals is being recognised as a cause of focal ischemia with increasing frequency after injury. Ischemia may thus be focal but it is frequently also global with ischemia from the low blood pressure or hypoxia that occurs following trauma (22,23). This type of global ischemia often produces the typical 'boundary zone' or 'watershed' infarct (Fig. 36.4). Ischemic and hypoxic brain damage thus predominate following trauma but are not the only mechanism of secondary neuronal damage. One of the other forms of secondary brain damage seen after head injury is due to infection. Lacerations of the brain and disruption from penetrating injuries are also forms of primary brain damage that are largely irreversible. Similarly, primary brain damage from diffuse axonal injury (DAI) has a different pathophysiology (vide infra). An understanding of these processes is needed in order to implement effective preventative and therapeutic strategies in head-injured patients in the critical care environment.

Primary brain damage

The classic and most common type of lesion is known as *diffuse axonal injury* (DAI) because of its diffuse nature and the fact that axons are primarily affected. There are characteristic pathological features originally classified by Strich (24,25) as gliding contusions and axonal retraction balls. It has subsequently been recognized that the changes which occur in axons are dynamic and may take hours to develop (26). The original lesions were recognized in patients with severe head injury (27) but dynamic axonal changes may progress through a swollen stage and may take place in mild head injuries too (28). Recent MRI studies in patients with mild and moderate head injury have confirmed that changes can be demonstrated in the frontal lobes (29). These changes were not previously visible with CT or with conventional MRI techniques.

Axonal retraction balls are recognized as the hallmark of primary diffuse axonal injury, but recent evidence suggests that these may be preceded by axonal swelling (Figs. 36.5 and 36.6). Later on Wallerian degeneration takes place as an end-stage process. The hope now is that some of these dynamic changes may be reversible if treated early enough.

Lacerations of tracts in the central nervous system do not, unfortunately, recover. This has been known to neurosurgeons for over a century now with percutaneous lobotomies, rhiszotomies, and cordotomies resulting in permanent division of important CNS fiber tracts. Their efficacy is testament to the permanent nature of such white matter tract disruption. So lacerations are true primary lesions that do not recover.

Contusions on the other hand often enlarge during the first 24 to 48 hours after injury, with the hemorrhagic components of the contusion enlarging, sometimes rapidly. Classic teaching was that this primary event was permanent and could not be affected by treatment, but modern thought has led to the development of the STICH(TRAUMA) trial in which patients with hemorrhagic contusions (minimum volume 10 ml of blood) were randomized to early surgery or initial conservative treatment. This trial was stopped with recruitment at 170 and mortality was significantly reduced by more than half from 32% with Initial Conservative Treatment to 15% in the Early Surgery group. This was accompanied by a significant benefit from Early Surgery at 6 months as measured on the Rankin Scale (30).

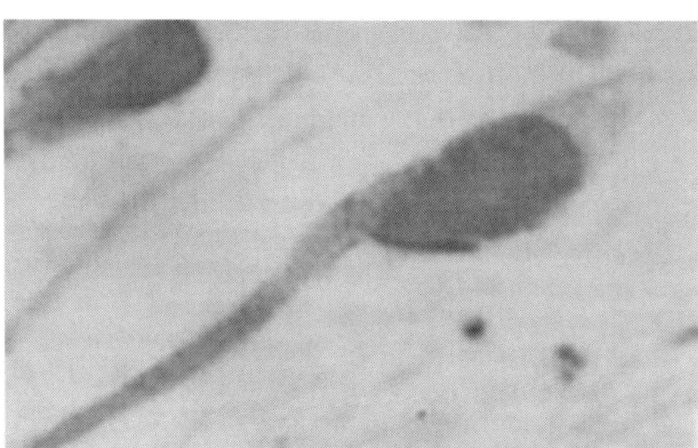

Fig. 36.5 Axonal retraction balls (reprinted with permission from Reilly and Bullock 2e). (See plate section for color version).

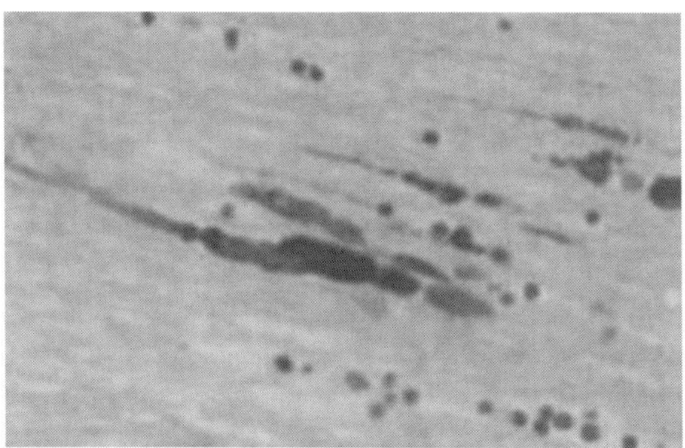

Fig. 36.6 Axonal swelling in the corpus callosum (reprinted with permission from Reilly and Bullock 2e). (See plate section for color version).

Brain injury and edema following trauma

With ischemic brain damage (IBD) there is secondary cytotoxic edema. This is best imaged with diffusion-weighted imaging (DWI) on MRI scanners but is seen after about 6 hours as low density on a CT scan (Fig. 36.7). The edema seen on CT and MRI reflects the development of neuronal dysfunction. This early cytotoxic edema is characterized by neuronal swelling that has been shown to have several pathological mechanisms. Firstly, mechanical deformation of cell membranes (neurons and astrocytes) leads to 'leaky' ion channels that allow rapid movements of water, sodium, and potassium (31,32). The aquaporin channels regulate water movement across cell membranes

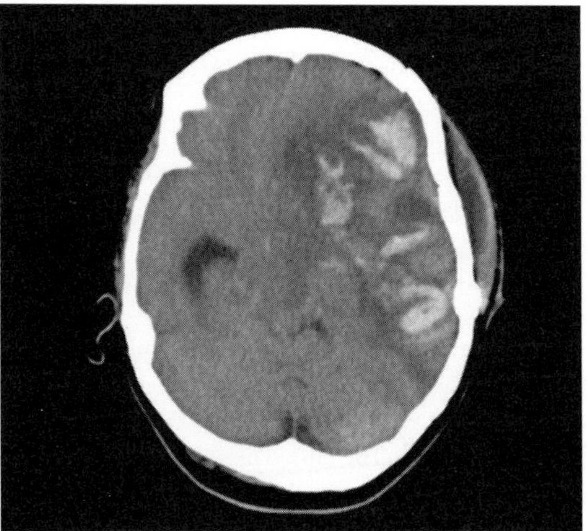

Fig. 36.7 Low-density lesions on CT represent cytotoxic edema.

and they too become dysfunctional after trauma (33). Secondly, neurotransmitters are released (34), affecting synaptic and axonal activity. Thirdly, ischemia and/or hypoxia can lead to the global or focal ischemic damage that has become so well recognized.

Global ischemic brain damage: Global ischemic damage results from low cerebral perfusion pressure (CPP), which can be due to hemorrhagic shock or rising intracranial pressure (ICP). The infarction and edema that occurs is seen in the classical arterial boundary zones or 'watershed areas'. Hypoxia at some point following the injury is also recognized by the late development of watershed infarcts on CT. All of this results in cellular swelling, which leads to localized pressures and deformity with brain shifts. As edema becomes worse, intracranial pressure rises and, with falling cerebral perfusion pressure, further ischemic damage takes place.

Focal ischemic brain damage: The pathobiological mechanisms with traumatic vascular occlusion are identical to those which occur with ischemic stroke. They are in the territory of large cerebral arteries and produce ischemic neuronal damage. Direct damage to the internal carotid artery in the neck may be due to acute flexion or extension (35) injury. Also direct trauma to the cervical carotid artery may result from safety belts. Intimal dissection and occlusion may result in occlusive thrombosis and distal embolization. Total occlusion of the internal carotid artery may produce hemisphere infarction. Carotid and vertebral artery damage due to fractures in the skull base and cervical vertebrae are relatively rare but have been recorded (36,37). The posterior cerebral artery may become occluded due to herniation of the uncus of the temporal lobe, resulting in a medial occipital infarct if it is unrelieved. The middle cerebral artery is sometimes damaged against the sharp edge of the sphenoid wing. In all these situations a classical large vessel infarct will become visible on CT or MRI.

Other forms of secondary brain damage

Infection is usually recognized about 5 days after the injury and takes the form of meningitis or a brain abscess. These conditions may follow a traumatic cerebrospinal fluid leak or a compound depressed skull fracture. The treatment of these two types of breaches to the dura that produce a portal for infection to enter the nervous system are described in the treatment sections below. Brain edema may follow infection and is usually of the vasogenic sort.

Hematomas may develop immediately or some hours after the primary injury and are characterized by deterioration in the level of consciousness and the development of focal neurological deficits. There are four types of hematoma that occur following trauma: extradural, subdural, intracerebral, and intracerebral with contusions. They may occur individually or in combination with each other. The treatment of each is also considered below.

Extradural hematomas

The extradural hematoma is classically associated with a lucid interval (a period of preserved consciousness reflects a minimal dose of primary brain damage). The bleeding is usually from a fracture of the skull and, typically, this crosses the middle meningeal artery. In fact, every skull fracture has a small extradural and a small, often matching, external subperiosteal hematoma because of bleeding from both sides of the fracture site. These may be very small initially, but with time the extradural and subperiosteal components enlarge. With the increased use of CT scanning following trauma, small extradural hematomas are often recognized and such patients should be carefully observed (Fig. 36.8). Larger extradural hematomas compress the brain and cause underlying ischemic neuronal damage if the pressure is unrelieved. Sustained brain shift leads to tentorial herniation with secondary compression of the posterior cerebral artery and an ipsilateral third cranial nerve palsy. At this stage the pupil dilates and surgery must be undertaken immediately to avoid permanent complications. Delay in evacuating the extradural allows secondary damage to occur and the outcome is much worse. In an observational study the delay time from first recorded deterioration in consciousness to operation was compared with the outcome and longer delays produced poorer outcomes. The mean delay in patients that had a good outcome

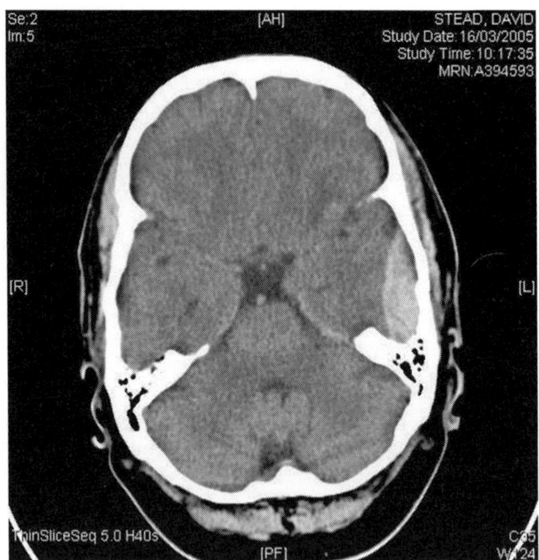

Fig. 36.8 A CT scan showing a small extradural hematoma.

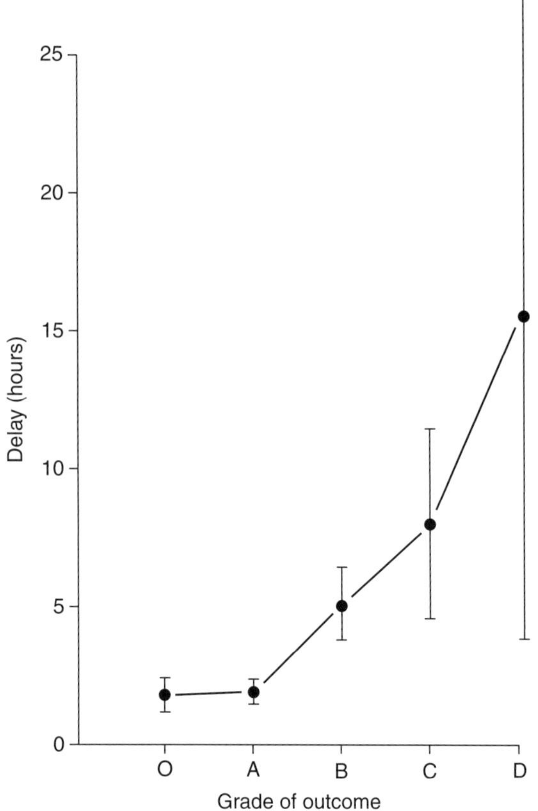

Fig. 36.9 Effect of delay on outcome in patients with acute extradural hematomas (Mendelow *et al.*).

was 1.9 hours whereas it was 15 hours in those who died (Fig. 36.9 (38)). Most triage guidelines recognize this short time required to diagnose and to treat extradural hematomas and the National Institute of Clinical Excellence (NICE) triage guidelines recommend a CT brain scan within 1 hour. Following motor vehicle accidents (MVA), extradural hematomas are almost always associated with diffuse axonal injury (DAI) (39). Such patients do not display the classic lucid interval and are in coma from the outset. This contrasts with the non-MVA where the DAI may not be present and the patient remains conscious or displays only transient concussion. Sometimes, when a fracture crosses a large venous sinus, a chronic venous extradural hematoma develops (40). Such chronic venous extradural hematomas may present days after the injury.

Subdural hematomas: The *acute* subdural hematoma is much less likely to have a lucid interval because it is usually, but not always, associated with more severe DAI as a manifestation of greater acceleration or deceleration forces. As such, it is more likely to follow a high-speed MVA. There is therefore no classical clinical picture as with the extradural hematoma and its correct diagnosis is dependent upon early CT scanning. This was made clear in studies from Richmond Virginia that evaluated the outcome in patients with acute subdural hematomas that were treated at different times after the injury (Fig. 36.10 (41)). The mortality rose sharply in patients that underwent surgery more than 4 hours after injury and was even less if surgery was undertaken within 2 hours of injury. The highest mortality (90%) was in patients in whom the delay was more than 6 hours from injury. This puts a huge burden upon all of those who evaluate and treat head-injured patients: rapid diagnosis is essential. Once again, the NICE Guidelines for the triage of head-injured patients were designed to minimize delays.

Chronic subdural hematomas (CSDH) are liquid and present three or more weeks after trauma, which is often minor or unrecognized. In about a third of

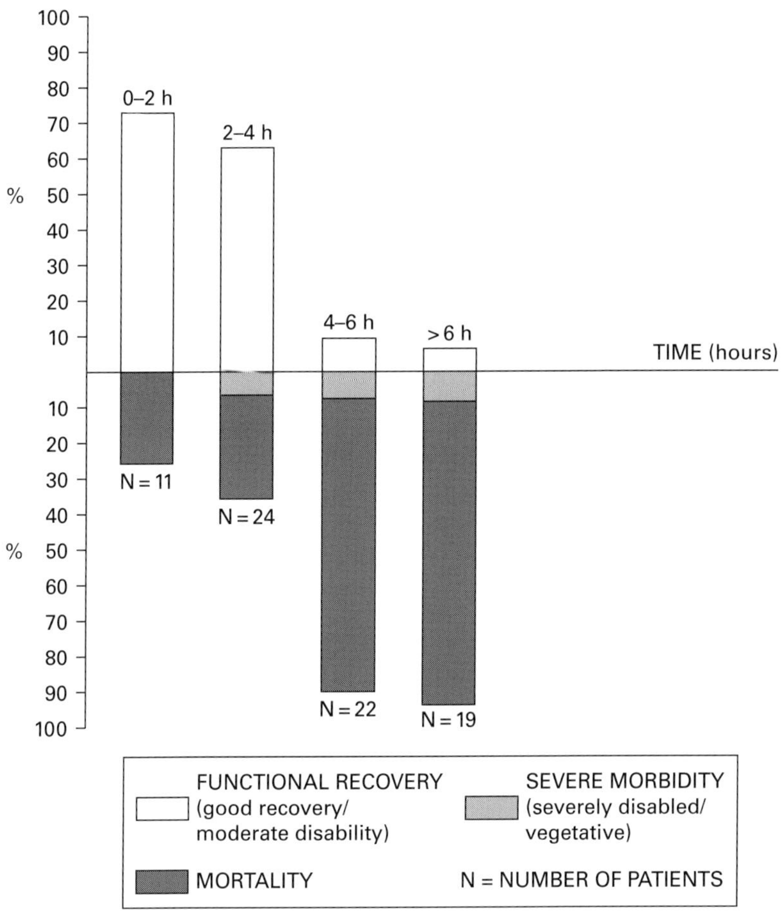

Fig. 36.10 The effect of delay on outcome in patients with acute subdural hematomas (41).

patients there may be no history of trauma at all (42,43). The liquefied blood looks like black oil and may be under pressure. It appears as a low-density surface lesion on CT scan that causes shift and enlargement of the contralateral ventricle. Between 1 and 3 weeks the clot may be subacute, in which case it slowly changes from hyperdense on CT to isodense and, finally, hypodense. The isodense subdural may not be obvious on CT but the shift and contralateral ventricular enlargement should lead one to suspect a CSDH. The shift that a CSDH causes may compress the contralateral cerebral peduncle against the tentorial edge. This 'notch' on the contralateral cerebral peduncle can be seen at autopsy and has become known as 'Kernohan's notch'. It may result in a hemiplegia or hemiparesis on the same side as the CSDH because the fibers in that cerebral peduncle cross over lower down in the medullary pyramid. Some have called this ipsilateral hemiparesis 'Kernohan's phenomenon'.

Intracerebral hematomas and contusions: Primary intracerebral hematomas in isolation are rare and constitute only 1.6% of all head-injured patients that are admitted to neurosurgery (44). More frequently intraparenchymal blood is associated with a contusion. Contusions result from sudden acceleration or deceleration forces that drive the brain onto immoveable ridges within the skull. The best known is the 'fronto-temporal' contusion on either side of the sphenoid wing. The crista galli damages the frontal lobes and 'bifrontal contusions' are a manifestation of this phenomenon as well. Often a contusion will be found on the opposite side of the head to an abrasion or laceration. This is the classic 'contra coup' lesion (45). Initially, the hemorrhagic component of the contusion may be small and there may just be several small hemorrhages. However, with time, the hemorrhages enlarge and coalesce. These enlarging parenchymal lesions then begin to behave more like mass lesions and appear as intracerebral hematomas on scanning. The delayed neurological deterioration that they produce was described by Oertel (46). Once there are more than three intracerebral hematomas, the prognosis is dismal (47). The ischemic brain damage surrounding the expanding hemorrhage may be considered as secondary damage (48) and as such, prevention of expansion may limit the ischemia. Many studies have described the toxic effects of the blood itself on the surrounding brain (5,49,50,51). Around the intracerebral hematoma there is penumbra of functionally impaired but potentially viable tissue. This has been shown experimentally and clinically (44). Therapeutic strategies (medical or surgical) aim to limit the amount of secondary ischemic brain damage that surrounds the clot. If there were no penumbra (as defined above) then therapeutic initiatives like the use of recombinant factor VIIa or tranexamic acid, will be likely to fail as would surgical initiatives like the STITCH (TRAUMA) trial. It may well be that such a penumbra exists in some patients but not in others. If that is the case, then these therapeutic initiatives may need to first identify the penumbra with CBF imaging before selecting those patients with a penumbra that may derive benefit from the treatment. Such selective imaging would be necessary if the ongoing trials turn out to be negative or neutral but would be unnecessary if they turn out positive results.

Imaging in head-injured patients: The rapid diagnosis of hematomas that need evacuation is very much dependent upon fast access to imaging, which is largely with the CT scan. MRI imaging has an important role to play but very few units around the world can provide immediate access to MRI. When early MRI is available, important information is forthcoming (52) but at present MRI remains a research tool within the first hours of TBI. This contrasts with its role in stroke where early MRI imaging is becoming more widespread. Most hematomas can be seen on CT as high-density lesions (Fig. 36.11). Diffuse axonal injury (DAI) may be difficult to see on CT with small petechial hemorrhages being the markers of gliding contusions that disrupt small capillaries as they course through large white matter tracts like the internal capsule (Fig. 36.12). Such lesions may be seen more easily on MRI and modern three Tesla MRI studies are revealing lesions and abnormalities that were previously undetected even in minor and moderate head-injured patients (53).

Prevention and treatment of secondary brain damage

Prevention of primary hypoxia and hypotension: Primary hypoxic damage occurs at the scene of the injury and may result either from the apnea that follows immediately after a blow to the head or as a result of chest injuries that produce global hypoxia like a tension pneumothorax. Primary ischemic brain damage is due to hypovolemic shock. Under all these circumstances, acute resuscitation using the Advanced Trauma Life Support (ATLS) principles will serve to minimize hypoxic and ischemic damage. More rapid availability of paramedic ambulance and helicopter services also improves primary resuscitation. Fine judgments need to be made by the personnel that work in these services in deciding whether to transport such casualties to the nearest hospital with resuscitation facilities or to take the patient to a more remote hospital that has neurosurgical facilities. In an observational study of patients in the Trauma Audit and Research Network (TARN) Patel *et al.* (54) showed that the mortality was halved when similar patients were transported directly to a hospital with neurosurgical facilities. In the UK there are only 36 such hospitals to serve about 300 major District General Hospitals, so the question is an important

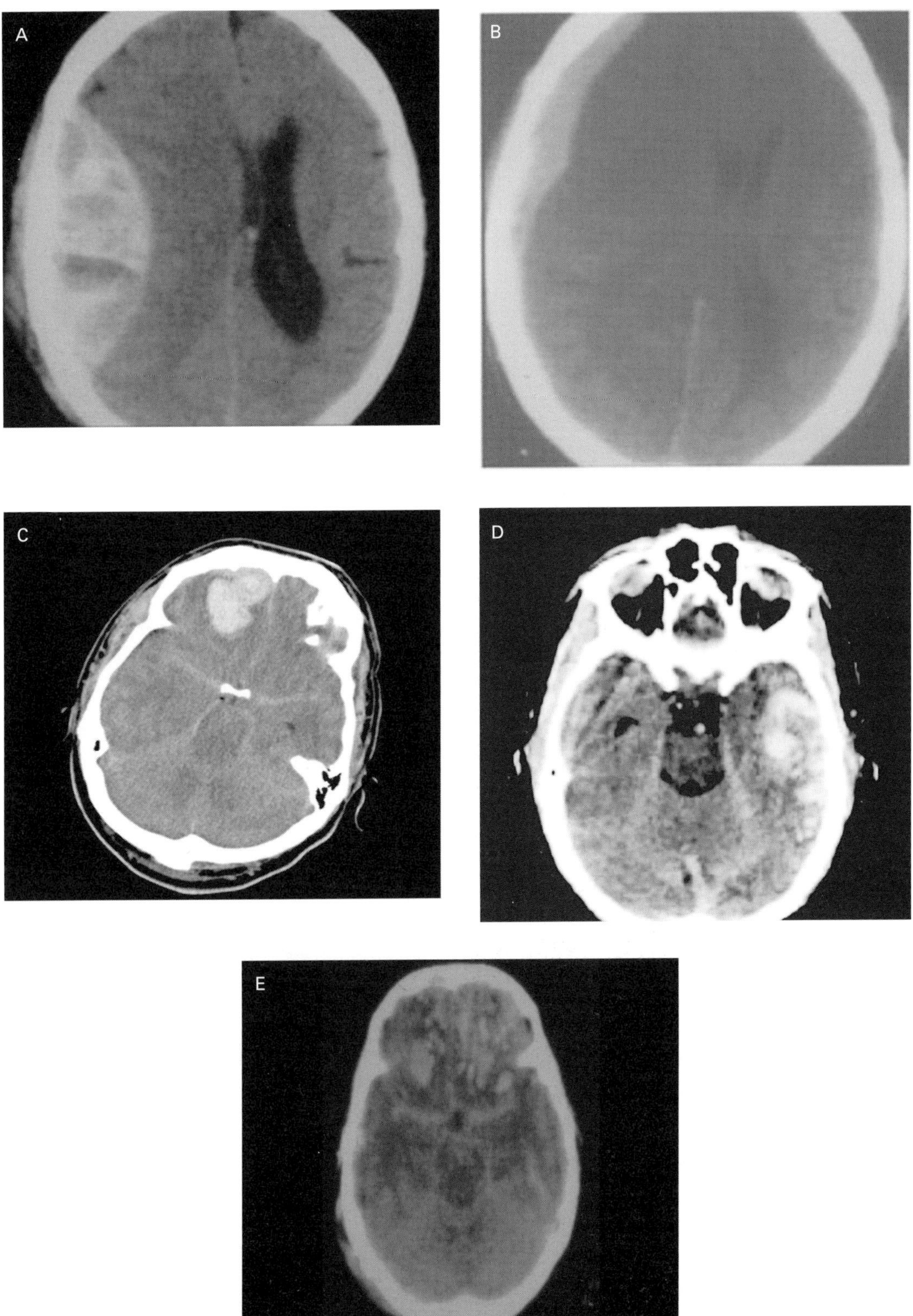

Fig. 36.11 Examples of traumatic hematomas on CT scan. A = extradural hematoma; B = subdural hematoma; C = right frontal intracerebral hematoma; D = left front-temporal hemorrhagic contusion; E = bifrontal contusions with multiple small hematomas.

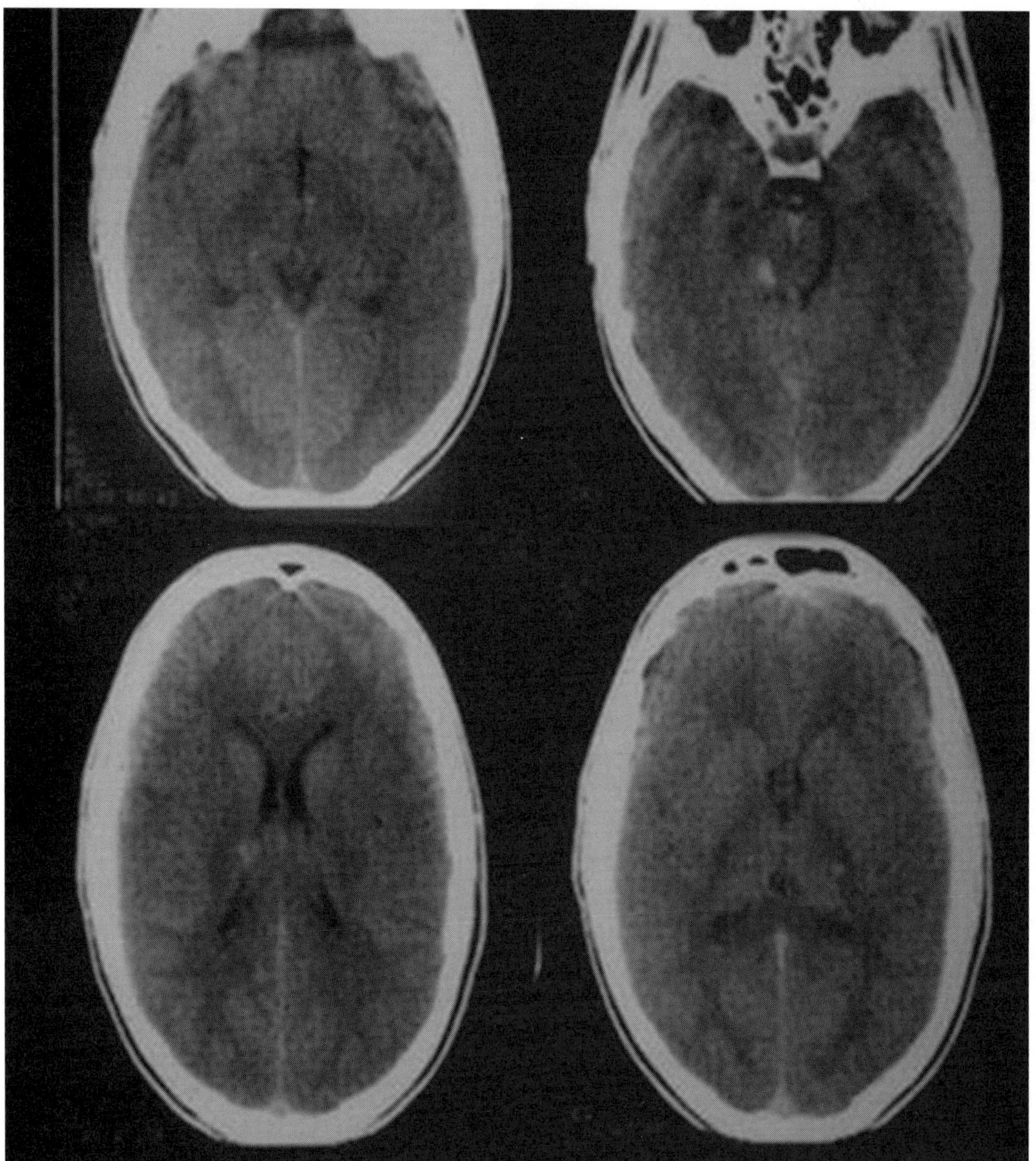

Fig. 36.12 CT showing petechial hemorrhages classical of DAI.

one. The HITS NS trial seeks to answer this question by the cluster randomization of ambulance services so that the outcome can be evaluated when patients receive one of these two options.

Prevention of secondary hypoxia and hypotension in critical care: Once the patient reaches a critical care environment, the primary objective is to avoid hypoxia and hypotension after injury and once again ATLS principles are paramount. The initial stabilization, however, should be rapid so that the head-injured patient who is not fully conscious can undergo CT scanning within an hour. This is to avoid delayed treatment of intracranial hematomas. The NICE Triage guidelines (55) set out the criteria for such imaging in adults and children. They also deal with the issues of imaging the spine after trauma.

Treatment of extradural hematomas

The rapid decompression required with an acute extradural hematoma cannot be over-emphasized (38) (see Fig. 36.9). Normally a craniotomy is made over the site of the hematoma but under emergency conditions, a linear incision with a simple burrhole will allow immediate decompression. Then the burrhole can be enlarged with bone nibblers to ensure more extensive evacuation of the solid extradural clot. Emergency decompression is the immediate priority. Hemostasis can be achieved later and many lives have been saved by expeditious decompression, packing the wound, and then transferring to a neurosurgical center. However, in the normal course of events, a frontotemporal skin flap is reflected and a craniotomy is cut with a craniotome. Skin flaps should be designed with a good blood supply and many standard text books illustrate the types of flaps that can be made (56). Bleeding from the middle meningeal artery is often encountered and this is also often associated with a fracture. Bone wax and Surgicell® with hitch sutures if necessary will usually stop the bleeding. Extradural hematomas are sometimes localized, particularly by the coronal and sagittal sutures and especially so in children. If there is extensive fracturing over a major venous sinus, then care should be taken to avoid further tearing of the sinus wall: packing with wet swabs over Surgicell® and elevation of the head end of the operating table will usually stop the hemorrhage and the wet swabs should prevent air embolism. A very large extradural hematoma may result in failure of the underlying compressed brain to re-expand after the clot has been evacuated. If so, elevation of the foot end of the operating table will encourage brain expansion and then a Poppen suture holding the center of the depressed dura to the center of the bone flap is sometimes used. Gentle gravity drainage is preferred to high negative pressure suction drainage. Chronic venous extradural hematomas (40) are sometimes located over the major venous sinuses and can often be evacuated through burrholes because their chronicity has rendered them liquid rather than solid.

Treatment of subdural hematomas

As with extradural hematomas, time is of the essence! Delayed evacuation of acute subdural hematomas results in an unacceptably high mortality (41) (Fig. 36.10) and by 4 hours from injury the clot should have been decompressed. As with the acute extradural hematoma, the first burrhole should be provided as soon as possible and the dura opened to release even 1 or 2 ml of blood because release of this small volume will immediately drop the intracranial pressure (Fig. 36.13) and restore the cerebral perfusion pressure towards normal. The craniotomy can then be completed. The flap size is usually larger with acute subdural hematomas because they are more extensive and tend to fill the subdural space, which is a potentially open space as compared with the extradural hematoma that dissects into a closed space because it has to strip the dura away from its attachment to bone. Looking from the left side, the 'trauma flap' is like a large question mark with the straight down section being just in front of the left ear extending down to the zygomatic process. This allows temporal decompression and relief

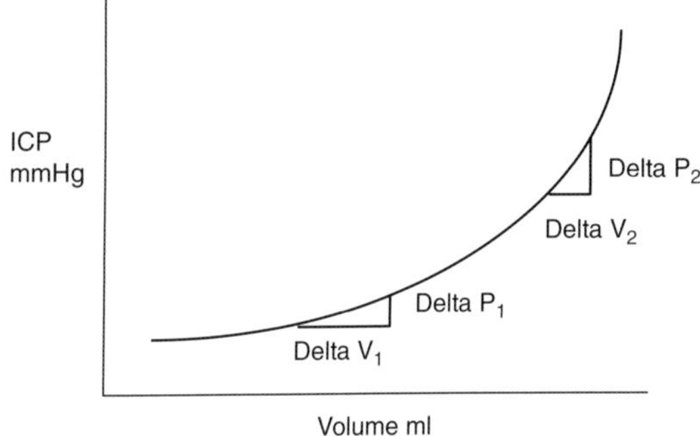

Fig. 36.13 Pressure volume relationship under different circumstances.

of the tentorial herniation that is often present due to the shift of the brain. Once the subdural hematoma has been removed, the brain may remain displaced and unexpanded, in which case head down tilt may help to re-expand it and will help to identify any undetected venous bleeders. By contrast, the brain will often swell up and start to herniate through the craniotomy opening, in which case more mannitol, hyperventilation, and head up tilt may alleviate the situation. If unrelieved by these maneuvers, then it may be prudent to leave the dura open with a covering of Surgicell® and the bone flap can be omitted when closing. As with extradural hematomas, a gravity drain in the sub-galeal space is often advisable.

Treatment of intracerebral hematomas

This is the greatest area of controversy because opinion is divided about whether to simply observe these patients and wait for clinical deterioration before embarking on surgery or rather to remove the hematoma prophylactically before deterioration occurs. The arguments in favor of early surgery are that secondary brain damage is avoided and that the late toxic effects of the hematoma on the surrounding brain are prevented (49–51, 57–67). The arguments against early surgery are that the surgery itself may inflict secondary brain damage and also that many of these hematomas are stable and that those patients with stable hematomas do not deteriorate from secondary damage. The problem is in knowing what to do with the individual patient. Intuitively some clots are in relatively silent areas of the brain and are surgically easily accessible as for example with hematomas in the right frontal lobe (Fig. 36.11C). By contrast, small hematomas in eloquent areas that are part of a contusion carry a higher risk of inflicting damage with surgery (Fig. 36.11D). Thus the intuitive reasoning that governs most neurosurgical practice will influence the decision about whether to operate or not. However, not all traumatic intracerebral hematomas are as clear-cut as in these two examples. It is those hematomas that are difficult to decide upon that are in the area of equipoise of most neurosurgeons. It is these patients that were randomized in the STITCH (TRAUMA) trial (http://research.ncl.ac.uk/trauma.STITCH/). This trial is now closed to recruitment of adult patients with one or two confluent hematomas of more than 10 ml within 24 hours of injury. Exclusion criteria include three or more such hematomas, extradural and subdural hematomas that require surgery and when surgery cannot be performed within 12 hours of randomization. The trial was stopped after 170 patients were enrolled because of poor recruitment in the UK where the funds originated. Results will be published in late 2013.

Treatment of cerebral contusions

Even greater controversy exists about the management of cerebral contusions. If there is an associated hematoma, then that can be managed according to the intuitive principles described above. These patients were eligible for randomization in the STITCH (TRAUMA) trial provided that there are no more than two hematomas of greater than 10 ml in volume. If there are no such hematomas, then internal decompression is seldom practiced. Internal decompression usually takes the form of a partial frontal or temporal lobectomy. This is often the best way to decompress a contusion that is associated with multiple small hematomas (Fig. 36.11E), although bifrontal lobectomy should be avoided at all costs because of the very severe morbidity associated with survival. An alternative to internal decompression in such cases is to do an external decompression with a decompressive craniectomy. The decompressive craniectomy should be large enough (at least 12 cm) to allow sufficient brain swelling and can be unilateral or bilateral. Sometimes a bilateral decompressive craniectomy can be performed, leaving a midline section of bone to protect the superior longitudinal sinus. With decompressive craniectomy, the dura is usually, but not always opened. Dural opening can take the form of a lattice-type opening to avoid massive herniation (68). A variation on the lattice duroplasty theme is to monitor ICP intra-operatively and to open segments of the dural lattice progressively until ICP is controlled below 20 mmHg. The lattices are initially opened over non-eloquent areas of brain such as the sub frontal region, thus avoiding eloquent cortical herniation of speech areas for example. The complete opening of dura is sometimes practised and techniques are described to prevent cortical venous obstruction at the edges: small pledgets of Surgicell® are placed on either side of emerging cortical veins to prevent their obstruction thus facilitating better venous drainage of the exposed cortex (69). The role of decompressive craniectomy is being explored in the Rescue ICP trial (www.rescueicp.com) and is considered below.

Treatment of raised ICP

The original concept of the Munro-Kellie doctrine was that the cranial cavity was incompressible so that the volume was fixed. The CSF, blood, and brain were in a state of equilibrium, so that a change in the volume of one could be compensated for by a change in volume of another. To a great extent this remains true and is useful in understanding how high ICP causes harm. As the volume of any of the components rises, either another component must reduce or brain shift will occur as ICP rises. The three structures through which they can shift are from one side of the falx cerebri to the other, through the tentorial hiatus or through the foramen magnum. Side to side shift occurs with unilateral lesions and can be seen in Figs. 36.11A–D. Tentorial herniation also occurs and the uncus of the temporal lobe herniates over the tentorial edge to compress the third nerve (causing pupillary dilatation), the posterior cerebral artery (causing a medial occipital infarct as shown in Fig. 36.11F), and the midbrain (causing vasomotor and visual changes and later secondary midbrain hemorrhage). Herniation of the cerebellar tonsils through the foramen magnum causes medullary compression with respiratory abnormalities including hyperventilation, Cheyne Stokes ventilation, hypoventilation, and eventually respiratory drive failure and apnea. If the ventricular volume increases, hydrocephalus occurs and the ICP will also rise. The perfusion of the brain with blood (cerebral blood flow = CBF) depends upon the cerebral perfusion pressure (CPP), which is the difference between the blood pressure and the intracranial pressure. CBF remains constant over a range of CPP from about 50 to 150 mmHg and this is known as cerebral autoregulation (Fig. 36.15). After head injury, this

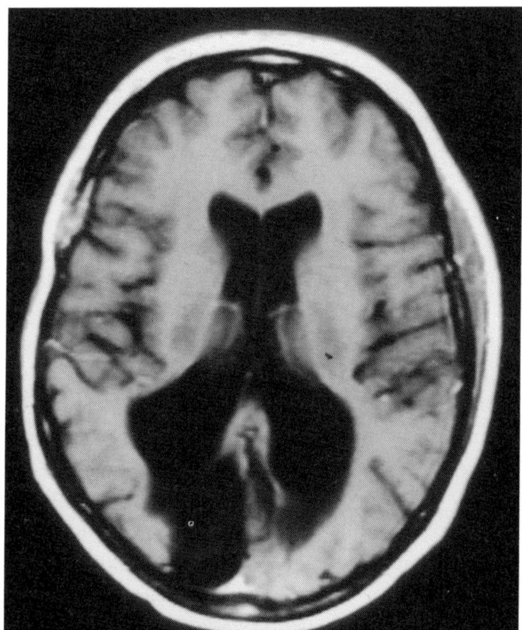

Fig. 36.14 Late MRI of a patient with delayed evacuation of an extradural hematoma that had caused uncal herniation with compression of the posterior cerebral artery and a medial occipital infarct.

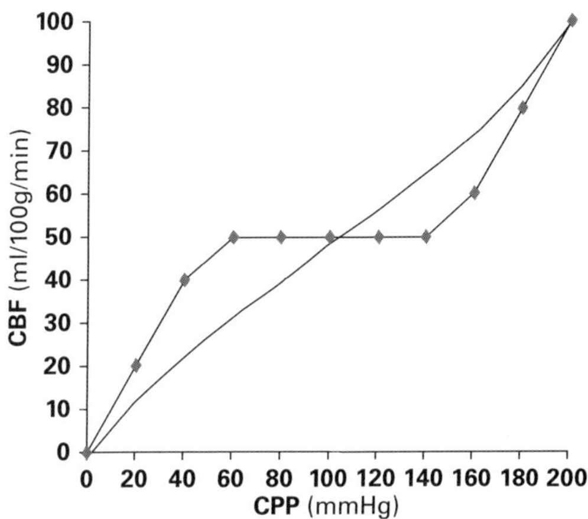

Fig. 36.15 The normal autoregulation curve (red dots) and how it alters after head injury (straight line). (CPP = BP – ICP). (See plate section for color version).

autoregulation phenomenon may be lost and the CBF becomes passively dependent upon the CPP. Under such circumstances, maintenance of an adequate blood pressure becomes even more important if CBF is to be maintained. The combination of high ICP and loss of autoregulation together make BP management one of the critical determinants of outcome in head-injured patients (70). Measurement of ICP with parenchymal brain transducers has become the normal method recently, although ventricular catheters can be used and they allow ventricular drainage as well. The difficulty is in getting into the ventricle when it is small and compressed as is often the case with severe head injury. Some doubt has recently been raised about the efficacy of ICP monitoring in ventilated patients with severe TBI compared with observation alone.

There are a number of effective methods to reduce elevated ICP. Many of these are obvious to neurosurgeons and neuroanesthetists who use them regularly to decrease the pressure when the dura is open at craniotomy. They also know how quickly the various maneuvers work. For example, simply tilting the table so that the head is higher will almost instantly reduce the amount of swelling by reducing the cerebral venous pressure. Other rapid methods include mild hyperventilation, which will have its effect within minutes. The use of hyperosmolar solutions like 20% mannitol will have their effect in about 20 minutes and the dieresis produced is easily monitored. Just these three maneuvers alone will often be enough to stop a tight brain from herniating through a dural incision. If a ventricular or a lumbar drain has been inserted as a pre-operative measure, then CSF drainage will have its effect within minutes as well. Sometimes a ventricular drain is inserted at operation because the brain is tight and retraction is difficult: again an effective method to reduce ICP rapidly. The question is whether or not these four simple maneuvers can be used effectively in the head-injured patient who is not in the operating theatre but rather in the critical care environment. The answer is intuitively ‘yes’ but each of the four methods may have adverse effects if used repeatedly for days at a time. Most doctors use these in a stepwise approach and they may reduce ICP and restore CPP in some cases. However, in many others ICP remains high and other methods are needed. These include barbiturates and decompressive craniectomy. The cumulative application of these various steps can be evaluated using the Therapy Intensity Level (TIL) methodology where the more interventions used, the higher the score (http://tbi-impact.org/cde/ see templates: TIL). There are currently three levels of TIL scoring: the basic score is 0 to 4, an intermediate score from 0 to 10, and a comprehensive score from 0 to 38. This methodology allows therapy that reduces ICP to be evaluated and compared in different studies.

While decompressive craniectomy has become widely practiced in some centers, its efficacy has only been fully and formally assessed in two high-quality prospective randomized controlled trials. The first decompressive craniectomy trial was in 27 children and showed that ICP was lowered and poor outcomes were reduced (71). The DECRA trial randomized 155 adult patients and ICP was promptly and significantly reduced but the outcome was worse in the decompressive craniectomy group (72). The Rescue ICP trial (www.rescueicp.com) seeks to resolve this controversy and 384 patients have been randomized to date. The cost per QALY of decompressive craniectomy for TBI was 17 900 Euros in a separate observational study (73) and even higher (125987 Euros per QALY) when the HAMLET trial evaluated the cost effectiveness of decompressive craniectomy in stroke patients randomized within 48 hours. The controversy about these trial results therefore continues (74), making it all the more important to complete the Rescue ICP trial as quickly as possible to produce a more robust conclusion about the role of decompressive craniectomy in severely head-injured patients.

Treatment of cerebrospinal fluid leaks

The vast majority of CSF leaks through the skull base are through the floor of the anterior cranial fossa. Anterior fossa fractures may manifest themselves as peri-orbital hematomas, sometimes known as ‘Panda eyes’ (Fig. 36.16). They may initially, or later, result in CSF leakage into the nasal cavity so that the patient presents with CSF rhinorrhea. Most such CSF leaks are self-

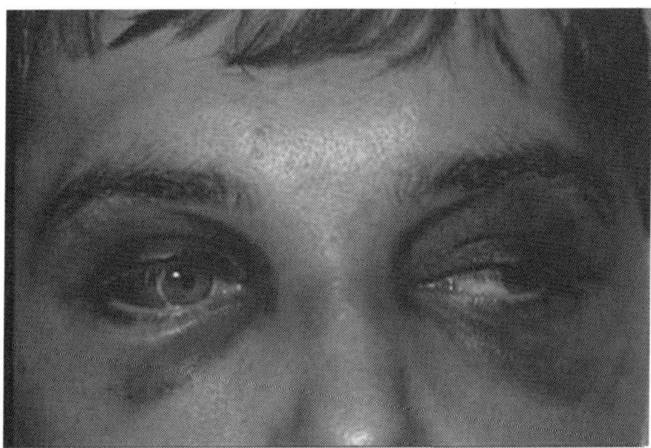

Fig. 36.16 Anterior fossa fracture with 'Panda eyes'.

limiting and stop within a week of the injury. By contrast CSF leaks from the ear (CSF otorrohea) are more difficult to repair, the fracture being through the petrous bone. For this reason, most neurosurgeons leave them for about 3 weeks to see if they are indeed self-limiting. Sometimes such a middle fossa fracture will leak into the middle ear and then down the eustachian tube into the nose, presenting with rhinorrhea rather than otorrohea. While waiting for spontaneous cessation it was once considered wise to use prophylactic antibiotics but now this practice is no longer recommended in the UK Microbiology guidelines! Rather, prophylactic antibiotics are recommended for elective clean surgical procedures while potential meningitis risk patients have such prophylaxis withheld! This somewhat anomalous recommendation is based on expert opinion (Class III evidence) rather than on Class I evidence. Intuitively the original wisdom appears correct and time will tell if the newer guidelines stand up to better evidence in years to come.

Once CSF rhinorrhea persists for more than a week or otorrohea for more than 3 weeks, then surgical repair is recommended. Before accurate imaging with contrast cisternography became available, it was taught that bifrontal approaches were required to ensure closure of the leak. This was usually achieved with a fascia lata graft or artificial dura. The problem was that these patients became bilaterally anosmic (a form of disability well characterized in the small notebook of head injury published by John Potter in 1968 in an epilogue in Appendix 1 called 'lost bouquets' (75). With cisternography it became possible to accurately identify the site of leakage (usually unilateral) so the patient retained the sense of smell on the normal side). The site of the leak can often be identified with high-resolution thin-slice imaging (76). Today, with nasal endoscopy and fluorescein cisternography, the site of the leak can be seen easily from below and an umbrella-like catheter inserted through it. The umbrella is then opened and withdrawn over a small pledget of muscle that becomes trapped (sometimes with glue) under the 'umbrella' thus sealing the leak without the need for a craniotomy (77,78). CSF otorrohea does not permit such endoscopic approaches and a middle fossa craniotomy with artificial dural grafting is the procedure of choice. This more major type of surgery is therefore postponed for up to 3 weeks to see if the otorrohea ceases, which it often does. In both CSF otorrohea and rhinorrhea, lumbar drainage for a few days is likely to increase the success of the surgical repair by temporally diverting CSF from the operative site.

Treatment of compound depressed fractures

The management of compound depressed fractures of the skull vault has, as its main goal, the prevention of secondary infection to consider. Surgical practice has been heavily influenced by military experience. In every war, surgeons have re-learnt that wide local debridement is essential if wound infection is to be avoided. This is because high-velocity missiles destroy a wide core of tissue by releasing kinetic energy as the skull is struck. This tissue is not viable and has to be removed. Clean grafting with pericranium or fascia lata with primary skin closure must be achieved, even if this necessitates the creation and rotation of skin flaps. This military principle has often been wrongly translated into civilian practice where small, uncontaminated, low-velocity, clean compound depressed fractures will often heal well without wide local excision and debridement. All that is required is that the skin is cleaned and the wound closed quickly. The few indications for wide local excision and extensive wound debridement and repair in civilian practice were well described by Van der Heever and Van der Merwe (79) as the following: severe contamination; in-driven fragments (e.g. brick); extensive skin loss with exposed brain. Many authors would add if the outer table of the skull is in-driven by more than 1 cm, then surgical repair is indicated. In practice, many civilian clean compound depressed fractures need only a good and rapid skin closure and antibiotic cover. This must be remembered when a major venous sinus is involved: more harm may result from the surgery if the depression is only slight. In all cases clinical judgment is necessary and secondary elevation and debridement can be practised if local infection does occur.

Treatment of CSDH

In general, chronic subdural hematomas are very different from acute head injuries because they present at least 3 weeks after what is often a minor or unrecognized injury. Nevertheless, they are sometimes included in databases and registers of head injuries because they are a form of head injury but usually present in the chronic phase. As such, they confound the outcome assessments from such databases unless they are removed, because the outcome is so much better than for the acute subdural hematoma. They occur at all ages and in about one third of chronic subdural hematomas there is no history of trauma (42,43). In the majority of patients the standard treatment is burrhole evacuation of the liquid clot, which is usually a thick, oily-looking fluid. This is washed out with saline or Hartmann's solution at 37°C. Recent evidence from a prospective randomized controlled trial has shown clot drainage from the subdural space through a catheter is associated with a better outcome and more effective drainage than with burrholes alone (80). Occasionally, when a chronic subdural hematoma is small and when the liquid clot has become more like cerebrospinal fluid, conservative management with a short course of dexamethasone may be effective (81). When the chronic subdural is associated with very thick membranes and frequent recurrences, it is sometimes necessary to perform a craniotomy to remove the membranes, although this is less frequent with modern management using catheter drainage of the subdural space. When removing the subdural catheter, it is important to avoid letting large quantities of air enter the subdural space. This can be avoided by placing the patient's head down and closing the drainage hole with a suture as soon as the catheter is removed.

Summary of prospective randomized controlled trials in head-injured patients

The vast majority of prospective randomized controlled trials in head-injured patients have been trials of pharmacological treatments and almost all of these have proven negative. These will not be summarized here for this reason, but some of the more important and some ongoing trials will be outlined.

The hyperbaric oxygen trial

In a prospective randomized controlled trial of hyperbaric oxygen (HBO_2) involving 69 patients, Rockswold *et al.* (82) showed that ICP was significantly lower with hyperbaric treatment and this ICP lowering effect persisted for hours after each treatment. There were also benefits from normobaric hyperoxia (NBH) but less so. The importance of this has been stressed by Bullock (83) and a phase III trial of NBH and HBO_2 in head-injured patients is warranted.

The CRASH I and II trials

The first CRASH trial (CRASH I) in patients with head injury revealed that high-dose steroids had an adverse effect on outcome with nearly 200 excess deaths in 10 000 patients randomized to steroids or placebo (84). The second CRASH trial (CRASH II) in patients with general trauma revealed a beneficial effect from tranexamic acid because of the effect on reducing blood loss (85).

The Rescue ICP trial (Multi-center prospective randomized trial of early decompressive craniectomy in patients with severe traumatic brain injury)
The rescue ICP trial has randomized 315 patients with an ICP in excess of 25 mmHg lasting for between 1 and 12 hours to decompressive craniectomy or best

medical treatment (86). The importance of the Rescue ICP trial is obvious given the ongoing controversy created by the DECRA trial result.

The DECRA trial (Multi-center prospective randomized trial of early decompressive craniectomy in patients with severe traumatic brain injury)
The DECRA trial completed recruitment in Australia in April 2010 and the final results were published in 2011 (72). While very successful at lowering ICP, the morbidity and serious mortality were higher in the surgical group than in those treated conservatively.
The decompressive craniectomy trials in children: In a small prospective randomized controlled trial in children, Taylor *et al.* (71) showed that there was a benefit from decompressive craniectomy but the number of children randomized in this trial was small, prompting the initiation of a further such trial in children: the SUDEN trial. The SUDEN trial has been very slow to recruit and is not yet complete.

The STITCH (TRAUMA) trial

This trial set out to randomize patients with traumatic intracerebral hemorrhage to early surgery or to initial conservative treatment. The trial's progress can be monitored on the website: (http://research.ncl.ac.uk/trauma.STITCH/). Patients with extradural or subdural hematomas that require surgical removal in their own right are excluded. Preliminary results show that mortality is more than halved with early surgery.

The Mission for Prognosis and Analysis of Clinical Trials in TBI (IMPACT)
Data from many of the prospective randomized controlled trials in head-injured patients have been pooled in the IMPACT database (87) . This has proved useful in deriving validated prognostic models and sets the stage for a new way to evaluate therapies in neurotrauma. This is achieved by setting standards for data collection in future randomized controlled trials. These are known as the common data elements and can be found on the IMPACT web site: http://www.tbi-impact.org/?p=home/news

Prognosis and outcome

The Glasgow Outcome Scale is universally accepted as the best classification of outcome in head-injured patients (88). There are five categories in the classic Glasgow Outcome Scale but an eight-point scale provides a wider breakdown of categories that lends itself to a prognostic-based outcome for clinical trials (89). Such a prognostic-based dichotomous outcome is also recommended in head-injured patients (90). There are many good prognostic models in head injury and the Brain Trauma Foundation developed these in the late 1990s: https://www.braintrauma.org/pdf/protected/prognosis_guidelines.pdf. Similarly the IMPACT prognosis calculator (http://www.tbi-impact.org/?p=home/news) provides a more modern prediction of outcome, albeit based on very much the same data as used by the Brain Trauma Foundation. Most such prognostic models come up with the same basic prognostic indices: age, the Glasgow Coma Score, pupillary dilation and reaction, hypotension, and CT indices of trauma.

Prediction of post traumatic epilepsy is also important and Jennett's monograph is one of the classics that is often quoted (91). More recent studies are now available (92,93).

Jennett also wrote about the vegetative state and produced another classic monograph in 2002. The definitions and descriptions that he uses make this the definitive statement on the medical issues. It also covers the legal and ethical dilemmas that any discussion about the vegetative state raises (94).

Summary of important guidelines

There are over 250 sets of guidelines on head injury management. Broadly speaking these can be divided into triage guidelines and guidelines for the management of severe head injury. Triage guidelines are useful for those hospitals and doctors practising away from large neuroscience centers and select those patients who should be referred for CT scanning and neurocritical care. The second edition of the United Kingdom's National Institute of Clinical Excellence guidelines for the triage, assessment, investigation, and early management of head injuries in infants, children, and adults (http://www.nice.org.uk/nicemedia/live/11836/36259/36259.pdf) are evidence-based and up-to-date. The management of severe head injury is best summarized in the Brain Trauma Foundation guidelines for the management of severe head injury (https://www.braintrauma.org/coma-guidelines/). These too are evidence-based and are currently in their third edition. They are currently available online, where other guidelines from the Brain Trauma Foundation are also available and include guidelines for pediatric head injury and military trauma. The European Brain Injury Consortium has also produced guidelines for the management of severe head injury. Many other head injury guidelines have been published, many in different languages that are more appropriate for local conditions. Nevertheless, those listed above are probably the most widely applicable and up-to-date.

Conclusions

Head injury is one of the most common diseases in the world and afflicts predominantly young males. The vast majority are mild, but even the most mild injury can prove fatal as was recognized in 400 BC by Hippocrates (http://classics.mit.edu/Hippocrates/headinjur.mb.txt). The most feared complication is the delayed development or expansion of a hematoma. Triage guidelines are designed to detect and prevent this and effective triage is likely to save more lives and to reduce disability to a greater extent than all the critical care expenditure will ever achieve in terms of reducing death and disability.

REFERENCES

1. Graham, D. I., J. H. Adams, *et al.* (1978). 'Ischaemic brain damage in fatal non-missile head injuries.' *Journal of Neurological Sciences* **39**:213–34.
2. Graham, D. I., I. Ford, *et al.* (1989). 'Ischaemic brain damage is still common in fatal non-missile head injury.' *Journal of Neurology Neurosurgery and Psychiatry* **52**(3):346–50.
3. Crompton, M. R. (1973). 'The pathology of subarachnoid haemorrhage.' *Journal of the Royal College of Physicians of London* **7**(3):235–7.
4. Jenkins A, Maxwell Wl, *et al.* (1989). 'Experimental intracerebral haematoma in the rat: sequential light microscopical changes.' *Neuropathology & Applied Neurobiology* **15**(5):477–86.
5. Jenkins, A., A. D. Mendelow, *et al.* (1990). 'Experimental intracerebral haematoma: the role of blood constituents in early ischaemia.' *British Journal of Neurosurgery* **4**:45–51.
6. Bullock, R. and H. Fujisawa (1992). 'The role of glutamate antagonists for the treatment of CNS injury.' *Journal of Neurotrauma* **9** Suppl 2:S443–62.
7. Stiell, I. G., G. A. Wells, *et al.* (2001). 'The Canadian CT Head Rule for patients with minor head injury. *Lancet* **357**(9266):1391–6.
8. Stiell, I. G., C. M. Clement, *et al.* (2005). 'Comparison of the Canadian CT Head Rule and the New Orleans Criteria in patients with minor head injury.' *JAMA* **294**(12):1511–18.
9. Ibanez, J., F. Arikan, *et al.* (2004). 'Reliability of clinical guidelines in the detection of patients at risk following mild head injury: results of a prospective study.' *Journal of Neurosurgery* **100**(5):825–34.
10. Fearnside, M. R. and D. A. Simpson (2005). Epidemiology. *Head Injury: Pathophysiology and Management.* P. R. Reilly and R. Bullock. London, Hodder Arnold: 3–25.
11. Tagliaferri, F., C. Compagnone, *et al.* (2006). 'A systematic review of brain injury epidemiology in Europe.' *Acta Neurochirurgica* **148**(3):255–68; discussion 268.
12. Vajkoczy, P., H. Roth, *et al.* (2000). 'Continuous monitoring of regional cerebral blood flow: experimental and clinical validation of a novel thermal diffusion microprobe.' *Journal of Neurosurgery* **93**(2):265–74.
13. Gupta, A. K., P. J. Hutchinson, *et al.* (1999). 'Measuring brain tissue oxygenation compared with jugular venous oxygen saturation for monitoring cerebral oxygenation after traumatic brain injury.' *Anesthesia & Analgesia* **88**(3):549–53.
14. Valadka, A. B., R. Hlatky, *et al.* (2002). 'Brain tissue PO2 correlation with cerebral blood flow.' *Acta Neurochirurgica* Supplement **81**:299–301.
15. Timofeev, I., M. Czosnyka, *et al.* (2011). 'Interaction between brain chemistry and physiology after traumatic brain injury: impact of autoregulation and microdialysis catheter location.' *Journal of Neurotrauma* **28**(6):849–60.
16. Zauner, A., E. Doppenberg, *et al.* (1997). 'Multiparametric continuous monitoring of brain metabolism and substrate

delivery in neurosurgical patients.' *Neurological Research* **19**(3):265–73.

17. Bullock, R., A. Zauner, *et al.* (1998). 'Factors affecting excitatory amino acid release following severe human head injury.' *Journal of Neurosurgery* **89**(4):507–18.
18. Hutchinson, P. J., M. T. O'Connell, *et al.* (2000). 'Clinical cerebral microdialysis: a methodological study.' *Journal of Neurosurgery* **93**(1):37–43.
19. Bouma, G. J. and J. P. Muizelaar (1992). 'Cerebral blood flow, cerebral blood volume, and cerebrovascluar reactivity after severe head injury.' *Journal of Neurotrauma* **9**(s1): s333–s48.
20. Schroder, M. L., J. P. Muizelaar, *et al.* (1995). 'Focal ischemia due to traumatic contusions documented by stable xenon-CT and ultrastructural studies.' *Journal of Neurosurgery* **82**(6):966–71.
21. Zauner, A., R. Bullock, *et al.* (1996). 'Glutamate release and cerebral blood flow after severe human head injury.' *Acta Neurochirurgica* Supplement **67**:40–4.
22. Kohi, Y. M., A. D. Mendelow, *et al.* (1984). 'Extracranial insults and outcome in patients with acute head injury – relationship to the Glasgow Coma Scale.' *Injury* **16**:25–9.
23. Gentleman, D. (1992). 'Causes and effects of systemic complications among severely head injured patients transferred to a neurosurgical unit.' *International Surgery* **77**(4):297–302.
24. Strich, S. J. (1961). 'Shearing of nerve fibres as a cause of brain damage due to head injury.' *Lancet* **ii**:443–8.
25. Strich, S. J. (1970). 'Lesions in the cerebral hemispheres after blunt head injury.' *Journal of Clinical Pathology* Supplement (Royal College of Pathologists) **4**:166–71.
26. Povlishock, J. T. and C. W. Christman (1995). 'The pathobiology of traumatically induced axonal injury in animals and humans: a review of current thoughts.' *Journal of Neurotrauma* **12**(4):555–64.
27. Adams, J. H., D. Doyle, *et al.* (1989). 'Brain damage in fatal non-missile head injury in relation to age and type of injury.' *Scott Medical Journal* **34**(1):399–401.
28. Oppenheimer, D. R. (1968). 'Microscopic lesions in the brain following head injury.' *Journal of Neurology, Neurosurgery & Psychiatry* **31**(4):299–306.
29. Cowie, R. A., A. D. Mendelow, *et al.* (2010). 'MRI in mild and moderate head injury'. British Neurosurgery Research Group, Dundee.
30. Mendelow, A. D., Gregson BA, *et al.* (2013). *Results of the STITCH(TRAUMA) Trial Part 2.* World Congress of Neurosurgery, Seoul, Korea.
31. Bowman, C. L., J. P. Ding, *et al.* (1992). 'Mechanotransducing ion channels in astrocytes.' *Brain Research* **584**:272–86.
32. Di, X., O. L. Alves, *et al.* (2003). 'Cytotoxic edema is independent of NMDA ion channel activation following middle cerebral artery occlusion (MCAO). An in vivo autoradiographic and MRI study.' *Neurological Research.* **25**(4):329–34.
33. Marmarou, A. (2007). 'A review of progress in understanding the pathophysiology and treatment of brain edema.' *Neurosurgical Focus* **22**(5):E1.
34. Delahunty, T. M., J. Y. Jiang, *et al.* (1995). 'Differential consequences of lateral and central fluid percussion brain injury on receptor coupling in rat hippocampus.' *Journal of Neurotrauma.* **12**(6):1045–57.
35. Stringer, W. L. and D. L. Kelly Jr (1980). 'Traumatic dissection of the extracranial internal carotid artery.' *Neurosurgery* **6**:123.
36. Eastman, A. L., D. P. Chason, *et al.* (2006). 'Computed tomographic angiography for the diagnosis of blunt cervical vascular injury: is it ready for primetime?' *Journal of Trauma-Injury Infection & Critical Care* **60**(5):925–9; discussion 929.
37. Eastman, A. L., V. Muraliraj, *et al.* (2009). 'CTA-based screening reduces time to diagnosis and stroke rate in blunt cervical vascular injury.' *Journal of Trauma-Injury Infection & Critical Care* **67**(3):551–6; discussion 555–6.
38. Mendelow, A. D., M. Z. Karmi, *et al.* (1979). 'Extradural haematoma – effect of delayed treatment.' *British Medical Journal* **1**:1240–2.
39. Gusmao, S. N. and J. E. Pittella (1998). 'Extradural haematoma and diffuse axonal injury in victims of fatal road traffic accidents.' *British Journal of Neurosurgery* **12**(2):123–6.
40. Stevenson, G. C., H. A. Brown, *et al.* (1964). 'Chronic venous epidural hematoma at the vertex.' *Journal of Neurosurgery* **21**:887–91.
41. Seelig, J. M., D. P. Becker, *et al.* (1981). 'Traumatic acute subdural hematoma: major mortality reduction in comatose patients treated within four hours.' *New England Journal of Medicine* **305**(25):1511–18.
42. Cameron, M. M. (1978). 'Chronic subdural haematoma: a review of 114 cases.' *Journal of Neurology, Neurosurgery & Psychiatry* **41**(9):834–9.
43. Nath, F., A. D. Mendelow, *et al.* (1985). 'Chronic subdural-hematoma in the CT scan era.' *Scottish Medical Journal* **30**:152–5.

44. Siddique, M. S., B. A. Gregson, *et al.* (2002). 'Comparative study of traumatic and spontaneous intracerebral hemorrhage.' *Journal of Neurosurgery* **96**:86–9.
45. Mitchell, P. (2011). 'Contre Coup Head Injury.'
46. Oertel, M., D. F. Kelly, *et al.* (2002). 'Progressive hemorrhage after head trauma: predictors and consequences of the evolving injury.' *Journal of Neurosurgery* **96**(1):109–16.
47. Choksey, M., H. A. Crockard, *et al.* (1993). 'Acute traumatic intracerebral haematomas: determinants of outcome in a retrospective series of 202 cases.' *British Journal of Neurosurgery* **7**(6):611–22.
48. Mendelow, A. D., R. Bullock, *et al.* (1984). 'Intracranial haemorrhage induced at arterial pressure in the rat: Part 2. Short term changes in local cerebral blood flow measured by autoradiography.' *Neurology Research* **6**:189–93.
49. Huang, F.-P., G. Xi, *et al.* (2002). 'Brain edema after experimental intracerebral hemorrhage: role of hemoglobin degradation products.' *Journal of Neurosurgery* **96**(2):287–93.
50. Keep, R. F., J. Xiang, *et al.* (2008). 'Blood-brain barrier function in intracerebral hemorrhage.' *Acta Neurochirurgica*. Supplement **105**:73–7.
51. Xi, G., Y. Hua, *et al.* (2001). 'Mechanisms of edema formation after intracerebral hemorrhage: effects of extravasated red blood cells on blood flow and blood-brain barrier integrity.' *Stroke* **32**(12):2932–8.
52. Firsching, R., D. Woischneck, *et al.* (2002). 'Brain stem lesions after head injury.' *Neurological Research* **24**(2):145–6.
53. Cowie, C., A. Blamire, *et al.* (2011). 'MRI in mild and moderate head injury.'
54. Patel, H. C., O. Bouamra, *et al.* (2005). 'Trends in head injury outcome from 1989 to 2003 and the effect of neurosurgical care: an observational study. [Erratum appears in Lancet. 2006 Mar 11;367(9513):816].' *Lancet* **366**(9496):1538–44.
55. Yates, D. W. (2007). Triage, assessment, investigation and early management of head injury in infants, children and adult. National Institute for Health and Clinical Excellence.
56. Jones, N., R. Bullock, *et al.* (2005). The role of surgery for intracranial mass lesions after head injury. *Head Injury: Pathophysiology and Management.* P. L. Reilly and R. Bullock. London, Hodder Arnold: 368–83.
57. Xi, G., Y. Hua, *et al.* (2000). 'Induction of colligin may attenuate brain edema following intracerebral hemorrhage.' *Acta Neurochirurgica* Supplement **76**:501–5.
58. Xi, G., Y. Hua, *et al.* (2002). 'Brain edema after intracerebral hemorrhage: the effects of systemic complement depletion.' *Acta Neurochirurgica* Supplement **81**:253–6.
59. Xi, G., J. Wu, *et al.* (2003). 'Thrombin preconditioning upregulates transferrin and transferrin receptor and reduces brain edema induced by lysed red blood cells.' *Acta Neurochirurgica* Supplement **86**:449–52.
60. Keep, R. F., G. Xi, *et al.* (2005). 'The deleterious or beneficial effects of different agents in intracerebral hemorrhage: think big, think small, or is hematoma size important?' *Stroke* **36**(7):1594–6.
61. Gong, Y., H. Tian, *et al.* (2006). 'Systemic zinc protoporphyrin administration reduces intracerebral hemorrhage-induced brain injury.' *Acta Neurochirurgica* Supplement **96**:232–6.
62. Xi, G., R. F. Keep, *et al.* (2006). 'Mechanisms of brain injury after intracerebral haemorrhage.' *Lancet Neurology* **5**(1):53–63.
63. Hua, Y., R. F. Keep, *et al.* (2007). 'Brain injury after intracerebral hemorrhage: the role of thrombin and iron.' *Stroke* **38**(2 Suppl):759–62.
64. Zhao, X., G. Sun, *et al.* (2007). 'Hematoma resolution as a target for intracerebral hemorrhage treatment: role for peroxisome proliferator-activated receptor gamma in microglia/macrophages.' *Annals of Neurology* **61**(4):352–62.
65. Zhao, X., Y. Zhang, *et al.* (2007). 'Distinct patterns of intracerebral hemorrhage-induced alterations in NF-kappaB subunit, iNOS, and COX-2 expression.' *Journal of Neurochemistry* **101**(3):652–63.
66. Hua, Y., R. F. Keep, *et al.* (2008). 'Deferoxamine therapy for intracerebral hemorrhage.' *Acta Neurochirurgica* Supplement **105**:3–6.
67. Zhao, X., S. Song, *et al.* (2009). 'Neuroprotective role of haptoglobin after intracerebral hemorrhage.' *Journal of Neuroscience* **29**(50):15819–27.
68. Mitchell, P., M. Tseng, *et al.* (2004). 'Decompressive craniectomy with lattice duraplasty.' *Acta Neurochirurgica* **146**(2):159–60.
69. Csokay, A., L. Nagy, *et al.* (2001). 'Avoidance of vascular compression in decompressive surgery for brain edema caused by trauma and tumor ablation.' *Neurosurgical Review.* **24**(4):209–13.
70. Mitchell, P., B. A. Gregson, *et al.* (2007). 'Blood pressure in head-injured patients.' *Journal of Neurology, Neurosurgery & Psychiatry* **78**(4):399–402.
71. Taylor, A., W. Butt, *et al.* (2001). 'A randomized trial of very early decompressive craniectomy in children with traumatic brain injury and sustained intracranial hypertension.' *Childs Nervous System* **17**(3):154–62.

72. Cooper, D. J., J. V. Rosenfeld, *et al.* (2011). 'Decompressive craniectomy in diffuse traumatic brain injury.' *New England Journal of Medicine* **364**(16):1493–502.
73. Malmivaara, K., R. Kivisaari, *et al.* 'Cost-effectiveness of decompressive craniectomy in traumatic brain injuries.' *European Journal of Neurology* **18**(4):656–62.
74. Hutchinson, P. J., P. J. Kirkpatrick, *et al.* 'Craniectomy in diffuse traumatic brain injury.' *New England Journal of Medicine* **365**(4):375s; author reply 376.
75. Potter, J. M. (1968). *The Practical Management of Head Injuries*. London, Lloyd-Luke (Medical Books) Ltd.
76. Lloyd, K. M., J. M. DelGaudio, *et al.* (2008). 'Imaging of skull base cerebrospinal fluid leaks in adults.' *Radiology* **248**(3):725–36.
77. Lee, T.-J., C.-C. Huang, *et al.* (2004). 'Transnasal endoscopic repair of cerebrospinal fluid rhinorrhea and skull base defect: ten-year experience.' *Laryngoscope* **114**(8):1475–81.
78. Cui, S., D. Han, *et al.* (2010). 'Endoscopic endonasal surgery for recurrent cerebrospinal fluid rhinorrhea.' *Acta Oto-Laryngologica* **130**(10):1169–74.
79. Van der Heever, C. and D. Van der Merwe (1986). 'Management of depressed skull fractures: selective conservative management of non-missile injuries.' *Journal of Neurosurgery* **71**:186.
80. Santarius, T., P. J. Kirkpatrick, *et al.* (2009). 'Use of drains versus no drains after burr-hole evacuation of chronic subdural haematoma: a randomised controlled trial.' *Lancet* **374**(9695):1067–73.
81. Bender, M. B. and N. Christoff (1974). 'Nonsurgical treatment of subdural hematomas.' *Archives of Neurology* **31** (2):73–9.
82. Rockswold, S. B., G. L. Rockswold, *et al.* (2010). 'A prospective, randomized clinical trial to compare the effect of hyperbaric to normobaric hyperoxia on cerebral metabolism, intracranial pressure, and oxygen toxicity in severe traumatic brain injury.' *Journal of Neurosurgery* **112**(5):1080–94.
83. Bullock, R. M. (2010). 'Editorial.' *Journal of Neurosurgery* **112**:1078–9.
84. Roberts, I., D. Yates, *et al.* (2004). 'Effect of intravenous corticosteroids on death within 14 days in 10008 adults with clinically significant head injury (MRC CRASH trial): randomised placebo-controlled trial.' *Lancet* **364**(9442):1321–8.
85. Collaborators, H. Shakur, *et al.* (2010). 'Effects of tranexamic acid on death, vascular occlusive events, and blood transfusion in trauma patients with significant haemorrhage (CRASH-2): a randomised, placebo-controlled trial.' *Lancet* **376**(9734):23–32.
86. Hutchinson, P. J., E. Corteen, *et al.* (2006). 'Decompressive craniectomy in traumatic brain injury: the randomized multicenter RESCUEicp study (www.RESCUEicp.com).' *Acta Neurochirurgica* Supplement **96**:17–20.
87. Maas, A. I., E. W. Steyerberg, *et al.* (2007). 'Prognostic value of computerized tomography scan characteristics in traumatic brain injury: results from the IMPACT study.' *Journal of Neurotrauma* **24**(2):303–14.
88. Jennett, B. and M. Bond (1974). 'Assessment of outcome after severe brain damage.' *Lancet* (1) **7905**:80–484.
89. Mendelow, A., G. Teasdale, *et al.* (2003). 'Outcome assignment in the International Surgical Trial in Intracerebral Haemorrhage.' *Acta Neurochirurgica (European Journal of Neurosurgery)* **145**:679–81.
90. Murray, G. D., D. Barer, *et al.* (2005). 'Design and analysis of phase III trials with ordered outcome scales: the concept of the sliding dichotomy.' *Journal of Neurotrauma* **22**(5):511–17.
91. Jennett, B. (1975). *Epilepsy After Non-missile Head Injuries.* London, William Heineman Medical Books Ltd.
92. Annegers, J., A. Hauser, *et al.* (1998). 'A population-based study of seizures after traumatic brain injuries.' *NEJM* **338**:20–4.
93. Englander, J., T. Bushnik, *et al.* (2003). 'Analyzing risk factors for late posttraumatic seizures: a prospective, multicenter investigation.' *Archives of Physical Medicine & Rehabilitation* **84**(3):365–73.
94. Jennett, B. (2002). *The Vegetative State.* Cambridge, Cambridge University Press.

Index

Page numbers in *italics* indicate tables

abscess, tretment-related, 310
access sites, endovascular, 121
acid-base balance, hypothermia and, 141–142
activities of daily living
  Barthel ADL Index, 74
  Modified Rankin Scale, 73
adenosine cardiac standstill, 444
airway
  compromised, intubation for, 288
  difficult, 289
Alberta stroke program early CT score (ASPECTS), 104
anemia
  cerebral blood flow affected by, 21
  after subarachnoid hemorrhage, 471–472, 481
anesthesia for intracranial angioplasty, 121
aneurysm
  clipping vs. coiling, 437, 459–461
  craniotomy for
    aneurysm rupture during, 443–444
    indications, 437–438
    microscopic approaches, 440–442
    minimally invasive, 440
    proximal control, 442–443
    repair techniques, 443–444
    surgical techniques, 439–440, 445
    timing and preparation, 438–439
  development, 424
  embolization
    coil, 111–112, 437–438, 448–450
    development of, 447
  endovascular therapy
    clinical trials, 459–461
    complications, 456–457
    periprocedural care, 455–456
    site of aneurysm and, 453–455
    techniques and devices, 447–453

incomplete treatment, 458–459
interventional treatment
indications for, 111
options and procedures, 111–112
location, 423
rupture, 423–424
during endovascular therapy, 456–457
and hydrocephalus, 146, 159
intraoperative, 439, 443–444
surgery for
decompressive, 96
Hunt and Hess scale of risk, 72
lumbar drainage in, 160
monitoring in, 40
angiography
of aneurysm, 447–448
for craniotomy, 438–439
postoperative, 458
in arterial malformations, 114
in cavernoma, 406
in cerebellar hemorrhage, 366–367
in cerebellar infarction, 212
in cerebral hemorrhage, 392
in cerebral venous thrombosis, 502–505
in cervical artery dissections, 227
four-vessel as baseline, 122
in intracerebral hemorrhage, 338
in intracranial stenosis, 122
pre- and intraoperative, in excision of AVMs, 389
in subarachnoid hemorrhage, 427–428
in vasospasm, 109
angiomas
classification, 114
endovascular therapy, 114
venous, 401
angioplasty
after thrombolysis in basilar artery occlusion, 201
balloon, 109
balloon selection, 123
complications, 125
postprocedural care, 125
prophylactic, 432
vs. stent-assisted, 122–123
techniques, 123–125
in vasospasm, 457, 472
for spasmolysis, 109–111
prophylactic, 467
in intracranial stenosis, 120
anoxic depolarization, 130
antibiotic-impregnated catheters, 151
antibiotics
prophylactic
in cerebrospinal fluid leak, 531
in ventilator-associated pneumonia, 307
for ventricular drainage, 150–151, 357
selective decontamination by, 433
strategies for use of, 311, *311*
anticoagulants
after basilar artery occlusion, 202
after cerebral venous thrombosis, 509–510
in cerebral venous thrombosis, 234–235
in cervical artery dissections, 227
endovascular therapy and, 121
in endovascular therapy, 452, 455
and hematoma expansion, 265–268
novel direct oral, 267–268
in pregnancy, 236
reversal, 265–266, *266*, 268
antiedema therapy, 82
barbiturates, 84–85
elevated head position, 85–86
hyperventilation, 85, 316
in intracranial hemorrhage, 86–87
osmotherapy, 82–84, 316–317
steroids as, 86
tromethamine, 85
antihypertensives, *248*, 249–251, *279*
in acute hypertensive response, 278–280
in intracerebral hemorrhage, 276–277
hematoma expansion and, 262–263, *264*, 268
immediately post-stroke, 280–282
stop vs. continue, 245–246
anti-inflammatory treatment
in posthemorrhagic edema, 86
prophylactic for delayed ischemia, *467*
antiplatelet medication
after endovascular therapy, 125
in endovascular therapy, 121, 455
and hematoma expansion, 265
in stenosis, 106, 107
after stenting, 107, 109
in stenting, 107
APACHE Scores, 68–69
arterial malformations, endovascular therapy for, 112–114
embolization techniques, 114–117
arteriovenous malformations, 394
radiosurgery for, 394–396
surgical excision, 387–389

arteriovenous malformations (cont.)
decision-making, 390–392
with hemorrhage, 392–393
unexpected, in craniotomy, 324, 392–393
arteritis
giant cell, 229
Takayasu, 229–230
ataxia
in cerebellar hemorrhage, 365
in cerebellar infarction, 209
autoregulation, cerebral, 4–5, 20–22, 243
head injury and, 530
in hypertension, 274
in intracerebral hemorrhage, 275

bacterial infection as cause of stroke, 228–229
balloon
angioplasty, 109
balloon selection, 123
complications, 125
postprocedural care, 125
prophylactic, 432
vs. stent-assisted, 122–123
techniques, 123–125
in vasospasm, 457, 472
embolization, 447
occlusion of parent artery in aneurysm, 448
barbiturates, 84–85
Barthel ADL Index, 74
basilar artery occlusion, 194–195
brainstem hemorrhage in, 378
clinical trials of thrombolysis, 198–200
diagnostics and imaging, 195–196
differential diagnoses, *196*
intensive care after, 202–203
symptoms, *195*
Bedside Shivering Assessment Scale, 137, *137*
Behcet's disease, 230
blood pressure, systemic
management
guidelines, *247*, 277–278, 282
in cerebellar hemorrhage, 370
in intracerebral hemorrhage, 262–263, *264*, 276–277, 280–282, 338
in subarachnoid hemorrhage, 430
stroke and, 243–245
target levels, 246
See also hypertension, hypotension
blood–brain barrier
in edema formation, 81, 82
hypothermia and, 130
metalloproteinases and, 130
osmotherapy and, 82
brain damage
ischemic, 518–519
primary, 519–520
prevention, 526
secondary, 521
ischemic, 520–521
brain symmetry index, 61
brain tissue oxygenation
cerebral perfusion pressure and, 39
and hyperventilation, 39
monitoring, 37–39
in intracranial hemorrhage, 41
in ischemic stroke, 40
by near-infrared spectroscopy, 63
neurochemical monitoring and, 39
in subarachnoid hemorrhage, 40, 468, 485
thresholds, 38–39
brainstem auditory evoked potentials, 212
for monitoring, 61
brainstem cavernoma, 382–383
brainstem compression, 367, 371
brainstem hematoma, 378
surgery in, 381–383
brainstem hemorrhage, 378–379
prognosis, 379–380
respiratory effects, 288
surgery in, 381

CADASIL, 232
calcium influx, hypothermia and, 130
calcium-channel blockers
in delayed ischemia, 465, 487
in vasospasm, 109, 110, 433, 465
Call–Fleming syndrome, 231–232
Canadian Neurological Scale, 71
capillary telangiectases, 400–401
carbon dioxide, cerebral blood flow modulated by, 21, 287
cardiac assist devices, 495
cardiac investigations after basilar artery occlusion, 203
cardiac rhythm
hypothermia and, 140, 141
subarachnoid hemorrhage and, 492
vasopressors and, 473
cardiopulmonary dysfunction, CNS-mediated, 490
cardiomyopathies, 492–493, 495

clinical features and diagnosis, 492–494
pathophysiology, 490–492
catecholamine surge, 491, 495
catheters
balloon, for intracranial angioplasty, 123
brain tissue oxygenation, 38
Camino, 8
cerebral microdialysis, 44, 46
cooling, 132
for intracranial angioplasty, 122
and hemorrhage risk, 8
and infection risk, 8, 308
intraventricular, 8
antibiotic-impregnated, 151, 357
placement, 148–149, 355
lumbar
complications, 163
placement, 159
in pressure monitoring, 162
micro-, for intracranial angioplasty, 124
urinary, and infection, 307–308
cavernoma, 400–402
clinical presentation, 408, 409–410
diagnostic imaging, 406–408
epidemiology, 402–404
histopathology, pathobiology and pathogenesis, 404–406
management, 410–413
surgical, 382–383, 413–415
-related intracranial hemorrhage, 408–410
central volume principle, 27
cerebellar hemorrhage, 363–364
complications, 367
diagnosis, 365–367
prognosis and outcome, 372–374, *373*
signs and symptoms, 364–365, *364*
treatment, 367–370
surgical, 370–371
ventricular drainage, 371
cerebellar infarction
combination therapy in, 183
course and outcome, 213–214
decompressive surgery in, 95, 182–183
diagnosis, 210–213
epidemiology and risk factors, 207
mortality, *219*
pathogenesis, 207–208
prognosis and outcome, 218–219, *220*
signs and symptoms, 208–210, *215*
treatment strategies, 214–218, *216*, 219–223
cerebral autoregulation, 4–5, 20–22, 243
head injury and, 530
in hypertension, 274
in intracerebral hemorrhage, 275
cerebral blood flow, 20
in acute ischemic stroke, 25
hyperventilation and, 85
in intracerebral hemorrhage, 275–276
in intracranial hemorrhage, 25
as marker of ischemia, 22–24
monitoring, 26–33, *27*
comparison of methods, *29*
indications for, 33
in subarachnoid hemorrhage, 25–26
in subarachnoid hemorrhage, 468
thresholds for ischemia, 22
cerebral cavernous malformation. *See* cavernoma
cerebral infarction, delayed, 429
cerebral ischemia, 22
cerebral blood flow as marker of, 22–24
delayed, 464–465
adjunctive therapies, 474
detection, 468–469
hemodynamic goals, *471*
hemodynamic interventions, 469–470, 472, 473–474
indications for treatment, 469
prevention, 464–465
microdialysis to detect, 44, *47*, 48–50, 468
cerebral perfusion pressure, 5, 20
brain tissue oxygenation and, 39
vs. intracranial pressure, 9
reduced, compensatory mechanisms, 22
cerebral vasospasm. *See* vasospasm
cerebral venous thrombosis, 233–234
causes, 506–507
clinical features, 502–505
diagnosis, 502–505
differential, 505–506
epidemiology, 501
intracranial pressure monitoring in, 12
malignant, decompressive surgery in, 96–97
outcome and prognosis, 507–508
recurrent, 509–510
risk factors, *506*
treatment, 234–235, 508–512
cerebrospinal fluid
altered dynamics after craniectomy, 98, 100
blockage of, and hydrocephalus, 146, 158
leaks, 530–531

cerebrospinal fluid (cont.)
  role in regulation of ICP, 3
  shunt, 152
  surveillance, 151
    antibiotic-impregnated catheter and, 152
  See also lumbar drainage, ventricular drainage
cerebrovascular malformations, 400–402
cerebrovascular reserve, 21
cervical artery dissection, 226–227
clipping of aneurysms, 443–444
  aneurysm rupture during, 443–444
  vs. coiling, 437, 459–461
  galvanic corrosion of clips, 445
clot burden
  and choice of treatment, 103
  high, recanalization in, 106
$CMRO_2$. *See* metabolic demand
coagulopathy, 237–238
  hematoma expansion and, 265–268
  hypothermia and, 142
  intracerebral hemorrhage and, 323, 338
  and ventricular drainage, 153
coil embolization
  development of, 447
  in aneurysm, 111–112, 437–438
    vs. clipping, 437, 459–461
    devices, 448–450
  of fistulas, 116
  stent-assisted, 450–453
coma
  airway compromise in, 288
  in basilar artery occlusion, 200
  causes, 287
  in cerebellar hemorrhage, 365
  in cerebral venous thrombosis, 501
  Glasgow Coma Scale, 66–68
    in cerebellar infarction, 210
    as predictor of extubation, 293
  microdialysis in, *48*, 50–51
combination therapy
  decompressive surgery and hypothermia, 185
  drugs and hypothermia, 135–136
  hypothermia and drainage, 183
  intraventricular fibrinolysis and drainage, 162
  thrombolysis and interventional therapies, 175–177
  thrombolysis and minimally invasive surgery, 315–318
complement in edema formation, 86
consciousness
  brainstem hemorrhage and, 379
  in cerebellar hemorrhage, 364, 367
  in cerebellar infarction, 210
  Glasgow Coma Scale, 66–68
    in cerebellar infarction, 209
    as predictor of extubation, 293
  respiratory drive and, 287
contra coup lesion, 524
contusions, cerebral, 520, 523–524
  treatment, 528–529
cooling
  invasive methods, 132–133, 186
  non-invasive methods, 132, 185–186
  optimal temperature, 186
  rewarming, 134
core temperature
  monitoring in cooling, 132
  regulation, 131
  and shivering, 136
  target, in hypothermia, 133
craniectomy, decompressive, 10, 90–92
  in cerebral contusions, 528–529
  clinical trials, 530, 532–533
  complications, 97–100
  converting craniotomy to, 324
  indications, 92–97
  suboccipital, 217, 371
  in traumatic brain injury, 14
cranioplasty, 91, 100
craniotomy
  in aneurysm
    aneurysm rupture during, 443–444
    indications, 437–438
    microscopic approaches, 440–442
    minimally invasive, 440
    proximal control, 442–443
    repair techniques, 443–444
    surgical techniques, 439–440, 445
    timing and preparation, 438–439
  for arteriovenous malformations, 387–389
    decision-making, 390–392
    with hemorrhage, 392–393
  decompressive
    in extradural hematoma, 527
    in intracerebral hematoma, 528
    in subdural hematoma, 527–528, 532
  in intracerebral hemorrhage, 323–326
  in prevention of hematoma expansion, 260–262
  suboccipital, 371
CSF. *See* cerebrospinal fluid

CT
in basilar artery occlusion, 195–196
in cavernoma, 407
in cerebellar hemorrhage, 366
in cerebellar infarction, 210–211
in cerebral venous thrombosis, 502–503
in cervical artery dissections, 227
in head injury, 524
Marshall classification, 69
in intracerebral hemorrhage, 338–339
of malignant MCA infarction, 182
to measure cerebral blood flow, 28, *30*
in subarachnoid hemorrhage, 426–428
in subdural hematoma, 523
CT perfusion to measure cerebral blood flow, 27, 28–31, *30*, 468–469

decompressive surgery, 90–92, 180
in cerebellar infarction, 182–183
in cerebral contusions, 528–529
in cerebral venous thrombosis, 509–510
clinical trials, 530, 532–533
complications, 97–100
in extradural hematoma, 527
indications, 92–97
in intracerebral hematoma, 528
clinical trials, 528
for ischemic stroke, 179
in malignant MCA infarction
clinical trials, 180–181, *180*
complications, 182
in subdural hematoma, 527–528
suboccipital, 217, 371
diaschisis, 23
diffuse axonal injury, 519–520
in hematoma, 522
disability
acceptability, 95
Modified Rankin Scale, 73
studies of, after decompressive surgery
in cerebellar infarction, 95
in hemispheric infarction, 92–95
dislocation, third ventricle, 59
dissection, cervical artery, 226–227, 521
dizziness, diagnostic value of, 208
drainage
lumbar, 163–164
complications, 162–163
intraoperative, 439
in intraventricular hemorrhage, 356–357
in subarachnoid hemorrhage, 159–161
in traumatic brain injury, 14
ventricular, 8, 145–147
in brainstem hemorrhage, 381
in cerebellar hemorrhage, 371
in cerebellar infarction, 183, 217
complications, 149–150
in intracranial hemorrhage, 11–12
in intraventricular hemorrhage, 353
insertion, 147–149
management, 150–152, 357
-related infections, 357
removal, 152
and risk of hemorrhage, 8
risk of infection, 309
thromboprophylaxis, 152–153
drugs
for control of shivering, 137
hypothermia alters pharmacokinetics, 139–140, *140*
dural opening in decompressive craniectomy, 91, 528
dysphagia, 299–300, 306

ECG
hypothermia and, 140
in subarachnoid hemorrhage, 492, 494
eclampsia, 236
edema
cytotoxic, 520
ischemic, 90
pathophysiology, 81
in malignant MCA infarction, 190–191
predictors of, 192
treatment, 192–193
perihemorrhagic
management, 315–318
pathophysiology, 81–82, 315
post-trauma, 520–521
pulmonary, 433
space-occupying
in cerebellar infarction, 207, *211*, 213–214, 218–223
diagnosis, 210–213
evoked potentials in, 61
predictors of, 192
signs and symptoms, 208–210
treatment, 192–193
See also antiedema therapy
EKOS ultrasound device, 175
electroencephalography, continuous, for monitoring, 60–61

electrolytes
  hypothermia and, 141–142
  subarachnoid hemorrhage and, 429, 433, 482
embolism, postoperative, 235
embolization
  balloon, 447
  coil
    in aneurysm, 111–112, 437–438
    vs. clipping, 437, 459–461
    development of, 447
    devices, 448–450
    of fistulas, 116
    stent-assisted, 450–453
  of arterial malformations, 112–114
    preoperative, 388
    before radiosurgery, 396
    techniques, 114–117
empyema, treatment-related, 310
endoscopic techniques for clot evacuation, 331, 332, 337
  in intraventricular hemorrhage, 356
endothelin antagonists in subarachnoid hemorrhage, 434, 466
endovascular therapy
  complications, 125
  in aneurysm
    clinical trials, 459–461
    complications, 456–457
    periprocedural care, 455–456
    site of aneurysm and, 453–455
    techniques and devices, 447–453
  in arterial malformations, 112–114
    embolization techniques, 114–117
  in basilar artery occlusion, 202
  in cerebral venous thrombosis, 509
  in intracranial stenosis
    antiplatelet therapy before, 121
    indications for, 120
  vs. medical management, 120
  postprocedural care, 125
  procedural considerations, 121–122
  techniques, 122–125
  in vasospasm, 457–458, 472–473
  See also interventional therapy
energy demand, 298
enteral nutrition, 299–301
  vs. parenteral, 301–302
epilepsy
  after cerebral venous thrombosis, 511
  cavernoma and, 408, 410
  surgery for, 413–414
  See also seizures
European Stroke Scale, 73
evoked potentials, for monitoring, 61
external lumbar drainage, 163–164
  complications, 162–163
  intraoperative, 439
  in intraventricular hemorrhage, 356–357
  in subarachnoid hemorrhage, 159–161
  in traumatic brain injury, 14
external ventricular drainage, 8, 145–147
  in brainstem hemorrhage, 381
  in cerebellar hemorrhage, 371
  in cerebellar infarction, 183, 217
  complications, 149–150
  insertion, 147–149
  in intracranial hemorrhage, 11–12
  management, 150–152, 357
  -related infections, 357
  removal, 152
  and risk of hemorrhage, 8
  risk of infection, 309
  thromboprophylaxis, 152–153
  in ventricular hemorrhage, 353

Fabry disease, 232–233
feeding. *See* nutrition
fever
  and intracerebral hemorrhage, 263–264
  after subarachnoid hemorrhage, 474, 481
fibromuscular dysplasia, 230
Fick principle, 20
  in monitoring of cerebral blood flow, 26–27
Fisher Grade Scale, 72
  Modified, *427, 465*
fistulas
  classification of Cognard, 116
  embolization, 114, 116–117
focal syndrome, 501
FOUR Score, 68

gait instability, diagnostic value of, 209
Glasgow Coma Scale, 66–68
  in cerebellar infarction, 210
  as predictor of extubation, 293
Glasgow Outcome Scale, 74–75
glucose
  microdialysis of, 50
  monitoring after subarachnoid hemorrhage, 484

glutamate release
  hypothermia and, 130
  and ischemia, 485
glycemic control
  hypothermia and, 138
  and intracerebral hemorrhage, 264, 302–303
  after subarachnoid hemorrhage, 433, 482
  in traumatic brain injury, 51
glycerol, 84
Graeb Score, *147*, 351, *352*
guidelines
  blood pressure management, 277–278, *277*, 282
  head injury, 517, 533–534
  insertion of ICP monitors, 13
guidewires for intracranial angioplasty, 123–124

handicap, Modified Rankin Scale, 73
head elevation as antiedema therapy, 85–86
head injury
  APACHE Scores, 68–69
  clinical trials, 532–533
  epidemiology, 517
  FOUR Score, 68
  Glasgow Coma Scale, 66–68
    in cerebellar infarction, 210
    as predictor of extubation, 293
  guidelines, 517, 533–534
  Marshall CT classification, 69
  primary brain damage in, 519–520
  prognosis and outcome, 533
  treatment, 527–532
  See also traumatic brain injury
headache
  in cerebral venous thrombosis, 501, 505
  diagnostic value of, 209
  differential diagnosis, 511
  in subarachnoid hemorrhage, 426
hematological disorders, 237–238
  and cerebral venous thrombosis, 506–507
  and infection, 309
hematoma
  expansion, 257–259, 276
    future strategies, 268–269
    pathophysiology, 259
    predictors, 259–260
    and prognosis, 350
    restricting, 260–268, 276–277
  extradural, 521–522
    treatment, 527
  intracerebral, 523–524
    treatment, 528
  subdural, 522–523
    chronic, 522–523, 532
    treatment, 527–528
hemicraniectomy, decompressive, 90–92, 180
  complications, 97–100
  in hemorrhagic stroke, 317
  indications, 92–97
  in malignant MCA infarction, *94*
    clinical trials, 180–181
    complications, 182
  in subarachnoid hemorrhage, 96
hemispheric infarction
  decompressive craniectomy in, 92–95
  See also malignant MCA infarction
hemispheric syndrome, 81
hemodilution, 471
hemorrhagic transformation, detection, 59
hemostasis, surgical, methods for, 324, 342, 388
  in intraoperative aneurysm rupture, 444
heparins, 508–509
herniation, 529
  brainstem, FOUR Score and, 68
  as cause of death in stroke, 90
  in cerebral venous thrombosis, 96
  after craniectomy, 98
  levels of, in space-occupying infarction, 191
  lumbar drainage and, 161, 162–163
  paradoxical, 99
  prevention, 530
herpes simplex encephalitis, 229
hibernation, 275
HIV, 309
hormonal therapy, cerebral venous thrombosis and, 512
Hunt and Hess scale, 72–73
hydrocephalus
  aneurysm rupture and, 146, 159
  in cerebellar hemorrhage, 367
  in cerebellar infarction, 182
  drainage in, 13
  posthemorrhagic, 158, 161–162
    drainage, 146–147, 159–161, 161–162, 353
hyperbaric oxygen, 532
hypertension
  acute hypertensive response, 274, 275
    antihypertensives in, 278–280
  induced, 469, 470
  in intracerebral hemorrhage, 274

hypertension (cont.)
hematoma expansion and, 262–263, 276
immediately post-stroke, 280–282
management, 262–263, *264*, 276–277
management, 245–251
guidelines, 277–278, 282
syndromes, in cerebral venous thrombosis, 501
hypertonic saline, 14, 83–84, 316–317, 433, 470
hyperventilation
brain tissue oxygenation and, 39
in control of intracranial pressure, 85
in regulation of intracranial pressure, 4, 21, 287
hypotension, 251
hypothermia, therapeutic, 129, 185
clinical application
hemorrhagic stroke, 135
ischemic stroke, 133–134
in combination therapy, 135–136
future directions, 134–135
to lower intracranial pressure, 15
mechanisms of action, 129–131, 185
modes of cooling
invasive, 186
non-invasive, 185–186
onset and duration, 186–187
physiology and physics of, 131
side effects, 136–139
during thrombolytic therapy, 134

imaging
in aneurysm, 447–448
for craniotomy, 438–439
of arterial malformations, 114
after basilar artery occlusion, 203
in basilar artery occlusion, 195–196
in cavernoma, 406–408
intraoperative, 414
in cerebellar hemorrhage, 366–367
in cerebellar infarction, 210–212
in cerebral venous thrombosis, 502–505
in head injury, 524
in ischemic stroke, 103
perfusion, after subarachnoid hemorrhage, 468–469
pre-/intraoperative, 388
in cavernoma resection, 414
in excision of arterionvenous malformations, 389
in intracerebral hemorrhage, 338–339
immune-modulating nutrition, 302
immunity in stroke patients, 306
immunosuppression
for cervical artery dissections, 227
hypothermia and, 139
infection
antibiotic strategies, *311*
as cause of stroke, 228–229
blood-borne, 308
catheter-related, 8, 308
urinary, 307–308
hospital-acquired, modifiable risk factors, 310, *310*
hypothermia and, 139
intracerebral hemorrhage-related, 308–309, *308*
lumbar catheter, 163
management, 310–312
postoperative, in decompressive surgery, 97
treatment-related, 309–310
urinary tract, 307–308
ventricular drain-related, 357
ventriculostomy-related, 150–152
wound, hypothermia and, 139
inflammation
in edema formation, 81, 82, 86, 315
effects after traumatic brain injury, 15
hypothermia and, 130
systemic inflammatory response syndrome, 308
and vasospasm, 467
interventional treatment
aneurysm, options and procedures, 111–112
arterial malformations, 112–114
embolization techniques, 114–117
in combination with thrombolysis, 175–177
ischemic stroke, 103
indications, 103–104, 106–107
options and procedures, 104–106, 107–109
vasospasm
indications, 109
options and procedures, 109–111
See also endovascular therapy
intracerebral hemorrhage, 257, 335
acute hypertensive response and, 274, 275
anticoagulants and, 265–268
coagulopathy and, 323
decompressive hemicraniectomy in, 96
extending to ventricles, 145–146, 161–162, 259, 337
hematoma expansion, 257–259, 276
pathophysiology, 259
predictors, 259–260
restricting, 260–268, 276–277

future strategies, 268–269
hypertension and, 274
pathophysiology, 274–275
preoperative management, 338–339
-related infection, 308–309, *308*
surgical removal, 336
craniotomy for, 323–326
effects of subgroup on, 321–323, 336
effects of timing on, 322, 325, 339–340
minimally invasive, 329–332, 336–337, 340–343
selection of patients, 320–321, 329
intracranial atherosclerotic disease.
as cause of stroke, 120
See also under stenosis
intracranial compliance, 4, 5
intracranial dynamics, 3–5
intracranial hemorrhage
antiedema therapy in, 86–87
arterial malformations and, 112
brain tissue oxygenation monitoring in, 41
cavernoma-related, 408–410
cerebral blood flow in, 25
intracranial pressure monitoring in, 11–12
intracranial pressure, 3
barbiturates and, 84–85
vs. cerebral perfusion pressure, 9
decompressive craniectomy in high, 91, 180
hypertonic saline and, 83–84
hyperventilation and, 85
hypothermia and, 129
mechanical ventilation in high, 287
monitoring, 3–8
in aneurysmal subarachnoid hemorrhage, 12–13
Brain Trauma Foundation guidelines, 13
in cerebral vein thrombosis, 12
complications, 8
during craniectomy, 92
in intracranial hemorrhage, 11–12
in ischemic stroke, 9–11
by lumbar catheter, 162
in traumatic brain injury, 13–15
treatment of raised, 529–530
tromethamine and, 85
ventricular drainage in high, 146, 150, 353
waveform, 5
intraventricular hemorrhage, 145–146, 348–349
clearance, 146–147, 161–162, 353–357
endoscopic techniques, 337
conventional therapies, 353
grading, 351
investigational therapies, 353–354
pathophysiology, 349
prognosis, 349–351
score, *350*, 351, *352*
intubation
in cerebellar hemorrhage, 370
indications for, in intracerebral hemorrhage, 286–288
options for, 288–290
ischemia
cerebral, 22
delayed, 464–465
microdialysis to detect, 44, *47*, 48–50, 468
cerebral blood flow as marker of, 22–24
continuous EEG to detect, 61
delayed cerebral
adjunctive therapies, 474
detection, 468–469
Fisher Grade Scale predicts, 72
hemodynamic goals, *471*
hemodynamic interventions, 469–470, 472, 473–474
indications for treatment, 469
prevention, 464–465
edema in, 90
pathophysiology, 81
excitotoxic, 130
hypothermia and, 130, 186
traumatic brain injury and, 518–519
ischemic brain damage, 520–521
prevention, 526

Kernohan's phenomenon, 523

lactate/pyruvate ratio, 46
as biomarker of ischemia, 48, 468, 485
LeRoux Scale, 351, *352*
leucocyte activity, hypothermia and, 130, 139
locked-in syndrome, 195
lucid interval, in hematoma, 521, 522
lumbar drainage, 158, 163–164
complications, 162–163
in intracranial hypertension, 161
intraoperative, 439
in intraventricular hemorrhage, 356–357
placement, 159
in subarachnoid hemorrhage, 159–161
in traumatic brain injury, 14
lumbar puncture, in subarachnoid hemorrhage, 428

malignant cerebral venous thrombosis, decompressive surgery in, 96–97
malignant MCA infarction, 90, 179, 190
  clinical features and prognosis, 190–191
  decompressive surgery in, 92–95, *94*
    clinical trials, 180–181, *180*
    complications, 182
  edema in
    predictors of, 192
    treatment, 192–193
  herniation in, 191
  hypothermia in, 185
  imaging and prediction of, 182
  signs and symptoms, *191*
Marshall CT classification for head injury, 69
matrix metalloproteinases
  in hematoma expansion, 269
  hypothermia and, 130
mean transit time, 27
MELAS, 233
meningitis, 229, 309–310
  antibiotic strategy, *311*
  ventriculostomy -related, 357
metabolic crisis
  biomarkers, 46
  glycemic control and, 51
metabolic demand
  cerebral blood flow related to, 20
    in intracranial hemorrhage, 25, 275–276
    in subarachnoid hemorrhage, 25
  measurement, 27
metabolic derangements after subarachnoid hemorrhage
  cerebral, 483–485, *486*, *496*
  systemic, 481–482, *486*, *496*
metabolic effects of hypothermia, 139, 141
microdialysis, 39, 44–47
  in subarachnoid hemorrhage, 48–50, 483–484
  in traumatic brain injury, 47–48
microemboli detection, transcranial Doppler for, 56
midline shift
  in head injury, 69
  in malignant MCA infarction, 179, 191
  ultrasonography to monitor, 59
mismatch, PI/DWI, 172–173
Modified Fisher Grade Scale, *427*, *465*
Modified Rankin Scale, 73, *94*
monitoring
  brain tissue oxygenation, 37–39
    in intracranial hemorrhage, 41
    in ischemic stroke, 40
    by near-infrared spectroscopy, 63
    neurochemical, 39, 44–47
    in subarachnoid hemorrhage, 40
  by continuous EEG, 60–61
  cerebral blood flow, 26–33, *27*
    comparison of methods, *29*
    indications for, 33
  continuous non-invasive, 54
  evoked potentials for, 61
  in subarachnoid hemorrhage, 470–471, 494
  intracranial pressure, 3–8
    in aneurysmal subarachnoid hemorrhage, 12–13
    during BP reduction, 278
    Brain Trauma Foundation guidelines, 13
    vs. cerebral perfusion pressure, 9
    in cerebral vein thrombosis, 12
    complications, 8
    during craniectomy, 92
    in intracranial hemorrhage, 11–12
    in ischemic stroke, 9–11
    by lumbar catheter, 162
    in traumatic brain injury, 13–15
  neuro-, in subarachnoid hemorrhage, *431*
  neurochemical, 39, 44–47
  ultrasonography for
    transcranial color-coded duplex, 58–60
    transcranial Doppler, 6, 55–57
Monro-Kellie doctrine, 3, 180, 529
mortality
  APACHE Score, 68
  in cerebellar hemorrhage, 372, *372*
  in excision of arteriovenous malformation, 390
  in subarachnoid hemorrhage, 425
motor effects of cerebellar infarction, 208
motor evoked potentials, 212
Moya Moya syndrome, 230
MR perfusion to measure cerebral blood flow, 27, *30*, 31, 468
MRI
  of arterial malformations, 114
  in basilar artery occlusion, 195–196
  in brainstem hemorrhage, 379
  in cavernoma, 407–408
    of brainstem, 382
  in cerebellar hemorrhage, 366
  in cerebellar infarction, 211–212
  in cerebral venous thrombosis, 503–504
  in cervical artery dissections, 226
  in evaluation for thrombolysis, 172–174

in head injury, 524
in prediction of edema, 192
in subarachnoid hemorrhage, 428
myocardial injury in subarachnoid hemorrhage, 493
myocardial performance, hypothermia and, 140–141

nausea, diagnostic value of, 208
near-infrared spectroscopy for monitoring of cerebral blood flow, 32, 63
neurogenic cardiopulmonary injury, 490
clinical features and diagnosis, 492–494
pathophysiology, 490–492
neurological deficits
basilar artery occlusion and, 194, 195
Canadian Stroke Scale, 71
in cavernoma, 408
in cerebellar hemorrhage, 365, *365*
in cerebellar infarction, 208
in cerebral venous thrombosis, 501, 507
delayed, 429, 464, 468
lumbar drainage and, 160
European Stroke Scale, 73
NIH Stroke Score, 70
Scandinavian Stroke Score, 70
neurological examination in cerebellar infarction, 210
neuromonitoring, 5–8, 44–47
neuromuscular blocking agents in control of shivering, 186
neurosonology. *See* ultasound
NIH Stroke Score, 70–71
in cerebellar infarction, 210
nutrition
efffect on prognosis, 297–298
enteral, 299–301
vs parenteral, 301–302
immune-modulating, 302
oral supplementation, 298–299
nystagmus in cerebellar infarction, 209

oligemia, 22, 26
Onyx embolic agent, 114, 453
opioids
to control shivering, 137
pharmacokinetics, hypothermia and, 140
oral contraception, cerebral venous thrombosis and, 512
osmotherapy, 82–84, 316–317
in brainstem hemorrhage, 381
outcome
after decompressive surgery, 181–182
in cerebellar infarction, 95, 183
in hemispheric infarction, 92–95
edema and, 81
in endovascular therapy, 114
Glasgow Outcome Scale, 74–75
Modified Rankin Scale, 73
nutrition and, 297–298
of thrombolysis, time window and, 170
overdrainage, herniation due to, 162–163, 164
Oxfordshire Community Stroke Project classification, 69–70
oximetry, brain tissue, 15
oxygen
consumption, cerebral metabolic
effects of hypothermia, 129
See also metabolic demand
extraction fraction (OEF), 20
in cerebral autoregulation, 22
in cerebral vasospasm, 25
in ischemic stroke, 24
saturation, cerebral blood flow and, 21
oxygenation, brain tissue. *See* brain tissue oxygenation

paralytic agents in rapid sequence intubation, 290
parenchymal lesions, 505–506
parenteral nutrition, 301–302
pbrO_2. *See* brain tissue oxygenation
penumbra, PI/DWI-mismatch and, 172–173
perfusion studies
CT to measure cerebral blood flow, 27, 28–31, *30*, 468–469
MR to measure cerebral blood flow, 27, *30*, 31, 468
transcranial sonography, 60
perioperative stroke, 235–236
PET to monitor cerebral blood flow, 27, *30*
pharmacokinetics, hyopothermia alters, 139–140, *140*
pneumonia
antibiotic strategies, *311*
aspiration, dysphagia and, 300
hospital-acquired, 306–307
ventilator-associated, 307
hypothermia and, 139
positive pressure ventilation, 291–292
in brainstem hemorrhage, 380
pregnancy
cerebral venous thrombosis in, 512
ruptured aneurysm in, 455
stroke in, 236–237
primary pontine hemorrhage, 378, 379
prognosis, 380
procoagulatory states, 237, 506

prognosis
  after decompressive surgery, 92–95, 181–182
  enteral nutrition and, 299–301
  Scandinavian Stroke Score for, 70
prophylaxis
  angioplasty as, 432, 467
  antibiotic
    in cerebrospinal fluid leak, 531
    in ventilator-associated pneumonia, 307
    for ventricular drainage, 150–151, 357
  thrombo-, for ventricular drainage, 152–153
prothrombotic conditions, 237, 506
proximal control, 442–443
pulmonary complications, 493–494
  See also cardiopulmonary dysfunction
pulmonary edema, 433, 492, 493–494

radiosurgery
  in arteriovenous malformations, 394–396
  for cavernoma, 415
radiotherapy for arteriovenous malformations, 396
re-bleeding
  in subarachnoid hemorrhage, 428
  See also hematoma expansion
recanalization
  in basilar artery occlusion, 196–202
  in cerebral venous thrombosis, 504
  indications, 103
  interventional treatment, 103
    indications, 103–104, 106–107
    options and procedures, 104–106, 107–109
  middle cerebral artery, timing and prognosis, 56
  outcome and, in basilar artery occlusion, 201
  rates, *56*
renal replacement therapy in ischemic stroke, 10–11
reocclusion, basilar artery, 202
respiratory drive
  brainstem hemorrhage and, 288
  intracerebral hemorrhage and, 286–287
  and mode of ventilation, 291
respiratory failure in intracerebral hemorrhage, 286
rewarming, 134
  electrolytes in, 141
risks of treatment, balancing, 390

saline, hypertonic, 14, 83–84, 316–317, 433, 470
salt-wasting syndrome, 433, 482
scales, 67
  APACHE Score, 68–69
  ASPECTS, 104
  Barthel ADL Index, 74
  Bedside Shivering Assessment, 137, *137*
  Canadian Neurological, 71
  CVT risk score, *508*
  European Stroke, 73
  Fisher Grade, 72
    Modified, *427*, *465*
  FOUR Score, 68
  Glasgow Coma, 66–68
  Glasgow Outcome Scale, 74–75
  Graeb Score, *147*, 351, *352*
  Hunt and Hess, 72–73
  IVH Score, *350*, 351, *352*
  LeRoux Scale, 351, *352*
  Modified Rankin, 73, *94*
  NIH Stroke Score, 70–71
  Oxfordshire Community Stroke Project classification, 69–70
  Scandinavian Stroke, 70
  Spetzler–Martin Grading System, 390, 395, *395*
  for subarachnoid hemorrhage, *427*
  Therapy Intensity Level, 530
  WFNS Grading for SAH, 71–72
Scandinavian Stroke Scale, 70
sedatives
  in brainstem hemorrhage, 380
  to control shivering, 132, 137, 186
  pharmacokinetics, hypothermia and, 140
  for rapid sequence intubation, 289–290
seizures
  in cavernoma, 408, 412
    surgery for, 413–414
  in cerebral venous thrombosis, 505, 511
  differential diagnosis, 505
  after subarachnoid hemorrhage, 434
sepsis, 308
  antibiotic strategy, *311*
shivering, 133, 136–138, 186
  Bedside Shivering Assessment Scale, 137, *137*
shunt
  infections, antibiotic strategy, *312*
  venous, in regulation of ICP, 4
  ventricular, 13, 152
SIADH, 482
sickle cell disease
  and infection, 309
  ischemic stroke risk, 57
sinking skin syndrome, 100, 182
skull fracture, depresssed, 531–532

somatosensory evoked potentials, 212
  for monitoring, 61
spasmolysis, 458, 472
  indications, 109
  options and procedures, 109–111
SPECT in monitoring of cerebral blood flow, 27
Spetzler-Martin Grading System, 114, 390, 395, *395*
spinal cord infarction, 237
statin therapy in subarachnoid hemorrhage, 434
stenosis, arterial
  intracranial
    balloon vs. stent-assisted angioplasty in, 122
    stenting vs. medical management in, 120
  stenting in, 106
    indications for, 106–107
    options and procedures, 107–109
stent, 106
  in aneurysm, 450–453
  -assisted coiling, 112
  devices, 107
  in failed thrombectomy, 106
  flow-diverting, 112, 453
  indications for, 106–107
  intracranial, 120
    placement, 125
    techniques, 123
  vs. medical management, 120
  options and procedures, 107–109
  -retriever, use for thrombectomy, 104
  for thrombectomy, 202
  Wingspan, 120
stereotactic aspiration
  in hematoma expansion, 261, 268
  of intracerebral hemorrhage, 331
  with fibrinolysis, 317, 331, 332
stereotactic evacuation of intracerebral hemorrhage, 329–332, 336–337, 340–343
steroids as antiedema therapy, 86
strokeectomy, 217
subarachnoid hemorrhage, 111, 146, 423, 425–426
  brain tissue oxygenation and, 40
  cardiopulmonary dysfunction in, 490
    cardiomyopathies, 492–493, 495
    features and diagnosis, 492–494
    pathophysiology, 490–492
    teatment, 495–496
  cerebral blood flow in, 25–26
  clinical presentation, 426
  complications of, 428–429
  decompressive craniectomy in, 96
  diagnosis, 426–428
  Fisher Grade scale, 72
  hydrocephalus after, 146, 159–160
  intracranial pressure monitoring in, 12–13
  lumbar drainage in, 159–161
  management, 494–495
    emergency department, 429–431
    intensive care, 431–434
    monitoring, 470–471
    novel strategies, 434–435
  metabolic derangements after
    cerebral, 483–485
    systemic, 481–482
  microdialysis in, 48–50, 483–484
  monitoring in, 494
  Moya Moya syndrome and, 230
  pathogenesis, 423–425
  pathophysiology of secondary injury, 480–481
  peri-mesencephalic, 424
  rare causes, *424*
  recurrent, 428
  WFNS Grading System, 71–72
surgery
  in aneurysm
    aneurysm rupture during, 443–444
    indications, 437–438
    microscopic approaches, 440–442
    minimally invasive, 440
    proximal control, 442–443
    repair techniques, 443–444
    surgical techniques, 439–440, 445
    timing and preparation, 438–439
  for arteriovenous malformations
    decision-making, 390–392
    with hemorrhage, 392–393
    radiosurgery, 394–396
    techniques, 387–389
  in brainstem hematoma, 382–383
  in brainstem hemorrhage, 381
  for cavernoma, 413–415
    radiosurgery, 415
  decompressive, 10, 90–92, 180
    in cerebellar infarction, 182–183
    in cerebral contusions, 528–529
    in cerebral venous thrombosis, 509–510
    clinical trials, 530, 532–533
    complications, 97–100

surgery (cont.)
converting craniotomy to, 324
in extradural hematoma, 527
in hemorrhagic stroke, 317
indications, 92–97
in intracerebral hematoma, 528
for ischemic stroke, 179
in malignant MCA infarction, *94*, 182
in malignant MCA infarction, clinical trials, 180–181, *180*
in subarachnoid hemorrhage, 96
in subdural hematoma, 527–528
suboccipital, 217, 371
in traumatic brain injury, 14
for intracerebral hemorrhage, 336
craniotomy, 323–326
effects of subgroup on, 321–323, 336
effects of timing on, 322, 325, 339–340
minimally invasive, 329–332, 336–337, 340–343
selection of patients, 320–321, 329
in intraventricular hemorrhage
minimally invasive, 356
in prevention of hematoma expansion, 260–262
sympathetic storm, 490
systemic inflammatory response syndrome, 308

Therapy Intensity Level score, 530
thermal diffusion flowmetry to measure cerebral blood flow, *30*, 31–32
thermoregulation, 131, 186
sedatives and, 137
thrombectomy
devices, 106
mechanical, 103, 104–106
in basilar artery occlusion, 201–202
thromboembolism
during endovascular therapy, 456
posthemorrhagic, 266
thrombolysis, 103
in basilar artery occlusion, 198–201
contraindications, *200*
blood pressure after, 246
Bridging Concept, 175
in cerebral venous thrombosis, 509
in cervical artery dissections, 227
clinical trials, 169–171, 174
based on MRI, 172–174
in combination therapies, 175–177
in combination therapy, 136
in hematoma expansion, 268
hypothermia and, 134
ongoing trials, 134–135
before interventional treatment, 104
intraarterial, 174–175, 198
clinical trials, 175
intraventricular, 147, 161
intraventricular combined with lumbar drainage, 162
intraventricular combined with ventricular drainage, 353–356
local intraarterial, 104
in failed thrombectomy, 106
and minimally invasive surgery, 317, 331, 332
in pregnancy, 237
thrombophilia, 237–238
thromboprophylaxis
for ventricular drain, 152–153
See also anticoagulants
time window
and choice of treatment, 103, 104
for decompressive surgery, 182
for surgery in hematoma, 521, 522, 527
in therapeutic hypothermia, 133
for thrombolysis
in basilar artery occlusion, 200–201
hypothermia and, 134
outcome and, 170
tracheotomy, 294
in brainstem hemorrhage, 380
transfusion in subarachnoid hemorrhage, 471–472
trauma, as cause of dissection, 226, 521
traumatic brain injury
brain tissue oxygenation monitoring in, 37–39
decompressive surgery in, clinical trials of, 533
epidemiology, 517
hemicraniectomy in, 98
intracranial pressure monitoring in, 13–15
ischemia resulting from, 518–519
managment, 517
Marshall CT classification, 69
microdialysis in, 47–48
triple-H therapy, 109, 432–433, 469, 471, 487
adverse effects, 473

ultrasonography
EKOS device, 175
intraoperative, 389
transcranial color-coded duplex, 55
for monitoring, 6, 55–57
transcranial Doppler, 54
in cerebellar infarction, 212

to measure cerebral blood flow, 32, 109, 467–468
for monitoring, 58–60
in vasospasm, 432
urinary tract infections, 307–308
antibiotic strategies, *312*
urokinase, 104

vasculitis as cause of stroke, 227–230
vasospasm, 480–481
and brain tissue oxygenation, 39, 40
continuous EEG to detect, 61
and delayed cerebral ischemia, 464–465
detection of, 467–468
diagnosis, 428
endovascular therapy in, 457–458, 472–473
Fisher Grade scale predicts, 72
grading criteria, *57*
interventional therapy, 109
indications, 109
options and procedures, 109–111
microdialysis in, 48
prevention, 464–465
by lumber drainage, 160–161
primary, 231–232
in subarachnoid hemorrhage, 25, 160–161, 431–432
novel strategies for, 434–435
transcranial Doppler to detect, 57, 109, 432
vegetative state, 533
venography in cerebral venous thrombosis, 502–505
venous angioma, 401
venous blood shunting in regulation of ICP, 4
ventilation, mechanical
in brainstem hemorrhage, 380
in cardiopulmonary complications, 496
indications for in intracerebral hemorrhage, 286–288
lung protective, 292
methods of, 288–290
specialized, 292
modes of, 291
parameters, 291
pneumonia and, 139, 307
positive end-expiratory pressure, 291–292
weaning, 292–294
ventricular drainage, 8, 145–147
in brainstem hemorrhage, 381
in cerebellar hemorrhage, 371
in cerebellar infarction, 183, 217
complications, 149–150
insertion, 147–149
in intracranial hemorrhage, 11–12
management, 150–152, 357
-related infections, 357
removal, 152
and risk of hemorrhage, 8
risk of infection, 309
thromboprophylaxis, 152–153
in ventricular hemorrhage, 353
ventriculitis, 309–310
ventriculostomy-related, 150–152, 357
ventriculostomy
endoscopic third, in cerebellar infarction, 218
See also ventricular drainage
vertigo, diagnostic value of, 208
viral infection as cause of stroke, 229
vitamin-K-antagonists and hematoma expansion, 265–266
volume status
after subarachnoid hemorrhage, 494–495
and triple-H therapy, 432
hypotension, 251
hypothermia and, 141
subarachnoid hemorrhage and, 433, 466, 469

warming in therapeutic hypothermia
rewarming, 134
skin-surface, 133, 137
weaning
from external ventricular drain, 152
from mechanical ventilation, 292–294
WFNS Grading System for SAH, 71–72
wound infection, hypothermia and, 139